THE CHEMICAL BASIS OF HEREDITY

Contribution No. 153 of the McCollum-Pratt Institute

A Symposium on
THE CHEMICAL BASIS
OF
HEREDITY

Sponsored by

THE
McCOLLUM-PRATT INSTITUTE
OF
THE JOHNS HOPKINS UNIVERSITY
with support from
THE ATOMIC ENERGY COMMISSION

Edited by

WILLIAM D. McELROY AND BENTLEY GLASS

BALTIMORE
THE JOHNS HOPKINS PRESS
1957

PREFACE

A Symposium on The Chemical Basis of Heredity was held at The Johns Hopkins University under the sponsorship of the McCollum-Pratt Institute on June 19-22, 1956. This volume consists of the papers and informal discussions presented at these meetings.

Biologists have long been concerned with the mechanism of duplication, and geneticists in particular have developed the concept that probably the only self-reproducing unit smaller than the cell is the gene. Chemical discoveries during the past ten years relating particularly to nucleic acid and chromosome structure, gene function, protein synthesis and enzyme action have provided a broad chemical and physico-chemical framework which makes speculation on the mechanism of duplication profitable. In the planning of the present symposium we attempted to bring together those geneticists, virologists, biochemists, physiologists, biophysicists, and physical chemists who have made important contributions to our understanding of the mechanism of self-reproduction with the hope that an exchange of ideas would be of value in eventually explaining "The Chemical Basis of Heredity".

In the planning of the Symposium the participants and members of the Institute contributed their time generously. It is a pleasure to acknowledge the important contributions of the following moderators: Dr. Bentley Glass (Part I), Dr. Boris Ephrussi (Part 2), Dr. S. Luria (Part 3), Dr. Roger Herriott (Part 4), Dr. Paul Doty (Part 5), Dr. Gerhard Schmidt (Part 6) and Dr. J. Lederberg (Part 7).

It is also a pleasure to acknowledge the important assistance of the Atomic Energy Commission in helping defray part of the expense of the Symposium.

October 10, 1956

W. D. McElroy, Director
McCollum-Pratt Institute

CONTENTS

ADDITIONAL PARTICIPANTS

R. L. Airth
Bruce Anderson
Hudson Ansley
Robert Austrian
Mordhay Avron
J. W. Bailey
Robert Ballentine
Claude F. Baxter
Paul Berg
T. N. Berlin
S. P. Bessman
David Bodian
G. L. Brown
J. W. Butler
Dan H. Campbell
H. Carlson
D. G. Catcheside
H. Chantrenne
Harold H. Clum
S. P. Colowick
C. Cooper
Helen Crause
R. O. Darrow
P. F. Davison
J. N. Davidson
C. DeLuca
Robert DeMars
R. D. DeMoss
D. Dennis
H. W. Dickerman
A. H. Doerman
K. O. Donaldson
Paul Doty
A. L. Dounce
Sterling Emerson
Boris Ephrussi

W. Epstein
L. H. Frank
R. Franklin
Joseph Gall
Bentley Glass
A. Goldin
A. A. Green
Maurice Green
L. Grossman
George O. Guy
David Harker
Zlata Hartman
Verl L. Hause
L. Hellerman
E. Y. Herbst
Roger M. Herriott
M. B. Hoagland
Alexander Hollander
David S. Hogness
Julian Huxley
A. T. Jagendorf
K. Bruce Jacobson
D. Kacser
Akira Kaji
Herman Kalckar
N. O. Kaplan
Francis T. Kenney
M. Kern
Bengt Kihlman
Murray V. King
David Krogman
T. Langan
R. S. Langden
Ennis C. Layne
Esther N. Lederberg
J. Lederberg

Part I

CELLULAR UNITS OF HEREDITY

THE ROLE OF THE NUCLEUS IN HEREDITY

George W. Beadle

*Division of Biology,
California Institute of Technology,
Pasadena, California*

Several factors have interacted to accelerate the advance of genetics in recent years. The widespread use of microorganisms, including viruses, has been one of these (10). Such material makes feasible the study of phenomena that occur with a frequency several orders of magnitude smaller than those that are investigated in higher forms. An increasing tendency for geneticists and biochemists to think about biological problems in common terms and to make use of each other's methods has also been important. Perhaps even more significant has been the formulation of the Watson-Crick hypothesis of deoxyribonucleic acid structure (5, 50). This has made it increasingly profitable for biologists and chemists to think, talk, and write about genetic units in terms of clearly defined chemical concepts. Symposia such as this, in which investigators from a variety of disciplines come together to exchange information and views, likewise play an important part.

I believe it will be useful to attempt, at the beginning of the Symposium, to summarize present knowledge about genetic material. I propose to do this briefly and simply, making use of those interpretations and hypotheses of gene structure and gene function that seem more probable to me. This is not easy, for there is much that we do not yet know and many points on which presently available evidence appears to be conflicting. I fully realize that my presentation will be colored by my prejudices and will suffer from my incomplete knowledge of certain lines of evidence.

The Gene as a Biological Unit

Beginning with Mendel and for some sixty years thereafter geneticists worked almost exclusively with higher plants and animals. The garden pea, maize, the jimson weed, the fruit fly, the mouse, and man

3

were some of the organisms that contributed importantly to the knowledge of classical genetics. The "factor" or "gene" of the genetics of this time was a unit of inheritance, detected only if it existed in two or more forms each with a characteristic developmental effect (37, 38).

In the second decade of this century it became clear that genes are carried in chromosomes and are arranged linearly. The many genes carried in a single one of the several kinds of chromosomes of a given species are "linked," i.e., transmitted from one generation to the next as a group. During chromosome pairing at meiosis, heterozygous linked genes may recombine through "crossing over" between homologous chromosomes. The frequency with which such recombination occurs for any two linked genes is a function of the distance between them and provides the basis on which linear genetic "maps" of gene loci are constructed.

Until recently it was widely believed that the process of crossing over does not alter individual genes—that it occurs between genes, not within them. The evidence on which this belief was founded is the basis for considering the gene to be an elementary biological unit, occupying a definite position in a chromosome (a locus), and transmitted intact from one generation to another.

In recent years evidence has accumulated that can be interpreted to mean that the gene is divisible by intragenic crossing over. The nature and significance of this evidence will make up an important part of this Symposium (2, 3, 4, 18).

The Chemical Nature of the Gene

Chromosomes are composed of deoxyribonucleic acid and protein combined in a way that is not yet completely understood (25, 32, 42). For many years it was assumed that genetic specificity was to be accounted for entirely in terms of the structures and configurations of proteins.

The demonstration that transformations in type specificities of pneumococcal bacteria can be brought about by highly purified preparations of deoxyribonucleic acid (DNA) first focussed attention on this substance as possible carrier of genetic information (1). Over the years it has become increasingly clear that DNA does indeed constitute the primary genetic material in this organism (11, 12, 23, 24).

In the phages (bacterial viruses), too, the evidence is strong that genetic continuity resides in DNA. In these relatively simple systems, infection of host cells is accomplished through the injection of phage DNA. Experiments in which DNA and protein are labeled with P-32 and S-35 show that the injected material is 97 per cent DNA and only 3 per cent protein (19). The protein coats remain outside. Although it remains conceivable that the protein injected plays some direct genetic role, it seems more probable that continuity of phage genetic material depends solely on DNA at this stage of the life cycle.

Unlike phages, tobacco mosaic virus contains ribonucleic acid (RNA). In the virus rod RNA is carried inside a cylindrical protein jacket (13, 14, 17, 30). No DNA is present. Obviously in this system the primary genetic information must be carried in the form of RNA, for RNA alone can bring about infection under certain conditions (14, 15). This conclusion is confirmed by the behavior of artificially reconstituted virus particles consisting of protein and RNA from genetically different strains. The progeny of such "hybrid" viruses are like the strain that contributed the RNA (14).

The evidence in higher forms is less decisive. By analogy with viruses, it is assumed as a working hypothesis that the primary genetic material is DNA rather than protein.

THE WATSON-CRICK HYPOTHESIS

The Watson and Crick hypothesis (5, 50) that the polynucleotide chains of DNA normally assume the configuration of a double helix in which chains are hydrogen-bonded together through complementary base pairs is strongly supported by evidence from x-ray diffraction patterns and from analytical data on base ratios (52). In the double helix, adenine (A) and thymine (T) form one base pair. Guanine (G) and cytosine (C) constitute the second pair. Since there are two ways in which a given base pair can be turned at a given level in the helix, there are four base pairs possible.

The Watson-Crick structure is attractive from a biological point of view because it provides a plausible basis for gene specificity, for gene replication, and for gene mutation.

Gene Specificity.

It is assumed that gene specificity resides in sequence of base pairs in a DNA double helix. If there were no restrictions as to the proportion in which base pairs occur or in the sequence in which they occur, the number of different DNA molecules possible is 4^n, where n is the number of base pairs. Thus it is clear that DNA provides an adequate basis for gene specificity.

Gene Replication.

The two complementary polynucleotide chains of the Watson-Crick structure provide a plausible basis for gene reproduction (50). It is postulated that the complementary chains separate and that each acts as a template for the synthesis of a new partner. Indicating the building blocks with the letters A, T, C, and G, the replication process can be schematically represented as follows:

$$
\begin{array}{ccc}
& & \begin{array}{c} \text{A} \ \text{C} \ \text{T} \ \text{G} \\ || \ \ || \ \ || \ \ || \\ \text{T}\_\text{G}\_\text{A}\_\text{C} \end{array} \\
\begin{array}{c} \text{A}\ \text{C}\ \text{T}\ \text{G} \\ || \ \ || \ \ || \ \ || \\ \text{T}\_\text{G}\_\text{A}\_\text{C} \end{array} \rightarrow \text{A}\ \text{C}\ \text{T}\ \text{G} \rightarrow & \\
& \text{T}\_\text{G}\_\text{A}\_\text{C} \rightarrow \begin{array}{c} \text{A}\ \text{C}\ \text{T}\ \text{G} \\ || \ \ || \ \ || \ \ || \\ \text{T}\_\text{G}\_\text{A}\_\text{C} \end{array}
\end{array}
$$

It is not at all clear in detail how this process might occur, a situation that accounts for the fact that the subject is dealt with in this Symposium (5, 6).

Since replication of genetic material never occurs in the absence of a living cell in which RNA and protein are present in addition to DNA, the possibility must be kept in mind that replication could be less direct than is suggested by the above simplified scheme. It is an impressive fact that DNA is the only large molecule so far known to have a structure that so plausibly provides for multiplication through replica formation.

Gene Mutation.

If genetic specificity does indeed consist in base-pair sequences in DNA molecules, mutation almost certainly consists in alteration of these sequences. Four types of such alteration are obviously possible, viz.: (a) substitution at one or more base-pair levels, (b) rearrangement of base-pair sequences, (c) duplication of one or more base pairs, and (d) deletion of base-pairs. Watson and Crick (50) have suggested a mechanism by which the first of these might occur. In terms of chromosomes, which are structures many times larger than DNA helices but in which genetic information may well be carried in the form of DNA, both inversions and deletions are known to occur.

Gene Function.

In whatever form it is carried, genetic information must obviously be made use of in the development and functioning of a living system. In bacterial viruses the DNA that is injected into the host cell somehow directs that the cell synthesize the protein material that is to constitute the coats of daughter viruses. These proteins differ from normal host proteins (19).

It seems probable that, whatever mechanism exists for translating DNA information into protein specificities, there are discrete segments of DNA that correspond to particular protein configurations. From the standpoint of function, such DNA segments may be defined as genes.

It has been postulated that in protein synthesis in general, RNA is directly involved in a template mechanism (9, 45, 46). On this view specific proteins are built up on RNA templates of corresponding specificities. It seems reasonable to suppose that such RNA templates are in turn somehow derived from the DNA segments that are the genes. In cellular forms genetic DNA is largely or wholly confined to the nucleus. The RNA which serves as templates for protein synthesis is largely but not wholly located in the cytoplasm.

GENETIC CROSSING OVER

In maize, *Neurospora, Drosophila,* and several other organisms in which conventional sexual reproduction occurs, crossing over occurs at meiosis at the time or shortly after paired homologous chromosomes are replicated. This is sometimes called the four-strand stage. At a given level only two of the four strands cross over. Thus in the double heterozygote represented as follows:

$$A\ B\ /\ a\ b$$

where A and a indicate alternate forms of one gene and B and b alternate forms of a linked gene, and alleles in one of the homologous chromosomes are placed on the same side of the solidus, the products that result from a single crossover between A and B are:

A	B
A	b
a	B
a	b

It is important to note that the reciprocal products *A b* and *a B* arise from a single crossover event. It is also significant that, with respect to a given gene pair, one or the other of the alternative forms is found in a given daughter chromosome. It does not happen with any appreciable frequency that the crossover goes through the region of the chromosome occupied by gene *A* in such a way that daughter genes are made up of parts of both *A* and *a*.

Genes may lie so closely together in the chromosome that crossovers occur between them with a very low frequency—for example, one per thousand daughter chromosomes.

The chromosomes of higher forms may consist of discrete segments consisting of DNA and protein joined linearly by divalent calcium ions (31). The evidence for this lies in the fact that chelating agents cause the dissociation of chromosomes into units about 4000 Å units long, possibly corresponding to individual genes. It has been suggested that conventional crossing over occurs exclusively at these connections— that is, between genes. This suggestion receives support in the observation that crossing over and chromosome rearrangements are increased in frequency under conditions of calcium deficiency (27, 47).

The Functional Test for Allelism

Genes that occupy different positions characteristically have different functions. Thus A may be necessary for the formation of one enzyme and B for another. In such cases the double heterozygote

$$A \quad b \ / \ a \quad B$$

will produce both enzymes, *a* and *b* being the inactive and recessive forms of the two genes.

Allelic forms of a single gene occupy corresponding loci in homologous chromosomes. They affect the same character presumably because they modify a single primary function of the gene. When two such mutant alleles of a single gene are recessive and are carried in homologous chromosomes, i.e.,

$$a \ / \ a'$$

the organism in which they occur is usually not normal.

The difference between the phenotypes of a double heterozygote involving two different genes and of a heterozygote for mutant alleles of a single gene provides the basis for the classical test for allelism. An $A\ b/a\ B$ genotype is $A\ B$ (normal) in phenotype whereas a/a' is a or a' (mutant) in phenotype. This test can be made in diploids, heterocaryons or, under special circumstances, in "haploid" bacteria (7, 18) or viruses (2).

There is some evidence that this test may occasionally break down in either of two ways:

First, in cases interpreted in terms of closely linked genes with related functions—for example, genes assumed to be required for the formation of enzymes that catalyze successive steps in a sequence of chemical reactions such as

$$\rightarrow\ P\ \rightarrow\ A\ \rightarrow\ B$$

—the so-called "trans" double heterozygote, $A\ b/a\ B$, may be unable to carry out the reaction sequence, whereas the "cis" heterozygote, $A\ B/a\ b$, does so in a normal way. Crossing over between such genes may be infrequent but in some cases is conventional in that it is associated with the expected crossovers for closely linked marker genes, and in that reciprocal crossover products are found to result from a single event (28). The inability of the trans heterozygote to function normally is referred to as one type of "position effect." It should be emphasized that in none of the cases in which this interpretation has been made have the assumed separate chemical steps been convincingly demonstrated. Consequently alternative interpretations are possible in terms of single genes in which intragenic recombination occurs (39).

Secondly, there are now known a number of cases in which it appears that alleles of a single gene complement each other in heterozygotes in such a way that a/a' functions normally or nearly so, whereas a/a and a'/a' fail to carry out a function dependent on the A gene (34, 35, 36, 40). It is not easy to understand how such alleles can be modifications of a single functional unit, but again it should be pointed out that alternative interpretations have not been excluded. For example, it may turn out that what has been assumed to be a single chemical step may prove to be two steps catalyzed by separate enzymes dependent on closely linked genes.

It is important to learn more about the reactions and enzymes involved in those situations that appear to involve complementary alleles of a single gene. Not only is such knowledge important for an understanding of gene action in cases that appear to be exceptional, but it is highly desirable to know whether the complementarity test is valid for identifying functional units of heredity. It is currently a widely used and convenient criterion for allelism and will probably continue to be useful at least as a first approximation.

TRANSMUTATION

The above account assumes that the gene as a functional unit is identical with the gene as a unit of recombination. If crossing over occurs within as well as between genes, this assumption of course cannot be correct. Recently phenomena have been observed that have been interpreted as indicating intragenic crossing over. They can, however, also be interpreted in terms of a process that differs significantly from crossing over.

If many mutants of a given gene, as defined in terms of position and function, are obtained through independent mutational events, it is found that reversions are obtained in a low frequency when two such mutant forms of the gene are carried in homologous chromosomes. Thus *a-1/a-2* may give rise to the *A* allele with a frequency higher than that expected from reverse mutation. This result suggests that the two mutants *a-1* and *a-2* represent modifications of the gene at different "sites" along its length and that crossing over can restore the normal form of the gene by recombining "good" ends. Using a linear model for a single gene, the postulated recombination would be of the following kind

$$A\text{-}1 \; a\text{-}2 \; / \; a\text{-}1 \; A\text{-}2 \; \rightarrow \; A\text{-}1 \; A\text{-}2$$

where *a-1* and *a-2* now represent modifications at non-overlapping sites within a single linear gene.

If the *A-1 A-2* condition were the result of conventional crossing over, the reciprocal *a-1 a-2* would be expected to be produced by the same event that produces the normal form of the gene, *A-1 A-2*. At the same time closely linked independent genes should show recombinations of particular types.

Tests made in situations of the following type

$$B \; A\text{-}1 \; a\text{-}2 \; c \; / \; b \; a\text{-}1 \; A\text{-}2 \; C$$

should give chromosomes carrying the normal forms of gene *A* that are always of the constitution

$$B \; A\text{-}1 \; A\text{-}2 \; C$$

The reciprocal product *b a-1 a-2 c* should be formed at the same time.

The simultaneous occurrence of such reciprocal products can be detected only if two or more products of meiosis are recovered.

Only a few tests have been made in a way that would simultaneously detect recombination of linked markers and the reciprocal products of crossing over.

Mary Mitchell (34, 35) has found that two mutants of a gene for pyridoxine synthesis in *Neurospora* show reversion in the *p-1 P-2/ P-1 p-2* condition but that reciprocal products are not necessarily found in a single set of products of meiosis. Furthermore, linked markers on opposite sides of the gene under study show recombination in only about half the reversions, and these are not always in the expected type. Thus from the heterozygote

$$a\ P\text{-}1\ p\text{-}2\ b/A\ p\text{-}1\ P\text{-}2\ B$$

four products of a single meiotic process were obtained of the following constitution:

$$a\ P\text{-}1\ p\text{-}2\ b$$
$$a\ P\text{-}1\ p\text{-}2\ b$$
$$A\ P\text{-}1\ P\text{-}2\ B$$
$$A\ p\text{-}1\ P\text{-}2\ B$$

Mutation of *p-1 P-2* to *P-1 P-2* would explain the result except that controls homozygous for *p-1 P-2* indicate a very much lower frequency of such mutation.

There are several other instances in which intragenic recombination may occur without close correlation with recombination for outside markers (16, 41, 44). In one of these, namely in *Aspergillus*, it has been demonstrated that reciprocal recombination products arise from what are almost certainly single recombinational events (41). In yeast, 3:1 segregations at several loci have been found under circumstances that strongly suggest the phenomenon described above for *Neurospora* (34, 35).

It has been suggested (34, 43) that a kind of miscopying during gene replication may account for results of this kind. One way of representing this is the following:

$$- - - - - - - - - \rightarrow \quad a\ \text{P-1}\ \text{p-2}\ b$$

$$\underline{a\ \text{P-1}\ \text{p-2}\ b} \qquad\quad \rightarrow \quad a\ \text{P-1}\ \text{p-2}\ b$$

$$\rightarrow \quad A\ \text{P-1}\ \text{P-2}\ B$$

$$\underline{A\ \text{p-1}\ \text{P-2}\ B} \qquad\quad \rightarrow \quad A\ \text{p-1}\ \text{P-2}\ B$$

This type of miscopying, in which a segment of one allele is copied twice and its partner is not copied at all, must be rare, if indeed this is the mechanism, it may well be limited to segments of only a few genes. This special type of recombination has been called gene conversion (29, 33, 41) but it is clearly not the same as the process postulated by Winkler to account for normal crossing over (53). Professor Horowitz (20) has suggested that a more appropriate term for it would be "transmutation."

Other explanations for transmutation have been offered. Conventional crossing over, with one of a pair of double crossovers occurring within a gene, has been suggested (41), but this does not account for the absence of reciprocal intragenic recombination products and requires that interference be strongly negative. H. K. Mitchell (33) has presented evidence that temperature shocks have quantitatively different effects on crossing over and transmutation in *Neurospora*, another observation indicating that these processes are basically different. He suggests that transmutation may result from the transfer of a functional group from one allele to another, but sees no necessity for assuming a linear arrangement of such groups.

All of the above interpretations imply that mutants of a given gene may occur at different sites. None is inconsistent with the view that genes consist of segments of DNA, each containing perhaps several hundred to several thousand nucleotides—enough to specify the configuration of a protein or other macromolecule.

Transmutation and Crossing Over

Whatever the mechanism of transmutation, its occurrence is somehow positively correlated with conventional crossing over. This is evident from the fact that when it occurs, crossing over between closely linked marker genes is higher than would otherwise be expected. It is reasonable to suppose that if the two processes are different, both depend on close association of homologous chromosomes in the region under study, and such proximity would be expected to favor their simultaneous occurrence (34, 35, 43).

Several investigations of the relations of chromatids involved in double crossing over indicate that two-, three-, and four-strand crossovers occur with the relative frequencies 1-2-1. In other words, the non-sister chromatids that take part in a crossover at one level do so at random with respect to those involved at a second level. For crossovers close together the data show an excess of two-strand doubles that is probably but not certainly statistically significant (51). If transmutation occurs in *Drosophila,* in which most of the data referred to were obtained, it is possible that this process could account for the observed excess doubles. The attached-X technique used in this organism involves recovery of two of the four products of a single meiotic process, but these are not sufficient in all cases to distinguish transmutation from conventional two-strand double crossing over.

FINE STRUCTURE OF THE GENE

Bacteriophage.

Benzer (2, 3, 4) and Streisinger and Franklin (48) have shown that for two genes in bacteriophages (bacterial viruses, or simply phage), reversions can be obtained from "crosses" in which the parent phages carry mutants that are of different origins but involve a single functional unit. It is assumed that intragenic recombinations occur by the same mechanism by which recombination in general occurs in phages. This may well be so, but it does not follow that this is the same mechanism by which conventional crossing over occurs in higher forms. In phages, recombination is presumed to involve DNA polynucleotide chains either as double helices or possibly as single chains. Reciprocal products are not produced by a single recombinational event. In higher forms, on the other hand, chromosome threads large enough to be observed under a light microscope, i.e., many orders of magnitude larger, undergo crossing over by a process that does lead to the production of reciprocal products from a single event.

The process by which recombination occurs in phages may be fundamentally like the mechanism of miscopying proposed by M. Mitchell (34) and by Roman (43), and both processes may differ basically from conventional crossing over. If this were so, it would not be necessary to assume that the last-named process is ever intragenic.

Salmonella.

Zinder and Lederberg (56) have show that temperate phages may carry genic material from a donor to a recipient bacterial cell. Such a carried fragment of bacterial genetic material may be incorporated into the genetic mechanism of the recipient cell, a process called transduction. It is probably fundamentally similar to transformation in pneumococci, but with the superficial difference that in one case naked bacterial DNA enters the recipient cell while in the other such DNA is carried by a phage particle and is injected into the recipient cell along with viral DNA. In the latter case the host survives if the phage DNA establishes itself in a lysogenic state in the recipient.

In both transformation and transduction the segment of DNA that is transferred appears to be small relative to the total genetic material. It is perhaps only a few genes in length on the average. Insertion of the donated segment may occur by a method essentially like the miscopying mechanism described above.

Demerec and his coworkers (7, 8) have made use of transduction in *Salmonella* for a study of fine structure of the gene. This work will be presented later in the present Symposium (18) and will therefore be reviewed only briefly here.

If a large series of independently occurring nutritional mutants requiring substance S for growth is established and classified as to what steps in the synthesis of S are blocked, it is in general found that those mutants that block a specific step are allelic genetically. Presumably all involve modification of a single functional unit, and therefore all interfere with the synthesis of a single enzyme. In some cases the genes necessary for successive steps in a chain of reactions are closely linked and may be arranged in the same order as are the steps in synthesis. Presumably proximity of such functionally related genes has a selective advantage (18).

Allelism or non-allelism is determined by frequency of cross transduction. Non-allelic mutants show a high frequency while allelic ones show a lower frequency. Alleles can be divided into subclasses: homoalleles, which show no cross transduction, and heteroalleles, which show a low frequency of cross transduction (terminology suggested by Roman, 43).

Heteroalleles can be arranged in linear order by the use of combinations in which transduction for three closely linked mutants is followed simultaneously. By this means it can be shown that a single functional unit—a gene—can be modified at many different levels and presumably in several ways. Some mutant alleles act like intragenic inversions in that they fail to give transduction with several heteroalleles but show back-mutation. Others appear to be deficiencies of gene segments in the sense that they fail to give cross transductions for several heteroalleles and fail to give back-mutations.

Yeast.

Roman (43) has obtained recurrent mutations of independent origin for a number of genes concerned with adenine synthesis in yeast. Heteroalleles are distinguished from homoalleles by the fact that relatively frequent reversions—assumed to result from intragenic recombination—are obtained from diploids in which heteroalleles are present, whereas such reversions—assumed to be mutations—are much rarer in the corresponding diploids in which homoalleles are present.

As in *Salmonella,* many heteroalleles of a single gene have been found in yeast.

GENES FOR TRYPTOPHAN SYNTHESIS IN NEUROSPORA

As pointed out above, there is good evidence for the occurrence of heteroalleles in *Neurospora* (16, 44). Yanofsky and Bonner (54, 55) have made a special study of the alleles of a gene (td^+) concerned in the synthesis of tryptophan synthetase. Of twenty-five independent occurrences of a mutant type in which tryptophan synthetase is inactive, all proved to be allelic. Heteroalleles are indicated by the fact that reversions are obtained in some combinations.

All mutants lack tryptophan synthetase activity. In some a serologically related substance is found—presumably an enzymatically inactive protein. This is found in small amounts in wild-type strains.

Enzymatic activity may be restored to a mutant strain by a "suppressor" gene—a mutant gene at a separate locus. Suppressors are found to be specific to particular heteroalleles. Thus, Suppressor-2 suppresses allele *td-2* but not *td-1, -3, -6,* or *-24.* Suppressor-6, on the other hand, suppresses *td-2* and *-6* but not *-1, -3,* or *-24.*

It seems possible that in a suppressible mutant a potentially active protein is modified in such a way that a normal metabolite acts as an inhibitor by combining with the protein at the site at which it is modified. If this inhibitor were not dissociable, it would be difficult to restore activity of the protein in vitro. In such a case a suppressor mutant might act by blocking the synthesis of the inhibitor. This hypothesis appears to be consistent with the fact that there may be several non-allelic suppressors of a given mutant allele and that suppressor genes are specific as regards alleles of the primary gene.

Gene Function

On the template hypothesis of gene function, it would be expected that qualitatively different gene products would result from different alleles. If RNA is an intermediate between genic DNA and such macromolecules as proteins, mutational modifications in DNA would result in corresponding alterations in both RNA and protein. So far no satisfactory way has been found to look for modifications in RNA. But for proteins genically controlled alterations have been found in a number of cases.

In man there are eleven qualitatively different forms of hemoglobin known (49). For each of the ten deviant proteins so far discovered, there is a corresponding mutant gene known. The mutant genes associated with S (sickle cell) hemoglobin and C hemoglobin appear to be alleles. The data are not sufficient to establish whether genes concerned with other hemoglobins are allelic to S and C, but so far as I know there are no facts that counter the assumption that all mutant genes associated with qualitative modifications of adult hemoglobin are alleles, as a simple form of the template hypothesis would predict.

In many cases loss of enzyme activity is associated with mutant genes, but only in a few cases has it been established that such loss of activity results from qualitative alterations in enzyme protein rather than from its complete absence (21).

Perhaps the most extensive study of such gene-controlled qualitative alteration in an enzyme is that reported by Horowitz and Fling (21, 22) for tyrosinase activity. Here the only difference so far discovered in the two enzymes associated with different alleles of a single gene are their thermostabilities and activation energies of thermal inactivation.

Although the evidence available is limited, it is consistent with the template hypothesis of gene action (22). For more detailed studies of this kind what is needed is experimental material in which both the fine structures of a gene and its corresponding enzyme can be investigated in detail.

In the case of tryptophan synthetase activity in *Neurospora*, 25 independently occurring mutants selected on the basis of a growth requirement for tryptophan that could not be satisfied with indole were found to be allelic (55). In the large series of nutritional mutants of *Salmonella* in the laboratory of Demerec (7, 18), it was found that in the great majority of cases in which it could be determined, mutants that blocked a single chemical reaction were allelic. These are the results to be expected on the assumption that the activity of a gene is limited to the control of a single macromolecule—the so-called "one gene— one enzyme" hypothesis as formulated by Horowitz (21). It further suggests that in many cases the total specificity of an enzyme, of which substrate specificity is a part, is referable to a single gene. For a fuller discussion of the "one gene—one enzyme" hypothesis the reader is referred to three papers in the recently held Henry Ford Hospital Symposium (21, 26, 55).

The apparent complementarity of alleles of a single gene, such as suggested for the pyridoxine and pyrimidine genes in *Neurospora* (33, 34, 35, 36), is not easy to understand. In these cases it appears that two mutant genes with non-overlapping defects are able to complement one another in function even though they are carried by separate nuclei in a heterocaryon. Clearly more needs to be learned about situations of this kind, particularly the nature of the enzyme or enzymes associated with heteroalleles that complement each other in this way. As suggested earlier, it is possible that in these cases distinct genes rather than complementary alleles at a single locus are involved.

RNA as Genetic Material

No configuration of RNA has yet been proposed that suggests a mechanism of replication like that postulated for DNA. Nevertheless, it is clear from the recent work on tobacco mosaic virus referred to above that RNA is capable of carrying primary genetic information in that virus. If the RNA of higher organisms is not regularly replicated in the absence of its DNA counterpart in the nucleus, how does the RNA of tobacco mosaic virus multiply in a tobacco plant host? Possibly it is capable of replication, in which case one would suppose it to differ in this important respect from the cytoplasmic RNA of higher plants and animals. A second possibility is that its information is transferred to DNA, made by the host cell under its influence, and that this DNA is then replicated. Following replication viral genetic information can be assumed to be transferred back to RNA, which serves to store it until the next round of infection.

Defining the Gene as a Localized Functional Unit

A series of recent investigations, including those summarized at this Symposium by Benzer (4) and by Hartman (18), makes it increasingly clear that there are localized regions of the genetic material characterized by specific functions. Their positions relative to one another are determined by the methods of genetics. Their functions are studied by the methods of both genetics and chemistry. They quite clearly correspond to the units that geneticists have long called genes. That these units can be resolved into subunits capable of separate mutation and of reassociation by some mechanism of intragenic recombination seems an inadequate reason to discontinue calling them genes.

In some respects the term *gene* in the above sense—a localized unit of genetic material with a specific function—is analogous to the term *enzyme* in chemistry. Biochemists have for many years found it useful to work with enzymes as physically discrete units with specific functions. This was so before their chemical nature was known and before any one of them was isolated in pure form. It remained so after it was discovered that some of them are made up of dissociable subunits. It has continued to be so in spite of evidence that some of the so-called insoluble enzymes are functional only when associated in a particular way with other enzymes. In much the same way the concept of function is useful in defining the gene. In neither case does it provide the basis for a complete definition. In the case of the gene a final definition will presumably await the working out of the complete chemical structure of the gene itself and its macromolecular products.

In the meantime it is far more important that we make use of all possible methods of learning more about the nature of the genetic material than that attempts be made to answer with finality questions of terminology. Evolution of definitions will continue to take place, and it will remain important that terms be clearly defined in particular instances if confusion is to be avoided.

Summary

For purposes of discussion and further investigation it seems useful to make the following assumptions:

The primary genetic material in all living systems appears to be nucleic acid, deoxyribonucleic acid (DNA) in all cellular forms and some viruses, ribonucleic acid (RNA) in some plant and animal viruses.

Genetic information consists in specific sequences of bases in DNA or RNA.

The gene is defined as a localized unit of nucleic acid with a specific function, in higher forms closely associated with proteins. The function is presumed to consist in the determination of the specificity of a nongenic macromolecule such as a protein.

In phages (bacterial viruses) the genetic material appears to consist of one continuous Watson-Crick double helix of DNA built up of possibly 200,000 base pairs.

The double helix of DNA of phage is presumed to be replicated by separation of complementary polynucleotide chains, each of which then serves as a template for the synthesis of partners. The details of the process are not yet understood. Presumably the mechanism by which DNA is replicated in higher forms is fundamentally the same as in phages.

The DNA of a phage consists of many genes.

Recombination of genetic material from DNA of different parental phages occurs by a process that gives only one genetic recombinant per event; that is, reciprocal recombination products are not formed simultaneously and by a single event.

Intragenic recombination in phages occurs with a relatively high frequency, but there is no basis for believing that intergenic recombination does not also occur.

It is not known whether in phage successive genes are contiguous or are separated by "spacer" segments of DNA. By analogy with higher organisms it seems likely that adjacent functional units do not overlap, but this possibility cannot be entirely excluded by existing experimental evidence.

In tobacco mosaic virus, RNA alone is capable of transmitting genetic information from one generation to another, but it is not known whether its RNA is replicated directly or indirectly via DNA, or possibly protein, as an intermediary.

In cellular forms primary genetic information can be assumed to be carried by DNA intimately associated with protein in the chromosomes.

In plants and animals in which conventional meiosis occurs, genetic recombination occurs by a process of crossing over. This occurs in the stage at which four strands of each chromosome are present, and single events involve two non-sister chromosome threads at random and in a way that leads to two daughter chromosomes of parental genetic composition and two reciprocal recombination chromosomes.

It is at present tenable to assume that conventional crossing over is always intergenic.

Gene mutation in all organisms is presumed to consist in alteration of nucleic acid structure through base substitution, inversion of intergenic segments, duplication of intragenic segments of one or more bases, or deletion of bases. Intragenic mutations of the above kind may occur at many levels, called "sites," within a single gene. Inversions or deletions are known to transcend the limits of a functional unit in higher organisms. They are then called chromosomal aberrations.

In *Neurospora, Aspergillus,* and yeast, intragenic recombination occurs by a mechanism that can be interpreted as miscopying of small segments of genetic material. This process differs from conventional crossing over in that a single event does not result in reciprocal products and also by the fact that it does not necessarily lead to a recombination of genetic markers close to and on opposite sides of the genes within which it occurs. It is proposed that this be called "transmutation."

Transmutation and crossing over are assumed to be distinct processes, positively correlated in occurrence because both depend on the proximity—or contact—of homologous chromosomes.

The mechanism by which intragenic crossing over occurs in the above organisms—and presumably also in higher forms such as *Drosophila*—may be the same as that by which recombinations arise in phage and by which donor cell DNA is incorporated into genetic material of the recipient cells during transformation and transduction in bacteria.

Genes of cellular forms may function by a process in which genetic information is transferred from DNA to RNA segments, which then serve as templates for construction of macromolecules such as proteins.

There are now several instances in which many mutants of independent origin, selected on the basis of their relation to a specific enzyme or a chemical reaction assumed to involve a single enzyme, are found to be allelic. Evidence of this kind suggests that many genes have as their function the transfer of specificity to an enzyme. In a number of instances it appears that the total specificity of an enzyme, of which substrate specificity is only a part, is derived from a single gene.

REFERENCES

1. Avery, O. T., McLeod, C. M., and McCarty, M., *J. Exptl. Med.*, **79**, 137 (1944).
2. Benzer, S., *Proc. Natl. Acad. Sci. U. S.*, **41**, 344 (1955).
3. Benzer, S., *Brookhaven Symposia in Biol.*, **8**, 3 (1956).
4. Benzer, S., this Symposium.
5. Crick, F. H. C., this Symposium.
6. Delbrück, M., and Stent, G., this Symposium.
7. Demerec, M., *Cold Spring Harbor Symposia Quant. Biol.*, **21**, in press.
8. Demerec, M., Blomstrand, I., and Demerec, Z. E., *Proc. Natl. Acad. Sci. U. S.*, **41**, 359 (1955).
9. Dounce, A. L., *Nature*, **172**, 541 (1953).
10. Emerson, S., *Handbuch der physiol.—und pathologisch.—chemischen Analyse*, 10 Aufl., Bd. II, 443 (1955).
11. Ephrussi-Taylor, H., *Cold Spring Harbor Symposia Quant. Biol.*, **16**, 445 (1951).
12. Ephrussi-Taylor, H., this Symposium.
13. Fraenkel-Conrat, H., and Williams, R. C., *Proc. Natl. Acad. Sci. U. S.*, **41**, 690 (1956).
14. Fraenkel-Conrat, H., and Williams, R. C., this Symposium.
15. Gierer, A., and Schramm, G., *Nature*, **177**, 702 (1956).
16. Giles, N. H., *Brookhaven Symposia in Biol.*, **8**, 103 (1956).
17. Hart, R. G., *Nature*, **177**, 130 (1956).
18. Hartman, P., this Symposium.
19. Hershey, A. D., *Brookhaven Symposia in Biol.*, **8**, 6 (1956).
20. Horowitz, N. H., pers. commun.
21. Horowitz, N. H., and Fling, M., in *Enzymes: Units of Biological Structure and Function* (Gaebler, O. H., ed.), p. 139, Academic Press, New York (1956).
22. Horowitz, N. H., and Fling, M., *Proc. Natl. Acad. Sci. U. S.*, **42**, in press.
23. Hotchkiss, R. D., in *Enzymes: Units of Biological Structure and Function* (Gaebler, O. H., ed.), p. 119, Academic Press, New York (1956).
24. Hotchkiss, R. D., this Symposium.
25. Kaufmann, B. P., and McDonald, M., *Cold Spring Harbor Symposia Quant. Biol.*, **21**, in press.
26. Lederberg, J., in *Enzymes: Units of Biological Structure and Function* (Gaebler, O. H., ed.), p. 161, Academic Press, New York (1956).
27. Levine, R. P., *Proc. Natl. Acad. Sci. U. S.*, **41**, 727 (1955).
28. Lewis, E. B., *Am. Naturalist*, **89**, 73 (1955).
29. Lindegren, C. C., *Science*, **121**, 605 (1955).
30. Lippincott, J. A., and Commoner, B., *Biochim. et Biophys. Acta*, **19**, 198 (1956).
31. Mazia, D., *Proc. Natl. Acad. Sci. U. S.*, **40**, 521 (1954).
32. Mirsky, A., *Cold Spring Harbor Symposia Quant. Biol.*, **21**, in press.
33. Mitchell, H. K., this Symposium.
34. Mitchell, M. B., *Proc. Natl. Acad. Sci. U. S.*, **41**, 215 (1955).
35. Mitchell, M. B., *Proc. Natl. Acad. Sci. U. S.*, **41**, 935 (1955).
36. Mitchell, M. B., and Mitchell, H. K., *Genetics*, **41**, 319 (1956).
37. Muller, H. J., *Proc. Roy. Soc. (London)*, B, **134**, 1 (1947).
38. Muller, H. J., *Brookhaven Symposia in Biol.*, **8**, 126 (1956).
39. Pontecorvo, G., *Advances in Enzymol.*, **13**, 121 (1952).
40. Pontecorvo, G., *Cold Spring Harbor Symposia Quant. Biol.*, **21**, in press.
41. Pritchard, R. H., *Heredity*, **9**, 343 (1955).

42. Ris, H., this Symposium.
43. Roman, H. L., *Cold Spring Harbor Symposia Quant. Biol.*, **21**, in press.
44. St. Lawrence, P., *Proc. Natl. Acad. Sci. U. S.*, **42**, 189 (1956).
45. Spiegelman, S., In *Enzymes: Units of Biological Structure and Function* (Gaebler, O. H., ed.), p. 67, Academic Press, New York (1956).
46. Spiegelman, S., this Symposium.
47. Steffensen, D., *Proc. Natl. Acad. Sci. U. S.*, **41**, 155 (1955).
48. Streisinger, G., *Cold Spring Harbor Symposia Quant. Biol.*, **21**, in press.
49. Thorup, O. A., Itano, H. A., Wheby, M., and Leavell, B. S., *Science*, **123**, 889 (1956).
50. Watson, J. D., and Crick, F. H. C., *Cold Spring Harbor Symposia Quant. Biol.*, **18**, 123 (1953).
51. Welshons, W. J., *Genetics*, **40**, 918 (1955).
52. Wilkins, M. H. F., *Cold Spring Harbor Symposia Quant. Biol.*, **21**, in press.
53. Winkler, H., *Biol. Zentr.*, **52**, 163 (1932).
54. Yanofsky, C., and Bonner, D., *Genetics*, **40**, 761 (1955).
55. Yanofsky, C., in *Enzymes: Units of Biological Structure and Function* (Gaebler, O. H., ed.), p. 147, Academic Press, New York (1956).
56. Zinder, M. D., and Lederberg, J., *J. Bacteriol.*, **64**, 679 (1952).

CHROMOSOME STRUCTURE

Hans Ris

*Department of Zoology, University of Wisconsin,
Madison, Wisconsin*

Introduction

THE STUDY of chromosome structure has been much hampered by the limitations of the optical microscope. As a result the interpretations of the microscopic images have been largely subjective, and the field has been plagued by speculative constructions which were set up to fill the gaps where direct analysis was impossible. The electron microscope has now moved the limits of direct visualization to the level of macromolecules, so opening the ways for a synthesis between morphology and chromosome chemistry. The purpose of this review is to look at some old problems of chromosome organization in the light of information gained by the new approach.

The study of chromosome structure went through a series of distinct phases. In the first phase, the essential features of chromosomes were discovered and the main problems of their organization, which occupy us still today, were recognized. Thus Flemming called attention to the longitudinal splitting of chromosomes during mitosis. Van Beneden, Herla, and Bonnevie described a longitudinal split in anaphase chromosomes which indicated that chromosomes contain more than one strand also in interphase. Pfitzner and Balbiani recognized the longitudinal differentiation of chromosomes into darker and more lightly staining segments. Baranetzky, Vejdovski, and Bonnevie discovered the helical structure during mitosis, and emphasized the coiling cycle of the chromonema. Roux interpreted the longitudinal splitting to mean that essential and specific materials, hereditary determiners, were lined up into a chromosome thread so as to assure constant association and equal distribution during cell division, a concept that was established experimentally some decades later by Morgan and his collaborators. Miescher and Kossel laid the foundation for a chemical study of chromosomes with the discovery of nucleic acids, protamines, and

23

histones. Thus in the years from 1880 to 1920 the basic problems of chromosome organization were outlined:

(1) How many strands are present in a chromosome and what is the nature of the elementary unit (chromonema, genonema)?

(2) What is the nature of the longitudinal differentiation along the chromosome (chromomeres, heterochromatin)? How are chromosome structure and chromosome chemistry related to the "reproductive" and "metabolic" aspects of the gene, to gene mutation and the crossing-over unit?

(3) What is the significance and mechanism of the coiling cycle during mitosis and how is it related to chromosome chemistry and chromosome function?

(4) What are the processes leading to the duplication of chromosomes or its subunits?

(For reviews of this period, see 38, 69, 75, 102.)

The next phase was occupied mainly with a detailed analysis of the structure, coiling cycle, and reproduction of chromosomes at the level of the light microscope and with relating this structure to the mutant gene and crossing-over unit. (Cytogenetic analysis of the banding pattern in dipteran salivary chromosomes and the chromomere pattern of pachytene chromosomes.)

The analysis of structure led mainly to controversy and a wealth of contradictory and undigestable observations. The limitations of the available methods were either naively ignored, or when realized, the urge for an integrated picture led to excessive speculative construction. The picture of the chromosome that became generally accepted in this phase is best represented by a diagram of Heitz (see Fig. 1). According to this model a mitotic chromosome consisted of two, or perhaps more, helically coiled chromonemata which were made of chromomeres (CH) of specific size and structure connected by interchromomeric fibers. This helical structure was surrounded by the kalymma or matrix (M). Heterochromatic regions (H) differed in the type of chromomeres they possessed and in characteristics of the matrix. Other specialized regions were recognized: the spindle attachment, kinetochore, or primary constriction (K); secondary constrictions (S.C.); and the nucleolar organizer. Some authors added a pellicle or membrane, others insisted on a single strand except in prophase. Perhaps the major achievement of this period in descriptive karyology was the analysis of the coiling cycle of chromosomes in mitosis and meiosis. The metaphase chromosome was shown to be compact and condensed because of its helical structure. This helix originated in prophase and was unravelled again in telophase. Where the chromosome contained more than one strand, the bundle might be coiled so that the subunits were freely separable (paranemic coil, Fig. 2a) or they might be intertwined (plectonemic coil, Fig. 2b). However, it was rarely possible to decide between these alternatives by microscopic observation.

The analysis of chromosome coiling was made possible through the introduction of certain pretreatments before fixation. These pretreat-

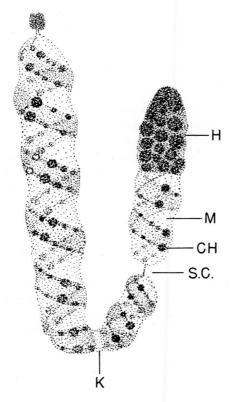

Fig. 1. Diagram illustrating the concept of chromosome structure most generally accepted in the past. CH, chromomere; H, heterochromatin; K, kinetochore or primary constriction; M, matrix; S.C., secondary constriction. (After Heitz, ref. 50.)

ments loosen up the helices and reveal the internal structure. These methods also disclosed a helical organization in the heterochromatin and suggested that morphologically these chromosome regions differ mainly in the degree of coiling from the euchromatic regions, which

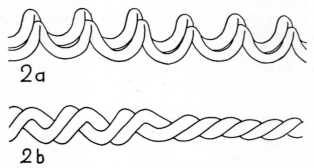

FIG. 2.   Diagram of paranemic (2a) and plectonemic (2b) coils of two strands. If drawn out the plectonemic coil turns into a relational coil (2b, right).

in turn become largely unravelled during telophase. A number of investigators furthermore became convinced that even the small chromomeres of leptotene chromosomes were in reality gyres of the chromonema helix. The chromonema was thus the basic unit and the longitudinal differentiation was essentially due, it was thought, to specific regional patterns of coiling.

The cytogenetic analysis, on the other hand, advanced rapidly despite these structural uncertainties, since at that level of analysis it made little difference what the finer structure of the specific chromosomal regions turned out to be. (For reviews of these aspects of chromosome structure, see 52, 54, 78.)

In the late 1930's the study of chromosomes entered a third phase with increased interest in the chemical constituents of chromosomes. New cytochemical techniques, especially cytospectrophotometry and the chemical analysis of isolated nuclei and chromosomes, permitted the recognition of the major chemical components of chromosomes and their quantitative relationships. The use of isotopes opened a way to the examination of the metabolic role of chromosomal constituents. So far two generalizations stand out as major results of this phase: (1) The absolute amount of DNA (deoxyribonucleic acid) per chromosome is remarkably constant from one cell to another within a species. In some groups of organisms variations between species may be large (amphibians), in others surprisingly small (mammals). The DNA molecule is also relatively constant metabolically. Synthesis is restricted to chromosome duplication (endomitosis or mitosis), and turnover appears to be practically absent, at least in mammalian tissues. (2) The non-histone protein fraction and RNA (ribonucleic acid), on the other hand, vary considerably from cell to cell, not only for whole nuclei, but also in isolated chromosomes. In cells with metabolically active cytoplasm (liver, pancreas, kidney) the chromosomes contain a good deal more of this fraction than in cells such as thymocytes or erythrocytes. In sperm nuclei this fraction may even be absent or at least undetectable with present methods (35). Both RNA and non-histone protein are very active metabolically. (For a review of these aspects of chromosomes, see reference 4.)

The intensive research into the chemical and biochemical properties of chromosomes has now given information in regard to the building blocks of chromosomes and together with results from other fields, especially from virology and the transformation and transduction phenomena in bacteria, has indicated possible relationships of these compounds to gene action and to gene mutation.

It now remained to relate the findings from the chemical analysis of chromosomes to the results of the cytological and cytogenetic studies. The aim of chromosome analysis is, of course, to integrate the chemical, biochemical, cytological, and genetic data into a unified picture of the chromosome as a functional unit, to understand chromosome structure and function in terms of the properties of the molecules of which it is made. Before any meaningful synthesis can be attempted, however, it is necessary to have more information about chromosome organization at a level between that of classical cytology and the molecular building blocks. Recent theoretical discussions on genes and chromosomes have unfortunately largely ignored this gap in our knowledge of chromosomes. Thus much print has been wasted in speculations on the distribution of DNA or protein in chromomeres or bands and interbands of salivary chromosomes, in heterochromatin and euchromatin, or on the relation of the molecular structure of DNA to chromosome duplication, crossing over, gene mutation, etc.

In the current and fourth phase of chromosome analysis this gap is being filled by the investigation of chromosome organization on the macromolecular level. The techniques of this phase are mainly polarizing microscopy, x-ray analysis, and electron microscopy, in combination with the methods of classical cytology and chemical analysis. Though this phase is only in its beginning, some information has already been gained which will have a profound effect on our picture of chromosome organization and which extends that picture to the level where a preliminary integration of structural and chemical information becomes possible.

Let us now look at the four basic problems of chromosome organization mentioned above and see what the recent analysis on the submicroscopic level can contribute to their understanding.

How Many Strands Are Present in a Chromosome and What is the Nature of the Elementary Morphological Unit?

It is generally accepted today that the chromosome is a multiple-stranded structure in all stages of the mitotic cycle (52, 63). This view is supported not only by direct microscopic evidence, but also indirectly by the results of certain experiments which can give information as to the subdivision of chromosomes. Thus chromosome breakage and recombination by chemicals (79) or by x-rays (55) reveal the subdivision of chromosomes below the chromatid level. The delayed effect of certain chemical mutagens (8, 109) is explained most satisfactorily if we assume a sorting out of subunits through successive mitoses until a recessive mutation that affected only one of the subunits is present in all strands of a chromosome. Similarly, the appearance of lethals in successive generations of *Amoeba proteus* after the incorporation of P^{32} into the chromosomes is best explained by postulating 16 strands per chromosome each of which can be affected independently by the decaying radiophosphorus (40a). There is, of course, no reason why the chromonema, which is defined as the unit strand visible in the light microscope, might not be further subdivided, as various authors in the past have pointed out. It is not the organization of the chromosome, but our prejudiced view of it which is determined by the limit of resolution of the light microscope. The electron microscope, with its greater resolving power, has now demonstrated that the "chromonema" of the light microscope is indeed further subdivided into strands of macromolecular dimensions. The preparation of chromosomes for electron microscopy presented at first some difficulties. Chromosomes are desperately small to the light microscopist. But in the electron microscope they made trouble by being too thick and dense, so that when prepared according to the usual cytological techniques they at first failed to show any details. To overcome this difficulty some investigators turned to suspensions of chromosomes isolated mechanically from various vertebrate tissues. The dangers of this approach are obvious: it is impossible to eliminate completely non-chromosomal contamination either from the material itself or from the media in which it is suspended, and there is no assurance that a structure observed is chromosomal in origin, nor does one know how the isolation procedure has modified the chromosomes on the level observed by the electron microscope. It is absolutely essential to have observational continuity from the level of the light microscope to the new level of organization revealed by the electron microscope. In the following discussion I shall consider only work that has followed this basic rule.

Yasuzumi, Odate, and Ota (116) were the first to show some reasonable detail in salivary chromosomes of *Drosophila virilis* by using a replica technique. The chromosome appears to be made of large numbers of fibrils which run mainly parallel to the long axis of chromosomes in the interband regions and are twisted and tightly packed together in the bands. The fibrils were reported to be about 500 Å thick. With ultrasonic treatment the X-chromosome in salivary glands of *Drosophila virilis* split up into a large number of fibrils about 200 Å thick (117).

Tomlin and Callan (108) published micrographs of a lampbrush chromosome from *Triturus*. They found a long thin fiber about 200 Å thick to which dense bodies (chromomeres) and structures resembling loops were attached. It is obvious from the photographs that the chromosome was greatly stretched and distorted during preparation. Ris (87, 89, 90) studied lampbrush chromosomes from *Triturus, Necturus,* and *Amphiuma*, pachytene chromosomes from spermatocytes of insects and plants, and leptotene chromosomes of *Lilium* (Fig. 14). These prophase chromosomes were found to consist of a bundle of microfibrils about 500 Å thick and more or less coiled. Guyénot and Danon (48) published micrographs of lampbrush chromosomes from oocytes of *Triton*. Though the chromosomes appear greatly distorted, it is evident that the loops consist of microfibrils similar to those described by Ris. Submicroscopic fibrils were demonstrated also in interphase nuclei of erythrocytes from *Sebastodes* which were broken by osmotic shock. They appeared to be associated in bundles (118). Similar fibrils were seen by Ris (88, 89) in squashed interphase nuclei from various animal and plant cells. These fibrils were about 200 to 300 Å thick. In the meantime Bernstein and Mazia (14, 14a) had isolated a nucleoprotein from sea-urchin sperm that consisted of fibers about 200-300 Å thick. Ris (88, 89) suggested that a fibril of this thickness represents the basic morphological unit of chromosomes. In mitosis these fibrils are duplicated, the sister strands remaining closely associated during the mitotic stages. These sister pairs then correspond to the 500 Å unit found in prophase chromosomes. The doubleness of this unit is visible in lampbrush chromosomes as well as in leptotene and pachytene chromosomes of plants and insects (89, 90; cf. Figs. 10, 14). Lafontaine and Ris (56) prepared stereoscopic photographs of lampbrush chromosomes isolated from the oocyte nucleus and dried according to Anderson's critical-point method. The three-dimensional structure of these chromosomes is well preserved in such preparations, which are especially favorable for the demonstration of the coiled microfibrils in the loops (Fig. 35).

To study chromosomes in the intact cell and for better resolution it was necessary to prepare ultrathin sections for electron microscopy.

In the last few years techniques have become available which yield sections down to 200 Å or less in thickness, and a wealth of interesting observations have been reported on the organization of the cytoplasm, but chromosomes and nuclei have generally failed to reveal any discernible organization (cf. 26). It is obviously difficult to piece together a three-dimensional image from random sections about 250 Å thick.

Fɪɢ. 3.   Electronmicrograph of a thin section through the head of a grasshopper sperm. Fixed in buffered osmium tetroxide (Palade). The arrows point to sections through chromosome fibrils which appear as double lines or circles. (Photo by C. M. S. Dass)   65,000 ×

Fɪɢ. 4.   Electronmicrograph of a thin section through an oocyte nucleus of *Triturus*. Arrows point to sections of chromosome fibrils.   65,000 ×

Fɪɢ. 5.   Electronmicrograph of a section through a nucleus of a rat pancreatic cell. Arrows point to chromosome fibrils. N, nucleolus; NM, nuclear membrane.   42,000 ×

Fɪɢ. 6.   Electronmicrograph of a section through a pellet of tobacco mosaic virus (TMV) fixed in buffered osmium tetroxide. The pellet was obtained through the courtesy of Dr. G. Pound, Dept. of Plant Pathology, U. of Wis. The arrows point to oblique sections through TMV particles. Note the similarity to sections of chromosome fibrils (the double lines and circles).   65,000 ×

Fɪɢ. 7.   Electronmicrograph of a section through a leptotene chromosome of *Lilium longiflorum*. Arrows point to sections of chromosome fibrils.   65,000 ×

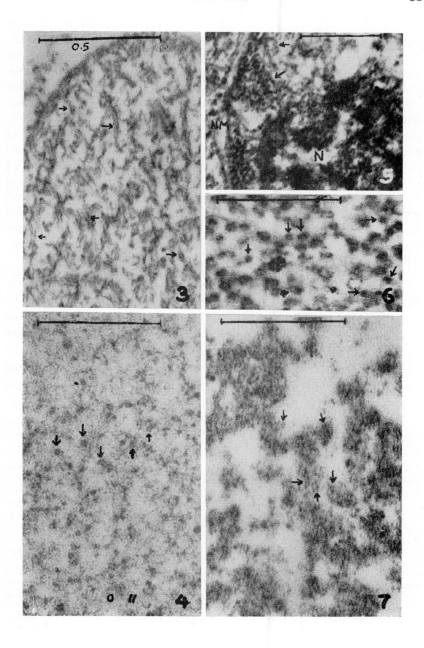

Furthermore, in a section through the interphase nucleus it is not at once obvious what is nuclear sap and what chromosomal material. To overcome this difficulty Lafontaine and Ris (56) prepared sections through isolated lampbrush chromosomes that were free from cytoplasm or nuclear sap. Since the structure of these chromosomes was already known from micrographs of whole chromosomes, it was possible to interpret the appearance in sections. As expected, these show short segments of chromosome fibrils, appearing as "granules" or shorter and longer "rods" about 500 Å thick. At higher magnifications these "rods" are seen to be double. Since the fibrils are helically coiled or at least much twisted and the sections are not much thicker than the fibrils themselves, only short pieces of the fibrils are present in a single section. Unless one knows the structure of the intact loop these are easily mistaken for granules, as for instance, in Gall's interpretation of loops. Chromomeres in sections showed a similar organization. This will be further discussed in the next part of this paper.

Sections through intact oocyte nuclei can now be interpreted. They show the "granules" and "rodlets" of the same dimensions and comparable electron density which correspond to sections through the microfibrils of loops and chromomeres. In addition a finely fibrous material, which is present between the chromosomes, probably represents the nuclear sap (Fig. 4). The sections through chromosome fibrils have a very characteristic appearance. Not only in lampbrush

---

Fig. 8. Tobacco mosaic virus protein from which the nucleic acid has been removed. Note the central hole, which in the intact virus is filled by the nucleic acid. (Photo by Williams, from Fraenkel-Conrat, 39.)   110,000 ×

Figs. 9, 11, 12. Electronmicrographs of sections through a somatic interphase nucleus from *Lilium longiflorum* (anther). Fixed in buffered osmium tetroxide; methacrylate removed with amyl acetate; shadowed with uranium. Note the sections through the chromosome fibrils which are about 200 Å wide and have a less electron-dense core. Cross sections through the fibrils (circles) are very similar in appearance to the TMV protein of Fig. 8. Arrows in Fig. 12 point to side views of sectioned fibrils, which appear solid, without any longitudinal split. (Cf. Figs. 3, 4, 7, and text.)   90,000 ×

Fig. 10. Electronmicrograph of section through a late prophase chromosome from a microsporocyte of *Lilium longiflorum*. Note the pairs of 200 Å fibrils (circles) corresponding to the units 500 Å wide seen in whole chromosomes (Fig. 14). End views of the fibrils again show the less electron-scattering core. It is assumed that these pairs of fibrils are the product of the latest duplication in the previous interphase.   42,000 ×

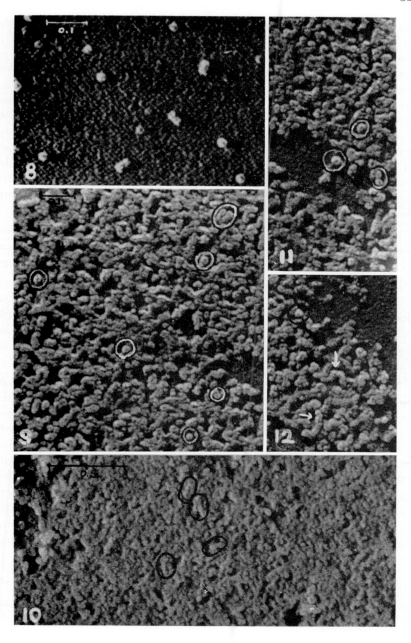

chromosomes, but in interphase nuclei of *Lilium, Tradescantia, Allium,* in liver, pancreas (Fig. 5), and testis of the rat, in leptotene (Fig. 7), pachytene, and metaphase chromosomes of *Lilium,* and in grasshopper sperm (Fig. 3), they appear as parallel double lines and circles. If the sections are shadowed with uranium after removal of the methacrylate, no split is visible in the 200 Å fibrils, but they seem to have a less electron-scattering "core," so that cross sections through the fibrils resemble doughnuts (Figs. 9, 11, 12). Since the contrast in micrographs of osmium-fixed material depends largely on the distribution of bound osmium, we must conclude that the outer layer of the fibrils has bound more osmium than the "core," either because the osmium did not penetrate, or because the "core" is chemically different and does not react with OsO_4 (90).

Gay (44) has sectioned salivary chromosomes of *Drosophila* and found fibrils 200 to 500 Å in thickness. Yasuzumi and Higashizawa (119) reported microfibrils 100-200 Å thick in sections through carp erythrocyte nuclei.

The electron-microscopic study of chromosomes thus leaves little doubt that the chromosome is subdivided into strands which are below the resolution of the light microscope. Furthermore, there is good evidence that a more or less coiled fibril about 200 Å thick is a universal structural unit of chromosomes.[1]

We must now turn to the question of how many such fibrils make up a chromosome. Exact numbers have not yet been determined. In the leptotene chromosome of *Lilium longiflorum* (Fig. 14) there seem to be about 8 subunits, in lampbrush chromosome loops of *Necturus* perhaps 16 (Fig. 34). Various observations suggest that the number varies not only between cells of an individual because of endomitosis (resulting in polytene chromosomes) but also in comparable chromosomes of different species. Variation in the number of subunits in chromosomes was suggested by Mirsky and Ris (73) to explain the great variations in DNA content of diploid nuclei in certain animal groups. Support for this view came from a comparison

---

[1] Some authors have used the term "chromonema" or "chromofibril" for these submicroscopic units. I think "chromonema" should be retained for the strand visible in the light microscope and stainable with basic dyes. "Chromofibril" is hybrid in origin and sounds awkward. I shall use here the phrase "elementary chromosome fibril" to indicate that it is considered to be the basic morphological unit of chromosomes.

of lampbrush chromosomes of various vertebrates (87, 89). There are great differences in the average thickness of loops in lampbrush chromosomes: in birds and fishes they are very thin; they increase in thickness from frog to *Necturus* and *Amphiuma*. The average size of the nuclei and the DNA content of the diploid nucleus increase in the same series (Figs. 17-20). If the structural unit in these chromosomes is the same and the coiling of the loops comparable, then we must assume a greater number of subunits in the thicker bundle. Similar size differences are found in chromosomes of mitotic or meiotic prophase of various species. We may expect to find few subunits in species with very tenuous chromosomes and low DNA content per nucleus, and more in groups with large chromosomes and high DNA per nucleus. Schrader and Hughes-Schrader (94) have recently reached similar conclusions in a study of chromosome numbers and DNA content of chromosomes in the genus *Thyanta*.

We must keep in mind, though, that variation in the number of strands is only one of several factors that can cause differences in the basic amount of DNA per nucleus from one species to another.

A further problem of great interest is the organization of the elementary chromosome fibril in terms of its molecular constituents. How are nucleic acids and proteins put together to form this fibril? A working hypothesis is suggested by the following considerations: Electron micrographs indicate that it is not further subdivided into finer strands (90; Figs. 9, 11, 12). The absence of any other persistent structure in chromosomes and the findings of Bernstein and Mazia (14, 14a) justify the assumption that the nucleic acids and proteins of chromosomes are located in the elementary chromosome fibril. The nucleoprotein which is best known structurally is the tobacco mosaic virus (TMV) particle, a rod about 3000 Å long and 150-200 Å thick. It appears that in this virus particle the RNA forms a "core" surrounded by a protein "shell" (39, 40, 49, 95).

Superficially, at least, the appearance of the chromosome fibril in electron micrographs is remarkably similar to that of the TMV particle (compare Fig. 8 with Figs. 9, 11, 12). After fixation with osmium the chromosome fibril has a less dense "core" very much like the RNA core of the virus. According to Bahr (9), OsO_4 reacts with proteins but not with nucleic acids. This would explain why, after OsO_4 fixation, the chromosome fibril is more electron-scattering on the surface than in the interior, if we assume that it is built like the TMV rods.

After fixation in formalin or ethanol the fibrils of lampbrush chromosome loops do not show this differentiation into a core and an outer shell (Fig. 35). If the DNA is removed enzymatically, there is no change in the morphological appearance of the fibril (90, 116). This would be expected if the nucleic acid was in the "core" of the fibril. Sections through TMV particles after osmium fixation look like sections through chromosome fibrils (compare Fig. 6 with Figs. 3, 4, 7; unpublished observations).[2] No doubt this hypothesis will be tested by a direct analysis of isolated chromosome fibrils with methods similar to those used on TMV particles.

WHAT IS THE NATURE OF THE LONGITUDINAL DIFFERENTIATION ALONG THE CHROMOSOME (CHROMOMERE, HETEROCHROMATIN)? HOW ARE CHROMOSOME STRUCTURE AND CHROMOSOME CHEMISTRY RELATED TO THE "REPRODUCTIVE" AND "METABOLIC" ASPECTS OF THE GENE, TO GENE MUTATION, AND TO CROSSING-OVER UNITS?

Genetic analysis has shown that the chromosome is differentiated along its length into specific regions which have characteristic developmental effects on cell and organism. It is still undecided whether these differences are due to relative position on a continuous structure (considering the chromosome fibril as a giant molecule) or whether genes are discrete and separate units with distinct borders (46, 77). Another question still debated is whether genes are separated by "non-genic" substance or border on each other.

The microscopic study of chromosomes had early revealed a morphological discontinuity along the chromosome in the form of thinner and thicker, lightly and more darkly staining, regions. The small basophilic granules, visible mainly in early prophase, are known as "chromomeres." The larger segments of chromosomes which remain contracted and deeply staining are differentiated as "heterochromatin" from the more diffuse and lightly staining "euchromatin." In the course of cytogenetic analysis this morphological discontinuity became identified with the genetic differentiation, most radically by Belling (13), who considered chromomeres to be physical counterparts of genes, hooked together by non-genic fibrils. The association of genetic

[2] I wish to thank Dr. G. Pound, Dept. of Plant Pathology, University of Wisconsin, for the tobacco mosaic virus pellets.

properties with the banding pattern of salivary gland chromosomes in *Drosophila* was often taken as proof for the identity of gene with band or chromomere. Now both genetic differentiation and morphological discontinuity must be expressions of some basic chemical and structural difference along the length of the chromosome, but there is no convincing evidence that genes correspond to either chromomeres or interchromomeres—nor to bands or interbands. The observation of McClintock (66), for instance, that deficiencies of interchromomeric regions have definite genetic effects supports the contention that a simple identification of genes with chromomeres or bands is much too naive. Before the significance of the morphological discontinuity can be appreciated we must have a better understanding of the structural and chemical differences between these chromosomal regions. Observations with the light microscope produced two opposing views: according to one the chromomeres (bands) and heterochromatin are radically different in organization from interchromomeric (interband) or euchromatic regions. The other view asserts that the chromonema is the structural unit in both and that differentiation is produced by a specific pattern of coiling.

Chromomeres.

It is widely accepted today that leptotene chromosomes are completely unravelled and display most clearly the real, ultimate chromomeres. Yet an increasing number of cytologists, working with relatively large chromosomes, have reached the conclusion that these ultimate chromomeres are really gyres of the new coil which appears at about this stage (25, 58, 59, 61, 63, 80, 85, 103, 106; cf. Fig. 15). They find that the chromonema in leptotene is rather uniform for considerable lengths, with no evidence of chromomeres (Fig. 13, arrows). Electron micrographs of leptotene chromosomes now fully support this view. In Fig. 14 we see a leptotene chromosome from *Lilium longiflorum*. It consists of several, possibly 8, strands which run longitudinally in the interchromomere regions and appear folded back and forth in the chromomeres. Though it is difficult to follow the fibrils here, it looks as if the bundle as a whole formed one or a few closely packed turns of a coil in these regions (CH in Fig. 14). Chromomeres appear to contain the same fibrils as interchromomeric segments and morphologically therefore differ mainly in the way these are arranged.

A discussion of chromomeres leads naturally to the specific banding pattern of salivary gland chromosomes. There are two main problems involved here: (1) What causes the great increase in width of these chromosomes? (2) What is the origin and structure of the bands and interbands? The evidence is conclusive today that these chromosomes are polytene, i.e., that they are made up of a very large number of strands which originate through endomitotic duplication without any separation of daughter chromosomes. X-radiation (98) and chemicals (15) applied to chromosomes at early stages produce partial breaks which become visible in chromosomes of later stages. In certain regions the chromosome may split up into numerous subunits (10, 11, 68). By micromanipulation it can be split up into many strands (27). The DNA content suggests that about 1000 times more strands are present in salivary gland chromosomes than in ordinary somatic chromosomes (53). Finally, in the electron microscope the polytene nature is directly visible (44, 116, 117, 120). The unit is a fibril 200-500 Å thick. Gay (44) has estimated that in mature chromosomes of *Drosophila melanogaster* there are 1000 to 2000 of these fibrils.

The nature of the crossbands presents a more difficult problem. According to the chromomere hypothesis, they are formed by a lateral association of the specific chromomeres on the chromonemata. Ris and Crouse (91), on the other hand, have suggested that the bands are the result of a specific coiling pattern formed by a bundle of chromonemata. In median-aged *Sciara* larvae chromonemata were visible which could be followed while twisting through the band and into the next interband. Pretreatment of salivary gland chromosomes with KCN, which is known to uncoil chromosomes, causes the bands

---

Fɪɢ. 13. Leptotene chromosomes of *Lilium longiflorum*. Feulgen-squash. The chromonema is Feulgen-positive along its entire length and of uniform thickness for considerable lengths (arrows). Compare region marked x with Fig. 14.   2500 ×

Fɪɢ. 14. Electronmicrograph of part of a leptotene chromosome of *Lilium longiflorum* fixed in 10% formalin. Feulgen-squash transferred to formvar film, shadowed with uranium. Arrows point to 500 Å fibrils that are visibly split (cf. Fig. 10). Chromomeres (CH) are places where the bundle of microfibrils is packed more tightly, possibly in one or two turns of a helical coil.   22,000 ×

Fɪɢ. 15. Leptotene chromosome of the grasshopper *Chortophaga*. Arrows point to gyres of the new helix which appear as chromomeres.   2700 ×

Fɪɢ. 16. Metaphase chromosome of *Tradescantia*, pretreated for 2 min. with .002 *M* KCN; aceto-carmine squash. Major and minor coils (arrow) are visible.   2700 ×

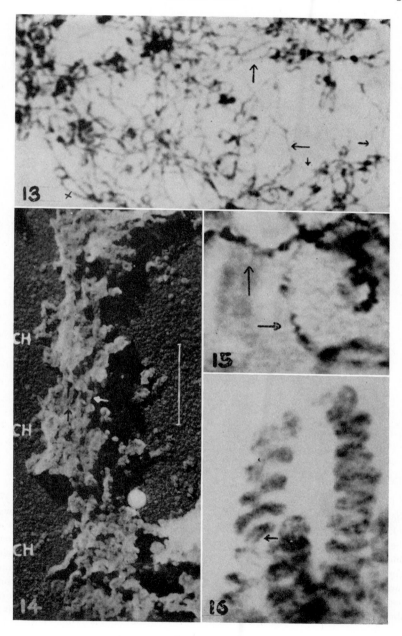

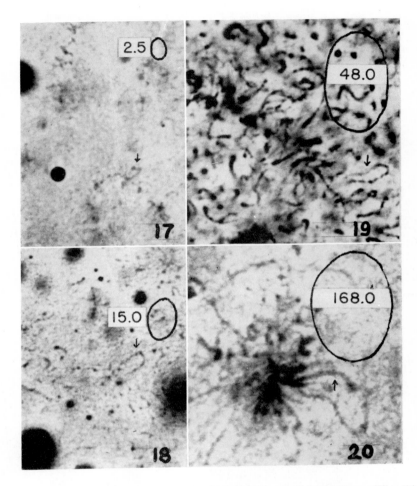

FIGS. 17–20. Sections through oocyte nuclei of the cat-fish *Ameiurus* (Fig. 17), the frog *Rana pipiens* (Fig. 18), the mud-puppy *Necturus* (Fig. 19) and the Congo eel *Amphiuma* (Fig. 20), to show lampbrush chromosomes. The numbers refer to the DNA content of diploid (erythrocyte) nuclei (times 10^{-9} mg.). The black outlines indicate the relative sizes of erythrocyte nuclei in the respective species. Correlated with the increasing DNA content is increasing nuclear volume in comparable cells and increase in width of lampbrush loops (chromatids). It is suggested that this is related to an increased number of elementary chromosome fibrils per chromatid.

1800 ✕

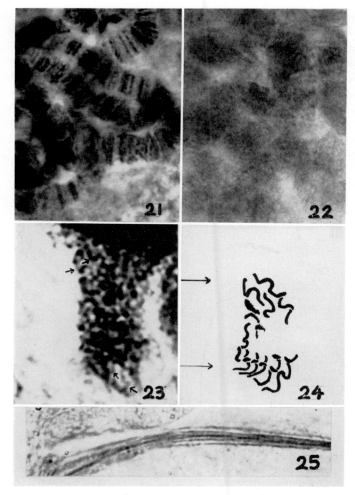

FIGS. 21–22. Salivary gland chromosomes of *Drosophila melanogaster* without and with pretreatment (0.002 *M* KCN). Aceto-orcein squash. After pretreatment with the uncoiling agent the banded structure disappears. Instead we find an irregular mass of twisted chromonemata. 1800 ×

FIGS. 23–24. Salivary gland chromosome of *Sciara*, pretreated with sodium bicarbonate (uncoiling agent) for 2 min. Arrows point to regions where coiled chromonemata twisting from band to band are visible. 2500 ×

FIG. 25. Salivary gland chromosome of *Sciara*, squashed in Ringer's solution before fixation with aceto-orcein. The greatly extended chromosome has lost its banded structure and has turned into a bundle of straight fibers. 1300 ×

to disappear and to be replaced by a mass of twisted fibers (Figs. 21, 22). Fig. 23 shows a treated chromosome at higher magnification. The arrows point to regions where the chromonemata are visible. If a polytene chromosome is stretched before fixing by squashing it between slide and coverslip, the bands disappear and the chromosome is transformed into a bundle of parallel chromonemata (Fig. 25).

The studies of Bauer and Beermann (10) on chironomids, on the other hand, have convincingly demonstrated that in the large chromosomes of older larvae the bands cannot be due to a coiling pattern of the kind suggested by Ris and Crouse (91). In the Balbiani rings the

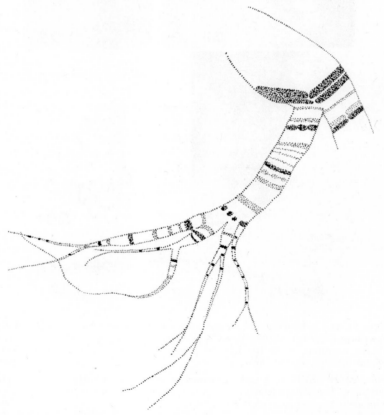

Fig. 26. Salivary gland chromosome of *Acricotopus lucidus* (a chironomid). In the nucleolar region the chromosome splits into many thinner subunits which still show the banding. After Mechelke (68, Fig. 27).

chromosome splits into progressively thinner strands which retain the banding pattern (Fig. 26). Yet Figs. 23 and 25 are difficult to understand if we believe that the chromonemata are stretched out and run parallel to the chromosome axis. Perhaps the two views can be reconciled if in early stages of development the chromonemata form relatively wide gyres in the bands, but later straighten out. The region in the bands might then look rather like the "chromomeres" in lily leptotene (Fig. 14, CH; compare this with Fig. 2, ref. 116). In this way smaller "chromomeres" previously hidden in the gyres would become visible and become oriented into bands. This could also explain the observed increase in the number of bands during the growth in length and width of these chromosomes. It seems that the structure of the bands cannot be resolved with the light microscope. We have seen earlier that the structural unit of chromosomes is a submicroscopic fibril. It is thus not surprising that the analysis with the light microscope has led to conflicting views and has not been able to give satisfactory answers to these structural problems. Electron microscopy has now supplied information which can provide at least a partial solution. Micrographs of whole chromosomes (44, 116, 120) show that the bands consist of microfibrils like those found in interbands, but are greatly twisted and closely packed together. In sections through bands of *Chironomus* chromosomes Beermann and Bahr (12) also found "closely packed thread-like elements." The exact three-dimensional arrangement of the fibrils in the bands remains to be worked out.

Schmitt (93) has approached the problem from a different angle. He has tried to explain the banding of salivary chromosomes on the basis of his experience with collagen. The periodicity in collagen is of the order of a few hundred Ångstrom units. The bands in salivary gland chromosomes, on the other hand, may be microns apart. On a submicroscopic level, the fibrils visible in the electron microscope do not show any cross striations. It is therefore unlikely that the organization of collagen has any bearing on the structure of polytene chromosomes or of any other chromosome.

Heterochromatin.

Heitz (50) defined as "heterochromatin" chromosome regions that remain condensed and darkly staining (heteropycnotic) throughout interphase. White (112) added the concept of negative heteropycnosis for chromosome regions that are lightly staining and less contracted during metaphase. The same region may be positively heteropycnotic at one time and negatively at another. The expression of heteropycnosis is often influenced by internal or external factors. In the X-chromosome of insects it may be expressed only in certain cells of the testis. Negative heteropycnosis of specific chromosome segments is produced by cold treatment (19, 28, 115). Heterochromatin usually refers to chromosome segments that are persistently heteropycnotic under any condition. But the degree of heteropycnosis may be quite variable even in these segments (36, 51, 59, 60, 99). What is the structural basis for this heteropycnosis? How does heterochromatin differ from euchromatin in organization? Analysis with the light microscope has indicated that one difference is the degree of spiralization of the chromonema. Heteropycnosis is characterized by differences in the relative width of the gyres, in the degree of packing, or by the presence of a double helix (51, 59, 99, 113, 115). Even in uniformly dense regions in prophase or interphase the coiled chromonema can be made visible by uncoiling agents such as dilute KCN (22, 23, 24, 61, 74, 85, 97). Figs. 27 and 28 show the chromocenters in a nucleus from *Amphiuma* spleen with and without pretreatment. The chromonema is certainly continuous from the euchromatin to the heterochromatin, and we have to determine now whether on a submicro-

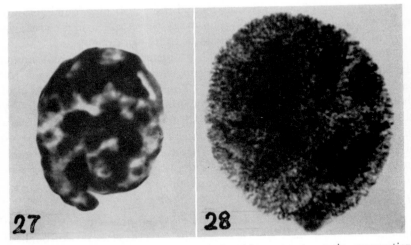

Figs. 27–28. Nucleus from spleen of *Amphiuma;* aceto-orcein preparation. The nucleus shown in Fig. 28 was pretreated with 0.002 *M* KCN for 2 min. The heterochromatin (chromocenters) visible in Fig. 27 has thus been unravelled into a mass of twisted threads.   1800 ×

scopic level it is organized differently in heterochromatin than in euchromatin. Electron micrographs of thin sections through the heterochromatin in lampbrush chromosomes ("chromomeres") and chromocenters of interphase nuclei reveal the same microfibrils that are found in euchromatic sections (Ris, unpub.). As far as structure is concerned, heterochromatin seems to contain the same basic unit as euchromatin, a fibril 200 Å wide, but it differs in the degree of packing either in the form of a system of coils or perhaps in a less regular fashion. It is probable that these fibrils are continuous throughout the chromosome, just as the unit on the level of the optical microscope, the chromatid or half chromatid is continuous. Direct evidence for this, however, is not yet available.

The information as to chemical differences between heterochromatin and euchromatin is still inconclusive. Cytochemical studies on structures of this size are extremely difficult. Since they are based ultimately on optical methods, the structure of the regions which are compared must be known before one can draw conclusions on chemical composition. The literature abounds with statements that chromomeres, bands, and heterochromatin are rich in nucleic acid, while interchromomeric regions, interbands or euchromatin are said to have little or no nucleic acid! Were we to remove the nucleic acid from these structures, we would find the same density distribution as before, and a protein stain would reveal that chromomeres or bands are richer in proteins than are interbands (67). In other words, such statements are absolutely meaningless until we know the structural organization of the regions involved and have more specific and sensitive cytochemical methods to study the *relative* composition of the parts in terms of DNA, RNA, and various types of protein. Equally empty are the often-used terms "nucleic acid charge," "nucleination," and "chromatization," since they were never based on actual chemical analysis.

Matrix.

Another element that is supposed to differentiate euchromatin from heterochromatin is the so-called matrix (see Fig. 1, M). This concept is difficult to define because various authors have used it in many different ways (cf. 50, 52). Generally it describes some non-genic chromosome material that accumulates around the chromosome thread, mainly during mitosis. It is said to be "achromatic," that is, free of nucleic acid; or "chromatic," and consisting mainly of DNA. It is supposed to surround the chromonema helix, or to be part of the helix itself, and accumulating specifically on chromomeres or heterochromatin (cf. 96). We do not have to consider the chemical interpretations here, since they are purely fictitious. We must however take a look at some morphological observations that seem to support the interpretation given in Fig. 1. In preparations of meiotic prophase one often finds the situation shown in Fig. 29. It represents micro-

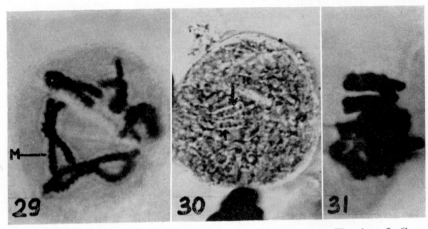

FIGS. 29–31. Smear of microsporocytes from *Trillium* sp. Fixation, LaCour 2BD. Staining: Figs. 29 and 31, Feulgen and fast green; Fig. 30: Millon reaction for protein. Note that the so-called matrix (M) is negative for protein (arrows, Fig. 30). It corresponds to a shrinkage space produced when the chromosomes shrink before fixation due to mechanical injury during the smearing (Fig. 29). In Fig. 31 the chromosomes have been fixed in the original extended state.   1800 ×

sporocytes from *Trillium* smeared and then fixed in an osmium fixative and stained with Feulgen and fast green. I have made some cytochemical tests on such preparations (obtained from C. L. Huskins) and found that the so-called matrix is negative for nucleic acids, proteins (Fig. 30), carbohydrates, and lipids; in other words, nothing is there except mounting medium. It is a shrinkage space and Fig. 30 explains how it was produced. According to Ris and Mirsky (92), chromosomes shrink when a cell is mechanically injured, or fixed in an acid fixative. Osmium fixatives preserve the chromosome in its extended state. In preparing a smear of microsporocytes some cells are injured, and the chromosomes shrink and are preserved as seen in Fig. 29. In other cells the chromosomes are fixed in the extended state, as shown in Fig. 31, filling the entire space which was occupied in the chromosomes of Fig. 29 by "chromonema" and "matrix." We have to conclude that the most suggestive evidence for a matrix was based on an artifact. Electron micrographs of sections through chromosomes never show any evidence for either a matrix or a membrane around the chromosome.

Particulate Organization of the Chromosome Fibril.

Mazia (65) and Ambrose (5, 6, 7) have independently produced evidence that the chromosome fibril might be formed by an end-to-end aggregation of rod-like particles. Bernstein and Mazia (14, 14a) prepared a native nucleoprotein from sea-urchin sperm which forms rods about 4000 Å long and 200 Å wide. It contains DNA, basic protein, and non-histone protein in similar proportions to those found in isolated whole chromosomes. The free particles appear under conditions that remove calcium and magnesium from the chromosomes. Mazia (65), therefore, concluded that bridges of divalent cations (Ca^{++}, Mg^{++}) link the particles together. Ambrose treated salivary gland chromosomes with agents known to break hydrogen bonds (phenol, urethane, or urea) and found that they dissolve the chromosomes. He postulated that the submicroscopic fibrils of chromosomes consist of rods linked end to end by hydrogen bonds. Ambrose, however, has not seen the macromolecular units or demonstrated that units of regular dimensions are actually produced by his treatment. Such evidence is limited so far to the nucleoprotein from sea-urchin sperm.

The presence of low-energy bonds linking segments of chromosomes is of special interest in regard to chromosome breakage, rearrangement, and crossing-over. Steffensen (100, 101) observed that spontaneous chromosome breakage was greatly increased in frequency by growing plants in media deficient for Mg^{++} or Ca^{++}. Such plants were also much more sensitive to x-rays than those grown under normal conditions. Levine (57) fed *Drosophila* larvae with excess calcium and reported a decrease in crossing-over. The feeding of a chelating agent (ethylenediamine tetraacetic acid) on the other hand increased crossing-over in the early egg-laying period. Feeding to the adult had no effect. Without a direct analysis of the calcium content of chromosomes, however, such experiments hardly prove a direct relation of Ca-links and crossing-over. Eversole and Tatum (33), working with *Chlamydomonas*, determined the intracellular concentrations of

Ca^{++} and Mg^{++} after treatment with ethylenediamine tetraacetic acid and $MnCl_2$ and compared them with the observed crossing-over frequency. Lowering of the Ca^{++} and Mg^{++} levels in these cells increased crossing-over considerably and treatment with Ca^{++} and Mg^{++} reversed that effect. It remains to be explained, however, how the breaking of links at 400 millimicron intervals in a multistranded bundle can produce the exactness of breakage and recombination that we must assume occurs in crossing-over.

Structural and Chemical Variations in Relation to Chromosome Function.

Physiological and biochemical studies of the cell nucleus strongly suggest that it plays an active role in the metabolism of the cell (3, 4, 64). RNA and non-histone protein are especially active metabolically, and their absolute amounts in chromosomes vary directly in relation to cell activity. There is convincing evidence that RNA as such, or perhaps as nucleoprotein, is transferred from the nucleus to the cytoplasm (47). Electron-microscopic studies suggest activity on the nuclear-cytoplasmic boundary and perhaps even transfer of particulate material (43, 105, 111). Is there any morphological expression of chromosomal activity? For some years now cytologists have known two types of chromosomes that are especially favorable for the study of this problem: the giant chromosomes in the oocytes of many vertebrates (lampbrush chromosomes), and the polytene chromosomes in dipteran larvae.

Lampbrush Chromosomes.

The chromosomes of many oocytes undergo a tremendous growth during the diplotene stage of meiotic prophase. They assume a characteristic brush-like apppearance that suggests a central axis with a series of smaller and larger granules of irregular, but rather specific shape ("chromomeres," heterochromatin) and sideloops (Fig. 33). The structure of these chromosomes has been much debated (see ref. 1). In 1945 I proposed that the loops were part of the continuous chromonema and not lateral secretions of the chromomeres, as was then generally believed (31, 32, 41, 48). While I first thought that the "chromomeres" were points of overlap of the chromonemata, I have since become convinced that they represent heterochromatic regions in which the chromonemata are tightly coiled (Fig. 33). I thus agree in essence with Alfert (1), who has also accepted the chromonemal

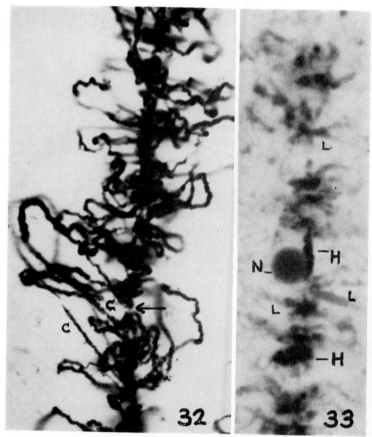

Fɪɢ. 32. Lampbrush chromosome of *Necturus,* isolated in sucrose, fixed in osmium tetroxide, and stained with iron-hematoxylin. Note the apparent central axis with the heterochromatic regions of various size and shape (chromomeres). The loops often proceed from one such region to the next, bridging a gap (arrow). The helix on the loops is visible at *c.*   1200 ×

Fɪɢ. 33. Section through oocyte nucleus of *Amphiuma,* showing lampbrush chromosome (iron-hematoxylin stain). Note series of heterochromatic regions (H) to which often small nucleoli (N) are attached. The bases of the faintly staining loops (L) are visible where they come out of the heterochromatin.   2500 ×

nature of loops. In Fig. 32, for instance, we can see clearly how the loop bridges a gap from one heterochromatic region to the next, but does not return to the point of origin. Both Callan (20) and Gall (42), who for years had opposed this view of the origin of loops, have now

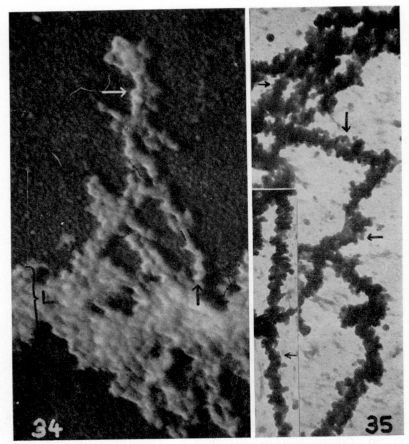

Fig. 34. Part of a loop from a lampbrush chromosome of *Necturus* (electron micrograph, uranium-shadowed). A few microfibrils have been accidentally pulled out of the bundle and are thus more distinctly visible. They are 500 Å thick (two parallel lines) and show a helical structure (arrows). L indicates the width of the loop (chromatid). The zig-zag of the bundle of fibrils corresponds to the flattened coil of the loop (cf. Fig. 32, *c* and Fig. 35, arrows).   34,000 ×

Fig. 35. Loops from a lampbrush chromosome of *Triturus*. This chromosome was isolated in 30% sucrose, washed in distilled water, and fixed in ethanol. It was then dried according to Anderson's critical-point method. Note the coiling of the bundle and the individual 500 Å fibrils (arrows). (Photo by J. Lafontaine.)
        22,000 ×

Fig. 36. Various degrees of "puffing" by a specific band of a salivary chromosome in *Chironomus*. After Beermann (11, Fig. 30).

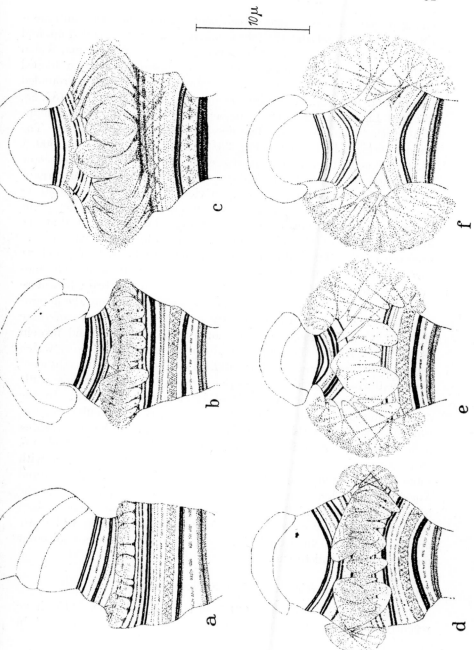

changed their conviction and agree that the chromonema is continuous through the heterochromatin (chromomeres), where it is coiled up, and into the loops. They believe, however, that this chromonema, which corresponds to a chromatid, since there appear to be two looped threads per chromosome, is a single submicroscopic fiber surrounded by granular material. The electron-microscopic studies of Ris (87, 88, 89) and Lafontaine and Ris (56), on the other hand, have demonstrated that the loops are bundles of submicroscopic fibrils. The bundle forms a helical coil (Fig. 35, arrows). The fibrils are 500 Å wide and consist of two subunits, each 200 Å thick. Stereoscopic micrographs prepared by Lafontaine and Ris (56) show this organization of loops especially clearly. In view of the similarity in structure of loops and more usual chromosomes such as the leptotene chromosomes of *Lilium*, there can no longer be any doubt that the loops are part of the chromonema. Especially significant is the presence of the 500 Å double fibrils which are typical of prophase chromosomes. Thin sections through the heterochromatin (chromomeres) indicate that they contain the same kind of fibrils, but more closely packed. Chemically, the loops differ markedly from the heterochromatic regions which are the only Feulgen-positive parts of these chromosomes. The loops seem to contain mainly RNA and protein (41). Furthermore, the loops are dissolved under conditions which leave the heterochromatin intact (32, 41). Treatment with ethylenediamine tetraacetic acid disperses the loops within a few seconds, while the heterochromatin is not affected by a short treatment. In the electron microscope we see in place of the loops an irregular mass of tangled fibrils 200 Å thick (unpub. observations). Prolonged washing in a large volume of ice-cold water causes the loops to break up. In electron micrographs the loops often look like a frayed rope with some of the strands broken. Pieces of microfibrils several thousand Ångstrom units long are scattered over the formvar film next to the loops (Lafontaine and Ris, unpub.). These observations would seem to support the view of Mazia and suggest that the loops, which are predominantly ribonucleoprotein, are also built of macromolecular particles linked end to end.

Puffs and Balbiani Rings in Polytene Chromosomes.

Beermann (11), Mechelke (68), and Breuer and Pavan (18) have recently described some remarkable structural changes in certain bands. Briefly, the essential points are these: at a definite stage in the development of the larvae specific bands on the polytene chromosomes greatly enlarge into structures known as "puffs," "bulbs," or "Balbiani rings" (Fig. 36). While this goes on in one type of cell the same band remains unchanged in others. A different band may show this puffing at another stage in development and in other cell types. The

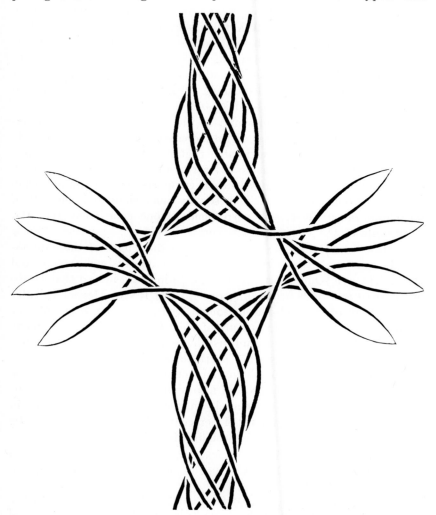

Fig. 37.   Diagram of structure in "puffs" and Balbiani rings. After Beermann (11).

puffs seem to be produced by a separation of the chromosome strands, which increase greatly in length and form lampbrush-like loops protruding laterally from the chromosome (Fig. 37). According to Breuer and Pavan (18), the puffing is associated with accumulation of basophilic but Feulgen-negative material.[3] Electron micrographs of thin sections through Balbiani rings (12) reveal twisting spongy threads about 250 millimicrons wide. At higher magnifications these show "spherical bodies" 250 Å thick surrounded by twisted fibrils about 100 Å wide. The "spherical bodies" look remarkably like sections through chromosome fibrils of other cells (Figs. 3, 4, 5, 7) with the same double lines and circles. Most likely, therefore, they represent sections through the elementary fibrils which in turn make up the bundle 250 millimicrons thick.

In lampbrush chromosomes and in the puffs of polytene chromosomes the chromonema seems to increase considerably in length. Beermann and Bahr (12) estimated that in puffs originating from a single band this must amount to at least five times their original length in the band and to about fifty times if compared with the same region of the pachytene chromosome. These very much elongated segments of the chromosome fibrils still correspond to one gene locus (cf. 91). If the rule of DNA constancy is correct and the histone here too is proportional to DNA (17), the increase in the length of the chromonemata must be caused by the addition of non-histone protein and RNA. The available information seems to indicate indeed that lampbrush loops and puffs are mainly protein and RNA. Morphologically they consist of typical chromosome fibrils. On the basis of our hypothesis of the internal structure of these fibrils, as discussed above, we might assume that in lampbrush loops and puffs the fibril has a core of RNA. If the fibrils are particulate, as Mazia has suggested, these units would have much in common with TMV particles. The relative concentration of RNA is also similar. In TMV it is about 6 per cent. The RNA associated with the non-histone protein in chromosomes varies from 7 to 14 per cent (70). This value may be too high, since some protein is probably lost during preparation.

Variations in the RNA-protein fraction of chromosomes in relation to nuclear activity have been observed in many cells (72), but nowhere

---

[3] The impression of Breuer and Pavan that there is an increase in absolute amount of DNA in the puffing band has to be substantiated by cytochemical determinations.

do they reach such extremes as in lampbrush chromosomes and puffs. In these chromosomes we can, therefore, correlate the chemical with visible morphological changes. The physical basis for the chemical variation appears to be a longitudinal growth of the chromonema (86), perhaps by adding ribonucleoprotein particles interstitially to the chromosome fibrils. In lampbrush chromosomes this takes place in many loci, in salivary chromosomes it is restricted to a few, at least to the extent that the result becomes visible microscopically. When the lampbrush loops and puffs decrease in size, some material must leave the chromosome. Perhaps ribonucleoprotein units are released from the chromosome into the cytoplasm. We would thus have a mechanism to transfer "information" from specific chromosome loci (genes) to regions of synthesis in the cytoplasm (ergastoplasm). Perhaps there is a genetic relationship between the chromosomal ribonucleoprotein particles and the particles seen in the ergastoplasm (cf. 81) which have been implicated as sites of protein synthesis.

The Coiling Cycle of Chromosomes

The spiral structure of chromosomes has been reviewed recently by Manton (62). There is no new information that would throw light on the mechanism of this cyclical structural change. Chromosomes reveal a whole hierarchy of helical systems superimposed on one another, even beyond the major and minor coil seen in the light microscope during meiosis (Fig. 16). Certain protozoa appear to be especially favorable for the study of such coiling systems (21). The helical arrangement also transcends the level of the optical microscope. In the electron microscope we see the coiling of the elementary fibril (Figs. 14, 34, 35), and beyond that we find the helical structure of nucleic acids (37, 110, 114) and proteins (82, 37). Future studies will have to show what relation exists between the helices on these different levels. Cytochemical investigations of coiled and uncoiled chromosomes, of heterochromatin and euchromatin, are needed now to show possible relationships between coiling and chemical composition.

Electron micrographs of thin sections through chromosomes have revealed a puzzling structure that possibly has bearing on chromosome coiling. Mid-prophase chromosomes in spermatocytes of the crayfish (76) and of several vertebrates (34) show a "core" in the chromosomal helix about 700 Å in diameter (Fig. 38). It is not clear yet whether this structure is present throughout the length of the chromo-

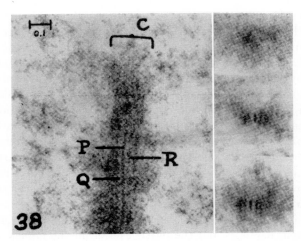

Fig. 38. Electron micrograph of a section through a prophase chromosome in a primary spermatocyte of the crayfish. The "core" within these chromosomes is shown in longitudinal and cross sections. P is a central dense structure less than 150 Å wide, bounded by less dense areas about 250 Å wide (Q). Beyond these are roughly parallel lines (R). From Moses (76, Figs. 2 and 4).

some or is restricted to certain segments. Morphologically it is very similar to the chromosomal fibers described by Porter (84). This suggests a possible relationship to the spindle attachment. If it extends throughout the chromosome at mid-prophase, i.e., at the time when the helical contraction of the chromosome takes place, it might serve as a core around which the chromonemata are coiled. By contracting it could change the loose coil of mid-prophase into the compact helix of metaphase.

Chromosome Reproduction

The most fascinating aspect of chromosomes is their duplication during mitosis and endomitosis. It is responsible for the continuity of genetic systems from one cell generation to another. It forms the bridge which links cells, individuals, and species into a continuous stream of life.

The reproduction of a chromosome consists of several distinct processes at different levels of organization. First, there must be a synthesis of the macromolecular components of chromosomes, nucleic acids, and proteins. The DNA is particularly interesting, because of its constancy and the fact that synthesis occurs only at the time of chromosome reproduction. This takes place at a certain period during interphase (104, 107). Little is known about the synthesis of chromosomal proteins, except that histones seem to be approximately doubled at the time when DNA is synthesized (2, 17). Certain observations in viruses and bacteria have indicated that there is a close connection between nucleic acids and the material responsible for genetic properties. This would imply that the synthesis of DNA is not only quantitatively exact, but also qualitatively exact in producing a true copy of the DNA molecule. The structure of this molecule has now suggested some interesting models for its replication. They will be discussed in a later section of this volume.

The chromosome, however, is not just a mass of DNA macromolecules. Models for DNA replication give no information about the duplication of the chromosome. Electron microscopic studies have now revealed a basic structural unit, the chromosome fibril. The second aspect of chromosome reproduction, therefore, on a submicroscopic level, involves the replication of this elementary fibril. In prophase chromosomes, after the synthesis of DNA and chromosomal protein has taken place, we find pairs of fibrils closely associated (Figs. 10, 14). Most probably these are the products of the latest duplication, which has resulted in the doubling of every elementary fibril of the chromosome. How is this duplication accomplished? If the nucleic acid turns out to be located in the core of the fibril, it will be simpler to make a connection between the process of DNA duplication and the duplication of the chromosome fibril. A scheme similar to that of Bloch (16), for instance, would first yield a fibril of double thickness. As this splits longitudinally, two relationally coiled fibrils are produced. Gay has found that in polytene chromosomes the microfibrils are indeed relationally coiled (44). At some later stage this must be changed into a paranemic coil so that the strands can separate. Now by coiling a pair of strands which are twisted around each other into a helix with a gyre for each relational twist, two separable helices are formed (16, Fig. 4). Perhaps the helical coiling of prophase chromosomes has the function of forming a paranemic (separable) helix of the double fibrils, and thus preparing their independence for the time when they become chromatids.

The third aspect of chromosome reproduction, on the level of the optical microscope, is concerned with the division of the bundle of microfibrils into chromatids, half-chromatids, and quarter-chromatids. The chromatids are the subunits which become the daughter chromosomes at anaphase.

The multistranded organization of chromosomes has important implications for the process of chromosome division. Unfortunately, they have been ignored in most recent discussions of this subject. The daughter chromosomes do not represent "old" and "new" chromosomes. They were separate units (chromatids) already at the time when new fibrils are synthesized and therefore, contain equally new and old strands. Depending on the number of subunits present, it will take several generations of chromosome divisions until newly formed microfibrils separate as daughter chromosomes (Fig. 39).

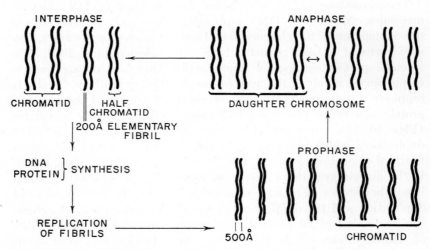

Fig. 39. Diagram illustrating the replication of elementary fibrils in relation to chromosome division. See text.

Summary

The organization of chromosomes has been discussed in the light of recent studies with the electron microscope. The major aspects of the picture emerging from this work are the following:

1. The basic morphological unit of chromosomes is a fibril approximately 200 Å thick. Based on comparisons with the particle of tobacco mosaic virus, a model for the organization of this fibril in terms of nucleic acids and proteins has been suggested.

2. Chromosomes are multistranded bundles of such fibrils. While the exact numbers present have not yet been determined, they are expected to be some power of two. This number appears to vary in different organisms, and it seems that this is one of the factors determining the variation of DNA content in chromosomes of different species.

3. Based on the structure of lampbrush chromosomes and of the "puffs" found in polytene chromosomes a working hypothesis is advanced, integrating morphological and chemical changes with chromosome function.

4. Chromosome reproduction is discussed on three levels: the synthesis of nucleic acids and proteins; the replication of the elementary chromosome fibril; and the splitting of the bundle of fibrils into units of higher order such as chromatids, half-chromatids, and quarter-chromatids. Because chromosomes are multistranded, daughter chromosomes at anaphase do not correspond to "old" and "new" chromosomes. The unit of replication is the submicroscopic fibril and not the chromosome as a whole. Both daughter chromosomes contain "old" and "new" fibrils and their chemical analysis cannot give any information about the chemical aspects of "old" and "new" strands within the same division cycle.

REFERENCES

1. Alfert, M., *Intern. Rev. Cytol.*, **3**, 131 (1954).
2. Alfert, M., in *Fine Structure of Cells*, p. 157, Noordhoff, Groningen (1955).
3. Allfrey, V. G., this volume.
4. Allfrey, V. G., Mirsky, A. E., and Stern, H., *Adv. in Enzym.*, **16**, 411 (1955).
5. Ambrose, E. J., *Bull. Soc. Chimie Biol.*, **37**, 1263 (1955).
6. Ambrose, E. J., in *Progress in Biophysics*, **6**, 25 (1956).
7. Ambrose, E. J., and Gopal-Ayengar, A. R., *Heredity,* **6** (Suppl.), 277 (1953).
8. Auerbach, Ch., in *Cold Spring Harbor Symposia Quant. Biol.*, **16**, 199 (1951).
9. Bahr, G. F., *Exptl. Cell Research*, **7**, 457 (1954).
10. Bauer, H., and Beermann, W., *Chromosoma*, **4**, 630 (1952).
11. Beermann, W., *Chromosoma*, **5**, 139 (1952).
12. Beermann, W., and Bahr, G. F., *Exptl. Cell Research*, **6**, 195 (1954).
13. Belling, J., *Univ. Calif. Publs. Botany*, **14**, 307 (1928).
14. Bernstein, M. H., and Mazia, D., *Biochim. et Biophys. Acta*, **10**, 600 (1953).
14a. Bernstein, M. H., and Mazia, D., *Biochim. et Biophys. Acta*, **11**, 59 (1953).
15. Bird, M. J., and Fahmy, O. G., *Proc. Roy. Soc. (London)*, B, **140**, 556 (1953).
16. Bloch, D. P., *Proc. Nat. Acad. Sci. U. S.*, **41**, 1058 (1955).
17. Bloch, D. P., and Godman, G. C., *J. Biophys. Biochem. Cytol.*, **1**, 17 (1955).
18. Breuer, M. E., and Pavan, C., *Chromosoma*, **7**, 371 (1955).
19. Callan, H. G., *Proc. Roy. Soc. (London)*, B., **130**, 324 (1942).
20. Callan, H. G., in *Fine Structure of Cells*, p. 89, Noordhoff, Groningen (1955).

21. Cleveland, L. R., *Trans. Amer. Philos. Soc.*, **39**, pt. 1 (1949).
22. Coleman, L. C., *Amer. J. Botany*, **27**, 887 (1940).
23. Coleman, L. C., *Amer. J. Botany*, **28**, 742 (1941).
24. Coleman, L. C., *Genetics*, **28**, 2 (1943).
25. Colombo, G., *Experientia*, **11**, 333 (1955).
26. Dalton, A. J., and Felix, M. D., *Ann. N. Y. Acad. Sci.*, **63**, 1117 (1956).
27. D'Angelo, E. G., *Biol. Bull.*, **90**, 71 (1946).
28. Darlington, C. D., and LaCour, L., *Ann. Botany*, NS, **2**, 615 (1938).
30. Denues, A. R. T., *Exptl. Cell Research*, **3**, 540 (1952).
31. Dodson, E. O., *Univ. Calif. Publs. Zool.*, **53**, 281 (1948).
32. Duryee, W. R., *Ann. N. Y. Acad. Sci.*, **50**, 920 (1950).
33. Eversole, R. A., and Tatum, E. L., *Proc. Nat. Acad. Sci. U. S.*, **42**, 68 (1956).
34. Fawcett, D., *J. Biophys. Biochem. Cytol.*, in press.
35. Felix, K., Fischer, H., and Krekels, A., *Progress in Biophysics*, **6**, 1 (1956).
36. Fernandes, A., *Bol. Soc. Brot.*, II ser., **25**, 249 (1951).
37. Feughelman, M., Langridge, R., Seeds, W. E., Stokes, A. R., Wilson, H. R., Hooper, C. W., Wilkins, H. F., Barclay, R. K., and Hamilton, L. D., *Nature*, **175**, 834 (1955).
38. Flemming, W., *Zellsubstanz, Kern, and Zellteilung*, Vogel, Leipzig (1882).
39. Fraenkel-Conrat, H., *Scientific American*, **194**, 42 (1956).
40. Fraenkel-Conrat, H., and Williams, R. C., *Proc. Nat. Acad. Sci. U. S.*, **41**, 690 (1955).
40a. Friedrich-Freksa, H., and Kaudewitz, F., *Z. Naturforsch.*, **8b**, 343 (1953).
41. Gall, J., *J. Morphol.*, **94**, 283 (1954).
42. Gall, J., *Brookhaven Symposia Biol.*, **8**, 17 (1955).
43. Gay, H., *Proc. Acad. Sci. U. S.*, **41**, 370 (1955).
44. Gay, H., Univ. Microfilms, Ann Arbor, Publ. #11, 407 (1955).
45. Geitler, L., *Chromosoma*, **1**, 554 (1940).
46. Goldschmidt, R. B., *Theoretical Genetics*, Univ. of Calif. Press, Berkeley (1955).
47. Goldstein, L., and Plaut, W., *Proc. Nat. Acad. Sci. U. S.*, **41**, 874 (1955).
48. Guyénot, E., and Danon, M., *Rev. Suisse Zool.*, **60**, 1 (1953).
49. Hart, R. G., *Proc. Nat. Acad. Sci. U. S.*, **41**, 261 (1955).
50. Heitz, E., *Z. indukt. Abst. u-Vererbungsl.*, **70**, 402 (1935).
51. Japha, B., *Z. Botan.*, **34**, 321 (1939).
52. Kaufmann, B., *Botan. Revs.*, **14**, 57 (1948).
53. Kurnick, N. B., and Herskovitz, I., *J. Cell. Comp. Physiol.*, **39**, 281 (1952).
54. Kuwada, Y., *Cytologia*, **10**, 213 (1939).
55. LaCour, L. F., and Rütishauser, A., *Chromosoma*, **6**, 696 (1954).
56. Lafontaine, J., and Ris, H., *Genetics*, **40**, 579 (1955).
57. Levine, R. P., *Proc. Nat. Acad. Sci. U. S.*, **41**, 727 (1955).
58. Linnert, G., *Chromosoma*, **3**, 400 (1949).
59. Linnert, G., *Chromosoma*, **7**, 90 (1955).
60. Lorbeer, G., *Jb. wiss. Botan.*, **80**, 567 (1934).
61. Makino, S., and Momma, E., *J. Morph.*, **86**, 229 (1950).
62. Manton, I., *Biol. Revs.*, **25**, 486 (1950).
63. Marquardt, H., *Planta*, **31**, 670 (1941).
64. Mazia, D., in *Trends in Physiol. and Biochem.*, (Barron, ed.), p. 77, Academic Press, New York (1952).
65. Mazia, D., *Proc. Nat. Acad. Sci. U. S.*, **40**, 521 (1954).
66. McClintock, B., *Genetics*, **29**, 478 (1944).
67. McDonough, E. S., Rowan, M., and Mohn, N., *J. Hered.*, **43**, 3 (1952).

68. Mechelke, F., *Chromosoma,* **5**, 511 (1953).
69. Miescher, F., *Die histochemischen und physiologischen Arbeiten,* Leipzig (1897).
70. Mirsky, A. E., *Cold Spring Harbor Symposia Quant. Biol.,* **12**, 143 (1947).
71. Mirsky, A. E., and Ris, H., *J. Gen. Physiol.,* **31**, 1 (1947).
72. Mirsky, A. E., and Ris, H., *Nature,* **163**, 666 (1949).
73. Mirsky, A. E., and Ris, H., *J. Gen. Physiol.,* **34**, 451 (1951).
74. Momma, E., *Cytologia,* **17**, 156 (1952).
75. Morgan, T. H., *The Physical Basis of Heredity,* Philadelphia, 1919.
76. Moses, M. J., *J. Biophys. Biochem. Cytol.,* **2**, 215 (1956).
77. Muller, H., *Brookhaven Symposia Biol.,* **8**, 126 (1955).
78. Nebel, B. R., *Botan. Revs.,* **5**, 563 (1939).
79. Oehlkers, F., and Marquardt, H., *Zeit. Ind. Abst. Vererb.,* **83**, 299 (1950).
80. O'Keefe, M., *Am. J. Botan.,* **35**, 434 (1948).
81. Palade, G. E., and Siekevitz, P., *J. Biophys. Biochem. Cytol.,* **2**, 171 (1956).
82. Pauling, L., *American Scientist,* **43**, 285 (1955).
83. Polli, E. E., *Chromosoma,* **4**, 621 (1952).
84. Porter, K. R., in *Fine Structure of Cells,* p. 236, Noordhoff, Groningen (1955).
85. Ris, H., *Biol. Bull.,* **89**, 242 (1945).
86. Ris, H., In *Symposium on Cytology,* p. 21, Michigan State College Press (1951).
87. Ris, H., *Genetics,* **37**, 619 (1952).
88. Ris, H., *Excerpta Medica,* **8**, 399 (1954).
89. Ris, H., in *Fine Structure of Cells,* p. 121, Noordhoff, Groningen (1955).
90. Ris, H., *J. Biophys. Biochem. Cytol.,* in press.
91. Ris, H., and Crouse, H., *Proc. Nat. Acad. Sci. U. S.,* **31**, 321 (1945).
92. Ris, H., and Mirsky, A. E., *J. Gen. Physiol.,* **32**, 489 (1949).
93. Schmitt, F. O., *Nature,* **177**, 503 (1956).
94. Schrader, F., and Hughes-Schrader, S., *Chromosoma,* **7**, 469 (1956).
95. Schramm, G., and Zillig, W., *Z. Naturforsch,* **10b**, 493 (1955).
96. Serra, J. A., in *Encyclopedia of Plant Physiology,* **I**, 445, Springer, Berlin (1955).
97. Shinke, N., *Cytologia Fujii Jub.,* Vol. **I**, 449 (1937).
98. Slizynski, B. M., *Genetics,* **35**, 279 (1950).
99. Smith, S. G., *Chromosoma,* **4**, 585 (1952).
100. Steffensen, D., *Proc. Nat. Acad. Sci. U. S.,* **39**, 613 (1953).
101. Steffensen, D., *Proc. Nat. Acad. Sci. U. S.,* **41**, 155 (1955).
102. Strasburger, E., *Zellbildung und Zellteilung,* Jena (1880).
103. Swanson, C. P., *Am. J. Botan.,* **30**, 422 (1943).
104. Swift, H., *Intern. Rev. Cytol.,* **2**, 1 (1953).
105. Swift, H., *J. Biophys. Biochem. Cytol.,* in press.
106. Taylor, J. H., *J. Hered.,* **40**, 87 (1949).
107. Thorell, B., in *Nucleic Acids,* Vol. II (Chargaff and Davidson, eds.), Academic Press, New York (1955).
108. Tomlin, S. G., and Callan, H. G., *Quart. J. Micr. Sci.,* **92**, 221 (1951).
109. Vogt, M., *Z. indukt. Abst. u.-Vererbungsl.,* **83**, 341 (1950).
110. Watson, J. D., and Crick, F. H. C., *Nature,* **171**, 964 (1953).
111. Watson, M., *J. Biophys. Biochem. Cytol.,* **1**, 257 (1955).
112. White, M. J. D., *Proc. Roy. Soc. (London)* B, **119**, 61 (1935).
113. White, M. J. D., *J. Genet.,* **40**, 67 (1940).
114. Wilkins, M. H. F., Stokes, A. R., and Wilson, H. R., *Nature,* **171**, 737 (1953).
115. Wilson, G. B., and Bothroyd, E. R., *Canad. J. Research,* **22**, 105 (1944).

116. Yasuzumi, G., Odate, Z., and Ota, Y., *Cytologia,* **16**, 233 (1951).
117. Yasuzumi, G., and Kondo, A., *J. Hered.*, **42**, 219 (1951).
118. Yasuzumi, G., and Yamamoto, Y., *Cytologia,* **18**, 240 (1953).
119. Yasuzumi, G., and Higashizawa, S., *Cytologia,* **20**, 280 (1955).
120. Yasuzumi, G., Deguchi, K., and Tomita, A., *J. Electronmicr.,* **3**, 20 (1955).

DISCUSSION

DR. GLASS: In respect to the proposal made through Dr. Beadle from Dr. Horowitz, I might comment that the term transmutation, just like the term conversion, has a historical connotation which makes it somewhat undesirable. Of course, there is nothing to prevent us from taking an old term and modifying it in the light of current usage, and if it really seems more appropriate—and it does—I really have no objection to it. To go back in the literature, the term transmutation was used in the early days in genetical work by the Russians, in particular by Timofeeff-Ressovsky, as a synonym for what the English and the American geneticists called ordinary mutation.

DR. H. W. LEWIS: I would like to point out to you, Dr. Ris, that you have read more than was intended into Dr. Schmitt's speculations on chromosome structure, and, consequently, perhaps you have misinterpreted Schmitt's view of the chromosome. Unless I have misinterpreted your remarks, it is your opinion that Schmitt has suggested that chromosome structure is like that of fibrous collagen and that the bands of the dipteran salivary gland chromosomes are analogous to the bands of collagen. This is not Schmitt's point of view. He did draw an analogy between chromosomes and other macromolecular systems but like any analogy it is useful only if we do not carry the comparison too far. Allow me to point out the salient features of Schmitt's analogy. In essence what he did was examine, with the view of seeking common denominators, biological entities whose structures on a macromolecular level we understand at least moderately. The biocolloids that Schmitt has had experience with include not only collagen, but also myosin, fibrinogen and keratin. What impressed him most is that it is the precise organization rather than the precise composition of the biologically functional unit that is of prime importance. Now, what are the factors responsible for this precise organization? They are factors which the physical biochemists are beginning to understand intimately and can be grouped into two categories. The first is what Schmitt calls the "built-in specificity" of the macromolecules and includes the specific composition and structure of the macromolecules such as the sequence of amino acids or nucleotides, the degree of polymerization, the position or direction of rotation of certain chemical groups, etc. The second group of factors are those which make up the environment in which the macromolecules interact, i.e., the presence or absence of certain substances, pH, ionic strength, etc.

Now, what common principles can we deduce from analysing the structure of the above-mentioned macromolecular systems? The most important point is that the properties we recognize in the system are a function of the manner in which the component macromolecules are integrated into the system as a whole and are not the properties of the component macromolecules. The biological and morphological properties of the system can be changed by changing the precise organization of the component macromolecules but the component macromolecules themselves remain unchanged. The second generalization that can be made is that the integration of the component macromolecular units is extremely sensitive to certain subtle changes in the environment while at the same time insensitive to other less subtle changes. Furthermore the mechanics of the integration of macromolecules into a biologically meaningful unit can be explained in terms of known physical-chemical phenomena; e.g., thermal agitation, van der Waals forces, hydrogen bonding, and electrostatic links influenced by such variables as ionic strength and pH.

Chromosomes are much more complex than the biological systems from which these generalizations have been derived. However, the different species of macromolecules that chromosomes are composed of, such as DNA, RNA, and proteins, as well as lipids and water, interact to form a polyelectrolyte biogel and from the physical-chemical point of view the same principles of organization may apply. This is as far as the analogy may be carried and still be useful. These general considerations are completely compatible with all known genetic and cytological phenomena, and in fact, viewing the genetic material from the level of integrating macromolecules may offer new understanding of its biological activity.

The final point I would like to make concerns the banding of the dipteran salivary gland chromosomes. In Dr. Schmitt's original published article he used the banded structure of collagen as an illustration of the fact that the properties of the system as a whole are not the properties of the component macromolecules of the system and that the properties of the integrated system are determined largely by the immediate environment. This does not mean that the origin of all banded structures in nature is the same. It should be overwhelmingly apparent that the banded structure of collagen and the banded structure of salivary gland chromosomes cannot be the same because collagen is composed of a single species of macromolecule, tropocollagen, while the characteristic banded structure of the chromosomes is due to alternating regions of high to low DNA ratio to other macromolecules. The concentration of DNA is not the same in the different bands and the manner in which the macromolecules are integrated into the organized system varies along the length of the chromosome, as indicated by the fact that the various bands have their own characteristic appearance. I may add, not as part of my argument to be sure, but as an aside to one of your comments, Dr. Ris, that the tropocollagen macromolecule in reference to the dimensions of the collagen bands one sees with the electron microscope is in the same order of magnitude as the DNA macromolecule with reference to the bands of salivary gland chromosomes.

DR. RIS: I don't think much is gained by such comparisons of completely unrelated things as the banding in collagen and the banding in salivary gland chromosomes. Before we can interpret the structure of these chromosomes on the molecular level we must have more information on the organization of bands and interbands in terms of chromosomal subunits, like the ones now studied in the electromicroscope. We also need more reliable data on the chemical composition of bands and interbands, especially with reference to the distribution of DNA.

DR. ALFERT: Dr. Bernard Nebel at the Argonne laboratory has had an ingenious idea to get at the submicroscopic structure of nuclear material. This has just been reported at Cold Spring Harbor and is interesting enough to be repeated here. Nebel made use of an old observation of Mrs. Schrader's, dealing with the spermatogenesis of some coccids: there are only two chromosomes which, at a certain stage, leave the nucleus and move into the sperm tail where they become lined up one behind the other. The nucleus remains as an intact vesicle free of chromatin. Nebel had the good idea to make electron microscopic studies of this system. There appear to be lots of strands and coils in such completely chromatinless nuclei. These pictures furnish a structural blank with which electron micrographs of other nuclei should be compared: the remaining structure in such "empty" nuclei has to be subtracted from that of chromatin-containing nuclei before one can get a good idea of the submicroscopic structure of the chromatin itself.

DR. RIS: What is the structure of the chromosomes in the tail?

DR. ALFERT: The chromosomes are in the tail surrounded by a mitochondrial sheath.

DR. RIS: What does the chromatin look like?

DR. ALFERT: Dr. Nebel didn't have detailed pictures of the fine structure of the chromosomes in the sperm tail. This work has just started and there will be more of it.

Another point is the question of coils vs. chromomeres. Dr. Herbert Taylor at the Columbia Botany Department has very good microscopic evidence that images of coils and chromomeres are interchangeable, depending on the pretreatment and handling of the living material. At one time you may see a definite chromomeric pattern, yet one can get a complex pattern of coils in the same chromosomes by slight changes in the preparation. This seems to bear out Dr. Ris' long-standing opinion on this particular subject.

DR. LEDERBERG: Did Dr. Ris give a best estimate of how many fibrils there are in the diplotene chromatid? How many degrees of subdivision do we have to cope with when dealing with crossing over?

DR. RIS: You'll have to tell me what animal you're working with, because the number seems to vary from one group of organisms to another. In Drosophila and corn for instance I think there are only very few. In salamanders, lily and Tradescantia there are rather many. As I said, in lily leptotene my guess would be eight microfibrils per chromosome.

DR. MAALØE: We have tried very recently to section bacteria, and we are not fully certain of what we see. One minor point concerning the interpretation that Dr. Ris gave to his structure: in the first place, we see a similar thing in bacteria when we get them imbedded in something that will not tend to destroy them in the process of polymerization of methacrylate. The other thing is that Dr. Ris says that according to Bahr you get the main contrast from the protein. I am afraid that is not true, for two reasons. In the first place, if you do not use osmium at all but use some other stain or some other fixative for the cell nearly all the elements that are in there should present themselves in the same contrast as they do if you use osmium. The second reason is that if you take phage and first agglutinate it to collect the particles, fix it with osmium, and then dehydrate, imbed, and section, then you get a picture which looks this way. You get a particle with a dark central core and with a faint halo around it, and measurements of the dark center show that this is probably the DNA-containing core of the particle. We know that for special reasons the DNA here must be packed very, very tightly. The thing is that the core here gives a very strong contrast in the electron microscope, whereas the protein shell around it gives a very dim contrast. In our reasoning the osmium is not responsible for contrast to a very appreciable extent. The contrasts that we do see would have to come mainly from phosphorus and sulfur atoms, as these would have to be heavier than the nitrogen, carbon, and oxygen atoms of the protein.

DR. RIS: If you fix lampbrush chromosomes with formalin, then the fibrils do not show this differentiation into core and outer shell. It is rather difficult to do this with sections because after formalin fixation much of the tissue is destroyed in the electron beam. Councilman Morgan has obtained pictures of formalin-fixed material, but he had to shoot in the dark at such low beam intensities that nothing was visible on the fluorescent screen. I haven't had the courage to do that yet. The use of electron stains is rather tricky and I have not had any success with chromosomes so far.

DR. BEADLE: I would like to ask Dr. Ris or someone else in the audience a question that has been bothering me and that I have not heard discussed. This is the report by Marshak that sea urchin eggs contain no DNA at certain stages. Can anybody explain this?

DR. ALFERT: They do contain DNA, but Marshak thinks that all of this is due to contamination by polar bodies and other nuclear material. The question is whether it is possible to account quantitatively for all the DNA present on the basis of such contamination.

DR. RIS: I have made some Feulgen preparations of mature sea urchin eggs before fertilization and there is no doubt that Feulgen positive material was present in nuclei. It was, however, very much dispersed and the reaction was rather weak. This is not surprising since the amount of DNA per diploid nucleus in the sea urchin is relatively small to begin with and the chromatin in these nuclei is much dispersed.

DR. J. A. V. BUTLER: I should just like to suggest that Dr. Ris' pictures are a little hard to reconcile with the chemical evidence of the composition of nucleoprotein. Davison and I have made analyses of nucleic acids and amino acid contents of carefully prepared nucleoproteins. They are very constant. There is nearly one basic amino acid to each phosphate group. Now there are 3 non-basic amino acids per phosphate group. It is probable that each basic amino acid is associated with a phosphate group, and if you pack these together it would be difficult to make a single thread of 200 Å units diameter.

DR. R. WILLIAMS: I would like to make a comment first of all regarding the remarks about the appearance of bacteriophage. Bernstein at Berkeley has done some differential staining of phage with osmium, and with iron in the absence of osmium. Interestingly enough, his results could hardly be more contrary to the picture shown by Dr. Maaløe that we have seen here; namely, Bernstein finds that in the presence of osmium the outer coating is dark, and the inner region is relatively light. In the case of the iron staining, the inner becomes quite opaque, and Bernstein has a fairly good stoichiometric relation between the amount of iron taken up and the amount of DNA in the phage head. I wanted particularly to ask Dr. Ris a question, and to make a comment concerning a remark that he made. I gather you concluded from the sections which were observed before the methacrylate had been removed that the holes in the otherwise complete discs represent where the nucleic acid is localized, but is unstained. I take it that in the picture in which the methacrylate had been removed we saw "doughnuts." In the latter case, surely, the origin of the contrast is not the same—that is, in the latter case, where the specimen had been shadowed, a hole that one sees in the center of the "doughnut" represents where something isn't. This means that before the methacrylate was removed that space was filled with methacrylate only, in order to show as a hole after the methacrylate had been removed. So in a way the matter seems contradictory; as though on the one hand you are maintaining that there is nucleic acid in the center of these circular objects, and on the other hand implying that there isn't anything in the center of the circular objects.

DR. RIS: I was puzzled by this myself. In formalin fixation you don't get these double lines. The fibril seems to be uniformly dense throughout with no hole in it. Now as to shadowing, I wonder whether you wouldn't agree that if you have osmium on the outside and no osmium in the center you still would get a greater contrast on the outside even after shadowing.

DR. WILLIAMS: I would have concluded from the amount of metal evidently put on during shadowing that it is very likely not so. Is there any possibility that material which perhaps initially filled the inside of the doughnuts has been removed during methacrylate imbedding following incomplete fixation with osmium? You might truly be looking at holes which were filled with nucleic acid to start with and, if it weren't fixed adequately, it would appear as a hole later on, having been washed out of the sample. It's a possibility.

DR. RIS: Perhaps this could happen. Of course, it is also possible that the chromosome fibril is hollow inside. I would like to emphasize that I did not conclude that the nucleic acid is in the core. This suggested itself because of the striking similarity in appearance of the chromosome fibril and tobacco mosaic virus where the nucleic acid was thought to be in the core. In view of the recent work of Dr. Franklin, however, the virus seems to have a hole down the middle, and the same could be true for chromosome fibrils.

DR. HUXLEY: Just a terminological point: I am rather sorry that Dr. Ris rejected the term chromofibril on the ground that it is hybrid. It seems to me that when you have discovered a definite unit like this you want a term which is not a descriptive term which could apply to almost anything like chromosome fibril, but something which you can define accurately. After all, there are quite a lot of hybrid words in common use. Perhaps if Dr. Ris stuck to this rule he could not use the word homosexual—perhaps he never does. He wouldn't be able to use the word automobile, or even macromolecule.

DR. RIS: The name "chromofibril" would to me at least imply a fibril that combines with dyes and becomes colored, which is meaningless in the electron microscope. Chromosome fibril on the other hand indicates clearly that it is a unit of chromosomes.

DR. DOUNCE: I would like to point out that the structure of these nucleoproteins of the chromosomes is very sensitive to pH and also to ionic strength. I wonder, if you think your interpretation is correct that the nucleic acid is surrounded by proteins, whether this might not be due to the action of the fixative, either because of the ionic strength or the pH of the preparation. If you combine DNA and protein, it seems logical that the protein should arrange itself in a shell around the DNA fibers—perhaps that's what you are seeing. On the other hand, if this structure were present in the nucleus originally, one would wonder why the DNAase would remove the DNA, because RNAase, which is a much smaller molecule, doesn't attack the tobacco mosaic virus, which seems to have a similar structure consisting of a nucleic acid thread surrounded by protein. In our own laboratory we have found that the action of DNAase on isolated nuclei is quite different at pH 6 than at pH 7 where there's not much complexing of proteins with the DNA. The DNAase depolymerizes the DNA quite readily at pH 7; but, although the enzyme tends to have a very rapid action at pH 6 in cleaving the DNA, possibly near the end of the fiber, from the residual protein, the DNA is not depolymerized, extensively. This indicates that at pH 6, where protein complexing begins, there may actually be a steric hindrance against the action of DNA-ase, owing to this protein shell around the DNA fiber. Dr. Ris, I wonder if you would care to comment on this.

DR. RIS: With whole chromosomes such as lampbrush chromosomes or meiotic prophase chromosomes we got the same picture after freeze-drying, fixation with ethanol, formalin or osmium. With regard to the action of DNA-ase, it should make a difference whether you first fix the preparation or not. In our case the material was always fixed first. After denaturation of the protein there may be enough holes so that the enzyme can get inside.

DR. DOUNCE: Did you use DNAase at pH 7 or thereabouts after fixation?

DR. RIS: Yes.

DR. BEADLE: I would like to ask Dr. Ris about the consistency of this picture of different numbers of ultimate units in the chromosome with the genetic data on the times at which mutations are expressed. If there were many units in sperms, for example, induced mutations ought to show us very small "fractionals" and this might be different in different organisms. In Drosophila mutations induced in sperms are not all expressed as "fractionals." There are some whole mutations, as though there were only one unit instead of many.

DR. RIS: Drosophila and corn are two organisms that seem to have very few units. You would have to work with something like lily or salamander in order to study such an effect. Then you also have to consider that the mutational event could affect more than one unit at a time, like a single x-ray hit, breaking a whole chromosome or a chromatid.

DR. ALFERT: There is a question whether such structures occur in sperm. The chemical composition of sperm chromatin is quite different from that of interphase chromatin, and the electronmicroscopic appearance of sperm chromatin is quite different. It has a crystalline and very regular appearance which is lacking in other nuclei. Maybe the material becomes arranged in a very different way just while it's being transported and cannot be directly compared with the chromosome structure in the active nucleus.

DR. DAVISON: I would like to ask Dr. Ris a question in regard to those electron micrographs. There was a section where you showed whole nuclei which seemed to be lacking in ordered structure, and I wondered, in view of that, whether you would retract your original identification of isolated interphase chromosomes with chromosomes visible at mitosis.

DR. RIS: Are you referring to the swelling, sliding, and contraction of the chromosomes?

Dr. DAVIDSON: No. Your work with Mirsky where you identified isolated products.

Dr. RIS: The pictures you saw can tell us really nothing about the existence of individual chromosomes such as are isolated mechanically from interphase nuclei. First, we deal with random sections through the nucleus, 25 millimicrons thick; secondly, the chromosomes have no distinct boundaries or membranes and are in a swollen state in the living nucleus and are fixed like this by the osmium fixative. Therefore, you could not expect to see definite structures corresponding to specific chromosomes in these pictures.

THE ELEMENTARY UNITS OF HEREDITY*

SEYMOUR BENZER

Biophysical Laboratory, Purdue University,
Lafayette, Indiana

INTRODUCTION

THE TECHNIQUES of genetic experiments have developed to a point where a highly detailed view of the hereditary material is attainable. By the use of selective procedures in recombination studies with certain organisms, notably fungi (14), bacteria (2), and viruses (1), it is now feasible to "resolve" detail on the molecular level. In fact, the amount of observable detail is so enormous as to make an exhaustive study a real challenge.

A remarkable feature of genetic fine structure studies has been the ability to construct (by recombination experiments) genetic maps which remain one-dimensional down to the smallest levels. The molecular substance (DNA) constituting the hereditary material in bacteria and bacterial viruses is also one-dimensional in character. It is therefore tempting to seek a relation between the linear genetic map and its molecular counterpart which would make it possible to convert "genetic length" (measured in terms of recombination frequencies) to molecular length (measured in terms of nucleotide units).

The classical "gene," which served at once as the unit of genetic recombination, of mutation, and of function, is no longer adequate. These units require separate definition. A lucid discussion of this problem has been given by Pontecorvo (13).

The unit of recombination will be defined as the smallest element in the one-dimensional array that is interchangeable (but not divisible) by genetic recombination. One such element will be referred to as a

* This research has been supported by grants from the American Cancer Society, upon recommendation of the Committee on Growth of the National Research Council, and from the National Science Foundation.

70

"recon." The unit of mutation, the "muton," will be defined as the smallest element that, when altered, can give rise to a mutant form of the organism. A unit of function is more difficult to define. It depends upon what level of function is meant. For example, in speaking of a single function, one may be referring to an ensemble of enzymatic steps leading to *one* particular physiological end-effect, or of the synthesis of *one* of the enzymes involved, or of the specification of *one* peptide chain in one of the enzymes, or even of the specification of *one* critical amino acid.

A functional unit can be defined genetically, independent of biochemical information, by means of the elegant *cis-trans* comparison devised by Lewis (12). This test is used to tell whether two mutants, having apparently similar defects, are indeed defective in the same way. For the *trans* test, both mutant genomes are inserted in the same cell (e.g., in heterocaryon form, or, in the case of a bacterial virus, the equivalent obtained by infecting a bacterium with virus particles of both mutant types). If the resultant phenotype is defective, the mutants are said to be non-complementary, i.e., defective in the same "function." As a control, the same genetic material is inserted in the *cis* configuration, i.e., as the genomes from one double mutant and one non-mutant. The *cis* configuration usually produces a non-defective phenotype (or a close approximation to it). It turns out that a group of non-complementary mutants falls within a limited segment of the genetic map. Such a map segment, corresponding to a function which is unitary as defined by the *cis-trans* test applied to the heterocaryon, will be referred to as a "cistron."

The experiments to be described in this paper represent an attempt to place limits on the sizes of these three genetic units in the case of a specific region of the hereditary material of the bacterial virus T4. A group of *"rII"* mutants of T4 has particularly favorable properties for this kind of analysis. Mutants are easily isolated. Recombinants can be detected, even in extremely low frequency, by a selective technique. The system is sufficiently sensitive to permit extension of genetic mapping down to the molecular (nucleotide) level, so that the recon and muton become accessible to measurement. The *rII* mutants are defective in the sense of being unable to multiply in cells of a certain host bacterium (although they do infect and kill the cell). The *cis-trans* test can therefore be readily applied.

GENETIC MAPS

Method of Construction.

The construction of a genetic map of an organism starts with the selection of a standard ("wild") type. From the progeny of the wild type, mutant forms can be isolated on the basis of some heritable difference. When two mutants are crossed, there is a possibility that a wild-type organism will be formed as a result of recombination of genetic material. The reciprocal recombinant, containing both mutational alterations, also occurs. The proportion of progeny constituting such recombinant types is characteristic of the particular mutants used. The results of crosses involving a group of mutants can be plotted on a one-dimensional diagram where each mutant is represented by a point. The interval between two points signifies the proportion of recombinants occurring in a cross between the two corresponding mutants. Usually, it is not possible to construct a single map for all the mutants of an organism; instead the mutants must be broken up into "linkage groups." A linear map may be constructed within each linkage group, but the mutant characters assigned to different linkage groups assort randomly among the progeny. The number of linkage groups, in some cases, has been shown to correspond to the number of visible chromosomes.

The procedure for constructing a genetic map for a bacterial virus is much the same (9). A genetically uniform population of a mutant can readily be grown from a single individual. Two mutants are crossed by infecting a susceptible bacterium with both types and examining the resulting virus progeny for recombinant types. Virus T4 has been mapped in some detail (3, 1), and behaves as a haploid organism with a single linkage group (18).

Relativity of Genetic Maps.

A genetic map is an image composed of individual points. Each point represents a mutation which has been localized with respect to other mutations by recombination experiments. The image thus obtained is a highly colored representation of the hereditary material. Alterations in the hereditary material will lead to noticeable mutations only if they affect some phenotypic characteristic to a visible degree. Innocuous changes may pass unnoticed, leaving their corresponding regions on the map blank. At the other extreme, alterations having a

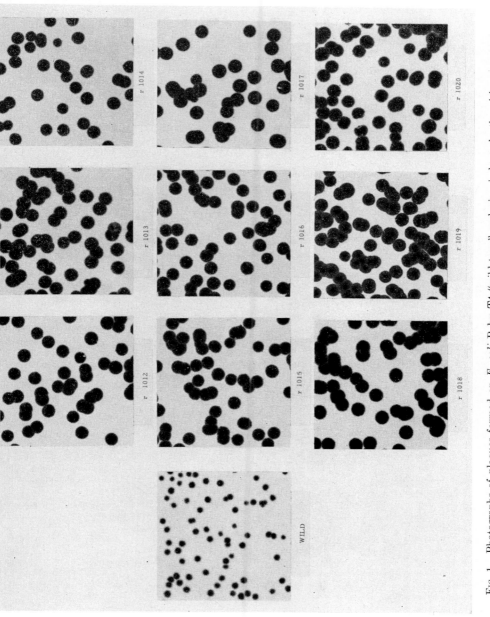

Fig. 1. Photographs of plaques formed on *E. coli* B by T4 "wild-type" and nine independently arising *r* mutants.

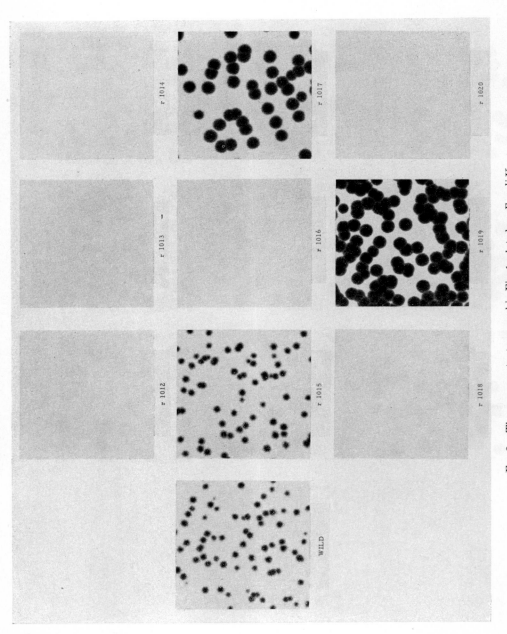

Fig. 2. The same mutants as used in Fig. 1, plated on *E. coli* K.

lethal effect will also be missed (in a haploid organism). The map represents, therefore, only cases which fall between these extremes under the conditions of observation. By varying these conditions, a given mutational event may be shifted from one of these categories (innocuous, noticeable, or lethal) to another, thereby appearing on, or disappearing from the map.

This effect may be illustrated by the "*r*" mutants of bacterial virus T4. Wild-type T4 produces small, fuzzy plaques on *Escherichia coli* B (Fig. 1). From plaques of wild-type T4, *r*-type mutants can be isolated which produce a different sort of plaque. Fig. 1 shows the plaques of nine *r* mutants, each isolated from a different plaque of the wild type in order to assure independent origin. The similarity of plaque type of these *r*'s on B disappears when they are plated on another host strain, *E. coli* K (a lysogenic K12 strain (10) carrying phage lambda), as shown in Fig. 2. Here, they split into three groups: two mutants form *r*-type plaques, one forms wild-type plaques, and the remaining six do not register. Thus, with B as host, all three types of mutation lead to visible effects, while with K as host, the effects may be visible, innocuous, or lethal.

When the same set of mutants is plated on a third strain, *E coli* S (K12S, a non-lysogenic derivative (10) of K12) or BB (a "Berkeley" derivative (17) of B) the pattern of plaque morphology is different from that on either B or K (Table 1).

TABLE 1

PLAQUE MORPHOLOGY OF T4 STRAINS (ISOLATED IN B) PLATED ON VARIOUS HOSTS

PHAGE STRAIN	BACTERIAL HOST STRAIN		
	B	S	K
wild	wild	wild	wild
r I	*r*	*r*	*r*
r II	*r*	wild	—
r III	*r*	wild	wild

If a genetic map is constructed for these mutants, using B as host, the three groups fall into different map regions, as indicated in Fig. 3. On strain S, the *rII* and *rIII* types of mutation are innocuous. Thus, if S had been used as host in the isolation of *r* mutants, only the *rI* region would have appeared on the map. On K as host, the *rIII* mutation is innocuous, and the *rII* mutation is (usually) lethal, so that only the

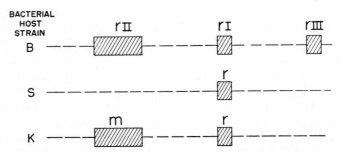

FIG. 3. Dependence of the genetic map of T4 upon the choice of host. Three regions of the map are shown as they probably would appear if *E. coli* strains B, S, or K were used as the host.

rI region would appear. Actually, a few *rII* mutants are able to multiply somewhat on K, producing visible tiny plaques. If K were used as host in the isolation and testing of mutants from wild-type T4, these mutants could be noticed and would probably be designated by some other name, perhaps "minute." The map would then appear as in the bottom row of Fig. 3. The distribution of points on the map within this "minute" region would be very different from those for the *rII* region using B as the host.

The appearance of a genetic map also depends on the choice of the standard type, which is, after all, arbitrary. For example, suppose an *r* form were taken as the standard type and non-*r* mutants were isolated from it. Then a completely different map would result. An example of this is to be found in the work of Franklin and Streisinger (5) on the $h \rightarrow h^+$ mutation in T2, as compared with that of Hershey and Davidson (7) on the $h^+ \rightarrow h$ mutation.

Another way in which the picture is weighted is by local variations in the stability of the genetic material. Certain types of structural alterations may occur more frequently than others. Thus, a perfectly stable genetic element (i.e., one which never errs during replication) would not be represented by any point on the map.

Determination of the Sizes of the Hereditary Units by Mapping.

Determination of the recon requires "running the map into the ground" (Delbrück's expression), that is, isolation and mapping of so large a linear density of mutants that their distances apart diminish to the point of being comparable to the indivisible unit. With a finite set of mutants, only an upper limit can be set upon the recon, which must be smaller than (or equal to) the smallest non-zero interval observed between pairs of mutants.

To determine the length of map involved in a mutational alteration, a group of three closely linked mutants is needed. Since map distances are (approximately) additive, a calculation of the "length" of the central mutation can be attempted (15) from the discrepancy observed between the longest distance and the sum of the two shorter ones, as shown in Fig. 4. The upper limit to the size of the muton would be

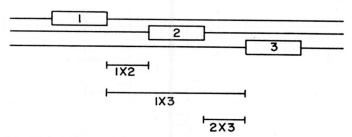

Fig. 4. Method for determining the "length" of a mutation. The discrepancy between the long distance and the sum of the two short distances measures the length of the central mutation.

the smallest discrepancy observed by this method, which can be determined accurately only if the three mutants are very closely linked. It should be noted that since the degree to which the genetic structure can be sliced by recombination experiments is limited by the size of recon, the size of the muton will register as zero by this method if it is equal to or smaller than one recon. A second method for determining the muton size is by the maximum number of mutations, separable by recombination, that can be packed into a definite length of the map.

For the cistron size, only a *lower* limit can be set with a finite group of mutants. The cistron must be at least as large as the distance between the most distant pair within it. Its boundaries become more sharply defined the larger the number of points which are shown to lie inside them.

Thus, the determination of the sizes of all three units requires the isolation and crossing of large numbers of mutants. The magnitude of this undertaking increases with the square of the number of mutants, since to cross n mutants in all possible pairs requires $n(n-1)/2$ crosses, or approximately $n^2/2$. Fortunately, however, the project can be shortened considerably by means of a trick.

The Method of Overlapping "Deletions."

Certain *rII* mutants are anomalous in the sense that they cannot be represented as *points* on the map. The anomalous mutants give no detectable wild recombinants with any of several other mutants which *do* give wild recombinants with each other. An anomalous mutant can be represented (Fig. 5) as covering a segment of the map. Reversion

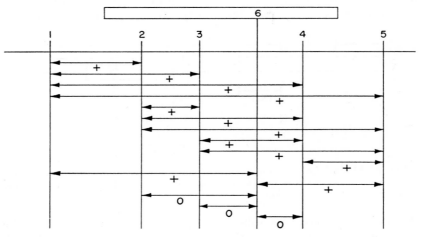

Fig. 5.   Illustration of the behavior of an "anomalous" mutant. Mutant no. 6 is anomalous with respect to the segment of the map indicated by the bar; it fails to give wild recombinants with mutants (nos. 2, 3, and 4) located within that segment. A + signifies production, and 0 lack of production, of wild recombinants in a cross.

of such an *rII* mutant has never been observed; also, no mutant which does revert has been found to have this anomalous character. The properties of an anomalous mutant can be explained as owing to the deletion (i.e. loss) of a segment of hereditary material corresponding to the map span covered. However, anomalous behavior and stability against reversion are not sufficient to establish that a deletion has occurred. Similar properties could be expected of a double mutant when crossed with either of two different single mutants located at the same points. An inversion also would show the same behavior. However, the occurrence of a deletion seems to be the only reasonable explanation in the cases of several of the *rII* mutants, since they fail to give recombinants with any of three or more (in one case as many as 20) well-separated mutants.

Whether a given mutation belongs in the region covered by a deletion can be determined by the appropriate cross. If wild recombinants are produced, the mutant must have a map position *outside* the region of the deletion. This eliminates the need to cross that mutant with any of the mutants whose map positions lie *within* the region of the deletion. The problem of mapping a large number of mutants is greatly simplified by this system of "divide and conquer." The mutants can first be classified into groups that fall into different regions on the basis of crosses with mutants of the deletion-type. Further crossing in all possible pairs is then necessary only within each group.

Suppose that three deletions occur in overlapping configuration, as shown in Fig. 6A. Fig. 6B represents the results that would be obtained

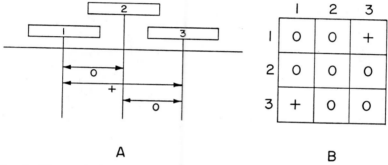

A   B

Fɪɢ. 6. The method of overlapping deletions. Three mutants are shown, each differing from wild type in the deletion of a portion of the genetic material. Mutants no. 1 and no. 3 can recombine with each other to produce wild type, but neither of them can produce wild recombinants when crossed to mutant no. 2. The matrix B represents the results obtained by crossing three such mutants in pairs and testing for wild recombinants; the results uniquely determine the order of the mutations on the map A.

in crosses of pairs of these three mutants. A diagonal element (representing a cross of a mutant with itself) is, of course, zero, since no wild recombinants can be produced. An overlap is reflected by the pattern of non-diagonal zeros. These results would establish a unique *order* of the deletions (without resort to the three-factor crosses that would ordinarily be necessary). With a sufficient number and appropriate distribution of deletions, one could hope to order a large length of map. The reader will note an analogy (not altogether without significance!) to the technique used by Sanger (16) to order the amino acids in a polypeptide chain by means of overlapping peptide segments.

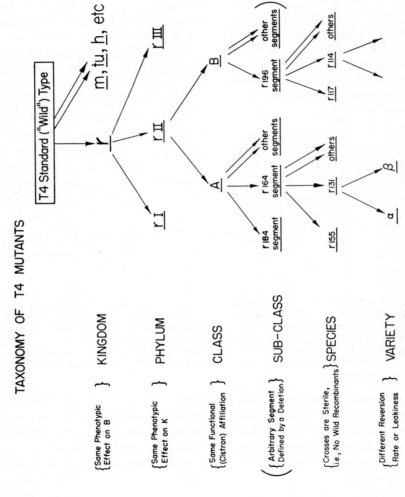

Fig. 7. Classification scheme for r mutants of T4.

MAPPING THE *rII* REGION OF T4

Taxonomy of r Mutants.

In classifying the mutants of T4, classical terminology may be conveniently used for the taxonomic scheme shown in Fig. 7. Mutants of the r "kingdom," isolated on B, can be separated into three "phyla" by testing on K. For the present purposes, our attention will be limited to mutants of the *rII* phylum, which are inactive on K.

A pair of *rII* mutants may be subjected to the *cis-trans* test. The *cis* configuration (mixed infection of K with double mutant and wild-type particles) is active, since the presence of a wild particle in the cell enables both types to multiply. The *trans* configuration (mixed infection of K with the two single mutants) may be active or inactive. If inactive, the two mutants are placed in the same "class." Since the members of a class fail to complement each other, they can be considered as belonging to a single functional group. On the basis of this test, the *rII* mutants divide into two clear-cut classes. The map positions of the mutants in each class have been found to be restricted to separate map segments, the A and B "cistrons."

Arbitrary sub-classes can be chosen (from among the available deletions) for convenience in mapping: mutants falling within the map region encompassed by a particular deletion form a sub-class.

Reverting mutants are considered as of different "species" if crosses between them yield wild recombinants. Among a group of mutants which have not yielded to resolution by recombination tests, "varieties" can in some cases be distinguished by other criteria (reversion rate or degree of ability to grow on K).

Procedures in the Classification of r Mutants of T4.

(1) Isolation of mutants

Each mutant is isolated from a separate plaque of wild-type T4 (plated on B) and freed from contaminating wild-type particles by replating. Stocks of mutants are prepared by growth on S (to avoid the selective advantage which wild type revertants would have on B). Mutants are numbered in the order of isolation, starting with 101 to avoid confusion with mutants previously isolated by others.

(2) Spot test on K

In this first test of a new r mutant, 10^8 particles are plated on K and then the plate is spotted with one drop (10^6 particles) of *r164* (a mutant having a "deletion" in an A cistron) and one drop of *r196* (a mutant having a deletion located in the B cistron). Typical examples of the results of this test are shown in Fig. 8. If the new mutant belongs either to the *rI* or the *rII* phylum, the plating bacteria will be completely lysed (except for a background of colonies formed by mutants of K which are resistant to T4), as typified by mutant *X* in Fig. 8.

Mutant *Y* in Fig. 8 is typical of a stable *rII* mutant. The background shows no plaques, indicating that the proportion of revertants in the stock is less than 10^{-8}. The spot of *r196* is completely clear, in contrast to the *r164* spot. This massive lysis is caused by the ability of mutant *Y* and *r196* to complement each other for growth on K. From this result, it may be concluded that mutant *Y* belongs to the A class. Within the *r164* spot, however, some plaques may be seen. These are due to wild recombinants arising from *r164* and mutant *Z* (by virtue of very feeble growth of *rII* mutants on K). Therefore, mutant *Y* is not in the subclass defined by *r164*.

The third test plate is typical of a reverting *rII* mutant. The stock contains a fraction 10^{-6} of wild-type particles which produce the plaques seen in the background. It is evident from the spot tests that the mutant *Z* belongs in the B class, and appears to lie within the *r196* subclass.

(3) Spot test on a mixture of K and B cells

Once the class of a new mutant is known, it can be tested on a single plate against several mutants of the same class. For this purpose, the sensitivity of the test may be increased enormously by the addition of some B cells (about one part in a hundred) to the K used for plating. The additional growth possible for the mutants on B cells enhances their opportunity to produce wild recombinants. This test gives a positive response down to the level of around 0.01 per cent recombination. A negative result does not, of course, eliminate the possibility that recombination occurs with a lower frequency.

(4) Preliminary crosses

A semiquantitative measure of recombination frequency may be obtained by mixedly infecting B with two mutants and plating the infected cells on K. B cells which liberate one or more wild-type particles can produce plaques. This method is convenient for preliminary testing for recombination in the range from 0.0001 to 0.1 per cent.

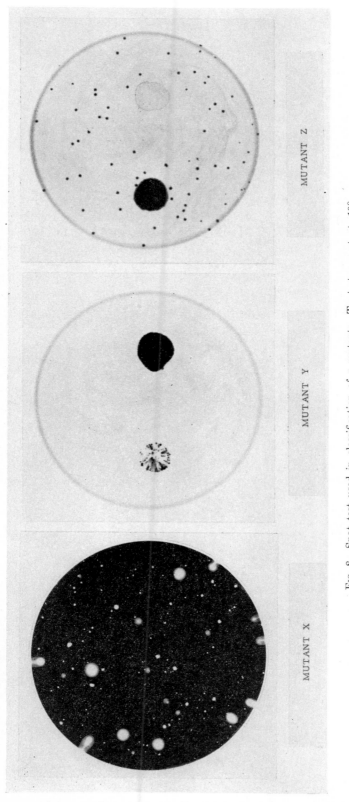

MUTANT X   MUTANT Y   MUTANT Z

Fig. 8. Spot test used in classification of r mutants. To test a mutant, 10^8 mutant particles are plated on bacterial strain K and the plate is spotted with one drop of $r164$ (left) and one drop of $r196$ (right). Mutants X, Y, and Z illustrate typical results. Mutant X is of the rI phylum. Mutant Y is a stable mutant of the rII phylum and the A class, but is not in the $r164$ sub-class. Mutant Z is a reverting mutant (wild-type plaques in background) of the rII phylum, B class, and $r196$ subclass.

With higher frequencies of recombination, approaching the point where a large fraction of the mixedly infected cells liberate recombinants, saturation sets in.

(5) Standard crosses

Standard measurements of recombination frequency are made in conventional crosses. B cells are infected with an average of three particles per cell of each phage. The infected cells are allowed to burst in a liquid medium, and the progeny are plated on K and on B to determine the proportion of wild-type particles. The reciprocal recombinant (double *rII* mutant) does not, in general, produce plaques on K, but since the two recombinant types are produced in statistically equal numbers (9), the proportion of recombinants in the progeny can be taken as twice the ratio of plaques on K to plaques on B (corrected for the relative efficiency of plating of wild type on these two strains, which is close to unity).

(6) Reversion rates

The reversion rate of a mutant is reflected in the proportion of wild-type particles present in a stock. This value is an important characteristic of each mutant, varying over an enormous range for different mutants. It may be less than 10^{-8} for "stable" (i.e., non-reverting) mutants or as high as several per cent. (For one exceedingly unstable mutant the proportion of revertants averages 70 per cent, even in stocks derived from individual mutant particles.) The precision with which a mutant can be localized on the map is inversely related to its reversion rate; only relatively stable mutants are useful for mapping. In the experiments here reported, it has been assumed that the reversion rate of a mutant is not altered during a cross; the reversion contribution is subtracted from the observed percentage of wild particles in the progeny. In most cases, this correction is negligible.

(7) "Leakiness" of *rII* mutants

rII mutants differ greatly in their ability to grow on K cells. A sensitive measure of this ability can be obtained by infecting K cells and plating them on B. Any K cell that liberates one or more virus particles can give rise to a plaque. The fraction of infected cells yielding virus progeny, which is a characteristic property of each mutant (when measured under fixed conditions), may vary from almost 100 per cent down to less than one per cent for different mutants.

Leakiness has the effect of limiting the sensitivity of K as a tool for selection of wild recombinants, thereby hampering the mapping of very leaky mutants.

TABLE 2

CLASSIFICATION OF AN UNSELECTED GROUP OF 241 *r* MUTANTS OF T4

The number of mutants in each classification is given in parentheses. An asterisk indicates that reversion of the mutant to wild type has not been detected. A few mutants (indicated as "not determined") could not be further classified due to excessively high reversion rate or leakiness.

Kingdom	Phylum	Class	Subclass	Species	Variety
r mutants (241)	rI (96)	IIA (73)	r164* (27)	1 sp. (20) / 1 sp. (2) / 4 sp. (1 ea.)	1 var. (11) / 1 var. (9)
			r184* (5)	1 sp. (2) / 1 sp. (2)*	1 var. (1) / 1 var. (1)* / 1 var. (1)
			r221* (4)	1 sp. (3)	1 var. (1) / 1 var. (1)
	rII (134)		r47* (4)	1 sp. (2)* / 1 sp. (1)*	
			r197* (2)	1 sp. (1)	
			others (29)	1 sp. (3)* / 1 sp. (2) / 1 sp. (2) / 1 sp. (2) / 1 sp. (2) / 1 sp. (2) / 1 sp. (2) / 14 sp. (1 ea.)	1 var. (1) / 1 var. (1) / 1 var. (1) / 1 var. (1)
			not determined (1)		
		IIB (60)	r196* (34)	1 sp. (21) / 1 sp. (9) / 3 sp. (1 ea.)	1 var. (19) / 1 var. (2) / 1 var. (5) / 1 var. (4)
			r187* (6)	1 sp. (3)* / 1 sp. (2) / 1 sp. (3)	1 var. (1) / 1 var. (1) / 1 var. (2) / 1 var. (1)
			others (16)	1 sp. (3) / 1 sp. (2) / 8 sp. (1 ea.)	
	rIII (11)		not determined (4)		
		not determined (1)			

Classification of a Set of 241 r Mutants.

A set of *r* mutants was isolated, using B as host, and given numbers from *r101* to *r338*; the mutants *r47*, *r48*, and *r51*, isolated by Doermann (3), were added to this set, making a total of **241** *r* mutants. These were analyzed according to methods already described.

The results are shown in Table 2. Of these mutants, **134** fell into the *rII* phylum. Each of these (with the exception of one very leaky mutant) could be assigned unambiguously to either of two classes on the basis of the test for complementary action of pairs of mutants for growth on K. Mutants within each class were crossed with stable mutants of the same class; those giving no detectable wild recombinants with a particular stable mutant were assigned to the same subclass. Mutants of each subclass were crossed in all pairs. When two or more mutants were found to be of the same species (i.e., showed, in a "preliminary" type cross, recombination of less than about 0.001 per cent, or less than the uncertainty level set by the reversion rate, whichever was greater), one was used to represent the species in further crosses. Those mutants not falling into any of the subclasses defined by the available stable mutants were crossed with each other in pairs. By these procedures, the classification was carried to the species level for the entire set of mutants, except for six highly revertible or leaky mutants whose subclass was not established.

Several of the species showed evidence of splitting into varieties distinguishable by reversion rate or degree of leakiness. Some mutant varieties recurred frequently (e.g., 19, 11, 9 times). These recurrences were far outside the expectation for a Poisson distribution, and are indicative of local variations of mutability. The fact that many species were represented by only one occurrence suggests that many other species remain to be found.

The 33 species found in the A cistron and the 18 species found in the B cistron are sufficient to define reasonably well the limits of each cistron. The minimum size of a cistron in recombination units is determined by the maximum amount of recombination observed in standard crosses between pairs of mutants within it. On the basis of the standard crosses performed so far, this value is about 4 per cent recombination for the A cistron, and 2 per cent for the B cistron.

Study of 923 r Mutants.

While the study of the foregoing 241 mutants yielded a good idea of the sizes and complexity of the A and B cistrons, it fell short of "saturating" the map sufficiently to provide the close clusters of mutants required for the determination of the sizes of the recon and muton. To this end, it was decided to isolate many more mutants. By confining attention to those falling into the *r164* subclass, a more exhaustive study could be made of a selected portion of the map.

In a group of 923 *r* mutants (*r101* through *r1020,* plus Doermann's three), 149 were found to belong to the *r164* subclass. Four of those were stable. The remaining 145 mutants separated into the 11 species shown in Fig. 9. One of the species accounted for 123 of the mutants! As shown in Table 3, this species included three varieties as distinguished by their reversion rates; two were of roughly equal abundance, while the third occurred only once.

Results of standard crosses between the mutants of the *r164* subclass are presented in Fig. 10. The smallest recombination distance, setting an upper limit to the size of the recon, is around 0.02 per cent (between

TABLE 3
Reversion Data for Mutants of the *r131* Species

The "reversion index" is the proportion of wild-type particles in a lysate prepared from a few mutant particles (to avoid introduction of any revertants present in the original stock) using S as host. The measurement is subject to large fluctuations due to the clonal growth of the revertants formed Therefore, four separate lysates are made for each mutant. Parentheses indicate extreme fluctuations. An asterisk indicates a background of tiny plaques (smaller than those produced by wild type) when the lysate is plated on K.

In addition to the examples listed in the table, 67 other mutants of this species are also of variety α, as judged by the proportion of revertants (from 0.2×10^{-6} to 4.0×10^{-6}) in single lysates; 45 additional mutants apparently are of variety β (having values from 300×10^{-6} to $4,000 \times 10^{-6}$).

The mutants of variety α give less than 0.001 per cent recombination with *r274.* For the more highly revertible mutants of variety β, this limit can only be set at less than 0.02 per cent recombination with *r274.* The mutant *r973,* of variety γ, gives less than 0.005 per cent (the limit set by background on K) recombination with *r274.*

	Mutant	Reversion Index (units of 10^{-6})			
variety α	r200	0.47	0.91	0.17	0.25
	r220	0.55	0.41	0.25	0.21
	r274	0.24	0.29	0.61	(10.)
	r930	0.17	0.66	0.19	0.21
	r1012	0.58	0.27	0.22	0.15
variety β	r245	420.	490.	490.	1120.
	r353	540.	530.	3900.	(500,000.)
	r376	520.	360.	1240.	450.
	r510	2000.	640.	460.	860.
	r888	610.	530.	250.	570.
variety γ	r973	0.01*	0.005*	0.005*	0.01*

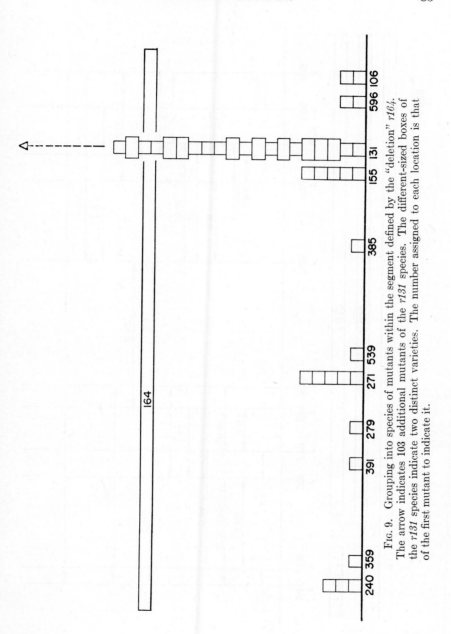

Fig. 9. Grouping into species of mutants within the segment defined by the "deletion" *r164*. The arrow indicates 103 additional mutants of the *r131* species. The different-sized boxes of the *r131* species indicate two distinct varieties. The number assigned to each location is that of the first mutant to indicate it.

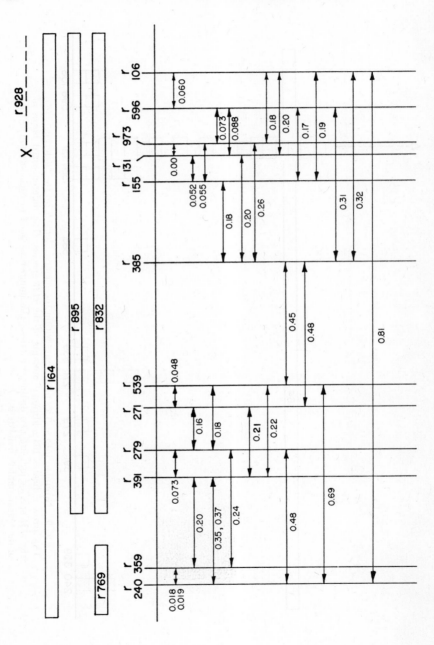

r240 and *r359*). Since only one interval has this value, the possibility of smaller values is not ruled out.

One procedure for measuring the size of the muton requires a group of three closely linked mutants in order to compare the long distance with the sum of the two shorter ones. If the central mutation has an appreciable size, there should be a discrepancy between these values. There are eight cases in Fig. 10 for which the distances have been measured for three adjacent mutants: 240-359-391, 359-391-279, 391-279-271, 279-271-539, 271-539-385, 385-155-131, 155-131-596, 131-596-106. The discrepancies for these groups are, reading from left to right, $+ 0.14$, $- 0.03$, $- 0.02$, $- 0.03$, $- 0.02$, $- 0.03$, $+ 0.03$, and $+ 0.05$ per cent recombination. The average of these values is $+ 0.01$, with an average deviation of ± 0.05. Since each measurement of recombination frequency is subject to experimental error of the order of 20 per cent of its magnitude, these determinations of mutation size (each derived from three measurements) are uncertain to plus or minus about 0.05 per cent recombination. Therefore, the latter is the smallest upper limit than can be set upon the size of the muton by these data.

Another measure of muton size can be attempted by finding the number of species that can exist within a given length of the map. As shown in Fig. 10, a map length of 0.8 per cent recombination includes 9 separable mutant species, or no more than 0.09 per cent per species. Both this determination and the previous one suffer uncertainty due to imperfect additivity of map distances ("negative interference"— see Discussion).

Stable Mutants.

Since the problem of mapping large numbers of mutants is greatly facilitated by the use of "deletions," particular attention has been paid to non-reverting mutants, in the hope of obtaining a complete set of

---

Fig. 10. Map of the mutants in the *r164* segment. The numbers give the percentage of recombination observed in standard crosses between pairs of mutants. The arrangement on this map is that suggested by these recombination values; it has not yet been verified by three-point tests. Stable mutants are represented as bars above the axis; the span of the bar covers those mutants with which the stable mutant produces no detectable wild recombinants. The stable mutant *r928* appears to be a double mutant having one mutation at the highly mutable *r131* location and a second mutation at a point in the B cistron. Mutants *r131* and *r973* are separated on the map so that the data for each can be indicated. Some of the data here given differ from (and supersede) previously published data based upon unconventional crosses which turned out to be incorrect.

overlapping deletions. Among the series of 923 r mutants, 72 stable *rII* mutants were found, 47 in the A cistron and 24 in the B cistron. One mutant *(r928)* was exceptional: it failed to complement mutants of either the A or B cistrons and therefore belongs to *both* classes.

The stable mutants of the B cistron have been crossed (by spot tests on K plus B) in all possible pairs. The results are shown in Fig. 11.

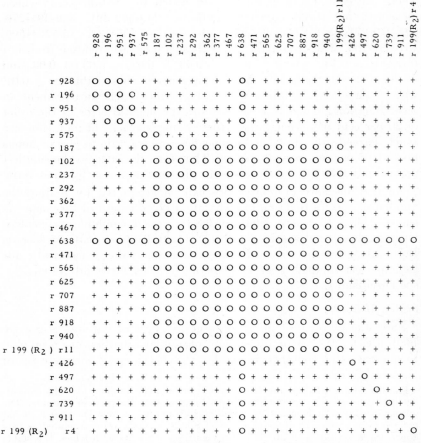

Fig. 11.   Recombination matrix for stable mutants of the B class. A + indicates production of wild recombinants (around 0.01 per cent recombination or more would be detected) in the cross between the indicated pair of mutants (by spot test on K plus B). All diagonal elements (self-crosses) are zero; non-diagonal zeros indicate overlaps. Two of the mutants are derived, not from the original wild type, but from a revertant of *r199*.

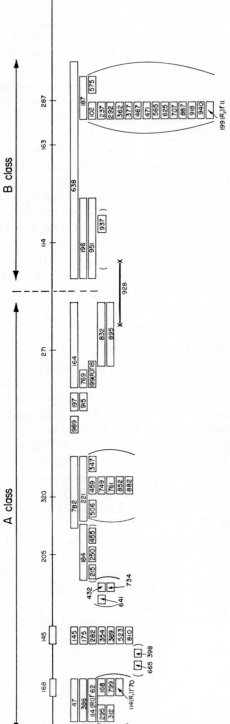

Fig. 12. Preliminary locations of stable *rII* mutants. Mutants producing no wild recombinants with each other are drawn in overlapping configuration. Pairs which produce small amounts are placed near each other. Since there remain some gaps, the order shown depends upon that established by Doermann (4) for the mutants shown on the axis. The scale is somewhat distorted in order to show the overlap relationships clearly. Brackets indicate groups, the internal order of which is not established. Ten stable mutants of the A class and six of the B class were not sufficiently close to any others to permit them to be placed on the map. (A class equals A cistron; B class equals B cistron.)

Overlapping relationships are indicated by non-diagonal zeros. Fig. 12 shows the genetic map representation of these results together with the results derived from an analysis (as yet incomplete) of the stable mutants of the A cistron. Unfortunately, gaps still remain in the map.

The mutant *r638* is of particular note. No B class mutant has been found that gives wild recombinants with it, so that it appears to be due to deletion of the entire B cistron. In spite of this gross defect, it is capable of normal reproduction on *E. coli* strains B and S.

In order to characterize a stable mutant of a "deletion" type, it is necessary to show that it gives no wild recombinants with at least three other mutants that do give recombination with each other (to exclude the possibilities that it is a double mutant or has an inversion). This criterion cannot be applied unless a suitable set of three mutants is available. Only some of the stable mutants (164, 184, 221, 196, 782, 638, 832, 895, 951) have as yet been shown to satisfy this criterion.

Stable mutations tend to occur "all over the map." However, as in the case of reverting mutants, certain localities show a strikingly high recurrence tendency, as illustrated by *r102*, et al., and by *r145*, et al.

DISCUSSION

Relation of Genetic Length to Molecular Length.

We would like to relate the genetic map, an abstract construction representing the results of recombination experiments, to a material structure. The most promising candidate in a T4 particle is its DNA component, which appears to carry the hereditary information (6). DNA also has a linear geometry (20). The problem, then, is to derive a relation between genetic map distance (a probability measurement) and molecular distance. In order to have a unit of molecular distance which is invariant to changes in molecular configuration, the interval between two points along the (paired) DNA structure will be expressed in nucleotide (pair) units, which are more meaningful for our purposes than, say, Ångstrom units.

Unfortunately, present information is inadequate to permit a very accurate calculation to be made of map distance in terms of nucleotide units. First, it is not known whether the probability of recombination is constant (per unit of molecular length) along the entire genetic structure. Second, there is the question of what portion of the total DNA of a T4 particle constitutes hereditary material (for a discussion

of this problem, see the paper by Delbrück and Stent in this volume). The result of Levinthal's elegant experiment (11) suggests a value of 40 per cent. Since the total DNA content of a T4 particle is 4×10^5 nucleotides (8), it would seem that the hereditary information of T4 is carried in 1.6×10^5 nucleotides. We do not know, however, whether the information exists in one or in many copies. If there is just one copy, and if it has the paired structure of the model of Watson and Crick (20), the total length of hereditary material should be 8×10^4 nucleotide pairs.

There are difficulties on the genetic side as well. The total length of the genetic map is not well established. The determination of this length requires a number of genetic markers sufficient to define the ends of the map. It also requires a favorable distribution of markers in order that the intervals between them can be summated; if the distance between two markers is sufficiently large, the frequency of recombination between them approaches that for unlinked markers and therefore loses its value as a measure of the linkage distance. Unfortunately, the linkage data presently available for T4 leave much to be desired. The experiments of Streisinger (18) indicate that the map of T4 consists of a single linkage group. Adding up the intervals between markers (corrected for successive rounds of mating according to the theory of Visconti and Delbrück, 19) leads to a total value of the order of 200 per cent recombination units. This estimate is very rough, since the number of available markers upon which it is based is small.

A further difficulty arises from the fact that the map distances measured in standard crosses are not quite additive: a large distance tends to be less than the sum of its component smaller distances. For distances of the order of 10 per cent recombination units and more, the deviations from additivity, referred to as "negative interference," can be accounted for by the Visconti-Delbrück considerations. However, a "negative interference" effect, not accountable for by their theory, persists, and apparently gets worse, at very small distances (4). This presents a serious obstacle for our purposes, since we are interested in knowing what fraction of the total map is represented by a small distance. According to preliminary data on this point, summation of the smallest available distances between *rII* mutants yields a total length for the *rII* region which is several fold greater than that found for crosses involving distant *rII* markers. If the total T4 map length could be obtained by a similar summation of small distances, the indications are that it might be of the order of 800 per cent recombination units in length.

Thus, there are plenty of uncertainties involved in relating the genetic map quantitatively to the DNA structure. The best we can do at present is to make a rough estimate based upon the following assumptions: (1) the genetic information of T4 is carried in one copy consisting of a DNA thread 80,000 nucleotide pairs long; (2) the genetic map has a total length of about 800 per cent recombination units; (3) the probability of recombination per unit molecular length is uniform. According to these assumptions, the ratio of recombination probability (at small distances) to molecular distance would be 800 per cent recombination divided by 80,000 nucleotide pairs, or 0.01 per cent recombination per nucleotide pair. That is to say, if two mutants, having mutations one nucleotide pair apart, are crossed, the proportion of recombinants in the progeny should be 0.01 per cent. This estimate is greater, by a factor of ten, than one made a year ago, in which it was assumed that all the DNA was genetic material and that the effect of negative interference was negligible. It should become possible to improve this calculation as more information becomes available.

The estimate indicates that the level of genetic fine structure which has been reached in these experiments is not far removed from that of the individual nucleotides. Furthermore, the estimate is useful in that it defines an "absolute zero" for recombination probabilities: if a cross between two (single) T4 mutants does not give at least 0.01 per cent recombination, the locations of the two mutations probably are not separated by even one nucleotide pair.

Molecular Sizes of the Genetic Units.

Recon: The smallest non-zero recombination value so far observed among the *rII* mutants of T4 is around 0.02 per cent recombination. If the estimate of 0.01 per cent recombination per nucleotide pair should prove to be correct, the size of the recon would be limited to no more than two nucleotide pairs.

Muton: Evidently, among the stable mutants, mutations may involve varied lengths of the map. The muton is defined as the *smallest* element, alteration of which can be effective in causing a mutation. In the case of reverting mutants, it has not been possible, so far, to demonstrate any appreciable mutation size greater than around 0.05 per cent recombination. This would indicate that alteration of very few nucleotides (no more than five, according to the present estimate) is capable of causing a visible mutation.

Cistron: A cistron turns out to be a very sophisticated structure. The function to which it corresponds can be impaired by mutation at many different locations. In the study of **241** *r* mutants, **33** species were found to be located in the A cistron, of which **6** were in the *r164* subclass. In extending the survey to **923** *r* mutants, the number of known species in the *r164* subclass was doubled. Consequently, it may be expected that about 60 A cistron species will be found—when the analysis of the **923** mutants is completed. Since many species are represented by only one occurrence, implying that many more are yet to be found, it seems safe to conclude that in the A cistron alone there are over a hundred "sensitive" points, i.e., locations at which a mutational event leads to an observable phenotypic effect. Just as in the case of the entire genetic map of an organism, the portrait of a cistron is weighted by considerations of which alterations are effectual. It should be fascinating to try to translate the "topography" within a cistron into that of a physiologically active structure, such as a polypeptide chain folded to form an enzyme.

REFERENCES

1. Benzer, S., *Proc. Natl. Acad. Sci. U. S.,* **41**, 344 (1955).
2. Demerec, M., Blomstrand, I., and Demerec, Z. E., *Proc. Natl. Acad. Sci. U. S.,* **41**, 359 (1955).
3. Doermann, A. H., and Hill, M. B., *Genetics,* **38**, 79 (1953).
4. Doermann, A. H., and collaborators, pers. commun.
5. Franklin, N., and Streisinger, G., pers. commun.
6. Hershey, A. D., and Chase, M., *J. Gen. Physiol.,* **36**, 39 (1952).
7. Hershey, A. D., and Davidson, H., *Genetics,* **36**, 667 (1951).
8. Hershey, A. D., Dixon, J., and Chase, M., *J. Gen. Physiol.,* **36**, 777 (1953).
9. Hershey, A. D., and Rotman, R , *Genetics,* **34**, 44 (1949).
10. Lederberg, E. M., and Lederberg, J., *Genetics,* **38**, 51 (1953).
11. Levinthal, C., *Proc. Natl. Acad. Sci. U S.,* **42**, 394 (1956)
12. Lewis, E. B., *Cold Spring Harbor Symposia Quant. Biol.,* **16**, 159 (1951).
13. Pontecorvo, G., *Advances in Enzymol.,* **13**, 121 (1952).
14. Pritchard, R. H., *Heredity,* **9**, 343 (1955).
15. Roper, J. A., *Nature,* **166**, 956 (1950).
16. Sanger, F., *Advances in Protein Chem.,* **7**, 1 (1952).
17. Stent, G. S., pers. commun.
18. Streisinger, G., pers. commun.
19. Visconti, N., and Delbrück, M., *Genetics,* **38**, 5 (1953).
20. Watson, J. D., and Crick, F. H. C., *Cold Spring Harbor Symposia Quant. Biol.,* **18**, 123 (1953).

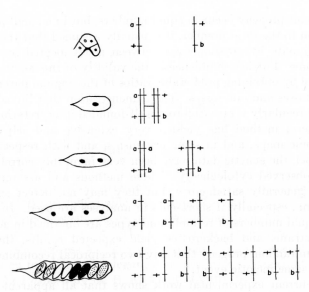

Fig. 1. A diagrammatic illustration of meiosis in *Neurospora*, showing the formation of all the products in a closed system. Normal ascospores are all black and varieties of shading are used here to indicate the four spore pairs, from left to right, as parental, double recombinant, wild recombinant, and parental. Tetrad segregation is shown at the right with a crossover between two linked genes. With close linkage this type of ascus is rare, but with crossing over as illustrated both recombinants are present.

represent loci separable by crossing over. Unfortunately, these mutants are self-sterile; and closely linked markers distal to the pyrimidine-3 locus are not available so that a complete analysis of this situation was not possible. The investigation was continued by making use of distinguishable alleles at the pyridoxine locus. Four alleles at this locus, are known, as are appropriately spaced markers (Fig. 2). Furthermore, the pyridoxine-requiring mutants are fertile in self crosses, and this system therefore permits a thorough and complete analysis of the origin of the apparent genetic recombinants that are produced. A summary of pertinent data obtained from observations of random progeny from crosses containing *pdx* and *pdxp* is given in Fig. 2. As shown, neither of these mutants gave rise to apparent recombinants in self crosses, but the heterozygous cross yielded non-pyridoxine progeny of four classes. Two of these represent parental and two represent crossover classes with respect to the marker genes.

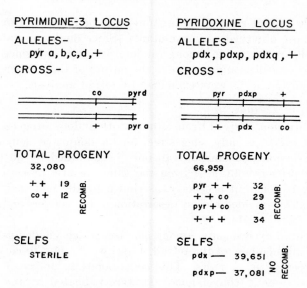

FIG. 2. Data from random progeny which are indicative of gene conversion. An association of conversion with crossing over is shown by the ratios of not-pyridoxine offspring. Markers are *co* (colonial) and *pyr* (pyrimidine 1).

These results, like those observed in studies of the pyrimidine-3 locus, are not compatible with a representation of *pdx* and *pdxp* as two loci separable by crossing over, since double crossovers within a short region would have to be as frequent as singles to yield the tabulated ratios of progeny. The data are consistent with the origin of the apparent recombinant forms through some form of mutation resulting from a process dependent on heterozygosity at the altered locus. In spite of this fact, it is clear that there is a relation between crossing over and the origin of the apparent recombinants. As shown by the data, nearly half of the non-pyridoxine offspring show that a crossover between the markers (*pyrd* and *co*) had accompanied their production, and the results indicate that an event that can lead to crossing over in the vicinity of the locus subject to mutation provides favorable conditions for consummation of the mutation.

These results from studies of random progeny demonstrated clearly that further analysis was needed to provide an adequate definition of the phenomenon. If the apparent recombinants had arisen by crossing over between two very closely linked but related genes (*pdx* and *pdxp*), then double mutant recombinants should also be found and in numbers equal to those observed as non-mutants. Since double mutants might not be easily recognizable among random progeny, and since proof of their existence still would not prove the nature of their origin, changes at the pyridoxine locus were examined by tetrad analysis.

Conversion in Tetrads.

The informtion derived from studies of random progeny such as that given above is only suggestive, and a definitive demonstration of the conversion phenomenon can only be obtained by an examination of all progeny obtained from the same meiotic process. This is technically tedious but necessary, as shown by the fact that it is this method that has yielded a clear description of the conversion phenomenon in *Neurospora* (14, 15).

In the initial experiments, among 585 asci which yielded germinated spores for all members of the tetrad, 4 asci were found to contain conversion types of spore pairs. This corresponds to approximately the same proportions of conversions that were indicated by the observations with random progeny. The parental genotypes used for this purpose are shown at the top in Fig. 3. Only two of the conversion asci obtained are used here for illustration. As shown in Fig. 3, the tetrad represented by ascus 1 contains three parental types and one in which *pdxp* has been apparently changed to wild-type. On the other hand, ascus 2 contains two pairs of phenotypically *pdxp* offspring, but one of the spore pairs expected to have the *pdx* phenotype has been replaced by a pair having a non-pyridoxine phenotype. Each ascus therefore

CROSS – Tetrad

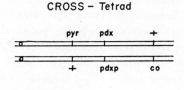

	PAIR 1	PAIR 2	PAIR 3	PAIR 4
ASCUS 1	pyr pdx +	pyr pdx +	+ + co	+ pdxp co
ASCUS 2	pyr pdx +	pyr pdxp +	+ + co	+ pdxp co

FIG. 3. Examples of gene conversion in tetrads. Each tetrad shows one apparent wild recombinant pair and three mutant pairs.

contains (pair 3 in each) one of the recombinant types that might be expected if *pdx* and *pdxp* were closely linked genes separable by crossing over. If this were true then each ascus would have the reciprocal recombinant double mutant with respect to *pdx* and *pdxp*. This leads to the dilemma illustrated in Fig. 4, where it is assumed for the

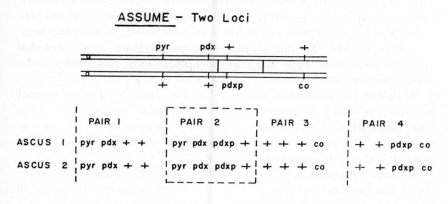

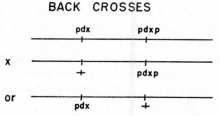

FIG. 4. Results of tetrad analysis expected if *pdx* and *pdxp* represented different genetic loci. The proof for the absence of a double mutant *(pdx pdxp)* in the tetrads is illustrated (see text).

moment that the two genes do represent different loci. As shown, the two asci described in Fig. 4 could be derived by the same two-strand double crossover (an improbable event) and the second pair in each case would be the double mutant in question. But, as already indicated, pair 2 of the first ascus has the phenotypic character of *pdx* and pair 2 of the second ascus has the phenotype of *pdxp*. Yet, by the assumption of two loci these two pairs should have identical gene constitutions. Obviously this renders the assumption of two loci improbable; but a still more exacting test that effectively eliminates the two loci concept has been carried out. All progeny from all aberrant tetrads that have been isolated (7 tetrads at present from a total of 1200 asci) were backcrossed or outcrossed. As shown at the bottom of Fig. 4, a back-cross of a double mutant to either parent would be equivalent to self-crosses which have been shown to give no apparent recombinants (Fig. 2). The results of these experiments demonstrated that all pheno-types correspond to genotypes. That is, all progeny with the *pdx* phenotype gave apparent wild recombinants in crosses to *pdxp* but none in crosses to *pdx*. In like manner, wild recombinants were obtained from progeny that were *pdxp* in phenotype only when they were crossed to *pdx*.

It should be noted that most of the asci isolated showed normal segregations of all of the markers present, including *pdx* and *pdxp*. The expected number showed crossover types with respect to the markers. Thus recombination by crossing over is the usual process even though exceptions occur.

As stated previously, only part of the available experimental evi-dence has been reviewed here. It is of interest to point out that gene conversion is also indicated in crosses heterozygous with respect to a third pyridoxine mutant *(pdxq)* and the wild allele. On the basis of all of these experimental findings it is considered here that *pdx, pdxp, pdxq,* and the corresponding non-mutant locus represent a series of alleles or similar genes at the same locus, in so far as crossing over is concerned. The findings are not consonant with the assumption of a gene cluster or a group of subgenes which are separable by crossing over, and they provide conclusive evidence for the existence of the gene conversion process in *Neurospora*.

Separation of the Crossing Over and Gene Conversion Processes

It has already been indicated that crossing over and gene conver-sion represent different phenomena but that crossover conditions favor simultaneous gene conversion. It is highly desirable to obtain a further understanding of this relationship and to provide means by which these processes can be studied separately. This is important from both theoretical and practical standpoints. In connection with the latter it is to be hoped that methods can be devised for distinguishing cross-ing over from gene conversion that will be applicable in organisms in which tetrad analysis is not possible. A step in this direction has been taken, though it is obviously a limited one at present, by studies of heat-shock effects on mutation, gene conversion, and crossing over in *Neurospora*. A review of the pertinent data obtained in recent studies on this problem follows.

Heat Shock and Mutation.

Experiments on the effects of heat shock on *Neurospora* were designed for purposes other than a study of gene conversion, but some of this background is important for the subsequent discussion. For example, data on the resistance to heat treatments of germinating conidia are summarized in Fig. 5. To obtain these results conidia from 4-day-old cultures of the colonial mutant C-102 (18) were suspended in 100 ml. of Fries minimal medium (1) (10^5 conidia per ml.) after filtration to remove bits of mycelium. The culture was aerated, and at each of the time intervals indicated in the figure a 1 ml. sample was removed and mixed quickly with 9 ml. of sterile water or medium that had been equilibrated at 60° C. Aliquots of hot suspension were removed after 30, 60, and 120 seconds in a water bath maintained at 60° C. These samples were pipetted directly into cold water for appropriate dilu-

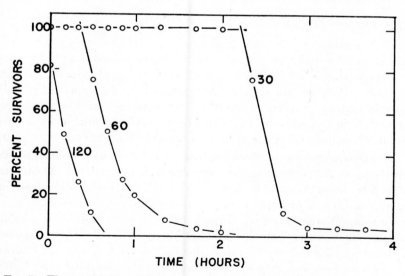

FIG. 5. The sensitivity of *Neurospora* conidia to heat treatments. Incubation time of conidia is indicated on the horizontal axis. The three curves show the percentage of survivors after heat treatments at 60° C. for 30, 60, and 120 seconds. The colonial strain C102 was used for the experiments.

tions and platings on minimal agar medium. Observations and counts were made after one-day and two-day incubations at 32° C.

The data show striking changes in the heat sensitivity of the conidia as germination is initiated. This is shown especially well by the curve representing the 30-second heat treatment, where the percentage of survivors drops very quickly after 2 hours, from 100 per cent to about 2 per cent. During the total 4-hour period no hyphae are produced, but the conidia swell to about twice the original diameter and presumably drastic biochemical changes are in progress. An additional observation of significance is that nearly all colonies were of normal size when survival was 100 per cent, but about 50 per cent of the colonies from cultures derived from periods of rapid killing grew very slowly for several days. Of about 100 of these which were isolated, all but 12 recovered normal growth rates in subcultures.

These experiments suggest that heat shock increases mutation rate and in addition causes a persistent but not a permanent destruction of systems that are essential for normal growth. The latter could be a cytoplasmic, nuclear, or combined effect. Also, the experiments demonstrate the need for careful timing in studies of mutation by heat shock.

Mutants from Ascospores.

Since conidia are usually multinucleate, crosses were made using heat-treated conidia or protoperithecia (wild strains), and the ascospores produced were plated and allowed to germinate on minimal medium. Progeny so derived are expected to be genetically pure. Visible mutants were then counted after a 16-hour incubation period according to the procedure that has been described previously for the isolation of mutants after treatment with ultraviolet radiation (10).

To prepare crosses conidia were treated at 60° C. as described above, although, so far, only pregermination periods of less than 20 minutes have been used. Treated conidia were pipetted directly into tubes containing 3-day-old protoperithecia on a standard crossing medium (25). Excess liquid was decanted. Protoperithecia were treated by placing cultures in a water bath maintained at 60° C. with a simultaneous addition of sufficient equilibrated, distilled water to cover the culture. Tubes were removed from the bath and the water decanted after different intervals of time. The cooled cultures were then fertilized with a water suspension of conidia of the opposite mating type. All cultures were then incubated for about three weeks to permit the formation of ascospores and their ejection from the perithecia. Random spores were then suspended in water, plated on minimal medium, and the total number and the number of visible mutants were determined by counting.

A summary of data obtained by administering a heat shock to conidia is given in Fig. 6. Each experimental point was obtained from counts

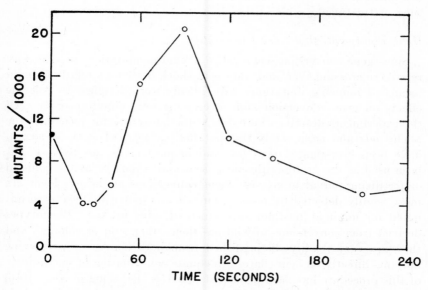

FIG. 6. Visible mutants produced by heat treatments of conidia of wild-type *Neurospora*. Counts of mutants were made from germinated ascospores obtained after fertilization of protoperithecia with conidia heated at 60° C. for the indicated periods of time. Each point was derived from a separate cross, and counts of 9,000 to 16,000 germinated spores were made for each.

of a total of approximately 9,000 to 16,000 progeny from each cross. Four independent experiments have been carried out and the results are qualitatively like those shown in the figure. In each case short treatments caused a reduction in the number of mutants observed, while longer treatments resulted in an increase. Morphological and nutritional mutants have been isolated from heated material, but these represent only a small proportion of the total, as has been observed previously following treatments with ultraviolet radiation (10, 17). The majority of mutants isolated were found to be lethals or to be unstable. Details will be considered elsewhere.

These results, which show a systematic variation in the proportion of mutants among the progeny obtained from crosses prepared from heat-treated conidia, are of particular interest in relation to the principal subject of this report. It should be noted that the heat treatments were applied prior to fertilization and thus prior to meiosis, but it is not necessarily true that mutants were eliminated or induced at the time of treatment.

Heat Treatments and Gene Conversion.

Since gene conversion seems to be a kind of mutation in some way related to crossing over, and since heat shock presents a relatively mild means of inducing mutations, experiments were designed to test the effects on gene conversion and on crossing over simultaneously. All the experiments described here deal with the pyridoxine locus and the alleles *pdx* and *pdxp*. Only the mutants *pyr pdxp* + and + *pdx co* have been investigated thus far, and in most cases *pyr pdxp* + has been used as the protoperithecial parent and + *pdx co* as the conidial or fertilizing parent in crosses. Gene conversions at the *pdx* locus are most readily detected by observations of ascospores that have germinated on minimal medium supplemented with uridine. Phenotypes derived from conversions to wild are then either wild or colonial, and they are very readily distinguished from both classes of pyridoxine mutants directly on agar plates. Adequate confirmation of the validity of this procedure has been presented (14, 15). By using progeny from the same crosses from which conversion frequency is determined, it is a simple matter to measure the extent to which crossing over occurs between the *pyr* and *co* marker genes. This is done by counts of ascospores germinated on minimal medium supplemented with pyridoxine. The map distances given here are based on counts of wild crossover types and the colonial parental type, among a total of 2,000 to 3,000 spores, for each determination.

A summary of data derived from heat treatments of *pyr pdxp* + protoperithecia is presented in Fig. 7. Results of two independent experiments on conversion are given. The lower curve is derived from data obtained from crosses made on cornmeal agar, and each point was determined from counts of a total of from 9,000 to 16,000 germinated spores. The upper curve is derived from data obtained from crosses made on synthetic medium (25) supplemented with uridine and pyridoxine, and from 9,000 to 23,000 progeny were counted to deter-

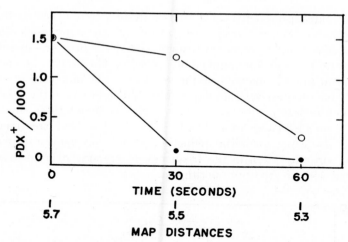

FIG. 7. The influence of heat shock on gene conversion and on crossing over. Protoperithecia were heated at 60°C. for the indicated periods of time. The two curves represent data on the production of apparent recombinants in two separate experiments. Each point was determined by counts of a minimum of 9,000 germinated ascospores. At 60 seconds the count for the upper point was 23,950 and the lower 13,054. Map distances after each treatment are indicated by the numbers below the graph. Crosses—*pyr pdxp* + protoperithecia × + *pdx co* conidia.

mine each point. At present the difference between these two conditions for crossing appears to be due to the fact that the synthetic medium promotes a continued formation of protoperithecia after the cross is made, while the cornmeal agar does not. On cornmeal agar no cross at all was obtained with heat treatments of protoperithecia longer than 60 seconds, while longer treatments with synthetic medium yielded secondary overgrowths and profuse crossing after a delay of several days. It appears that the protoperithecia present at the time of treatment are rendered non-functional by 90-second heating if either medium is used.

Crossover data as well as conversion figures are included in Fig. 7. As shown, there is no significant change in the map distance between the *pyr* and *co* markers as a result of the heat shock treatments. These results provide an effective supplement to the direct genetic data that demonstrate a distinction between gene conversion and crossing over phenomena (14-16, 19).

Further evidence, with a significant variation, was obtained by observations of progeny from crosses made using heat-treated conidia and untreated protoperithecia. In this system it is expected that all perithecia are derived from fertilization of surviving nuclei of the treated conidia, and secondary growth and subsequent crossing do not contribute a significant number of progeny. The results of one such experiment are summarized in Fig. 8. Two other independent experiments gave qualitatively similar results, but in one case the maximum frequency of loss of the *pdx* mutant was only about three times that of the control. These experiments indicate that heat treatments of conidia also cause an initial reduction in the conversion rate without making any alteration in the frequency of crossing over, just as was observed with treated protoperithecia.

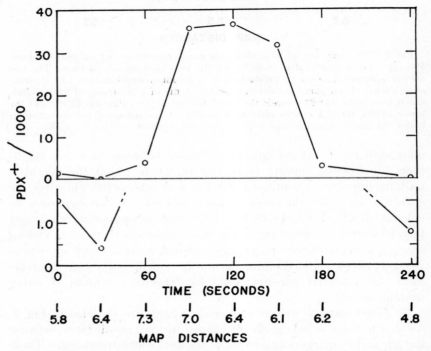

Fig. 8. The influence of heat shock on gene conversion and crossing over. Conidia were heated at 60°C. for the indicated periods of time just prior to fertilization of protoperithecia. The graph is divided to show both reduction and increase in the numbers of apparent recombinant progeny. Each point was determined by counts of from 9,300 to 16,500 germinated ascospores. Map distances between the *pyr* and *co* markers as determined after each treatment are given below the graphs. Crosses: *pyr pdxp* + protoperithecia × + *pdx co* conidia.

Present data are inadequate to establish with certainty the nature of the phenomena that give rise to the very large increase and subsequent decrease of pyridoxine-independent progeny from crosses derived from heat treatments longer than 60 seconds. Limited information indicates that conversion rather than random back-mutation is involved. The greatest increase in pyridoxine independence is in the *pyr*-containing parental type and not in the *co*-containing type. This is in spite of the fact that it was the *co* parent that was subjected to heat treatment. Random mutation induced in this fashion seems unlikely and if it occurred, half of the progeny in one perithecium should be pyridoxine-independent. Although only a small number of individual perithecia have been examined thus far, 38, none has yielded a high percentage of pyridoxine-independent progeny, whereas 1 to 3 might have been expected. One complete ascus containing 3 pyridoxine pairs and 1 non-pyridoxine pair was observed, and an excess of conversion-type recombinants was found to be well distributed among the perithecia examined. Further analysis is required before the nature of this phenomenon can be described satisfactorily.

The data reported above demonstrate one method by which gene conversion at the pyridoxine locus can be separated from crossing over. In addition they raise the interesting question of mechanism. The heat treatments were given before fertilization, and yet it has been shown that conversion must occur during meiosis. This occurs several hours or days after fertilization, and a delayed effect of the heat treatment seems likely even though it is possible that potential converting genes are eliminated at the time of treatment. The latter explanation cannot apply to the experiments with conidia that gave rise to numerous changes at the *pdx* locus which resided in the untreated parent in the crosses. Here, some sort of delayed effect must be operative. It is of interest to consider some possible mechanisms which might result in the observed changes.

THE MECHANISM OF CONVERSION

There remain, at present, a great many potentially informative experiments that should contribute to an understanding of the mechanism of gene conversion. However, it seems quite obvious that this kind of change must be intimately related to mutation in general and to the processes of gene reproduction and function. Unfortunately, these are not well known, and indeed generalizations with respect to any one of these problems cannot be justly made without reservations. For example, it is not necessary that two genes function by the same process or undergo mutation by the same mechanism.

In spite of these reservations it is perhaps of value to present some suggestions which may be of use in directing experimental endeavors. These suggestions have at present no factual support. They are purely speculative.

Gene structure from the chemical standpoint is a matter of great importance, but structure only provides a basis for function. It is therefore the primary contention of this discussion that problems of mechanism concerned with genes can only be resolved in terms of metabolic processes. Thus, the immediate biochemical environment of a gene is as much a part of the hereditary unit as are the molecular structures that are fixed by direct attachment to chromosomes. It is assumed here that the biochemical environment includes various diffusible substances of low molecular weight as well as high molecular weight materials such as enzymes. Although the metabolic systems associated with genes may be more specialized than those outside of the nucleus, it is to be expected that the same biochemical principles are applicable. Perhaps transfer reactions involving diffusible substances and enzymes are especially prominent in gene-associated metabolism. It is not assumed here that template mechanisms or designation of structure of macromolecules in a single operation are necessarily a part of a metabolic-genic process. Nor is it assumed here that there is necessarily a linearity of functional portions of a gene.

With these postulates in mind it is a relatively simple matter to devise schemes, based on analogies with well-established biochemical systems, which can account for gene conversion. In addition they can be rationalized into a unitary picture which can describe, in the same system, the processes of mutation, gene reproduction, the production of agents that control metabolic reactions, and a variety of other more specific genetic phenomena. However, the principal interest here is gene conversion; and it is not the intent of the present discussion to speculate at length on a general basis. This can be done in good time and more realistically if and when a sound basis for the basic principle (the existence and nature of gene-associated metabolic systems) becomes established.

In relation to gene conversion the subsequent discussion considers two possible variations on the theme of gene-associated metabolic systems.

1. It is assumed that heterozygous crosses in which conversion occurs involve genes which have complementary functional groups whose specificities increase the rate of mutation by group transfer, mediated by a metabolic system that is always present. This proposal is more or less an amplification of the copying schemes that have been suggested (9, 14).

2. It is assumed that a pair of genes which give rise to conversion do not necessarily carry complementary structures, but that their structures are such as to influence the localized metabolic system to produce mutational changes. This can be visualized in terms of a relative lack of specificity of functional groups in transfer reactions or in terms of localized accumulations or deficiencies of parts of the gene-associated metabolic systems.

Diagrammatic descriptions of these postulates are indicated in Figs. 9 and 10. Fig. 9 refers principally to the first suggestion, but the second is included if E, or R, are relatively non-specific or have type reaction specificities. It is considered also that it is possible for E_1R_1 to react directly with G to give GR_1 if conditions of the metabolic system are suitable (direct mutation). In part C of Fig. 9 the reaction of activated R_1 to give a new gene is considered to be limited by spatial factors, and the reaction requires that the two components be in intimate adjacent positions, perhaps such that an intermediate bridge can be formed in the reaction. No such limitation is proposed for transfer of R to the diffusible CA component, and this can proceed at a rapid rate.

The diagram of Fig. 10 is directed more specifically at gene conversion than is Fig. 9, but only the minimum of complexity is considered. That is, transfer of only one functional group by action of only one enzyme is shown. The solid arrows indicate transfer by activation through existing complementary groups in the heterozygous system, while no such change can occur in the homozygous situation (postulate 1). The broken arrows indicate reaction without activation (spontaneous mutation). In accordance with postulate 2 it is considered that the heterozygous situation may influence the relative concentrations of components of the metabolic system such that the reaction (spontaneous mutation) will occur more frequently (or less). The notion that such an altered metabolic system may provide an especially active R group by its own interactions is also included here. In addition it is considered possible that the transfer of R groups can be equivalent to

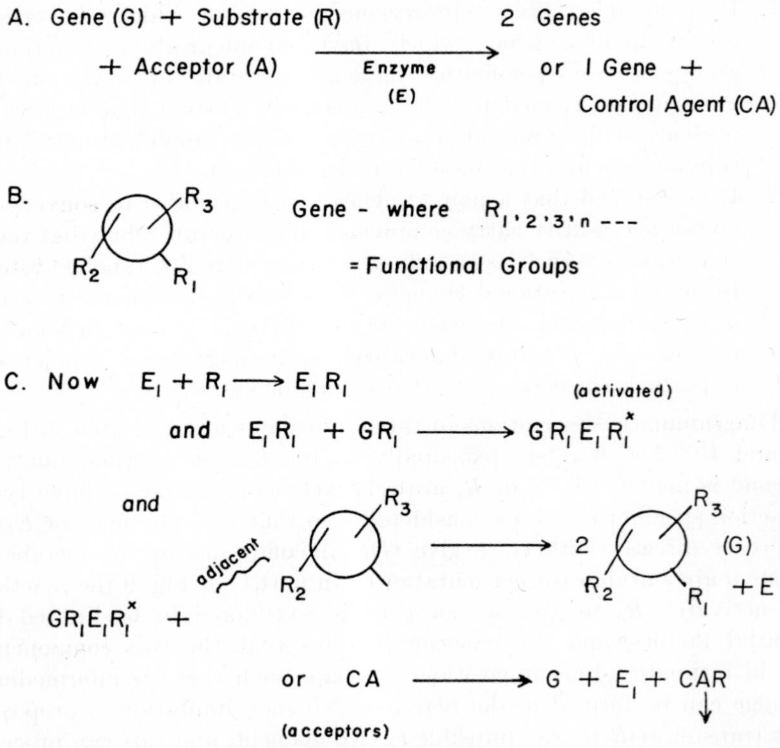

A. Gene (G) + Substrate (R)   2 Genes

  + Acceptor (A) $\xrightarrow{\text{Enzyme} \atop \text{(E)}}$ or I Gene +

                Control Agent (CA)

B.   Gene - where $R_{1,2,3,n}$ ---

        = Functional Groups

C. Now $E_1 + R_1 \longrightarrow E_1 R_1$ (activated)

  and $E_1 R_1 + GR_1 \longrightarrow GR_1 E_1 R_1^x$

  and

$GR_1 E_1 R_1^x +$ $\longrightarrow$ 2   (G) $+E$

   or CA $\longrightarrow$ G + E_1 + CAR

  (acceptors)

Fig. 9. A scheme indicating a possible mechanism for participation of presumed metabolic systems in the processes of gene mutation and function. A detailed description of the suggested scheme is given in the text.

alterations of existing structures with respect to spatial configuration but still under the influence of gene-associated metabolic systems.

These speculations, which consider that a metabolic halo is as much a part of a gene as is the chemical structure of the gene itself, can only be of value if such systems can be found and investigated on an experimental basis. This may be difficult since relatively few molecules of reacting components may be all that are needed in one nucleus. Nevertheless, a positive approach to the problem is indicated.

THE SIGNIFICANCE OF GENE CONVERSION

It is premature and difficult to assess the significance of gene conversion in relation to current concepts of genetic mechanisms, and it

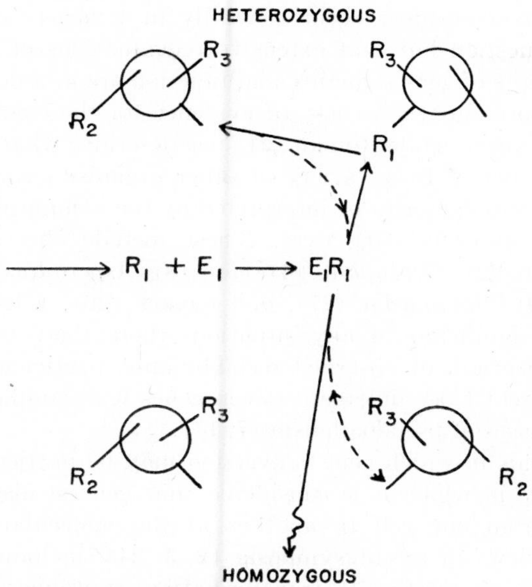

FIG. 10. A scheme indicating some suggestions concerning mechanisms of gene conversion. A detailed description of the proposal is given in the text.

seems clear that the most important problem in this connection is to devise ways and means for the recognition of conversion. The method described here is not generally applicable, since tetrad analysis is not possible in many organisms. Unfortunately, the heat-shock effects described here are not definitive since they are surely dependent on particular physiological states, and they are only useful in the situation described, where crossing over and gene conversion can be observed simultaneously. However, this may be a general approach that can be developed. That is, if other possible influencing factors such as radiation and chemical treatments can be shown to produce independent and different effects on crossing over and conversion, a generalized procedure for distinguishing the two processes might result. An approach of this kind appears to be worth trying, but the application of such a method would be expected to yield results limited by unavoidable assumptions. Obviously the method of choice for the detection of conversion would be one based on a knowledge of the precise mechanism of the process, but the author is not prepared to predict just how this can be attained at the present time.

If gene conversion does occur generally in a variety of organisms, there is no question but that extensive reevaluations of a number of existing concepts of gene structure and function are in order. Lindegren (12, 13) has presented a variety of evidence for the existence of gene conversion in yeast, while Roman (21) has described what appear to be similar phenomena. In a variety of other organisms some data presented can as satisfactorily be interpreted by the assumption of conversion as by that of crossing over. These include observations upon *Neurospora* (6, 22), *Drosophila* (4), corn (8), *Aspergillus* (20), *Escherichia coli* (9), *Bombardia* (27), and mosses (26). Clearly, conversion can be significant in any situation where there is uncertainty regarding the origin of observed recombinants, particularly in situations of apparent close linkage between genes with similar phenotypic effects or in cases of pseudoallelism (7, 11).

General fields in which gene conversion may be particularly important are those in which it is considered that genetic material can be transferred from one cell to another at the molecular level. [See numerous reviews in recent symposia (2, 3, 24), including this one.] Genetic studies in relation to transformation, transduction, and virus reproduction are included here, and it is possible that much of bacterial genetics should be also included. In these situations, where it appears that only chemical specificity or potential for orientations is supplied by a donor, materials to be oriented and metabolic systems concerned with the functioning of the donated material must be supplied by host cells. It would appear that this is an ideal situation for conversion, and such an interpretation would eliminate the apparent necessity for considering multitudinous crossing over in very small distances. However, to switch interpretations is no better than to switch nucleotides, in the absence of definitive experiments. At the present time the demonstration of the existence of gene conversion can only serve as a warning for caution in interpretations, reinforcing that already issued by Sturtevant (23).

REFERENCES

1. Beadle, G. W., and Tatum, E. L., *Am. J. Bot.,* **32**, 678 (1945).
2. *Brookhaven Symposia Biol.,* **8** (Mutation), 1955.
3. *Cold Spring Harbor Symposia Quant. Biol.,* in press.
4. Demerec, M., *Genetics,* **13**, 359 (1928).
5. Emerson, S., *Handbuch der physiologisch- und pathologisch-chemischen Analyse,* 10 Aufl., Bd. II, 443, Springer-Verlag, Berlin (1955).
6. Giles, N. H., *Brookhaven Symposia Biol.,* **8**, 103 (1956).

7. Green, M. M., *Am. Naturalist,* **89**, 65 (1955).
8. Green, M. M., *Proc. Natl. Acad. Sci. U. S.,* **42**, 73 (1956).
9. Laughnan, J. R., *Genetics,* **37**, 375 (1952).
10. Lederberg, J., *J. Cell. Comp. Physiol.,* **45** (No. 2), 75 (1954).
11. Lein, J., Mitchell, H. K., and Houlahan, M. B., *Proc. Natl. Acad. Sci. U. S.,* **34**, 453 (1948).
12. Lewis, E. B., *Am. Naturalist,* **89**, 73 (1955).
13. Lindegren, C. C., *J. Genetics,* **51**, 625 (1953).
14. Lindegren, C. C., *Science,* **121**, 605 (1955).
15. Mitchell, M. B., *Proc. Natl. Acad. Sci. U. S.,* **41**, 215 (1955).
16. Mitchell, M. B., *Proc. Natl. Acad. Sci. U. S.,* **41**, 935 (1955).
17. Mitchell, M. B., *Compt. Rend. Lab. Carlsberg,* in press.
18. Mitchell, M. B., and Mitchell, H. K., *Proc. Natl. Acad. Sci. U. S.,* **39**, 606 (1953).
19. Mitchell, M. B., and Mitchell, H. K., *Proc. Natl. Acad. Sci. U. S.,* **40**, 436 (1954).
20. Mitchell, M. B., and Mitchell, H. K., *Genetics,* in press.
21. Pritchard, R. H., *Heredity,* **9**, 343 (1956).
22. Roman H., *Cold Spring Harbor Symposia Quant. Biol.,* in press.
23. St. Lawrence, P., *Genetics,* **40**, 599 (1955).
24. St. Lawrence, P., *Proc. Natl. Acad. Sci. U. S.,* **42**, 189 (1956).
25. Sturtevant, A. H., *J. Cell. Comp. Physiol.,* **45** (No. 2), 237 (1955).
26. Symposium on Genetic Recombination (Oak Ridge), *J. Cell. Comp. Physiol.,* **45** (No. 2) (1955).
27. Westergaard, M., and Mitchell, H. K., *Am. J. Bot.,* **34**, 573 (1947).
28. Winkler, H., *Die Konversion der Gene,* Gustav Fischer, Jena (1930).
29. Zickler, H., *Planta,* **22**, 573 (1934).

GENE CONVERSION AND PROBLEMS OF ALLELISM*

PATRICIA ST. LAWRENCE AND DAVID M. BONNER

Dept. of Microbiology, Yale University,
New Haven, Conn.

AT THE PRESENT TIME contributions to an understanding of the genetic material are derived from three rather different approaches: analysis of inheritance phenomena; studies of the function of genes in determining the phenotype; and investigations of the chemical constitution of the gene. All three methods of attack seem to converge in studies of allelism. In fact, a precise knowledge of the relationships which may exist between alleles of a gene—in any terms from molecular to morphogenetic—is an essential requirement of satisfactory genetic theory. The advances of the past decade, however, have revealed so many unexpected aspects of allelic relationships that even to define the term allele is difficult. To provide a basis for discussion, the point of view adopted in this paper will be that two mutants are allelic if the mutations involved occur in a restricted chromosomal area and affect one and the same biochemical reaction.

Emphasis upon the functional aspect of allelism rather than on the classical aspect of hereditary behavior is not entirely arbitrary. In many organisms alleles of a locus have generally been shown to determine similar phenotypes. Furthermore, the field of biochemical genetics has provided abundant evidence that genes control specific metabolic reactions. Thus, for example, twenty-five tryptophan-requiring strains of *Neurospora crassa*, all representing mutations in a limited chromosomal area, have been shown to differ from wild-type strains in their ability to perform the tryptophan synthetase reaction—the coupling of indole and serine to form tryptophan (26). Only two of the mutants are capable of any growth in the absence of exogenous tryptophan. The enzyme responsible for the coupling reaction, tryptophan synthetase, is readily detected in extracts of wild-type strains, but no

* The original investigations described from the authors' laboratory were supported in part by the Atomic Energy Commission (Contract No. At (30-1) 1017), and in part by the American Cancer Society on recommendation of the Committee on Growth.

114

appreciable enzymatic activity has been found in extracts of twenty-four of these *td* mutants (26). Therefore the *td* mutants are clearly allelic, in the sense defined above, since a direct correlation between an alteration within a limited chromosome area and the ability to perform a specific metabolic reaction has been shown.

Nevertheless, some of the *td* mutants may be distinguished from others, and it is probable that increasingly sensitive methods of analysis will reveal additional differences between the remaining mutants. Four mutants exhibit a partial restoration of enzymatic function and of ability to grow on minimal medium if they carry a suppressor muta-tion (26). In some cases, the action of the suppressors appears to be specific, and an elevation of tryptophan synthetase activity is shown only by the mutant strain in which the suppressor originated. It is therefore clear that mutant alleles may lead to different alterations of a metabolic reaction.

It should be emphasized, however, that observations of a rather direct correlation between a biochemical alteration and allelic differ-ences do not rule out the possibility that other types of relationships between genes and enzymes may exist. It is not clear at present whether all parts of the genetic material control specific biochemical reactions nor, indeed, to what extent all enzymes and biochemical reactions are under genetic control. In most instances the material selected for study and the methods employed militate against recognition of any minor effects on other enzymes in addition to the one under immediate investigation. Indeed, so compelling is the evidence of biochemical genetics, that, if an apparent case of one gene controlling two enzymes were to occur, it would probably be classified as involving secondary effects of a primary mutation or be ascribed to two closely linked genes. Experimental discrimination between these possibilities is clearly exceedingly difficult.

It is furthermore not clear at present whether the rather direct and quantitative gene-enzyme relationship characteristic of the *td* alleles is sufficient to explain the generally observed pleiotropic effects of allelic systems in higher organisms. Many examples are known of gene and allele clusters which appear to function in a highly organized way in the determination of complex phenotypes (10, 11). It is quite likely that factors which govern gene and enzyme organization in different tissues and at different times may modify considerably the expression of gene-enzyme relationships.

For these reasons, determination of the precise nature of the metabolic alterations in many allelic systems, especially in higher organisms, is difficult. Nevertheless, in the absence of knowledge about enzymes or reactions, indirect methods may provide information concerning the functional similarity between mutants. There is, however, no general agreement on the interpretation of the experimental observations, and recent investigations may alter previous concepts.

The method most widely employed in haploid organisms is based upon the concept that a heterocaryon formed between two mutants blocked in different reactions will grow without any exogenous supplement. The growth of such a heterocaryon would not be expected in the absence of the required growth factor if the same reaction was blocked in each mutant. Although experimental observations in general support these conclusions, preliminary evidence obtained by Giles (6) suggests that some adenine-requiring mutants which lack the same enzyme do form heterocaryons on minimal medium. The general usefulness of this method for assessing functional relationships of alleles is therefore somewhat dubious.

Similar uncertainty is present in interpretations of the functional relationship between mutants in organisms with a prolonged diploid phase. Here a comparison of the phenotypes associated with different arrangements of the mutants (the *cis:* a $a'/+ +$ with the *trans:* $a +/+ a'$) is the method employed. Comparisons of this type have been made with several series of alleles in *Drosophila,* and in each case the *cis* arrangement is phenotypically non-mutant whereas the *trans* is mutant. According to Lewis (12, 13) and Green (8), these observations indicate that the mutants control related, specific, and sequential reactions. Moreover, the normal alleles controlling these steps must be located in close spatial proximity (i.e., on the same chromosome), or else the reaction sequence fails and the mutant phenotype is observed. This interpretation implies a complex gene-enzyme organization of the type previously mentioned. On the other hand, some investigators (7, 17) have suggested that the mutants affect a single biochemical reaction which can only proceed if the integrity of the functional chromosomal area is maintained. Present observations do not permit a decision between these two alternatives for any case in *Drosophila,* but the existence of a diploid phase in the life cycles of yeast and *Aspergillus* suggests that an experimental test is possible with mutants known to exhibit identical biochemical deficiencies.

Although a rigorous demonstration of the functional similarity of alleles cannot be given in many cases, emphasis on this aspect of allelism is of great heuristic value. It is, however, limited. The question may be asked: what information may be derived from studies of the physiological relationships of alleles concerning the nature of the limited chromosome region which controls a single biochemical function?

Evidence from many studies, among them those of the *td* mutants, clearly shows that alterations of a limited chromosomal region may result in similar but not identical phenotypic changes. Pontecorvo (18) has presented a picture of a functional area with multiple mutational sites and has used this as a means of estimating the size of the functioning region. It should be pointed out that speculations concerning the nature of the genetic material derived from the study of altered phenotypes may be unwarranted extrapolations. The fact that the tryptophan synthetase reaction is impaired in all of the 25 *td* mutants would not appear to provide information about the extent, type, or position of either the genetic changes or the functional area. If there is indeed a discrete region of the chromosome which controls a single metabolic step, the assumption that mutations affecting this reaction occur only within the confines of the region would not seem justified at present.

In order to examine the physical properties of the functional units, attention must be focused upon the behavior of alleles in inheritance. Unfortunately, to our knowledge, no case has yet been described in which a biochemical study such as that performed in the *td* series has been accompanied by a satisfactory analysis of crosses between the same alleles. Studies combining both approaches are under way in some laboratories, but information already obtained requires consideration.

The pioneer work of Green (8) and Lewis (12, 13) with a number of mutants in *Drosophila* has demonstrated that very infrequently crossing over occurs between mutants which appear allelic when tested in *cis* and *trans* arrangements. Roper (23) has reported that in the fungi, non-mutant progeny are occasionally obtained following crossing over between phenotypically similar biotin-requiring mutants of *Aspergillus*. These mutants are allelic in the sense that heterocaryons and *trans* diploids are phenotypically mutant.

In the majority of cases, however, the origin of rare, non-mutant progeny from crosses between physiologically similar mutants cannot be correlated so precisely with crossing over. The experimental results obtained in a number of instances appear to resemble the observations initially reported by Giles (4, 5) for crosses between inositol mutants of *Neurospora*. Crosses of the mutants carrying suitable markers gave rise to infrequent inositol-independent progeny, although none were recovered from crosses of two strains of the same mutant. Analysis revealed that the marker constitution of the majority of these isolates was compatible with their origin by a crossover between the parental mutants. A small but significant number of isolates were shown, however, to have a marker constitution indicating that crossing over had occurred in the opposite direction. In addition, isolates carrying the parental combinations of markers were recovered in high frequency. Similar observations with adenine mutants have been reported by de Serres (25) in *Neurospora* and by Pritchard (20) in *Aspergillus*.

Four niacin-requiring strains of *Neurospora*, the *q* mutants, provide an even more extreme example of a lack of correlation between crossing over and the origin of non-mutant progeny (24). There is some evidence to suggest that these mutants are blocked in the same metabolic reaction, and no niacin-independent progeny were recovered from "selfs" (i.e., crosses of two strains of the same mutant). Although the particular mutants used in a cross determined both the frequency and the marker constitution of the rare non-mutant isolates obtained, in some crosses progeny with either one of the parental marker combinations and either one of the recombinant marker constitutions were recovered in high frequency. The data appeared incompatible with the assumption that the niacin-independent isolates arose as the result of a crossover between the *q* mutants.

Whenever prototrophic progeny arise as the result of crossing over between two closely linked mutants, the reciprocal crossover type, a double mutant, should be recovered within the same tetrad. From crosses of two pyridoxine mutants of *Neurospora*, Mitchell (15) has recovered several asci with some non-mutant spores. None of the other spores in the asci were of the double mutant type. This analysis constitutes direct proof that prototrophic progeny may arise from crosses between mutants by some process other than crossing over. She has termed this phenomenon gene conversion.

Although a similar direct proof of gene conversion is absent in all the cases described above, it would appear reasonable to assume (especially in the case of the *q* mutants) that gene conversion also occurs in them. In some cases, as has been mentioned, the occurrence of non-mutant progeny is clearly correlated with crossing over, but by no means all of the isolates give evidence of origin in this manner. Nevertheless, an increase in recombination between markers is frequently observed. Pritchard (20) has suggested that crossing over within limited regions of the chromosome is vastly increased and that non-mutant progeny with unexpected combinations of markers are actually the result of multiple crossing over within a very short region. Attempts to extend this explanation to other data are unsatisfactory (24).

At the present time, the assumption that crossing over and gene conversion are mutually exclusive is not justified. It would appear more likely that both processes occur in any given cross, but with widely varying frequencies. In organisms in which tetrad analysis is feasible, it is possible to determine experimentally whether asci of the gene conversion type and asci of the crossover type occur in the same cross. It is hoped that some diligent investigator will undertake this arduous task.

A further question may be raised concerning the occurrence of gene conversion in organisms in which such a direct test is not possible. A precise correlation between crossing over and the appearance of wild-type progeny is evident in all published studies with *Drosophila*. As Green (9) has pointed out, however, if gene conversion occurs at a very low frequency in *Drosophila*, it would be difficult to detect with the populations generally examined in such experiments.

In maize, Laughnan's study (10, 11) of the origin of the A^d allele of the A locus has shown a high degree of correlation between the occurrence of the A^d phenotype and of crossing over within a very short segment of the chromosome. Not all occurrences of A^d can be related to such crossovers, however, and it may be suggested that gene conversion is responsible for the appearance of these exceptions.

It is clear that in studies such as this, gene conversion cannot be readily distinguished from mutation. In fact, gene conversion may be a particular type of mutation which occurs only under special circumstances. The term mutation, or reversion, has indeed been used to describe phenomena which resemble gene conversion. For example, Roman (21) has reported that the reversion frequency of diploid cells of *Saccharomyces* containing two adenine alleles of different origin is higher than that observed in diploids homozygous for either allele.

The similarity between the behavior of the mutant reddish in *D. virilis*, described by Demerec (3) some time ago and attributed by

composition of hereditary units (and this includes chromosomes as well as genes) is not yet sufficient to define these in chemical terms. It is hoped that the phenomena described in this paper may point out some of the properties which the future genetic material must possess.

REFERENCES

1. Benzer, S., *Proc. Natl. Acad. Sci. U. S.,* **41**, 344 (1955).
2. Bernardini, M., Adelberg, E. A., and St. Lawrence, P., unpub.
3. Demerec, M., *Genetics,* **13**, 359 (1928).
4. Giles, N. H., *Cold Spring Harbor Symposia Quant. Biol.,* **16**, 283 (1951).
5. Giles, N. H., *Brookhaven Symposia Biol.,* **8**, 103 (1955).
6. Giles, N. H., *Cold Spring Harbor Symposia Quant. Biol.,* in press.
7. Goldschmidt, R. B., *Proc. Natl. Acad. Sci. U. S.,* **36**, 365 (1950).
8. Green, M. M., *Am. Naturalist,* **89**, 65 (1955).
9. Green, M. M., *Proc. Natl. Acad. Sci. U. S.,* **42**, 73 (1956).
10. Laughnan, J. R., *Genetics,* **37**, 375 (1952).
11. Laughnan, J. R., *Am. Naturalist,* **89**, 91 (1955).
12. Lewis, E. B., *Cold Spring Harbor Symposia Quant. Biol.,* **16**, 159 (1951).
13. Lewis, E. B., *Am. Naturalist,* **89**, 73 (1955).
14. Lindegren, C. C., *Science,* **121**, 605 (1955).
15. Mitchell, M. B., *Proc. Natl. Acad. Sci. U. S.,* **41**, 215 (1955).
16. Mitchell, M. B., *Proc. Natl. Acad. Sci. U. S.,* **41**, 935 (1955).
17. Pontecorvo, G., *Symposia Soc. Exptl. Biol.,* **6**, 218 (1952).
18. Pontecorvo, G., *Advances in Enzymol.,* **13**, 121 (1952).
19. Pontecorvo, G., and Roper, J. A., *Heredity,* **10**, 124 (1956) (abstract).
20. Pritchard, R. H., *Heredity,* **9**, 343 (1955).
21. Roman, H., *Genetics,* **40**, 592 (1955) (abstract).
22. Roman, H., *Cold Spring Harbor Symposia Quant. Biol.,* in press.
23. Roper, J. A., *Advances in Genet.,* **5**, 208 (1953).
24. St. Lawrence, P., *Proc. Natl. Acad. Sci. U. S.,* **42**, 189 (1956).
25. de Serres, F. J., *Cold Spring Harbor Symposia Quant. Biol.,* in press.
26. Yanofsky, C., and Bonner, D. M., *Genetics,* **40**, 761 (1955).

GENE FUNCTION AND ENZYME FORMATION

SIGMUND R. SUSKIND*

*Department of Microbiology,
New York University College of Medicine,
New York, N. Y.*

THE NATURE OF THE functional genetic unit and the extent and manner in which it mediates protein formation present problems at once both fundamental and challenging. The work to be reported here was undertaken in an attempt to define more clearly the action of a specific genetic locus (*td*) relevant to the formation of a single enzyme, tryptophan synthetase (indole + serine $\xrightarrow[\text{pyridoxal phosphate}]{\text{enzyme}}$ tryptophan) in *Neurospora crassa* (14, 16).

Evidence will be given for the existence of certain serologically active proteins closely related to tryptophan synthetase, which are present in a number of allelic tryptophan-requiring mutants (*td* mutants) of *Neurospora* lacking the enzyme (13). The possible role of these proteins in tryptophan synthetase formation, and the manner in which they may contribute toward our understanding of the functional organization of a genetic unit will be briefly discussed.

In studies on the genetic control of tryptophan synthetase formation in *Neurospora*, Yanofsky (15) found that two allelic tryptophan-requiring mutants (*td*$_1$ and *td*$_2$), unable to utilize indole, lacked the enzyme, tryptophan synthetase, which is necessary for tryptophan formation. Similar results have been reported by Mitchell and Lein (9) and by Hogness and Mitchell (7), using strain *td*$_1$. Yanofsky (15) concluded, from a number of experiments, that the absence of enzyme activity in the mutants appeared to result from an effect of mutation on the formation of the enzyme itself. He also observed (15) that a

* Postdoctoral Fellow of the National Cancer Institute, National Institutes of Health, Public Health Service. Present address: McCollum-Pratt Institute, the Johns Hopkins University, Baltimore, Md.

123

second mutation (a suppressor) at another locus could partially restore enzyme formation in mutant td_2, and that the enzyme formed in this suppressed mutant strain appeared to be normal when judged by several criteria (15, 18). Of considerable importance was the fact that the td_2 suppressor gene (Su_2) had no effect on strain td_1 (15), a relation clearly demonstrating that although td_1 and td_2 were considered to be allelic, they behaved differently with regard to the property of specific suppressibility.

More recent work by Yanofsky and Bonner (17, 18, and unpub.) with over twenty-five independently occurring td mutants has strengthened the conclusion that functional differences exist within the td locus. As shown in Table 1, these mutants, allelic by recombi-

TABLE 1

SUPPRESSOR SPECIFICITY AT THE td LOCUS

td Mutant	Suppressor gene			
	$Su_{2, 2a, 2b, 2c, 2d}$	Su_3	Su_6	Su_{24}
td_1	—	—	—	—
td_2	+	—	+	—
td_3	—	+	—	+
td_6	—	—	+	—
td_{24}	—	+	—	+

A (+) indicates suppression. The data in this table are adapted from Yanofsky and Bonner (18).

nation and heterocaryon tests, can be divided into four distinct groups on the basis of their susceptibility to specific suppressor mutations. No linkage was found between the td locus and the suppressor genes. However, while striking specificity of a given suppressor gene for a particular td mutant is evident, it can also be seen in the table that a number of non-allelic suppressor genes exist, each of which has a similar effect with respect to the restoration of tryptophan synthetase formation for the td_2 allele. This seemingly anomalous situation, initially suggesting two levels of specificity, can be resolved if one supposes that the role of suppressor genes may be concerned with repair of minor enzyme damage or with control of certain quantitative aspects of enzyme formation. Attempts to demonstrate the presence of a "suppressor substance" by heterocaryon tests and biochemical analysis have thus far been unsuccessful (Yanofsky and Bonner, unpub.). It would seem, therefore, that genetic responsibility for the major steps in tryptophan synthetase formation resides in the *td* locus itself, and most important, that different areas within this locus may be altered in specifically different ways, detectable by suppressor tests.

Since mutations at the *td* locus appear to exert their effect at the enzyme-forming level, an effort was made to obtain further information on the complexity and function of this locus by additional means. Immunological technics were employed to screen the mutants for the presence of proteins which were serologically related to tryptophan synthetase, but which possessed no enzymatic activity. The usefulness of this approach, which provides a most sensitive and specific method for detecting similarities and differences between proteins, has been elegantly demonstrated by the classical work of Cohn and Torriani on the β-galactosidase system in *Escherichia coli* (3).

Using partially purified preparations of wild type *Neurospora* tryptophan synthetase as antigen, rabbit antibody was obtained which quantitatively and completely neutralizes enzyme activity (12, 13, and unpub.). This neutralization reaction is unaffected by either indole, serine, tryptophan, or pyridoxal phosphate, and is complete within a few seconds or less.

On testing extracts of several of the *td* mutants for their ability to react with and remove anti-tryptophan synthetase, it was found (Table 2) that a number of the mutant preparations did indeed contain serologically active, though enzymatically inert material (designated CRM). Two of the mutants, strain td_1 and strain td_2, were selected for more detailed examination, since preliminary results (13) indicated that strain td_2 contained CRM while strain td_1 did not. Hence, these two mutants, allelic by recombination and heterocaryon tests, appear to differ not only in their susceptibility to specific suppressor mutations, but also with respect to their ability to synthesize a protein serologically related to tryptophan synthetase. Whether any inherent relationship exists between suppressor susceptibility and the presence or absence of CRM remains to be seen.

Experiments employing partially purified preparations of strain td_2 have provided some information concerning the nature of the serologically active component (12, and unpub.). CRM appears to be closely related to tryptophan synthetase in several of its properties (Table 3). It follows the same fractionation pattern as the enzyme, and it elicits anti-enzyme formation when injected into rabbits. The

TABLE 2

PROPERTIES OF *Neurospora crassa* STRAINS

Strain	Reaction effected by genetic block	Tryptophan requirement	Tryptophan synthetase	CRM
Wild type (5256A)	In + Se $\xrightarrow[\text{B}_6\text{ - P}]{Tsase}$ Tr	0	$++++$	$+$
td_1	In + Se $\xrightarrow{\quad/\quad}$ Tr	$+$	0	0
td_2, td_3, td_6, td_7	In + Se $\xrightarrow{\quad/\quad}$ Tr	$+$	0	$++++$
td_{24} (temperature-sensitive)	In + Se $\xrightarrow[25°C.]{\quad/\quad}$ Tr	$+$	0	$+$
	In + Se $\xrightarrow[30°C.]{\quad/\quad}$ Tr	0	$+$	$++++$
$td_1 Su_2$	In + Se $\xrightarrow{\quad/\quad}$ Tr	$+$	0	0
$td_2 Su_2$, $td_3 Su_3$, $td_6 Su_6$	In + Se $\xrightarrow{\quad/\quad}$ Tr	0	$+$	$++++$

In, indole; Se, serine; Tr, tryptophan; B$_6$-P, pyridoxal phosphate; CRM, serologically active protein.

TABLE 3

SUMMARY OF THE PROPERTIES OF TRYPTOPHAN SYNTHETASE AND td_2–CRM

Properties	Tryptophan synthetase	CRM
Enzyme activity	$+$	0
Fractionation behavior (use of protamine SO$_4$, ammon. SO$_4$, and alumina gel)	about 70-fold	same
Antigenicity	$+$	$+$
type of antibody formed	anti-enzyme	same
action of antibody	complete neutralization of enzyme activity	same
absorption of anti-synthetase or anti-CRM serum	complete	complete
dialysis effect on serological stability	unstable to dialysis	stable to dialysis

enzyme neutralization curves obtained with anti-CRM serum are indistinguishable from those found with anti-synthetase serum. Furthermore, both antigens are equally effective in absorbing all of the anti-synthetase or anti-CRM from a given antiserum. It initially seemed that the only difference between the proteins was the absence of enzyme activity in CRM. However, we have recently found that the enzyme and CRM can be readily distinguished from one another by their behavior upon prolonged dialysis. CRM is stable when dialyzed, whereas the enzyme itself is inactivated both enzymatically and serologically by this treatment.

On subjecting preparations of strain td_1 to more intensive scrutiny, our earlier observation regarding the absence of CRM in this strain was verified. Purification of extracts of td_1 was carried out, following the same procedure ordinarily employed for the enzyme and CRM. Such fractions on testing proved to be serologically inactive (activity less than 0.2% of that present in td_2). In addition, injection of rabbits with td_1 preparations failed to elicit anti-enzyme formation. These findings have proved of considerable value, since td_1 fractions are now being used to absorb anti-enzyme serum, removing other antibodies, and giving a serum which appears, from quantitative tests, to be directed specifically against tryptophan synthetase and its related proteins.

At present we do not know whether the serologically active proteins found in the other td mutants are similar to td_2-CRM, nor do we have any evidence for the physiological role of CRM. Although detailed quantitative data are not yet available, recent observations may shed some light on these problems. As seen in Table 2, the wild-type strain also contains a CRM-like protein which is present in low concentration (about 10% of the enzyme). Furthermore, a temperature-sensitive mutant, td_{24} (17, 18), which forms small amounts of enzyme at 30° C., but none at 25° C., also forms five- to six-fold greater quantities of CRM at 30° C. In addition, suppressed mutant strains form both enzyme and considerable amounts of CRM (13), while interestingly enough, the unsuppressible strain, td_1, even when carrying the Su_2 suppressor gene, forms neither enzyme nor CRM.

Hence we are faced with several interesting possibilities concerning the identity of CRM in the different strains, including the likelihood that it may be a normal protein constituent whose rate of synthesis is controlled by mutations affecting the td locus. The relationship of

CRM to tryptophan synthetase, whether it be a specific precursor, an altered, closely related, or inactivated enzyme, or an accumulated shunt product, now appears subject to experimental test. Studies by Lerner and Yanofsky (unpub.) on indole biosynthesis and linkage in *E. coli* suggest that a CRM-like protein may catalyze one of the steps in indole formation, and furthermore, that the gene controlling this step appears to be closely linked to the coli *td* locus. We have been unable, so far, to assign an enzymatic role of this sort to the *Neurospora* CRM.

In conclusion, the evidence bearing on the nature of the *td* locus supports the view that a specific chromosomal area, intimately concerned with the formation of a single enzyme, may consist of a number of functionally related interdependent component parts, albeit the entire area remains indivisible by cross-over tests. Since one is able to examine the relationship between structure and function at this locus in precise enzymatic and serological terms, it would appear that we are in a position to determine whether different and specific CRM proteins are formed as the result of damage to particular areas within the *td* locus. Perhaps it will be possible to correlate the information obtained with the specific action of certain suppressor genes on enzyme formation, and so to provide further insight into the organization and function of the genetic material (1, 2, 4-6, 8, 10, 11, 17).

ACKNOWLEDGMENT

The author would like to express his deep appreciation to Dr. A. M. Pappenheimer, Jr., for his interest and many helpful discussions during the course of the immunological work.

REFERENCES

1. Benzer, S., *Proc. Natl. Acad. Sci. U. S.,* **41**, 344 (1955).
2. Bonner, D. M., *Cold Spring Harbor Symposia Quant. Biol.,* **21**, in press.
3. Cohn, M., and Torriani, A. M., *J. Immunol.,* **69**, 471 (1952).
4. Demerec, M., in *Enzymes: Units of Biological Structure and Function* (O. H. Gaebler, ed.), p. 131. Academic Press, New York (1956).
5. Demerec, M., *Cold Spring Harbor Symposia Quant. Biol.,* **21**, in press.
6. Green, M. M., *Proc. Natl. Acad. Sci. U. S.,* **42**, 73 (1956).
7. Hogness, D. S., and Mitchell, H. K., *J. Gen. Microbiol.,* **11**, 401 (1954).
8. Mitchell, M. B., *Proc. Natl. Acad. Sci. U. S.,* **41**, 215 (1955).
9. Mitchell, H. K., and Lein, J., *J. Biol. Chem.,* **175**, 481 (1948).
10. Pontecorvo, G., *Cold Spring Harbor Symposia Quant. Biol.,* **21**, in press.
11. St. Lawrence, P., *Genetics,* **40**, 599 (1955).
12. Suskind, S. R., *Federation Proc.,* **15**, 616 (1956) [abstract].

13. Suskind, S. R., Yanofsky, C., and Bonner, D. M., *Proc. Natl. Acad. Sci. U. S.*, **41**, 577 (1955).
14. Umbreit, W. W., Wood, W. A., and Gunsalus, I. C., *J. Biol. Chem.*, **165**, 731 (1946).
15. Yanofsky, C., *Proc. Natl. Acad. Sci. U. S.*, **38**, 215 (1952).
16. Yanofsky, C., in *Methods in Enzymology* (S. P. Colowick and N. O. Kaplan, eds.), Vol. 2, p. 233. Academic Press, New York (1955).
17. Yanofsky, C., in *Enzymes: Units of Biological Structure and Function* (O. H. Gaebler, ed.), p. 147. Academic Press, New York (1956).
18. Yanofsky, C., and Bonner, D. M., *Genetics*, **40**, 761 (1955); **40**, 602 (1955) [abstract].

DISCUSSION

DR. BEADLE: I would like to say that I don't want to get into any argument with Benzer about terminology. If he wants to call a functional unit a cistron that's all right with me. I would like to say, however, that I agree that his is a very beautiful work.

I would like to point out that sometimes when you convert a physicist to a biologist you get into certain difficulties. There is a deficiency in his hierarchy of taxonomic categories. He omitted the genus.

DR. BENZER: It was an oversight—it was in my notes. The category was taken care of. I was going to reserve it for the small segment which consists of a group of elements which go together to determine the specificity of one amino acid, giving the new slogan "One genus, one peptide hypothesis."

DR. LEDERBERG: Dr. Mitchell, do you know of any examples of aberrant crossing over—that is to say, tetrads which show non-reciprocal numbers of crossovers between the two peripheral markers?

DR. MITCHELL: The pyridoxine case is the only one so far which has appropriate markers and in which the mutants can be selfed. There are several other possibilities which haven't been analyzed by isolation of tetrads. The markers used for the pyridoxine locus have always segregated normally.

DR. BEADLE: I would like to ask Dr. Benzer this question: In your *rII* units, did you have markers outside this area that were followed simultaneously?

DR. BENZER: No. Doermann and his group are doing experiments where they watch the segregation of outside markers, and he can answer your questions on that point.

DR. BEADLE: If I remember correctly, in a report that was made at Cold Spring Harbor, by Streisinger and Franklin, there was a marker on one side, and this did not show a high correlation with the recombinant event in the *h* region, but instead gave a high negative interference.

DR. DOERMANN: Yes, that's correct, but it depends a little on circumstances. We have done quite a few crosses with Benzer's *rII* material, and it seems clear that this question of negative interference depends on the distance between the two or three markers in which we are interested. For example, we may do three-factor crosses which require the double crossover for production of the recombinant which can be selectively scored. When the outside markers in such a cross are far apart, say, four recombination units, we find 6 to 8 times as many double recombinants as expected from two-factor crosses involving these loci; when the outside markers are located close together, say one recombination unit or less, we find 30 or 40 times the expected number. I think that Edgar has convincingly shown that this particular type of negative interference, namely, that restricted to short regions, is a result of recombination in a special type of structure which seems to be characteristic of the T-even phages. It appears in Edgar's experiments as though recombinants are formed by replication in the partially heterozygous region of the so-called residual heterozygotes discovered by Hershey and Chase. Multiple crossing over is unusually frequent in such material. Since such heterozygous regions appear to be rather short, the probability of observing multiple crossovers is increased over the usual expectation as the markers involved are closer and closer together. I think that Franklin and Streisinger's experiments are an exact parallel. They cross mutant h_1+ and h_2+ which are very closely linked. In addition the h_2+ strain is marked with a rather distantly linked tu, while the h_1+ carries $tu+$. Assuming the order h_1+, h_2+, tu, you'd expect the h_1h_2 recombinant to carry the tu marker more frequently than $tu+$. In fact, Franklin and Streisinger found 50 per cent of the h_1h_2 recombinants carrying tu and 50 per cent carrying $tu+$. In our experiments it is clear that a similar situation is observed when the two r markers are closely enough linked; when the r markers are moved a little farther apart, then the linkage with the outside markers is maintained.

Dr. GLASS: I suspect there are a good many biochemists who have heard about negative interference for the first time from your remarks. Could you tell us briefly what you mean by negative interference?

Dr. DOERMANN: I guess we ought to start with positive interference. In the classical material a crossover in one region inhibits an additional crossover in an adjacent region. This has been called interference, more specifically positive interference, and may be expressed as the coefficient of coincidence. We let P_1 be the probability of crossover in one region and P_2 the probability of crossover in an adjacent region. On the assumption the crossover in region I is independent of that in region II, we expect P_1P_2 to be the probability of double crossover. The coefficient of coincidence is the frequency of observed double crossovers divided by the frequency expected. If the coefficient of coincidence is less than one, we say we find positive interference. If it is greater than one we call it negative interference.

Dr. BEADLE: What is the status of reciprocal recombination products? Do you get them under certain circumstances?

Dr. Doermann: I don't know of any case where it's clear that you do get reciprocal products.

Dr. Beadle: The assumption is that the single event gives one recombination product.

Dr. Doermann: The assumption is that, but I don't think we know.

Dr. Spiegelman: There are two comments I would like to make concerning the aberrant asci discussed by Dr. Mitchell. If one examines the results of crosses in the bacterial viruses by means of mass lysates, reciprocal recombinants are found in roughly equal proportions. However, this apparent accordance with genetic expectation is the statistical smoothing over of a rather different situation. Analysis of the products derived from single bursts reveals that they do *not* contain reciprocal recombinants. Thus, what is a rare exception in the Ascomycetes is the rule in the bacterial viruses. To search for a unique explanation of the aberrant tetrads which ignores the virus data would, to my mind, miss the cardinal point emphasized by the two sets of data. The intriguing possibility suggests itself that size is the crux of the matter. Thus, whenever experiments with classical or neo-classical material can be arranged by suitable selective devices to study small regions, the data become paradoxical when compared to the statistical norm predicted by classical genetic calculations. The operation of a sort of copy-choice mechanism suggests itself as one immediate possibility.

An important contribution emerged at the recent meeting at Cold Spring Harbor which I should like to note. Those of you familiar with genetic literature will recall the announcement by Lindegren in 1952 of his historical aberrant ascus. It involved a cross in yeast of an adenineless by a wild type. Among many normal asci, one was found yielding 3 negatives to 1 positive. Many, including myself, did not take this single ascus seriously since it could have arisen as the result of a mutation from plus to minus. It should be noted that available information on the stability of this locus made this possibility unlikely, but did not eliminate it. Herschel Roman reported on a reinvestigation of this question and has isolated a number of such aberrant asci involving the same locus. Using somatic recombinations in diplophase, he has shown that independent isolates of adenineless in this region are different since they exhibit recombinations. He then used this device to test whether the three negatives of an aberrant ascus are identical or different. In all cases examined, he finds that the extra negative is identical genetically to the one which went into the cross. This eliminates the possibility that these exceptional segregations can be explained in terms of rare independent mutations.

Dr. Hotchkiss: The question of non-reciprocal *vs.* reciprocal recombinations seems very important to me. I was looking at it a little differently, in terms of the size of the entities involved, inasmuch as small fragments of genome cannot contribute reciprocally to make progeny.

First, let me suggest that the size-distinctions of which Dr. Benzer was trying to make us aware are well illustrated by what goes on in his two-car garage. When, by dint of some handyman's work, the parts of two defective automobiles are put together to make one functioning one—let's say the two-inch-long condenser of one is put into the distributor of the other—Dr. Benzer was, I thought, trying to preclude some boy looking through the window from reacting, "My gosh, I never knew that a Ford car was really only two inches long." When such terms as pseudo-alleles or non-identical alleles (of some use for referring to the whole mutant gene, containing a changed element) are used, as they often are, for the changed element itself, the subunit, they name the part for the whole and obscure the relationship. It is only when so misunderstood that these beautiful new experiments seem to threaten the place of the old-fashioned, semi-autonomous gene—a unit of function which in the appropriate cellular environment can initiate a complete biochemical operation.

Of course, one can make another kind of mistake in interpretation. I think both Dr. Benzer and Dr. Mitchell would have liked my grandfather, who one day was trying to take an alarm clock apart. The clock wasn't functioning, and when he opened it, he found a dead fly inside. He turned to me and said, dryly, "No wonder the clock isn't working; the engineer is dead."

The essential point in these recombinations is that the size factor controls both reciprocality and the rules of frequency. When you are trying to interact two complete chromosomes you have a distance of a few hundred Å units involved, and so the possibility for this large, not altogether flexible, entity to bend back and interact twice within a short distance is reduced. From such a picture most of the facts of crossing over can be rationalized. In most of these new, "unorthodox" recombinations, however, you are trying to challenge whatever passes for a chromosome with a fragmented bit of genome. We presented evidence at the Henry Ford Hospital symposium on enzymes, that this is the kind of thing that is happening in transformation. It certainly looks as though this is what happens in the transductions used by Demerec and, from the results, apparently also in recombinations in phages or bacteria.

When a small fragment exchanges with an organized, intact section of genome, not only is the smaller part precluded from forming progeny, but every incorporation is the analogue of a "double crossover," requiring one breakage (or substitution) at each end. Accordingly, the probabilities of various exchanges are different than on a crossover model, and more in line with those actually observed. When far enough apart, the exchanges of markers require two transformations and are either independent or mutually inhibitory ("positive interference"). At closer distances the opportunity for one given event would depend not only upon linkage distance, but in 3-factor crosses, the factor of probable size of incorporated fragment enters importantly.

There are indications in transformation that large DNA fragments are not incorporated intact as readily as small ones, as seems reasonable. Here, then, we can see why in the close sequence, ABC, the region B may be introduced without disturbing A or C, far more often than expected, and in fact almost as often as it exchanges with A or C alone. On a crossing-over model, this result is interpreted as the troublesome "negative interference."

DR. CHARGAFF: I would like to ask Dr. Benzer one question. He made an estimate of the size of his units, and if I remember correctly he said that they could be one nucleotide or perhaps not more than a handful of nucleotides. Now, what does that leave us in chemical terms? Out of the chain of DNA, for instance, which has probably no repeating units that we can recognize, the removal or exchange of, say, one guanylic acid in a certain place is what you call this unit of yours; or do you think it could include the whole surroundings or habitat of this particular nucleotide? In other words, if you have one adenylic acid which is flanked on either side by five guanylic acids, is this adenylic acid equivalent to one which is next to another adenylic acid? How can you make an estimate as precise as one or two nucleotides?

DR. BENZER: The estimate is not precise. What we don't know is whether recombination is proportional to length regardless of the specific bases which are present. Suppose that recombination happens because of breaks in the backbone, with uniformity of bond strength between the nucleotides. If this assumption is correct (you have to make some assumption like this in order to set the order of magnitude) when you get very closely linked markers the recombination distances should be quantized into suitable multiples of a basic unit. This is very optimistic.

THE ROLE OF THE CYTOPLASM IN HEREDITY

DAVID L. NANNEY

Zoology Department, University of Michigan,
Ann Arbor, Michigan

INTRODUCTION

Definition of Terms.

BEFORE ATTEMPTING to assess the role of the cytoplasm in heredity, it is necessary to make clear what will be meant by the term *heredity* in the discussion. Many terms in their usage become encrusted with secondary attributes, and a stripping away of nonessentials may be useful in clarifying underlying concepts. Such a term is *heredity*. In common usage it has been endowed with connotations which restrict its usage to phenomena studied by certain techniques. Usually *heredity* refers to the transmission of specificities by sexual (or parasexual) means from one generation to the next. It implies breeding experiments and the analysis of genetic recombination.

An older and broader interpretation may be useful, however, in bringing together phenomena of fundamental similarity without restriction as to analytical devices. The term may be used to describe the more general capacity of living material to maintain its individuality (specificity) during proliferation. In this sense, hereditary mechanisms are any mechanisms which assure the continuity of specificity during the material dilution accompanying growth—regardless of whether a gamete or gemete-like phase is included in the growth process, and regardless of whether differences in specificity can be analyzed by genetic recombination. This definition—unlike the more common definition—includes the transmission of specificity within the soma of multicellular organisms or within clones of unicellular organisms. *Heredity,* in this sense, is a type of homeostasis, similar to physiological homeostasis but implying more, since it includes regulation during protoplasmic increase. Nevertheless, a single mechanism might serve simultaneously as a physiological and as an hereditary regulator. It is to be understood that the term as we will use it implies nothing about the mechanisms whereby specificity is maintained.

While heredity—in this sense of the perpetuation of specificity—is universally characteristic of protoplasm, so also are the variations in specificity which arise through the occasional failure of the hereditary mechanisms and which are in their turn perpetuated by these mechanisms. It would be useful to employ the term *mutation* for these alterations if it had not been so narrowed in its evolution. In its oldest sense "mutation" refers to any alteration in specificity which is heritable, and implies nothing regarding either the mechanisms or the materials involved in the change. With the identification of some mutations with particular chromosomal alterations, the concept has been restricted. "Mutation" now usually implies alterations transmitted through sexual reproduction and in particular alterations associated with chromosomal changes, either microscopic or submicroscopic. This class of hereditary modifications shares certain common attributes—rarity, irregularity, and a low degree of specificity between inducing agent and the changes observed—and those modifications which fail to manifest these attributes are dismissed as not being "true" mutations. The frequent and regular alterations occurring in cell lineages (particularly in embryonic development), often in response to specific stimuli, are thus excluded from consideration, and the problems they raise are deposited on the doorstep of the embryologists. Since it is unreasonable to expect a term so firmly entrenched as "mutation" to acquire the necessary connotations (or lack of connotations) needed for present purposes, we will simply substitute the term "hereditary modification," emphasize the lack of any particular implication as to the materials involved, and apply the term to any variation in an hereditary specificity which becomes in its turn hereditary.

Finally, I wish to take the liberty of extending the term *cytoplasm* in the title of this paper to permit a discussion not only of the cytoplasm proper, but also of the nucleoplasm. The cell is usually divided into two portions—the nucleus and the cytoplasm—but the nuclear portion is promptly reduced to mean chromosomes (or more recently, DNA), and the residual nucleoplasm is left out of consideration. By discussing the nucleoplasm in conjunction with the cytoplasm we are at least reminded of its existence. It is also evident that some more or less direct communication occurs between the cytoplasm and the nucleoplasm and that their properties, from a genetic point of view, may not be greatly different. This taxonomic invasion of the nucleus by the cytoplasm may also be viewed as a reciprocation for the extension of the nucleus into the cytoplasm—as witnessed by such terms as plasma*gene,* cyto*gene,* and *gen*oid. This deliberate confusion of the boundaries between the nucleus and the cytoplasm is based on a dissatisfaction with a classification of genetic systems in terms of geography alone and on the belief that such systems are more profitably discussed with reference to mechanisms.

Concepts of Genetic Mechanisms.

Two concepts of genetic mechanisms have persisted side by side throughout the growth of modern genetics, but the emphasis has been very strongly in favor of one of these and a synthesis between the two has not yet been achieved. The first of these we will designate as the "Master Molecule" concept. This concept presupposes a special type of material, distinct from the rest of the protoplasm, which directs the activities of the cell and functions as a reservoir of information. In its simplest form the concept places the "master molecules" in the chromosomes and attributes the characteristics of an organism to their specific construction; all other cellular constituents are considered relatively inconsequential except as obedient servants of the masters. This is in essence the Theory of the Gene, interpreted to suggest a totalitarian government. Refinements in the concept may be introduced in various ways to accommodate special situations. Thus, any sophisticated view requires that organic specificity be a function not only of the intrinsic capacities of the system, but also of the environmental circumstances in which it exists. Other observations require that the "master molecules" be not restricted to the nucleus, but that they may in some instances occupy stations in the cytoplasm.

The second concept of a genetic mechanism is one which is more difficult to describe, and one for which experimental evidence is harder to obtain. This concept we will designate as the "Steady State" concept. By the term "Steady State" we envision a dynamic self-perpetuating organization of a variety of molecular species which owes its specific properties not to the characteristics of any one kind of molecule, but to the functional interrelationships of these molecular species. Such a concept contains the notion of checks and balances in a system of biochemical reactions. In contrast to the totalitarian government by "master molecules," the "steady state" government is a more democratic organization, composed of interacting cellular fractions operating in self-perpetuating patterns. The possible details of such patterns

are almost unlimited—at least theoretically—and any meaningful discussion on a practical level must be directed at some particular system.
We will return to this problem later. We may note in passing, however,
that the "master molecule" and the "steady state" concepts are not
mutually exclusive and that both may be required for an orderly functioning organization.

The Role of the Cytoplasm in Sexual Heredity

Regardless of which of the above genetic concepts one embraces, the
cytoplasm must be accorded some role as genetic material. The best
understood examples of cytoplasmic transmission associated with
sexual processes are those involving "master molecules." One may cite
as examples of such cytoplasmic genetic determinants *sigma* (the CO_2
sensitivity factor in *Drosophila,* 14, 15) and *kappa* (the killer factor in
Paramecium, 2, 29, 30). One may mention also the "plastogenes"
presumably responsible for plastid characteristics in higher plants (10,
24), the statistical particles called forth to explain somatic segregation
of pollen sterility (23), and the particulates associated in various ways
with the enzymatic constitution of yeast (8, 28). On less convincing
evidence genetic properties are accorded to such entities as mitochondria, kinetosomes, blepharoblasts, and other similar cellular
organelles (16). Many of these studies have been reviewed repeatedly
(2, 5, 7, 8, 12, 30, 35), and no attempt will be made here to offer critical
evaluations of them individually. Although the evidence for genetic
continuity for some of these elements may be questioned, the existence
of a class of cytoplasmic particulates, showing great diversity of structure, function, and probable origin, but alike in controlling hereditary
traits, is firmly established. The chief problem is, therefore, not to
determine whether elements in the cytoplasm have genetic functions,
but rather to assess the extent of their distribution and their general
significance.

This problem requires some consideration of the *relative* roles of the
nucleus and the cytoplasm in heredity. We may ask—for example—
what are the relative frequencies of traits with chromosomal and cytoplasmic bases? This is not an easy question to answer. It is certainly
clear that the vast majority of *published* reports deal with traits at least
formally explicable by chromosomal inheritance; whether the ratio of
the two kinds observed in the literature is an accurate reflection of
the ratio in nature is another matter. We are all aware that many

considerations—both conscious and unconscious—are involved in the selection of traits to study and are cognizant of the non-randomness of the published accounts. Certain types of traits are more likely to be examined and certain types of results are more likely to be reported. One may argue, moreover, that these biases systematically prejudice judgment in favor of chromosomal inheritance.

The biases begin with a decision as to which traits should be studied. From the beginning of genetics attention has been focused on clear alternative characteristics which can be readily distinguished and enumerated. A chromosomal mechanism is admirably suited for the transmission of just such traits. While continuous variations may also be explained by chromosomal mechanisms, a satisfactory analysis is difficult when variations do not fall into discrete classes. Yet, a cytoplasmic basis can also explain continuous variation by the more or less random partitioning of one or more kinds of cytoplasmic elements. Thus, those traits without discrete classes—perhaps those most likely to involve a cytoplasmic mechanism—are deliberately excluded from study.

Even after the study of a trait is initiated, further sources of bias may appear. Unlike the clear operational approach to Mendelian characters, the establishment of a cytoplasmic basis is a devious and often inconclusive process of elimination. When differences in reciprocal crosses are encountered, for example, one must first eliminate the possibilities of differential fertilization, differential viability, preferential chromosome elimination, and many other possible vagaries of chromosome behavior, a task which may be beyond the ability of the investigator or impossible to undertake with certain types of material. When identical results are observed in reciprocal crosses and particularly when simple numerical ratios are obtained, these lengthy and often painful sequences are considered unnecessary—even though, as Ephrussi has pointed out (8), differences in reciprocal crosses need not be associated with cytoplasmic inheritance and, conversely, identity of reciprocal crosses does not automatically exclude a cytoplasmic basis. It is perhaps only natural that investigations of "messy" characteristics are discontinued before publication and that investigators move on to traits more readily analyzed. If this is, in fact, a correct evaluation of the practices of biologists, the role of the chromosomes in heredity may be seriously overemphasized. On the other hand, one would like to believe that the rule regarding the cherishing of exceptions is not only an ideal but a widespread practice, and that traits which raise real problems of interpretation by deviating from Mendelian patterns receive a disproportionate amount of study. If this is true, the ratio between cytoplasmic and chromosomal bases might be biased in the other direction. A resolution of this problem involves an analysis of the pressures to which scientists are subjected and the motivations of the investigator. Such an analysis is beyond the scope of this paper and the competence of the author, but remains essential for a completely satisfactory answer.

At the theoretical level one factor involved in assessing the genetic role of the cytoplasm is the relative efficiency of cytoplasmic as opposed to chromosomal mechanisms. It has been suggested, for example, that potentialities associated with chromosomes are more likely to be transmitted with precision than potentialities associated with the cytoplasm —simply because of the elaborate mechanisms evolved for the equal distribution of the chromosomes. Hence, any potentiality necessary for the maintenance of life would be forced by natural selection into a chromosomal niche and any genetic system remaining in the cytoplasm, being unreliable, would involve relatively inconsequential potentialities. First it may be pointed out, however, that a cytoplasmic mechanism is not necessarily an imprecise mechanism, though it might require a greater material investment by the cell in order to make it equally efficient with a chromosomal mechanism. The random assortment of, say, a thousand cell particulates will assure an approximate identity of daughter cells, almost as reliably as a mitotic spindle. If for some other reason (such as for a required heterocatalytic function) this amount of material was required anyway, the argument for economy is without force. It is true that many of the analyzed systems of cytoplasmic inheritance are less precise than chromosomal mechanisms (i.e., hereditary modifications occur in them frequently), but this may again be a matter of selection of traits—for it is these variations which in many cases permit the analysis of a cytoplasmic system.

This argument does not, of course, prove the indispensible nature of cytoplasmic genetic particles, but merely suggests that such particulates cannot be ruled out by *a priori* considerations. Moreover, the difficulties of detecting *essential* cytoplasmic elements are formidable. A lethal gene in a chromosome can be studied in a straightforward manner, simply because a recessive lethal can be carried in a heterozygous state and its effect can be tabulated numerically following

dent with cellular differentiation was a rarely observed phenomenon and in any case failed to provide sufficient nuclear constitutions to account for more than a small fraction of the observed cell types. Moreover, studies directed at this particular point by Roux, Hertwig, Spemann, and others failed to provide evidence for any nuclear alterations during development in some forms. We may mention briefly in this connection the famous experiments of Spemann on newt eggs (32). Spemann constricted fertilized eggs with a ligature, thereby separating the cytoplasm into two portions, one with and one without a nucleus. After a series of nuclear divisions one of the daughter nuclei might escape into the non-nucleated cytoplasm and there continue its divisions. If the nuclei had undergone any irreversible differentiation in hereditary capacities during these early divisions, abnormal development might be expected in the initially non-nucleated portion of the egg. However, a normal—if somewhat retarded—twin developed. It was concluded, therefore, that nuclear differentiation did not occur during these early nuclear divisions and that some other hereditary mechanisms must be involved in differentiation. It should be noted, however, that this experiment tested only the equivalence of nuclei during the early cleavage stages, i.e., before irreversible cellular changes of any kind could be detected. In spite of this fact, such experiments were sufficient to convince most biologists that somatic and germinal heredity involved separate and distinct mechanisms and must be treated as independent problems. More specifically, the interpretation evolved that, since germinal heredity was primarily a nuclear function and since somatic heredity must have a different basis, somatic variation and heredity were primarily under the control of the cytoplasm.

This opinion did not of course solve the problems of cellular differentiation and heredity, but only left a vacuum which had to be filled with something. A major effort to fill this vacuum involved the extension of the "master molecules" into the cytoplasm. By postulating various kinds of "master molecules," assorting at cell division, multiplying at various rates, responding differentially in different environments, and interacting with each other in various patterns of competition and cooperation, model systems of considerable explanatory value were provided (7, 17, 27, 30, 33, 35). While this interpretation has great merit as a theoretical scheme, it also has some inherent weaknesses; it has not been accepted with enthusiasm, and relatively little evidence has been obtained for it as a general phenomenon. Recently, moreover, the basic premise of a cytoplasmic interpretation has been challenged by studies which show the early work on nuclear differentiation to have been interpreted prematurely. King and Briggs (11) have taken up the studies of the early embryologists, but using modern methods of investigation have tested the hypothesis of nuclear equivalence at later stages of development—at times when irreversible cellular changes were known to have occurred. This was accomplished by removing nuclei from embryonic cells at various times during development, injecting these nuclei into enucleated eggs, and following the course of differentiation. While their results with nuclei from early cleavage stages corroborates the earlier experiments, nuclei from progressively later stages of development were progressively less capable of maintaining normal development, and the types of developmental anomalies were correlated with the location of the nuclei in the original embryo. Moreover, the anomalies detected with nuclei from differentiated cells were reproduced upon successive serial transfers, i.e., they were hereditary (4). Although the conclusion that nuclear differentiation had occurred may be criticized on technical grounds—for it has not yet been possible to eliminate the injection of some cytoplasm with the nuclei—these experiments do not stand alone, and taken in conjunction with other studies support the notion that at least some of the hereditary modifications encountered in development have a nuclear basis. In particular, the Lederbergs (13) have shown that long-lasting but impermanent variations in *Salmonella* serotypes have physical bases intimately associated with the bacterial "chromosome." It might appear, therefore, that the dichotomy between germinal and somatic inheritance, between cytoplasmic and nuclear bases, was after all a mistake, and that investigations may now converge with a unified perspective on the few remaining problems.

These few remaining problems, however, on careful examination are neither so few nor particularly small. Simply because some examples of cellular differentiation involve nuclear alterations, we must not conclude that all such differentiation has a nuclear basis. We must avoid another premature conclusion in our search for parsimony. Moreover, several characteristic features of hereditary modifications in embryonic development are without explanation in the customary frame of reference for nuclear modifications. For example, the changes involved in embryonic development may occur at a very rapid rate, as opposed to the usually slow rate of "mutations." These changes are,

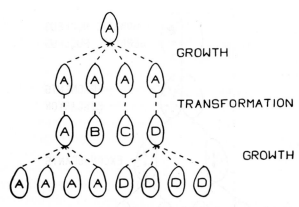

Fɪɢ. 2.   Schematic representation of intraclonal inheritance and intraclonal variations in antigenic specificity in *Paramecium aurelia*.

surface antigens (Fig. 2). If the clone is subjected to any of several injurious substances (antibodies, enzymes, physical or chemical agents), some or all of the cells may alter their surface specificities (i.e., undergo transformation), either in the same or in different ways, depending upon the conditions. When the cells are returned to standard conditions of growth, these new specificities are then maintained for long periods of time, i.e., they are hereditary. They may be altered again, however, by exposing the cells to environmental stress. When a single clone is studied exhaustively, it is found to have a limited number of potentialities which differ from those of other clones and which are controlled by nuclear genes. In spite of having several potentialities, only one specificity is normally expressed at a single time in a single cell. The expression of any one potentiality precludes the expression of the others.

This differentiation of a clone into a number of cell types, each expressing its own specificities and transmitting its properties to its progeny, is analogous in many ways to the differentiation in a developing organism. The chief difference lies in the relative ease of reversal of the serotype differentiations; but this, as pointed out elsewhere (21), may be a secondary attribute geared to the economy of a unicellular organism.

The physical basis for the serotype variations is elucidated through crosses of differentiated cells derived from a common source, a procedure not available yet for studying differences in somatic cells in multicellular organisms. As an example we may consider crosses between clones of serotypes A and B (Fig. 3). The results of such crosses depend strongly upon whether cytoplasmic exchange occurs during conjugation. In the absence of cytoplasmic exchange the nuclei in the conjugating cells become identical, but the two cells retain their initial antigenic properties and yield exconjugant clones of the original types. When extensive cytoplasmic exchange occurs (Fig. 4) the two cells become alike in their serotypes and produce exconjugant clones of the same type—either both of serotype A or both of serotype B.

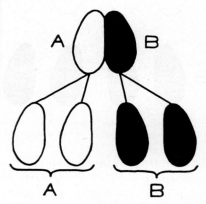

FIG. 3.   The transmission of antigenic specificities through conjugation in *Paramecium aurelia* when no cytoplasmic exchange occurs.

These observations establish that the hereditary differences characterizing the clones are due, in part at least, to differences in the cytoplasm. The failure to obtain cells of mixed types indicates that the mechanisms responsible for the perpetuation of different types are antagonistic; the differentiation to one type excludes differentiation to another. The variations are, in short, interdependent. Before considering possible explanations for these phenomena, other similar systems should be mentioned.

A second system which shows many of the characteristics of the serotype system, but which also involves some new features, is that associated with mating-type inheritance in the so-called Group B varieties of *P. aurelia*, of which variety 4 is again an example (2, 20, 29, 31). The two mating types in variety 4 are designated as mating types VII and VIII. As in the serotype system, cells with the same

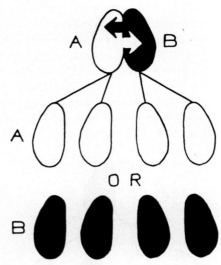

Fig. 4. The transmission of antigenic specificities through conjugation in *Paramecium aurelia* when extensive cytoplasmic exchange occurs.

genes may manifest different surface specificities, and these cellular characteristics are transmitted with even greater reliability in vegetative growth. The transmission of mating types through conjugation is also very similar to the transmission of serotypes through conjugation (Fig. 5). In the absence of cytoplasmic exchange, each cell usually

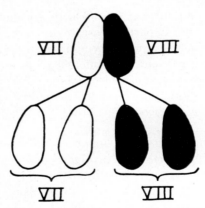

Fig. 5. The transmission of mating-type specificities through conjugation in the Group B varieties of *Paramecium aurelia* when no cytoplasmic exchange occurs.

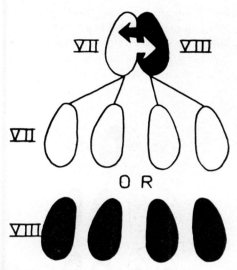

Fɪɢ. 6. The transmission of mating-type specificities through conjugation in the Group B varieties of *Paramecium aurelia* when extensive cytoplasmic exchange occurs.

retains its original type. When cytoplasmic exchange occurs (Fig. 6), the two cells usually become alike, either both of type VII or both of type VIII, depending upon the temperature. As in the case of the serotypes, these observations demonstrate that the perpetuation of a cellular type depends at least in part upon a cytoplasmic mechanism. Furthermore, since in most cases the two types are mutually exclusive, the systems leading to the manifestation of the different types are antagonistic. If this were the only information available, the serotype and the Group B mating type systems would appear different only in relatively minor details. The mating-type specificities, once established, are extremely stable, whereas the serotypes are relatively labile and may be reversed under some conditions. The serotype system also contains a greater variety of potentialities than the mating-type system, but this difference is probably trivial.

Other information, however, shows that more is involved in the mating-type system than a cytoplasmic mechanism. This conclusion is derived from an elegant experiment by Sonneborn (31). A number of years ago Sonneborn observed that under some circumstances the anlage of the new somatic nuclei either abort or are temporarily suppressed in their development, and that when this happens the fragments of the old somatic nucleus begin to develop and are segregated among the daughter cells as the functional somatic nuclei (Fig. 7). If the new somatic nuclei are only suppressed, a fraction of the cells in an exconjugant clone receives a new somatic nucleus and another fraction receives the old fragments. In the absence of cytoplasmic exchange, nuclear regeneration yields the same results as

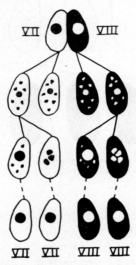

Fig. 7. The transmission of mating-type specificities through conjugation accompanied by macronuclear regeneration in the Group B varieties of *Paramecium aurelia*.

normal conjugation without cytoplasmic exchange. When both regeneration and cytoplasmic exchange occur, on the other hand, a new result is observed. At high temperatures, when only cytoplasmic exchange occurs, the two exconjugants regularly yield clones of mating type VIII. When both cytoplasmic exchange and regeneration occur, those cells receiving the new somatic nuclei behave as expected, i.e., they become mating type VIII, regardless of which exconjugant was their source. Those cells receiving fragments of the old somatic nucleus from the type VIII cell are also maintained as mating type VIII, but the cells receiving fragments from the original type VII cell become mating type VII (Fig. 8). These observations clearly contradict a simple cytoplasmic basis for the mating types, and in fact strongly support the notion of a nuclear basis. The mating type of a cell is maintained by even a fragment of the nucleus from a differentiated cell; and when nuclei of diverse origin are separated at cell division, the mating types are also separated.

We have previously indicated, however, that the perpetuation of mating types involves the cytoplasm. The interaction of these two components—the nucleus and the cytoplasm—may be understood as

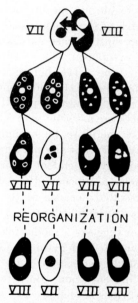

Fig. 8. The transmission of mating-type specificities through conjugation in the Group B varieties of *Paramecium aurelia* when both macronuclear regeneration and cytoplasmic exchange occur.

follows. Newly developing somatic nuclei are differentiated as to which mating type they will control, and this differentiation is usually irreversible. A major factor in determining the course of nuclear differentiation is the cytoplasmic environment. The cytoplasmic environment normally found in a type VII cell is conducive to the establishment of type VII nuclei, and that found in type VIII cells promotes the formation of type VIII nuclei. When the two kinds of cytoplasm are mixed, one suppresses the other, and the somatic nuclei are determined alike in the two members of a pair.

The next question this experiment both raises and answers is the relationship between the nuclear and the cytoplasmic determinants. To what extent is the cytoplasmic condition dependent on the nucleus? If the cytoplasm is independent, all the sublines of these clones should have the same kind of cytoplasm—that established at the previous conjugation. If the nuclei in addition to controlling the mating types also determine the cytoplasmic constitution, the two kinds of cytoplasm should be separated as the two kinds of nuclei separate. The cytoplasmic conditions responsible for specific nuclear differentiation were examined by allowing each of the subclones to undergo another process of nuclear reorganization (in this case autogamy) and to develop new somatic nuclei in their cytoplasm. The results observed were clear: clones showing mating type VIII before reorganization produced progeny showing mating type VIII, and clones showing mating type VII before reorganization produced type VII progeny. Hence, the cytoplasmic constitutions were assorted in precisely the same manner as were the nuclei and must, therefore, be strongly dependent upon them. We must not forget, however, that the nuclear constitution, during its early development, is equally dependent upon the cytoplasm. Similar nuclear differentiation may also occur in the serotype system, but this can scarcely be demonstrated because of the relative lability of the serotypes as compared with the mating types.

This particular system suggests a model for differentiation in higher forms involving both nuclear and cytoplasmic elements. Local cytoplasmic and environmental circumstances are responsible for directing the course of nuclear differentiation. Both the initial and the subsequent cytoplasmic conditions are, however, strongly dependent upon the initial and subsequent nuclear conditions.

Finally we come to a third type of system, resembling in many particulars the system just discussed, and like it involving mating-type differentiation and inheritance. Two patterns of mating-type determination in *P. aurelia* have been reported, that in the Group B varieties just described and that in the Group A varieties, which will be illustrated by variety 1 (2, 20, 29). This variety contains mating types I and II. As in the previous systems, cells with the same genic constitution may manifest different traits, and breed true for these traits in vegetative reproduction. When crosses are made between the two types, either or both types may appear among the progeny of a single pair and the distribution of these types comprises a pattern designated

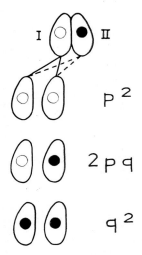

Fɪɢ. 9. The transmission of mating-type specificities through conjugation in the Group A varieties of *Paramecium aurelia*. P represents the probability that a particular caryonide will manifest mating type I and q represents the probability for a type II caryonide.

as "caryonidal inheritance" (Fig. 9). If both types are produced by a particular exconjugant, they are normally separated at the first fission after conjugation—at the same fission at which the new somatic nuclei are separated. Caryonides, in other words, are usually pure for a particular mating type, but sister caryonides from the same exconjugant are often different. Sister caryonides are no more often alike than caryonides from different exconjugants or even different pairs; the distribution of mating types among caryonides corresponds to the distribution expected by chance alone. The precise correlation between the distribution of new somatic nuclei and of new mating types, in both normal and atypical situations, leads to the conclusion that the somatic nuclei control the mating types. However, since the source of the cytoplasm in which they develop has no influence on the nuclear conditions established, no specific cytoplasmic direction of nuclear differentiation can be demonstrated. Presumably the factors determining the pattern of nuclear differentiation are largely intrinsic, and the cytoplasm is of relatively little significance.

In spite of their differences, these three systems of inheritance share many properties:

(1) The initial genic constitution of a clone determines a spectrum of possible phenotypes, but does not dictate which of these will be expressed. (This conclusion is well established for the serotypes and the Group A mating types, but genic factors have not yet been discovered for the Group B mating types.)

(2) The establishment of one of the available phenotypes excludes the establishment of the other phenotypes; mixed types are only rarely observed.

(3) When one of the possible phenotypes is established, it becomes an hereditary characteristic of the clone and is reproduced with great reliability.

The essential difference in the systems lies in the location of the mechanisms of perpetuation. The serotype "homeostat," according to available information, is restricted to the cytoplasm; the Group B mating types are perpetuated by a dual system with one part in the cytoplasm and one part in the nucleus. The Group A mating-type homeostat is located strictly in the nucleus. These three systems may be summarized as follows (Fig. 10). The serotype system possesses a cytoplasmic mechanism which selects one of the nuclear potentialities for manifestation. This cytoplasmic mechanism not only dictates which of the potentialities of an old nucleus is realized but maintains the same sort of pattern when new nuclei develop in the same cytoplasm. The Group B mating type system also has a cytoplasmic component,

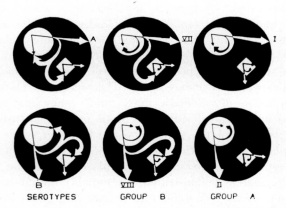

Fig. 10. Schematic summary of three systems of cellular heredity in *Paramecium aurelia*. The white circles represent the old macronuclei; the white squares represent newly developing macronuclei; and the arrows represent various internuclear and intranuclear systems of communication.

but in addition has an intranuclear mechanism for perpetuating a choice. The cytoplasmic mechanism is under the direct control of the mature nucleus and is responsible for the establishment of a specific intranuclear mechanism in the new nuclei, but it has no effect on other mature nuclei. The Group A mating-type system dispenses entirely with the cytoplasmic mechanism and each nucleus independently develops its own intranuclear mechanism of perpetuation. In short, the serotype system possesses an internuclear communications system; the Group B mating-type system has both an internuclear and an intranuclear communications system; and the Group A system has only the intranuclear mechanism. In spite of these differences, one is impressed by the many similarities and is stimulated to find a common physical basis—either in terms of master molecules or of steady states.

Such a common mechanism may be found in the concept of self-perpetuating metabolic patterns, as described in general terms by Wright (36), and as applied specifically to the serotype system first by Delbrück (6). According to this concept, the environment and the genic constitution of a cell potentiate a series of biochemical pathways leading to the manifestation of certain surface specificities. The various pathways are, however, not independent but interlocked; the establishment of one of the pathways results in the inhibition of the others. No information is available concerning the mechanism of the inhibition, but models for this are not hard to find. The reaction products in one sequence, for example, might antagonize parallel steps in another sequence. All the observations available concerning the systems discussed are formally explicable on such a basis, particularly if freedom is permitted in locating the essential reaction sequences. In the Group A system they would be restricted to the nucleus; in the Group B system they would also be located in the nucleus, but the inhibitory agents could spill forth into the cytoplasm; in the serotype system the reactions could be distributed uniformly throughout the cell, or at least the inhibitors would be freely diffusible. So conceived, antagonistic biochemical pathways provide a mechanism both for integrating cellular activities and for transmitting specificities in vegetative growth.

This scheme has the advantages of simplicity and uniformity; its disadvantages lie in the difficulty of obtaining critical evidence against alternative explanations. The serotypes can still be interpreted in terms of plasmagenes (2), particularly of plasmagenes dependent on nuclear genes for their specificity (35). The mating types can still be formally explained by some peculiar shuffling of master molecules within and between nuclei. The somatic nuclei of the ciliated protozoa present many problems and a genetic analysis of differentiated somatic nuclei is as difficult here as a genetic analysis of somatic nuclei in higher forms. Final judgment must await more information.

In the past few years I have been directing my attention to a detailed analysis of a system of mating-type differentiation in *Tetrahymena,* which may be less refractory in certain respects than those discussed above.* In this system the process of differentiation is not restricted to a short period of time, but is extended under some circumstances over hundreds of cell generations. This extension in time, coupled with a variety of cellular specificities, provides possibilities of analysis not available in the mating-type systems of *Paramecium.* Since these studies provide certain insights into the problems of nuclear differentiation, I would like to summarize them briefly.

Variety 1 of *T. pyriformis* is known at the present time to contain a total of seven mating types, any one of which can mate equally readily with each of the others, but not with itself. Certain crosses may produce all the seven known types; other crosses yield six of the types, and still other crosses five. The potentialities for the mating types are inherited in simple Mendelian fashion (21). I will restrict my remarks to crosses within a series of strains which are homozygous for the same mating type alleles and which yield at conjugation the five mating types, I, II, III, V, and VI. The distribution of these types among the caryonides is analogous to the distribution of types in the Group A varieties of *P. aurelia.* The cells within a single caryonide—under certain circumstances—are pure for one of the mating types, but sister caryonides are in most cases of different mating types. The mating types, in other words, are normally separated at the same cell division at which newly formed somatic nuclei are separated, and only at this cell division. This observation suggests that developing somatic nuclei are differentiated as to which mating type they will control. The fact that sister nuclei developing in the same cytoplasm show no correlation in mating type (and no correlation with the parental mating type) indicates that no specific cytoplasmic condition influences the course of nuclear differentiation. These observations, therefore,

* This work was supported by grants from the National Science Foundation.

demonstrate the existence of a system of nuclear differentiation similar to that in the Group A varieties of *P. aurelia,* but of greater complexity.

The newer insights come from an analysis of the deviations from this pattern. Under certain conditions—specifically, when exconjugant clones are not allowed to starve—differentiation is not completed immediately, and many clones maintain two or more potentialities over long periods of time (22). These incompletely differentiated clones can be detected as "selfers," clones within which conjugation can occur if the culture is allowed to starve. From such clones one may in the course of time obtain subclones which have completed the differentia-tion; this process of differentiation may be accelerated by starving the cells periodically. During the past year Dr. Sally Lyman Allen and I have undertaken a series of experiments analyzing the course of differentiation in these partially differentiated clones. It is our hope that information regarding the way the hereditary states are estab-lished will provide an understanding of their physical bases, just as a study of mutagenesis in conventional genetic work provides an under-standing of the nature of "mutations."

The first observations regarding these unstable clones concern the potentialities which are associated in them. These potentialities are defined by the types which can be obtained from the clones when they have been stabilized. Although as many as four types have been obtained from certain unstable clones, most of the clones have only two detectable potentialities, in one of the many possible combinations. Whatever may be their physical basis, therefore, certain of the unstable states—specifically, those with only two potentialities—are more stable than others. The larger the number of residual potentialities, the less likely is a clone to maintain it; the only completely stable condition is that in which only one potentiality is maintained. Even among the clones with dual potencies, differences in stability—based upon which potentialities are present—may be detected. Thus, almost any combi-nation of potentialities may be observed in young clones (60 to 100 fissions after conjugation), but the association of potentialities in the clones which persist in the unstable state for hundreds of fissions becomes progressively less random. The persistent unstable clones ("metastable clones") are almost exclusively clones with the potential-ities for types I and VI. These observations suggest that interactions among the various gene-controlled potentialities exist and that the interactions are not uniform; some of the antagonisms are quickly resolved, and others are maintained for long periods of time under constant growth conditions.

A second series of observations, primarily on the I-VI metastable clones, demonstrates that within a single clone a large and perhaps continuous array of nuclear states occurs. If the vegetative progeny produced from a single cell through eight to ten fissions are examined, some will be stabilized to one of the possible types, some additional ones may be induced to stabilize by starving them in distilled water, and some will remain in the unstable state (Fig. 11). In such a short

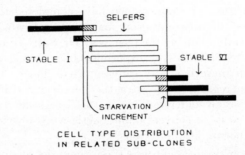

CELL TYPE DISTRIBUTION
IN RELATED SUB-CLONES

Fig. 11. Representation of the cell types found in small subclones of selfing caryonides in *Tetrahymena pyriformis*. The black portion of the bars represents the cells which are stable for a mating type and which breed true in subsequent growth. The hatched portion represents those cells which can be forced to stabilize by starvation in distilled water. The white portion represents the cells which cannot be stabilized by any known method.

period of growth only one of the two potentialities is normally stabilized. Different subclones derived from the same source after a larger number of fissions may stabilize at different types, and those stabilizing at the same type will differ in the fraction which have stabilized. Since the behavior of the individuals in such a subclone reflects the nuclear state in the cell beginning the clone, and since a continuous array of subclones is observed, the simplest interpretation of these phenomena is that a continuous array of nuclear conditions exists. Moreover, since the stabilization within a small subclone is normally to either one type or the other, we must conclude that the nuclear state conducive to the stabilization to one type is not favorable to the establishment of the other; a spectrum of nuclear states exists, varying from that readily stabilized to type I, through that not stabilized with ease to either type, to that prone to frequent stabilization at type VI. Once a cell is stabilized no known method for restoring the instability exists, but in the course of time the various kinds of unstable nuclear conditions are interconvertible.

Another method for studying the nuclear states in subclones reinforces the previous conclusion and also provides information on the rate of change of the unstable states. As in the previous experiments, subclones are initiated from single cells and a number of cells are isolated from each subclone. These derived cultures are then maintained in serial isolations, and their behavior in the course of time is recorded (Fig. 12). The cultures from some subclones may stabilize

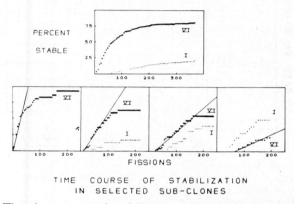

TIME COURSE OF STABILIZATION
IN SELECTED SUB-CLONES

Fig. 12. The time course of stabilization in various subclones of unstable caryonides maintaining the specificities for types I and VI. The upper graph is based on 1200 single cell isolations; the lower graphs are based on 60 or less.

very rapidly to type I; those from others may stabilize very rapidly to type VI; those from still others may stabilize only very slowly, and the two types will appear at approximately the same rate (Fig. 13). The fact that both types do not appear at a rapid rate within a single subclone establishes again a correlation between the rate of stabilization and the quality of the stabilization. A high initial rate of stabilization to I is correlated with a low initial rate of stabilization to VI, and vice versa. Regardless of the differences in the *initial* rates of stabilization, eventually the rates of stabilization to the two types become equivalent. The time required for these rates to become equivalent, however, depends upon the initial rates. Those with high initial rates to one type may require several hundred cell divisions; those with low and nearly equal rates may reach equivalence by 50 to 100 fissions. Presumably, by the time the rates are equivalent the

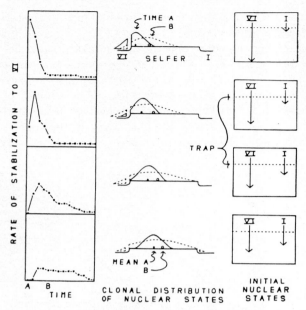

Fig. 13. A summary and interpretation of the observed rates of stabilization of unstable cells in *Tetrahymena pyriformis*. Each of the graphs on the left represents the rates of stabilization in time of subclones derived from a common source. The center diagrams suggest an interpretation in terms of a continuous spectrum of nuclear states, the extreme variants of which are permanently stabilized. The diagrams on the right represent the relative probabilities of stabilization to the types I and VI as arrows of different lengths.

still unstable daughter nuclei are distributed at random throughout the entire array of nuclear states.

These observations on *Tetrahymena* may be summarized briefly (Fig. 14). Initially a new somatic nucleus possesses a spectrum of potentialities conferred on it by its genes; in a short period of time certain of these potentialities have been discarded and only two remain; depending upon which two potentialities are present, this condition is resolved either rapidly or slowly by the exclusion of one of the remaining types. With some paired potentialities a reasonably stable intermediate condition can be maintained over long periods of time, and will show constant fluctuations in both directions until the nuclear state reaches a "point of no return," after which the state becomes fixed and is maintained indefinitely.

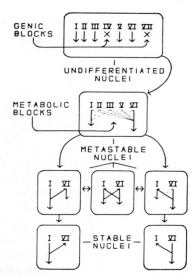

FIG. 14. An interpretation of the progressive restriction of mating-type potentialities in *Tetrahymena pyriformis,* based on the concept of competitive biochemical pathways.

These studies demonstrate a class of hereditary variations which
arise gradually over extended time intervals, unlike the discrete,
temporally localized alterations characterized usually as "mutation."
While these variations are in some instances associated with the nuclei,
very similar, and perhaps essentially identical, variations have cytoplasmic bases, or even bases in both nucleus and cytoplasm. A
geographical distinction between these bases does not appear particularly useful. While no compelling evidence for any particular mechanism can yet be advanced, these hereditary mechanisms can be conceived
at least as well in terms of self-maintaining biochemical patterns as in
terms of master molecules—either nuclear or cytoplasmic.

If such an interpretation can be more firmly established, some
reconciliation between the two classes of hereditary mechanisms will be
in order. Such a reconciliation has, of course, been implicit in the previous discussions. Reverting to our earlier allusions concerning protoplasmic governments, the master molecules could impose constitutional
limitations on the protoplasm; all those activities provided for in the
"constitution" would be possible, but the possible activities in any cell
far outnumber the realized activities. The biochemical antagonisms

would be mechanisms for selecting among those possibilities and integrating them into a smoothly operating whole. Some of these antagonisms would be located within the nuclei (or even within the chromosomes; if localized within the chromosomes and stable enough to persist through gametogenesis, they would mimic "gene mutations" and would be operationally indistinguishable from them). Other antagonisms would spill into the cytoplasm and yield cytoplasmic differentiation. Some might even pass beyond the cell boundaries in multicellular aggregates or organisms and, by creating "fields" of influence, cause associated cells to differentiate in similar patterns. In those cases where cell populations with different developmental histories are brought into close association, these intercellular influences might bring about special alterations in one or both of the populations, and thus provide a model for induction. In such a manner the entire organism would be integrated, and the role of the genetic determinants in the various differentiated tissues would be comprehensible. It appears unlikely that the role of the genes in development is to be understood so long as the genes are considered as dictatorial elements in the cellular economy. It is not enough to know what a gene does *when* it manifests itself. One must also know the mechanisms determining which of the many gene-controlled potentialities will be realized. In so far as these homeostatic mechanisms perpetuate a given specificity, they are "hereditary" mechanisms, and their physical basis is a part of the physical basis of inheritance.

REFERENCES

1. Avery, O. T., MacLeod, C. M., and McCarty, M. Studies on the chemical nature of the substance inducing transformation of pneumococcal types. Induction of transformation by a desoxyribonucleic acid fraction isolated from Pneumococcus Type III. *J. Exptl. Med.*, **79**, 137–158 (1944).
2. Beale, G. H., *The Genetics of Paramecium aurelia*, 179 pp. Cambridge, at the University Press (1954).
3. Boveri, Th. Ueber Differenzierung der Zellkerne während der Furchung des Eies von *Ascaris megalocephala*. *Anat. Anz.*, **2**, 688–693 (1887).
4. Briggs, R., and King, T. J., pers. commun.
5. Caspari, E., Cytoplasmic inheritance. *Advances in Genet.*, **2**, 1–66 (1948).
6. Delbrück, M. (See Discussion after Sonneborn, T. M., and Beale, G. H., Influence des gènes, des plasmagènes et du milieu dans le déterminisme des caractéres antigénique chez *Paramecium aurelia* variété 4.) Unités biologique données de continuité génétique. *Colloq. intern. centre natl. recherche sci. (Paris).* **7**, 25–36 (1949).
7. Darlington, C. D. Heredity, development and infection. *Nature*, **154**, 164–169 (1944).
8. Ephrussi, M. *Nucleocytoplasmic Relations in Microorganisms*, 127 pp. Clarendon Press, Oxford (1953).

9. Haldane, J. B. S. *The Biochemistry of Genetics,* 144 pp. George Allen and Unwin, London (1954).

10. Imai, Y. The behavior of the plastid as a hereditary unit: the theory of the plastogene. *Cytologia, Fujii Jubilee* Vol., 934–947 (1937).

11. King, T. J., and Briggs, R. Changes in the nuclei of differentiating gastrula cells, as demonstrated by nuclear transplantation. *Proc. Natl. Acad. Sci. U. S.,* **41**, 321–325 (1955).

12. Lederberg, J. Cell genetics and hereditary symbiosis. *Physiol. Revs.,* **32**, 403–430 (1952).

13. Lederberg, J., and Lederberg, Esther M. Infection and heredity. In *Cellular Mechanisms in Differentiation and Growth,* 14th Growth Symposium (Dorothea Rudnick, ed.). Princeton Univ. Press, Princeton (1956).

14. L'Héritier, Ph. Sensitivity to CO_2 in Drosophila—a review. *Heredity,* **2**, 325–348 (1948).

15. L'Héritier, Ph. The CO_2 sensitivity problem in Drosophila. *Cold Spring Harbor Symposia Quant. Biol.,* **16**, 99–112 (1951).

16. Lwoff, A. *Problems of Morphogenesis in Ciliates,* 103 pp. John Wiley & Sons, New York (1950).

17. Medawar, P. B. Cellular inheritance and transformation. *Biol. Revs.,* **22**, 360–389 (1947).

18. Michaelis, P. Interactions between genes and cytoplasm in Epilobium. *Cold Spring Harbor Symposia Quant. Biol.,* **16**, 121–129 (1951).

19. Mitchell, M. B., and Mitchell, H. K. A case of "maternal" inheritance in *Neurospora crassa. Proc. Natl. Acad. Sci. U. S.,* **38**, 442–449 (1952).

20. Nanney, D. L. Mating type determination in *Paramecium aurelia,* a study in cellular heredity. In *Sex in Microorganisms* (D. H. Wenrich, ed.), pp. 266–283. A.A.A.S. Symposium, Washington (1954).

21. Nanney, D. L. Caryonidal inheritance and nuclear differentiation. *Am. Naturalist,* **90**, 291–307 (1956).

22. Nanney, D. L., and Caughey, P. A. An unstable nuclear condition in *Tetrahymena pyriformis. Genetics,* **40**, 388–398 (1955).

23. Owen, F. V. Cytoplasmically inherited male sterility in sugar beets. *J. Agr. Research,* **71**, 423–440 (1945).

24. Rhoades, M. M. Plastid mutations. *Cold Spring Harbor Symposia Quant. Biol.,* **11**, 202–207 (1946).

25. Rizet, G. Les phénomènes de barrage chez *Podospora anserina.* I. Analyse génétique des barrages entre souches S et s. *Rev. Cytol. Biol. végétales,* **13**, 51–92 (1952).

26. Sager, R. Mendelian and non-Mendelian inheritance of streptomycin resistance in *Chlamydomonas reinhardti. Proc. Natl. Acad. Sci. U. S.,* **40**, 356–362 (1954).

27. Spiegelman, S. Differentiation as the controlled production of unique enzymatic patterns. *Symposia Soc. Exptl. Biol.,* **2** (Growth) 286–325 (1948).

28. Spiegelman, S. The particulate transmission of enzyme-forming capacity in yeast. *Cold Spring Harbor Symposia Quant. Biol.,* **16**, 87–98 (1951).

29. Sonneborn, T. M. Recent advances in the genetics of Paramecium and Euplotes. *Advances in Genet.,* **1**, 263–358 (1947).

30. Sonneborn, T. M. The cytoplasm in heredity. *Heredity,* **4**, 11–36 (1950).

31. Sonneborn, T. M. Patterns of nucleocytoplasmic integration in Paramecium. *Proc. 9 Intern. Congr. Genet., Caryologia,* **6** (Suppl. I), 307–325 (1954).

32. Spemann, H. *Embryonic Development and Induction.* 401 pp. Yale Univ. Press, New Haven (1938).

33. Waddington, C. H. The genetic control of development. *Symposia Soc. Exptl. Biol.,* **2** (Growth), 145–154 (1948).
34. Weismann, A. *Das Keimplasma. Eine Theorie der Vererbung.* Jena (1892).
35. Wright, S. The physiology of the gene. *Physiol. Revs.,* **21,** 487–527 (1941).
36. Wright, S. Genes as physiological agents. *Am. Naturalist,* **79,** 289–303 (1945).

Discussion

Dr. Kacser: I would like to make a point of correction in defense of Dr. Beale, who is not here. I work in the room next door, and I take it upon myself to interpret his reactions. I think Dr. Nanney implied that Dr. Beale favors the Delbrück steady state hypothesis. I don't think that if he were here he would agree to that. There are certain difficulties with the hypothesis and certain consequences appear to be absurd if one takes them to the logical conclusion, and this gives rise to serious doubts. I think the alternative explanation is contained in his book, so I think it should be made clear that all is not well with the steady state system.

Dr. Glass: Do you think that Dr. Beale favors the hypothesis of the master molecule?

Dr. Kacser: I wouldn't like to speak for Dr. Beale now, but I think there are alternatives to the master molecule, which is reproduced in the same sense that a nuclear gene is reproduced. An alternative system may be concerned with the establishment of certain solid phases in the cytoplasm which can be perpetuated as such. Strictly speaking it should not be described as steady state, because the term steady state applies to a homogeneous chemical system which is in dynamic equilibrium. The solid phases, of course, do not stand in dynamic equilibrium with their metabolic brothers, and therefore they don't enter the steady state system in the same way as the rest of the metabolic products.

Dr. Nanney: I had no intention of setting forth in any great detail any particular model for the serotype system and I certainly do not wish to put words in Dr. Beale's mouth. When I used the term "steady state," it was as a broad general term, intended to encompass all those hereditary mechanisms which do not depend entirely on "self-duplicating" particles for perpetuation. While in a strict sense Beale's model may not be a steady state model, it falls into the class of mechanisms to which I was trying to draw attention. Perhaps my use of the term "steady state" in this imprecise manner was unfortunate, and some more generally acceptable term should be adopted. What I have tried to do is to emphasize that all hereditary differences may not be due to differences in the DNA.

Dr. Luria: I would like to point out that at the present stage it may be disadvantageous to oppose two such concepts, because what we are talking about is a matter of gene function. What is relevant is whether the phenomena of cytoplasmic inheritance can be explained by interaction of gene activities at the level of primary gene functions or at late stages of function in the cytoplasm. Take, for example, the suggestion mentioned by Beadle this morning that you can have a mutant producing a certain gene product which is affected by a product of another gene. We may also think of a gene directly susceptible to inhibition by the product of another gene. Interactions of genes as units of function may occur at the level of the primary gene products within the chromosome, at the level of one late gene product interacting with the primary product of another gene, or finally by interaction between very late gene products. I think there are too few data for distinguishing in chemical terms between these possibilities.

DR. POTTER: I understood Dr. Nanney to say that he favored both concepts and that the final view would probably incorporate both views, which I certainly would want to go along with. I think there is a necessity here to take into consideration the fact that if we translate this into biochemical terms the synthesis of DNA appears to be irreversible, so this sort of gets into the master molecule line and is not a steady state phenomenon. The building blocks that go into DNA seem to stay as DNA and do not go back into the acid soluble pool. On the other hand, there is every reason to believe that there is a whole hierarchy of dissociation constants between the various RNA types that are formed and the nucleotide pool which enters into each one of them. I think that all the studies which have to do with the economics of scarcity in this system are what bring forth the differentiation, in that the RNA molecules which have the greatest pulling capacity for the 4 building blocks which they use finally take dominance over those which have less affinity for these building blocks. I had to say RNA molecules—someone had to say it some time in this symposium.

DR. LEDERBERG: I would like to punctuate those remarks in the same direction. I would be very much interested if anyone here could furnish the model for an experiment with which one could decide between the models. I don't think that would be possible, because they are models of different kinds. The steady state is essentially a mathematical one, and the master molecule is essentially either a political or a particulate model, whatever you want to call it. They are neither exclusive nor non-exclusive—they are descriptions of different kinds of things that are going on. It is a lot like asking whether it is more correct to say that the George Washington Bridge is made of steel or whether the cables take the form of a catenary.

DR. POTTER: It's not something you can't talk about. You have some molecules that pull in the building blocks and don't dissociate, whereas other molecules can take them in and give them back. Isn't that right? Or is that relevant? I would like to hear Dr. Nanney's opinion.

DR. NANNEY: I am in agreement with Dr. Lederberg's comments so long as he uses the term "steady state" in its strict sense, i.e., as a mathematical concept. I do not on the other hand agree that experimental distinctions are impossible between mechanisms involving "autocatalytic particles" and mechanisms which lack such particles. As Dr. Luria implied, what is required is a more detailed knowledge of the biochemistry of the various systems. Since the systems about which I have spoken have been studied primarily from a "biological" point of view, we have no direct information that RNA or any other compound is involved. We would like very much to know what chemical reactions are involved in these particular patterns of determination, but we have only begun such an analysis. Perhaps in 5, 10 or 15 years we can talk about the particular biochemical sequences or of the molecules involved. This was one of the main reasons for shifting study to Tetrahymena, which can be grown more easily in a controlled biochemical environment than can Paramecium. I am hesitant at the present time, however, to speak in more than general terms about what the mechanisms might be.

Part II

ROLE OF THE NUCLEUS, NUCLEIC ACIDS AND
ASSOCIATED STRUCTURES IN CELL DIVISION
AND PROTEIN SYNTHESIS

SOME PROBLEMS IN THE CHEMISTRY OF MITOSIS

DANIEL MAZIA*

Department of Zoology, University of California, Berkeley

THE PRECISION OF THE mechanisms of heredity depends not only on the exact replication of the genetic material but also on the just distribution of the products. Each daughter cell must receive a full representation of the genes present in the parent cell. The most familiar solution to this distribution problem—the mitotic cycle—imposes radical requirements on the design of the cell. Indeed, the only reason for discussing mitosis in a symposium on the chemical basis of heredity is to relate the genetic material to the reproductive process at the level of the whole cell.

The most obvious feature of the design of the cell for mitotic reproduction is the assembly of large numbers of genetic units into a small number of packages: chromosomes. This is especially striking when we consider that a chromosome in a plant or animal cell may contain upwards of 10^3 units the size of a DNA molecule,[1] and later, as we have heard here, may itself contain a large number of genetic activities as defined by recombination data. We have no basis for imagining a mechanism whereby such large numbers of units could be distributed properly if they were free, but do understand the principle whereby they are distributed if they are aligned in small numbers of chromosomes.

The essential point of the design of the chromosome for mitosis is the presence of a specialized body which is variously termed the *centromere, kinetochore,* or, more descriptively, the *point of spindle fiber attachment.* We cannot state positively that this body is not composed of genetic material, for we know nothing about its structure or chemistry. But we do know that it is indispensable, and it appears

* This work was aided by the Office of Naval Research (on Contract Nonr-22(24)) and by the American Cancer Society, through the Committee on Growth, National Research Council. The report includes the products of collaboration with Mr. John D. Roslansky and Dr. Robert Hersh, of the University of California, and Mr. Robert E. Kane, of Johns Hopkins University, which will be published more fully elsewhere.

[1] The calculation assumes a particle weight of 10^7 for DNA, a weight of 10^{-6} micrograms for the chromosomal material of the nucleus, and a complement of 50 chromosomes.

that it arrogates entirely the functional operations of the chromosome during mitosis. Genetic material can be distributed to daughter cells only if it is attached to a kinetochore, and the kinetochore will carry out its functions whether or not it is accompanied by its normal retinue of genetic material. Thus, the plant or animal chromosome is not merely an array of genes, but rather an array of genes attached to a kinetochore. Beyond the fact that the duplication of the kinetochores seems to be as exact as the duplication of the genetic material, we cannot say what it has in common with it. If we recall Stern's (16a) summary of genetic evidence that the genes function only between divisions and the evidence (discussed by Mazia, 11) that the physiological and biosynthetic activities of the nucleus are in abeyance during mitosis, we arrive at an interesting hypothesis: that *during division the role of the genetic material is passive;* it is taken along for the ride! I am afraid that this is a rather negative contribution to a symposium on the chemical basis of heredity, but it does provide a fragment of the time-perspective that we need so badly.

A further expression of chromosome organization in relation to mitosis is the condensation into compact bodies that the very term chromosome ordinarily connotes. In most kinds of cells, we cannot see the interphase chromosome, and imagine a highly uncoiled and extended thread. The fact that the chromosomes condense in preparation for mitosis makes very good sense in terms of the sheer mechanical task of moving them about precisely.

The exact mitotic distribution of the genetic material is not to be comprehended entirely in terms of chromosome structure and behavior. The best-organized chromosomes will not, in cells as we know them, distribute themselves correctly without the occurrence of a major transformation in the structure of the entire cell: the formation of the *mitotic apparatus.* This term is applied (12) to the entire ensemble of chromosomes, centrioles, spindle, and asters. The precision of the distribution of genetic material depends on the polarity and alignment of the mitotic apparatus to the extent that a number of fairly rigorous "rules" may be discerned. Since the available information about the physics and chemistry of the mitotic apparatus has been reviewed fairly recently (11), I shall concentrate, in this presentation, on questions that have been opened since the writing of the review mentioned, my theme being the relation of mitosis to the chemistry of the cell as a whole.

Isolation of the Mitotic Apparatus; Newer Developments

The mitotic apparatus is a conspicuous feature of the dividing cell. It represents a large part of the cell volume and contrasts optically with the rest of the cell because it does not include mitochondria or other large particles, and hence appears as a clear area. With phase contrast and polarization optics many of the details that were originally discovered in fixed and stained cells may now be seen in the mitotic apparatus of the living cell. In fixed and stained material, the spindles and asters have been designated as the "achromatic figure" because they stain less intensely with basic dyes than the chromosomes and, often, than the background cytoplasm. Nevertheless, they are basophilic, and recent studies employing basic stains (2, 17), and ultraviolet absorption (19) have led to the conclusion that the mitotic apparatus contains ribonucleoproteins. This is a point to which I shall return.

Obviously, the machinery of mitosis involves the structural and chemical differentiation of a large part of the cell, and the problem is made more interesting by the fact that the apparatus vanishes between divisions. Part of the task of trying to understand mitosis is to investigate in more detail than is permitted by optical methods alone what sort of structure the mitotic apparatus is, and we have approached this problem through the mass isolation of the mitotic apparatus from populations of dividing cells.

A method for isolating the mitotic apparatus from dividing sea urchin eggs was described by Mazia and Dan in 1952 (12). The procedures have been modified since that time, but are still based on the principle of selective solubilization: the dispersion of the cytoplasm by chemical agents that do not disrupt the mitotic apparatus. The cells used in this work were the eggs of the sea urchins *Strongylocentrotus purpuratus, S. franciscanus*, and *Arbacia punctulata*.

The first problem in developing the isolation procedure was to find a means of arresting the cells with minimum disturbance of the mitotic apparatus. This was solved by the use of 30 per cent ethanol at — 10° C., and such a treatment is the first step in all of the methods we have used. Thus far, we have found that direct treatment of the living cells with dispersing agents does not preclude the rapid breakdown of the mitotic apparatus that is commonly observed when the cell is insulted. Recently, we have attempted to substitute glycerol at low temperature for ethanol at low temperature, since Hoffmann-

Berling (4) has found that the mitotic apparatus of various vertebrate cells in tissue culture could be preserved in this way. Unfortunately, this treatment did not work with sea-urchin eggs. The mitotic apparatus of the much larger sea-urchin egg apparently broke down before the cells could equilibrate with the glycerol.

Mazia and Dan had used H_2O_2 and sodium dodecyl sulfate as a dispersing agent. Later, I reported a procedure employing the much gentler detergent, digitonin, without the use of peroxide. Most of the chemical work has been done with mitotic apparatus isolated by the digitonin method, which has been described elsewhere (10). The assumption that digitonin is in fact an agent that may disperse cell structures without denaturing biochemically active proteins has been substantiated in a number of cases. Most recently, Lehninger (7) has described the use of digitonin to disrupt mitochondria into smaller particles that retain the capacity for oxidative phosphorylation.

In evaluating the digitonin method, there are good reasons for assuming that neither the treatment with subzero ethanol nor with digitonin is likely to produce biochemical inactivation. A much more serious criticism of the method—as of most isolation methods—is that the organelle we are isolating is likely to include, in the living condition, important soluble components that will be washed away. Thus, we may claim that we have isolated the mitotic apparatus as a *structure* by a relatively gentle method, but cannot claim that the isolation preserves all of the functionally significant constituents.

We cannot begin to be satisfied with a cytochemical isolation procedure until the structures we are dealing with are isolated in media that approach the normal intracellular environment in composition. Even in the case of well-established methods such as the isolation of nuclei and mitochondria in sucrose solutions, one cannot help wondering why one fails when he uses electrolyte media that match the supposed composition of the intracellular aqueous environment. We have worked continuously toward a method of isolating the mitotic apparatus in an electrolyte solution and without the aid of a detergent, and have very recently found an unusually interesting condition for success. Earlier, we had found that the use of KCl or KCl-versene solutions gave poor isolation of the mitotic apparatus. Mechanical homogenization was required, and what was recovered was fragments containing mitotic apparatus heavily contaminated with coagulated cytoplasm. We have now found that a normal constituent of the cell, added to the KCl solution, serves as a dispersing agent comparable in effectiveness to digitonin: that constituent is ATP!

This finding came about partly as a byproduct of studies of the reaction of the mitotic apparatus to ATP and partly under the influence of the observations (summarized by Weber and Portzehl, 20) that ATP in high concentrations serves as a "plasticizing" agent for the structural elements of muscle. The eggs are transferred from the subzero 30 per cent ethanol to a medium containing 0.15 M KCl, 0.01 M phosphate buffer and 0.01 M ATP, the final pH being 7.0. In this medium the eggs are dispersed by manual shaking, about as with digitonin, and the mitotic apparatus is set free. The mitotic apparatus may then be purified simply by centrifugation in the same medium or in the KCl-phosphate buffer without ATP. The ATP is clearly serving as a dispersing agent; without it the eggs are coagulated and tough, with it they are soft and tend to disperse.

The structure of the mitotic apparatus isolated by the ATP method is not greatly different from that obtained with digitonin (Fig. 1). The chromosomes tend to be dissolved, for reasons that we do not yet understand, but this is not a disadvantage for most of our studies, which are concerned with the other parts of the mitotic apparatus.

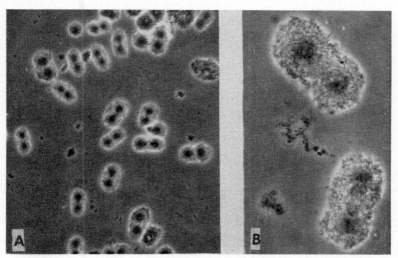

FIG. 1. Mitotic apparatus isolated from *S. purpuratus* eggs by the ATP method. Phase contrast photographs of figures suspended in 0.1 M KCl dissolved in 30 per cent glycerol.

A. 125 ×   B. 500 ×

The most striking feature of the material isolated with the ATP method is its sensitivity to the ionic environment. In water, these mitotic apparatus swell to the point where they almost vanish from view under phase contrast. On addition of electrolyte, they shrink progressively. The effects are all reversible. This is a most interesting property in view of various proposals, in the past, that swelling mechanisms played an important part in mitosis. The ATP method has been developed only recently and has been exploited very little. It seems worthy of mention at this time because it frees us from the degree of artificiality introduced by the presence of detergents. The ATP concentration used may seem high, but in fact it is only slightly higher than that which is believed to exist in resting muscle (15) and in other tissues (8).

CHEMICAL CHARACTERIZATION OF THE MITOTIC APPARATUS: THE NUCLEOTIDE CONSTITUENT

The first results of the analysis of the isolated mitotic apparatus were hardly surprising. It turned out that it consisted largely of proteins. Since many of the chemical results have been discussed elsewhere (10), I shall merely sketch the picture as it now stands.

(1) The mitotic apparatus may be dissolved by means that split disulfide bonds. Ordinarily, we use alkaline thioglycollate. While the results have been interpreted as indicating intermolecular S-S bonding, there are alternative explanations of the solubility properties. For instance, the thioglycollate could be competing with the protein for S-N bonds such as have been postulated recently by Barany (1) in the case of the polymerization of actin (cf. also, Mazia, 9, discussion following paper).

(2) The protein obtained by dissolving the mitotic apparatus in thioglycollate seems to be relatively homogeneous by the standards applied thus far. It is completely precipitated at pH 4.5 and gives an electrophoretic pattern containing one major component and a minor, faster-moving component which is interpretable as the same protein whose mobility is increased by the binding of nucleotide.

(3) The mitotic apparatus isolated with digitonin contains a considerable quantity of nucleotide. Estimated as RNA by perchloric acid extraction and ultraviolet absorption, it amounts to 2-3 per cent of the mass of the whole mitotic apparatus. The full complement of chromosomal DNA that is present in the isolated material represents so small

an absolute quantity compared with the mitotic apparatus as a whole that it is insignificant for these analyses.

The question of RNA and the mitotic mechanism has acquired increasing significance as microscopic cytochemical methods have been applied to the study of mitosis. The studies of Jacobson and Webb (5), of Walker and Yates (19), of Stich (17), and of Boss (2) describe interesting changes in "RNA" during mitosis as observed by staining and ultraviolet microscopy, and have evoked some challenging speculations. The possibilities are important enough to stimulate a closer examination of the "RNA" of the mitotic apparatus. As I stated in an earlier paper (10), the material ". . . is presumed to be RNA because it may be extracted with cold 5 per cent perchloric acid, but it has not yet been subjected to nucleotide analysis." Most workers employing staining or ultraviolet absorption methods are willing to make a similar qualification.

Dr. Robert Hersch has undertaken a study of the nucleotides of the isolated mitotic apparatus. The starting material was isolated by the digitonin method; the objection to the newer ATP method in this connection is obvious. The perchloric acid extract, which showed the typical nucleotide absorption spectrum, was concentrated and subjected to paper chromatographic analysis using several solvent systems.[2] ATP, ADP, and RNA that had been subjected to the same perchloric acid treatment as the mitotic apparatus, and hydrolyzed RNA were tested at the same time.

A single nucleotide component was obtained under conditions where RNA was resolved into constituent nucleotides. At the present moment this nucleotide has not been identified unequivocally. On the basis of its migration on paper with several solvents, it could be ADP, cytosine monophosphate, or uridine monophosphate. We are particularly interested in the possibility that it may be ADP. In control experiments, Dr. Hersch has found that ATP is largely converted to ADP by the same perchloric acid treatment that was applied to the nucleotide of the isolated mitotic apparatus. Hence, if the nucleotide he is recovering is ADP, it would be possible that the mitotic apparatus contains ATP.

Pending the exact identification of the nucleotide component of the isolated mitotic apparatus, we may doubt whether it is RNA.

[2] The systems that gave the best separations were those suggested in Pabst Laboratories (Milwaukee, Wis.) Circular No. OR-10, entitled "Ultraviolet Absorption Spectra of 5'-Ribonucleotides", January, 1956.

We may imagine the protein of the mitotic apparatus to contain at least 2 per cent of single nucleotide in a form that is bound so firmly that it is not removed by the preliminary extraction of the eggs with 30 per cent ethanol nor by the subsequent treatment with digitonin and the successive washings that are used to remove the digitonin and the cytoplasmic particles. From a cytochemical point of view, it is possible that the material that has been identified in the past as RNA by staining or ultraviolet absorption could be, to an important extent, a protein-bound nucleotide such as ATP. Obviously this would be a matter of great interest in connection with the movements that are the essence of mitosis. If we are dealing with a system containing contractile proteins, comparable to muscle proteins, as has long been imagined and has been demonstrated by the work of Hoffmann-Berling, the binding of nucleotide would seem to be a requirement, although we would not necessarily predict such firm binding that it would withstand the procedure used in isolating the mitotic apparatus. The apparent shifts in nucleotide concentration within the mitotic apparatus during anaphase movement, such as have been described by Boss (2), might be interpretable in terms of local contractile events. I do not wish to introduce excessive speculation at this time, but only to point out that the picture of the protein of the mitotic apparatus as it now emerges does bring its chemistry a little closer to functional expectations.

QUANTITATIVE RELATION BETWEEN MITOTIC APPARATUS AND CELL

Microscopically, the mitotic apparatus is a conspicuous body, occupying a large part of the volume of the cell. There is no evidence of a differentiated membrane, but the gel mass is solid enough to prevent the intrusion of mitochondria and other particles and to be manipulated. Clearly it involves more substance than just the fibers that we can see; it is a region where part of the cell substance has separated from the rest, and this is one reason for formulating its structure as that of a gel upon which fibrous orientation and condensation have been imposed by kinetochores and centrioles.

The isolation of the mitotic apparatus made it possible to deal with the question: how much of the cell's protein is invested in it (13)? The experimental approach is merely to determine the protein content of one mitotic apparatus and compare it with that of the cell. Technically, it has not been feasible actually to analyze a single mitotic figure, nor did sampling methods for counting large numbers prove to be reliable.

We fell back on a compromise: the analysis of small numbers that could be counted directly and yet could be analyzed for protein by sensitive methods that are now available. Table 1 gives the results of

TABLE 1

PROTEIN CONTENT OF WHOLE *Strongylocentrotus purpuratus* EGGS AND OF
MITOTIC APPARATUS ISOLATED FROM THESE EGGS

A. *Eggs (unfertilized)*

Number analyzed	Total protein (10^{-5} mg.)	Protein per egg (10^{-5} mg.)
40	285	7.1
86	480	5.6
65	460	7.2
33	219	6.6
95	530	5.6
19	134	7.0
39	280	7.2
85	490	5.8
581	680	5.0
136	295	5.1

average: 6.2×10^{-5} mg. protein per egg

B. *Isolated mitotic apparatus*
(metaphase and anaphase stages)

Number analyzed	Total protein (10^{-5} mg.)	Protein per mitotic apparatus (10^{-5} mg.)
410	300	.73
303	240	.79
221	160	.76
512	360	.70

average: $.72 \times 10^{-5}$ mg. protein per mitotic apparatus

Fraction of cell protein in mitotic apparatus $= \dfrac{.72}{6.2} = 11.6\%$.

a series of such determinations. The data presented the mitotic apparatus at metaphase and anaphase of the first cleavage of *Strongylocentrotus purpuratus*. The populations are not perfectly homogeneous with respect to the stage of mitosis, and we might expect, from visual evidence, that a group containing more of the later stages would contain more material. Thus the results are somewhat variable, but it appears that in the sea urchin egg about 10 to 12 per cent of all of the protein in the cell is invested in the mitotic apparatus. This figure, it should be noted, includes the asters.

These values should not have occasioned as much surprise as they did. The mitotic apparatus does occupy a large part of the volume of the dividing sea-urchin egg, and is even larger, relative to the whole cell, in other cases. Either the mitotic apparatus has a very low density and high water content, or else it must account for a goodly proportion of the cell's substance. But we now have evidence from interference microscopy that the mitotic apparatus of the sea-urchin egg has about the same concentration of dry matter as does the granule-free cytoplasm (14), and more recent results of x-ray absorption studies on plant cells show that the material density of the mitotic apparatus is not greatly different from that of the cytoplasm generally. Therefore, in considering the origin of the mitotic apparatus, we are concerned with cell proteins in large amounts.

One consequence of this fact is that it casts doubt on the simple, commonly assumed notion that the nucleus carries the substance of the mitotic apparatus and delivers it to the cytoplasm when the nuclear membrane breaks down. This seems to be excluded in the case of the sea-urchin egg, where the mitotic apparatus involves eight times as much protein as could be contained in the nucleus if the latter were solid protein. The evidence does not exclude the possibility that the protein of the mitotic apparatus is ultimately synthesized in the nucleus nor that the nucleus directly contributes some important constituent. Certainly, we are required to account somehow for the close correlation between nuclear events and the appearance of the mitotic apparatus.

SYNTHESIS VS. ASSEMBLY OF THE PROTEIN OF THE MITOTIC APPARATUS

Now that we know that the mitotic machinery may implicate 10 per cent or more of the protein of the dividing cell, we are bound to ask whether the cell makes this much extra protein during division or whether it assembles preexisting protein to form the mitotic apparatus. The older cytologists gave considerable thought to the latter possibility, proposing that the cell contained a fibrous component—an "archoplasm" (3) or "kinoplasm" (18)—that congregated and oriented itself at the time of division under the influence of the mitotic centers.

There is every reason to conclude that there is no *net* synthesis of proteins in cells during division. The sea-urchin egg with which we work is a poor object on which to test this, because the possibility of a net gain of "active" protein at the expense of storage protein cannot be ruled out experimentally, but there is adequate evidence from other cases. I have summarized this evidence elsewhere (13).

If we can exclude the production of extra protein to form the mitotic apparatus, we face several alternatives. (1) The protein of the mitotic apparatus may exist in the cell before division in a pool of some kind, and the formation of the mitotic apparatus may be merely an assembly process. (2) The protein of the mitotic apparatus may be made available by disassembly of structures in the interphase cell that are made of the same protein. Possibilities (1) and (2) are the same in so far as they do not require that the dividing cell carry out a synthesis of protein molecules, but demand only intermolecular assembly and disassembly. Both are in harmony with the classical hypothesis mentioned above. Experimentally, if either (1) or (2) is correct, we may expect to find in the cell before division an adequate amount of protein that is qualitatively identical with the protein of the isolated mitotic apparatus. This should, according to the first alternative, be recovered as soluble protein before division and disappear from the soluble phase as the mitotic apparatus forms. The second alternative, which implies a pool of soluble protein that is being depleted and replenished in the course of the formation of the mitotic apparatus, is more difficult to deal with.

A third possibility is the actual breakdown of preexisting protein and a total synthesis of mitotic-apparatus protein from the products. This is probably excluded if we can identify the protein of the mitotic apparatus in the cell before division, and it becomes the most likely hypothesis if we fail to do so.

Our experimental approach, therefore, has been to study the behavior of the soluble proteins of the cell through the division cycle and to search among the proteins of the interphase cell for components that resemble those of the isolated mitotic apparatus. Obviously, we are faced with a formidable haystack and with some uncertainty as to whether we can recognize the needle. The only thing in our favor is that it is a large needle, since the mitotic apparatus does demand at least 10 per cent of all the protein in the cell. All of the experiments have been done with sea-urchin eggs. In venturing to describe these experiments, I am taking advantage of the liberties encouraged in a symposium—all of the work is current, none complete. As long as the chemical characterization of the mitotic apparatus is incomplete, all we can do is to fingerprint it chemically as best we can, and seek the same prints among the proteins of the cell before and during division. For example, we had found that the protein obtained by dissolving the mitotic apparatus of the sea urchin egg could be precipitated nearly quantitatively at pH 4.5. Extraction of the unfertilized egg (following exposure to 30 per cent ethanol at $-10°$ C.) yielded a large amount of soluble protein (nonsedimentable at 100,000 g in 30 minutes in the Spinco Model L centrifuge) that was precipitable at this pH. If this protein fraction included components that were to become the mitotic apparatus, it might follow that some part of the fraction would be lost during division, since the mitotic apparatus is insoluble under the conditions of extraction.

Mr. Robert Kane and I have made a preliminary study of this question, using eggs of *Arbacia punctulata*. The procedure, briefly, was to stop the eggs at various stages of the first two division cycles by immersion in the subzero 30 per cent ethanol, then to extract them with water at pH 7-8 and precipitate the desired fraction at pH 4.5. The precipitate was redissolved in phosphate buffer at pH 7 and studied by analytical ultracentrifugation. The results are shown in Fig. 2. It is evident that there are two major components (on a particle-weight basis) and that the lighter one (sedimentation constant, about 7) is changing during the mitotic cycles observed. Shortly after fertilization, the peak splits, and then it gradually flattens out as the mitotic apparatus forms. The peak reappears as the cells go into the interphase between the first two divisions. This is shown in Fig. 2, which displays the picture at the time when half of the eggs have completed their cleavage. We interpret the sharp peaks as representing those eggs which are in interphase, and the fact that there is an additional hump in front of it is taken to mean that some of the eggs are proceeding into the second division. In other words, the situation is equivalent to a combination of those represented in Figs. 2B and 2C. This result would be expected if the eggs were imperfectly synchronized, as they are in fact.

We think that these experiments are telling us that a protein component having at least one property in common with the protein isolated from the mitotic apparatus is aggregating as the mitotic apparatus forms, reappears in its original state as the mitotic apparatus breaks down when division is completed, and reaggregates when the mitotic

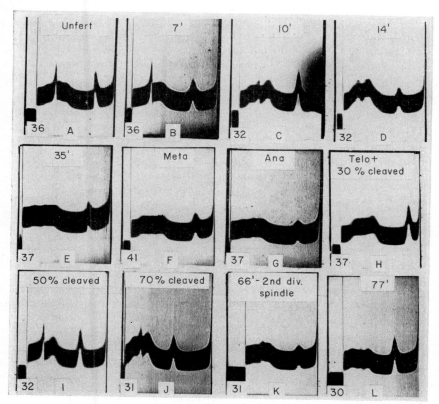

FIG. 2. Sedimentation patterns of soluble protein fraction of *Arbacia punctulata* eggs at various stages. Proteins precipitable at pH 4.5, redissolved in phosphate buffer, 0.1 *M, p*H 7.5. Duration of centrifugation at 59, 780 R.P.M. in Spinco analytical ultracentrifuge shown in lower left corner of each frame. Time following fertilization, or mitotic stage, shown over each frame.

apparatus forms for the next division. The results do support the idea of the formation of the mitotic apparatus through an assembly of preexisting material, but do not prove it. It is conceivable that we are seeing some change in the soluble proteins that parallels the mitotic cycle—and this would be interesting in itself—but one not necessarily concerned directly with the formation of the mitotic apparatus.

If we are observing the transition of preexisting protein into the mitotic apparatus, it does not automatically follow that the mechanism is as simple as the removal of soluble protein from a static pool and the restoration of that pool. The ultracentrifuge records show us the aggregation of one component in the course of the formation of the mitotic apparatus, but do not in themselves tell us how much of the cell's protein is soluble nor whether soluble protein is incorporated into the mitotic apparatus.

Recently we have studied the soluble and insoluble proteins of the eggs of *Strongylocentrotus purpuratus* in the course of the first division. The term "soluble" must here, as in all cases where the estimation depends on the extraction of killed cells, be referred to conditions of the experiment and can have only questionable meaning when referred to the intact cell. In this case, the procedure used to arrest the cells and to extract them was essentially identical to that used in the ultracentrifuge experiments. The results were as follows:

Stage	*Per cent soluble*
Unfertilized	46
Metaphase	49

From these results, it cannot be concluded that there is any appreciable change in the total amount of insoluble protein when the sea-urchin egg forms its mitotic apparatus. Yet our visual observations assured us that we were not dissolving the mitotic apparatus in the course of these extractions, and the chemical results I have described earlier have told us that the mitotic apparatus involves over 10 per cent of the protein of the cell. Obviously the situation is not so simple as the mere withdrawal of protein from a soluble pool.

At this time the most reasonable conclusions seem to be the following. (1) Since there is no net synthesis of proteins during division, the mitotic apparatus is formed by assembly of proteins already existing in the cell. The pool of free amino acids in the *S. purpuratus* egg, which has been measured by Kavenau (6), does not amount to 10 per cent of the total amino acids of the cell, and therefore cannot provide for the synthesis of the complete mitotic apparatus. (2) The ultracentrifugation experiments suggest that there is a pool of a soluble protein component in the cell before division which aggregates as the mitotic apparatus forms and reappears as the mitotic apparatus breaks down. (3) Since the amount of protein entering the mitotic apparatus is not reflected by a corresponding decrease in total soluble proteins, it would seem that other cytoplasmic structures are dissociating as the mitotic apparatus forms.

Since we are postulating that the protein of the mitotic apparatus exists in soluble form to some extent in the cell before division, it should be possible to isolate the proposed "precursor" from the unfertilized egg. We have a few criteria to go by. The protein should have a sedimentation constant of about 7, should be an asymmetric protein capable of forming fibers, should contain bound nucleotide, and should be present in an amount no less than 10 per cent of all the protein in the cell. We have found a protein meeting these requirements and isolable in a simple way. The eggs are first immersed in 30 per cent ethanol at $-10°$ C. and extracted with water or 0.1 M KCl. If $CaCl_2$ is added to the extract to a final concentration of 0.05 M, a fibrous precipitate forms. Indeed, it is so fibrous that it can be spun on a rod (like precipitated DNA, although it contains no DNA) and removed from the container as a wound-up mass. The protein readily dissolves when the Ca^{++} is removed. It contains 2 per cent of nucleotide. The redissolved structure-protein sediments as a monodisperse system with the same sedimentation constant as the slow peak in Fig. 2. We can extract 10 to 12 per cent of the protein of the egg as this fraction. Thus our search for the "precursor" to the mitotic apparatus has led us to this cytoplasmic "structure-protein" having the expected properties. While it is interesting in itself in the light of the history of attempts to isolate "structure-proteins" from cells other than muscles and similar specialized types, we are still a long way from proof that our protein is in fact identical with that of the mitotic apparatus.

The Major Problems of Mitosis

The isolation of the mitotic apparatus has made accessible for chemical study the problems of the brute chemistry of mitosis, and what I have described is the beginnings of that study. We have been able to consider, if not to solve, some questions regarding the construction work the cell must perform in order to carry out mitotic cell division. From the standpoint of the chemical basis of heredity, however, the main problems of mitosis are those involving the distribution of chromosomes, and the study of the gross chemistry of the mitotic apparatus in this relation can only tell us what sorts of matter the process involves and not how it is accomplished. Before we can go much further, several obvious barriers of ignorance have to be penetrated. The first and most important is the problem of the kinetochore.

Every thought about the precision of the mitotic separation of the chromosomes takes us back to the kinetochore, yet we know absolutely nothing about its chemistry. A second and related problem is that of the mitotic centers. In the case of animal cells we can at least identify definite centrioles, but in plant cells where the mitotic process is so similar that we must postulate some kind of polar differentiation we can ordinarily see no definite centrioles. If we could understand how a polarized fibrous connection is made between the kinetochores and the centers, we could begin to imagine how the chromosomes are separated correctly. Behind this problem lies the problem of how the kinetochores align themselves so precisely at metaphase.

The problem of the mechanism of chromosome movement is proving more amenable to attack because it is taking its place as part of the more general problem of cellular contractile mechanisms. Perhaps the outstanding advance in this connection is Hoffmann-Berling's (4) demonstration of spindle elongation (an important component of the mitotic movements) in glycerine-extracted cells ("anaphase models") under the action of ATP. Now that we have reason to think that the mitotic apparatus contains nucleotide-proteins, it is conceivable that we can find further analogies to better-understood contractile mechanisms. We shall probably understand how chromosomes move to the poles before we know how they align themselves for the movement.

Finally, we shall have to face the problems of the initiation and termination of mitosis. As has been pointed out (11), completion of chromosome duplication is a condition of mitosis but is not an immediate stimulus. Now that it seems likely that much of the mitotic apparatus may be of cytoplasmic origin, we shall have to explain how the formation of the mitotic apparatus is coordinated with the behavior of the chromosomes. And in the end we have to understand the methods whereby the mitotic apparatus breaks down once the chromosomes have separated, and the chromosomes are reconverted to their functional interphase state.

REFERENCES

1. Bárány, M., *Biochim. et Biophys. Acta*, **19**, 560 (1956).
2. Boss, J., *Exptl. Cell Research*, **8**, 181 (1955).
3. Boveri, T., *Zellen-Studien*, Heft 2, p. 62. G. Fischer, Jena (1888).
4. Hoffmann-Berling, H., *Biochim. et Biophys. Acta*, **15**, 226 (1954).
5. Jacobson, W., and Webb, M., *Exptl. Cell Research*, **3**, 163 (1952).
6. Kavenau, J. L., *J. Exptl. Zool.*, **122**, 285 (1953).

7. Lehninger, A. I., in *Enzymes: Units of Biological Structure and Function* (O. H. Gaebler, ed.), Academic Press, New York (1956).
8. Lepage, G., *Cancer Research*, **8**, 193 (1948).
9. Mazia, D., in *Symposium on Glutathione* (S. Colowick, et al., eds.), Academic Press, New York (1954).
10. Mazia, D., *Symposia Soc. Exptl. Biol.*, **9**, 335 (1955).
11. Mazia, D., *Advances in Biol. and Med. Phys.*, **4**, 69 (1956).
12. Mazia, D., and Dan, K., *Proc. Natl. Acad. Sci. U. S.*, **38**, 826 (1952).
13. Mazia, D., and Roslansky, J., *Protoplasma*, **46** (in press).
14. Mitchison, J. M., and Swann, M. M., *Quart. J. Micr. Sci.*, **94**, 381 (1953).
15. Mommaerts, W. F. H. M., *Muscular Contraction, A Topic in Molecular Physiology*, Interscience Publishers, New York (1950).
16. Schrader, F., *Mitosis*, Columbia Univ. Press, New York (1953).
16a. Stern, C., *Am. Naturalist*, **72**, 350 (1938).
17. Stich, H., *Chromosoma*, **6**, 199 (1954).
18. Strasburger, E., *Histologische Beiträge VI. Ueber Reduktionstheilung, Spindelbildung, Centrosomen und Cilienbildner im Pflanzenreich.* G. Fischer, Jena (1900).
19. Walker, P. M. B., and Yates, H. B., *Proc. Roy. Soc. (London)*, B, **140**, 274 (1952).
20. Weber, H. H., and Portzehl, H., *Progr. Biophys.*, **4**, 60 (1954).

SOME CYTOCHEMICAL CONTRIBUTIONS TO GENETIC CHEMISTRY

Max Alfert

*Department of Zoology and its Cancer Research Genetics Laboratory,** *University of California, Berkeley 4, California*

THE TOPICS UNDER discussion in this symposium bear witness to the rapid advances made during the last decade in genetic chemistry. Cytochemical studies, dealing with the characterization of substances in their natural locations within cells, have in the past contributed in two important ways to the body of work which resulted in the recognition of the genetic significance of deoxyribonucleic acid (DNA). The first of these consists in the contributions of Caspersson (17) and Brachet (15), who have drawn attention to the biological importance of nucleic acids at a time when there was little interest in these substances, and who developed methods for the study of their distribution in biological materials. Secondly, there should be mentioned the cytochemical establishment in more recent years of characteristic quantitative relationships between DNA and the chromosomes, leading to what has become known as the "constancy hypothesis of nuclear DNA." While Caspersson's, Brachet's, and their associates' work is too well known to warrant a review in this place, something might profitably be said about the history and present status of the constancy hypothesis.

Constancy of Nuclear DNA

The first but limited evidence for the view that the amount of nuclear DNA parallels the number of chromosome sets in different cells of a species was based entirely on analytical biochemical data and resulted from a comparison of the average DNA content of haploid sperms and diploid somatic mammalian nuclei by the Vendrelys (52). Ris and Mirsky (42) subsequently correlated, for a similar comparison, chemi-

* The work reported from this laboratory is supported by cancer funds of the University of California.

cal and cytochemical techniques, for the latter purpose using the Feulgen reaction in conjunction with a microspectrophotometric procedure developed by Pollister (e.g., 41) as a modification of Caspersson's method. Swift (46) in turn worked out a simple and convenient microspectrophotometric measuring technique (photometry of nuclear cores) which permitted him to obtain more accurate data on nuclear Feulgen-DNA content than had previously been possible. Except for a relatively few applications of two more recent and potentially more precise measuring techniques, the two-wave-lengths, method of Ornstein (36) and of Pätau (38), and the squashing-scanning method used by Deeley, Richards, Walker, and Davies (19), Swift's procedure has been applied by a vast majority of workers since 1950 and has led to the collection of numerous data (see 47 and 50 for recent reviews of these). Since then, correlated chemical and cytochemical studies have also been done in a few more cases (e.g., 28), but the quantitative cytochemical methods *alone* have permitted an extension of our knowledge about nuclear DNA content into situations inaccessible to chemical analysis: this is the case when nuclei in heterogeneous cell populations are to be analyzed and where the resolving power of the microspectrophotometric method is essential, as for measurements of different meiotic stages in a gonad (e.g., 48) or of individual pronuclei in fertilized eggs (e.g., 1). In a number of cases different and independent cytochemical procedures, such as direct ultraviolet microspectroscopy of living cells (53), ultraviolet absorption and basic staining of fixed nuclei (21), autoradiography (34, 49), and interference microscopy (23) have been satisfactorily correlated with Feulgen-DNA measurements.

The general body of data demonstrates that the DNA contents of individual nuclei fall into well-defined groups whose means form simple series that correspond to the numbers of chromosome sets present in the nuclei. When the chromosomes duplicate in preparation for mitosis or in the course of endomitotic cycles which may result in polyploid or polytenic conditions, the nuclear DNA content increases correspondingly. In the absence of chromosome duplication, the average nuclear DNA content appears to be relatively stable, however, even during marked physiological alterations of cells whose nuclear size and protein content may thereby be greatly affected (cf. 5, 44).

Aside from *apparent* variations due to the measuring technique (cf. 19), true variations in DNA content among individual nuclei within a group must be expected on the basis of the widespread occurrence of aneuploidy in various tissues (see 10 for review). Whether or not there occur additional "functional variations" in nuclear DNA content will remain an open question until such a case is proved. The necessary requirements to provide such proof and the general problems involved in the evaluation of microphotometric data have been discussed most explicitly by Pätau and Swift (39). In the past, apparent exceptions from DNA constancy have been reported in a few cases but could not be confirmed in subsequent studies (cf. 7, 19, 30, 37, 47); recently two new suggestions of this type have been made (9, 27), and further work is needed to assess their significance. It is important to remember in this connection that deviations in Feulgen stainability from the ordinary pattern require an independent method of confirmation before they can be attributed unequivocally to aberrant behavior on the part of DNA.

It should also be mentioned that, while quantitative constancy may to some persons appear to be an expected attribute of the hereditary material, it is certainly not a sufficient criterion to establish the genetic role of DNA. As recently discussed by Goldschmidt (24), a completely inert chromosomal frame-substance might also exhibit this type of behavior. Other lines of research have, however, provided good reasons to attribute genetic activity to DNA (e.g., 25).

At any rate, the currently available biochemical and cytochemical evidence relating to the quantitative behavior of DNA represents a fundamental cellular characteristic of much more general significance than that attributed formerly to mere numerical relationships among chromosome sets. It permits us to estimate the extent of chromosomal replication in cases where chromosome counts cannot be made; and, in conjunction with chromosome counts a knowledge of the nuclear DNA content now allows a clear-cut distinction between polyploid and polytenic conditions of nuclei. Thus we have gained a powerful tool for the study of evolutionary relationships among karyotypes (26, 43), and for the establishment of doubtful cell lineages (40).

CYTOCHEMICAL PROPERTIES OF NUCLEAR NUCLEOPROTEIN COMPLEXES

If one assumes that chromosomal DNA represents the repository of the cell's genetic information, the next problem becomes that of determining how this information is passed on to other cell regions and put into action. These questions, and some possible solutions, have recently been reviewed (22). Such transfers of genetic information must involve some sort of interaction among DNA and other nuclear components; any detectable changes in chromosomal nucleoprotein complexes, whether they be on a microscopic (11, 31) or a cytochemical level, may be of importance in this respect. Here again, in the study of protein fractions associated with DNA, cytochemical evidence has supplemented and in some instances advanced beyond the available biochemical information. A case in point is the period of DNA duplication which normally precedes mitosis: since the currently favored model of DNA structure (54) appears to solve some of the formerly most puzzling aspects of the replication process, the behavior of other nuclear components has not commanded much attention (except in some theoretical considerations, e.g., 12, 16). However, quantitative cytochemical data from animal (13) and plant nuclei (4) indicate that a basic protein fraction doubles in amount precisely at the same time as DNA. These findings suggest that one should think in terms of the replication of a nucleohistone complex rather than of DNA alone.

The cytochemical properties of nucleohistone complexes in proliferating animal cells have furthermore been shown to differ significantly from those of nondividing, physiologically active cells. This was demonstrated by Bloch and Godman (14), who determined the dye-binding characteristics of individual tissue nuclei microphotometrically, after sequential application of three different staining techniques to the same preparation. In this fashion information on nuclear DNA content (by the Feulgen reaction), on the basophilia of the DNA, i.e., the number of exposed, stainable phosphate groups (by methyl green staining), and on the acidophilia of histones associated with DNA (by fast green staining at elevated pH, according to the procedure of Alfert and Geschwind, 6) has been obtained simultaneously. The results show that the interphase chromatin of proliferating cells is more basophilic and that its associated histones are more acidophilic, per unit DNA, than is the case for cells which have stopped dividing but continue to grow and presumably function in a specific way. A schematic representation of these findings is given in Fig. 1. These data have been interpreted to indicate that nuclei, after they cease to proliferate, increase in size by acquiring a non-histone protein fraction which combines with DNA-phosphate groups and with basic end-groups of histones in such a way as to prevent their binding of methyl green and fast green dye ions. At present we can only guess that the protein

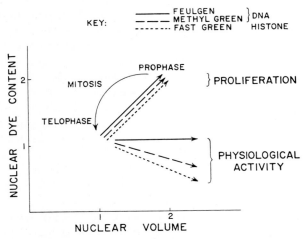

FIG. 1. A schematic representation of the dye-binding capacities of liver nuclei from young rats (14).

fraction(s) which modifies the staining behavior of the nucleohistones is perhaps related to the so-called "residual protein" of Mirsky and Ris (33). This fraction is quantitatively most prominent in nuclei of physiologically active cells and exhibits a rapid turnover when nuclei are engaged in protein synthesis (8).

Changes in the acid-dye-binding capacity of nuclear histones can generally be interpreted in two different, but not mutually exclusive ways. On the one hand, there may occur changes in the physical associations within nucleoprotein complexes leading to different degrees of staining inhibition without chemical changes in the amount or composition of the histones; on the other hand, it is possible that histones themselves change in quantity or composition and thereby become more or less acidophilic. The staining differences between proliferating and physiologically active nuclei discussed above have been interpreted in terms of varying degrees of staining inhibition, for reasons given in greater detail by the authors (14; see also 2).

In other cases similar staining differences can be correlated with available biochemical data to indicate actual changes in composition of the basic proteins. This is notably true for various types of sperm cells known to contain proteins of very basic character (e.g., 20, 51). Such basic sperm proteins, unless they are lost during the staining procedure because of their great solubility (e.g., the protamines of salmon sperm, cf. 3) exhibit a correspondingly greater acidophilia than somatic histones (6). Cytochemical methods, moreover, permit going beyond the mere recognition of this chemical difference and make it possible to determine at which stage of maturation the sperm proteins acquire their more pronounced basic character. This problem, unanswered for more than three-quarters of a century since Miescher's pioneering work (32), has been the subject of three recent independent studies (3, 29, 51). It appears that the modification of sperm proteins occurs after the completion of meiosis, at a late stage of spermiogenesis when the sperm chromatin condenses.

Where biochemical data are not yet available for comparison, it is sometimes possible to use auxiliary tests in the attempt to interpret cytochemical findings. This becomes necessary if we want to distinguish between the previously mentioned alternative explanations of changes in the stainability of histones in a case such as, for instance, the pycnotic degeneration of nuclei. When nuclei undergo this very common pathological condensation, their relative acidophilia increases markedly, similar to that of sperm. The underlying mechanisms responsible for this change are, however, different in these two systems, as can be most simply demonstrated by the effect of the acetylation of protein amino groups (35) on acidophilia: the acid-dye-binding capacity of ordinary histones is greatly decreased after acetylation, while the stainability of extremely arginine-rich sperm proteins is not noticeably affected. Such a comparison is shown in Figs. 2 and 3. The stainability of pycnotic nuclei lining an ovarian follicle is decreased to an extent similar to that of surrounding normal nuclei; in the testis, spermatogenic and connective tissue nuclei lose most of their acidophilia upon acetylation, while nearly ripe sperm nuclei do not. This observation reinforces our previous conclusion (2) that pycnotic degeneration leads to a dissociation and "unmasking" of stainable groups of histones, rather than to their conversion into more basic proteins, as is the case in sperm formation.

A correlation, which will require further extension into more than the few cases reported here, may be proposed as follows: the nuclear histones of physiologically active cells are less acidophilic (by reason of either of the mechanisms mentioned) than the basic proteins associated with DNA during times of physiological inactivity—for instance, when chromatin is just being transported, as in mitosis or in preparation of sperm for delivery to the egg. Such a notion would fit into the

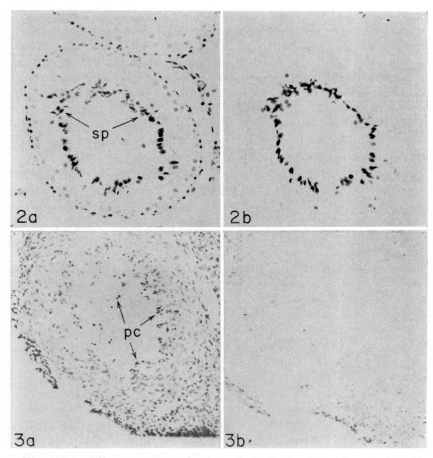

Figs. 2 & 3. Adjacent sections of guinea pig testis (2a, 2b) and ovary (3a, 3b), fixed in neutralized 10 per cent formalin, and stained for basic nuclear proteins (6). Wratten F filter, × 200 (photographed by Mr. Victor Duran).

Figs. 2a and 3a: Controls (sp = sperm, pc = pycnotic nuclei).

Figs. 2b and 3b: Terminal amino groups abolished by acetylation of the sections (cf. 3) prior to staining.

general schemes proposed by the Stedmans (45) or by Danielli (18), who regard histones as regulators of the genetic activities of chromosomes. Presumably the dye-binding capacities of histones provide a measure of actual or potential interactions between charged groups of these proteins, DNA, and chromosomal non-histone proteins.

Cytochemical methods can rarely give definite answers to problems of cell physiology. However, staining differences of the types described, quantitated by microphotometric techniques, tell us something about physicochemical interactions among components of nucleoprotein complexes. Such cytochemical techniques lend themselves easily for exploratory studies and can provide important clues to the biochemist as to when and where it would be most profitable to exert his skill for the application of more precise analytical methods. The biophysicist, in turn, may attempt to correlate such cytochemical dye-binding data with the molecular schemes derived from other lines of investigation (cf. 55).

REFERENCES

1. Alfert, M., *J. Cell. Comp. Physiol.*, **36**, 381 (1950).
2. Alfert, M., *Biol. Bull.*, **109**, 1 (1955).
3. Alfert, M., *J. Biophys. Biochem. Cytol.*, **2**, 109 (1956).
4. Alfert, M., and Bern, H. A., quoted by Alfert, M., in *Fine Structure of Cells*, pp. 157–163. Noordhoff, Groningen (1955).
5. Alfert, M., Bern, H. A., and Kahn, R. H., *Acta Anat.*, **23**, 185 (1955).
6. Alfert, M., and Geschwind, I. I., *Proc. Natl. Acad. Sci. U. S.*, **39**, 991 (1953).
7. Alfert, M., and Swift, H., *Exptl. Cell Research*, **5**, 455 (1953).
8. Allfrey, V. G., Mirsky, A. E., and Osawa, S., *Nature*, **176**, 1042 (1955).
9. Bayreuther, K., *Chromosoma*, **7**, 508 (1956).
10. Beatty, R. A., *Intern. Rev. Cytol.*, **3**, 177 (1954).
11. Beermann, W., *Chromosoma*, **5**, 139 (1952).
12. Bloch, D. P., *Proc. Natl. Acad. Sci. U. S.*, **41**, 1058 (1955).
13. Bloch, D. P., and Godman, G. C., *J. Biophys. Biochem. Cytol.*, **1**, 17 (1955).
14. Bloch, D. P., and Godman, G. C., *J. Biophys. Biochem. Cytol.*, **1**, 531 (1955).
15. Brachet, J., *Arch. biol. (Liège)*, **53**, 207 (1942).
16. Butler, J. A. V., *Radiation Research*, **4**, 20 (1956).
17. Caspersson, T., *Skand. Arch. Physiol.*, **73**, Suppl. 8 (1936).
18. Danielli, J. F., *Cold Spring Harbor Symposia Quant. Biol.*, **14**, 32 (1949).
19. Deeley, E. M., Richards, B. M., Walker, P. M. B., and Davies, H. G., *Exptl. Cell Research*, **6**, 569 (1954).
20. Felix, K., *Experientia*, **8**, 312 (1952).
21. Frazer, S. C., and Davidson, J. N., *Exptl. Cell Research*, **4**, 316 (1953).
22. Gamow, G., Rich, A., and Ycas, M., *Advances in Biol. and Med. Phys.*, **4**, 23 (1956).
23. Gelfant, S., and Clemmons, J. J., *J. Cell. Comp. Physiol.*, **46**, 529 (1955).
24. Goldschmidt, R. B., *Theoretical Genetics*, Univ. California Press, Berkeley (1955).
25. Hotchkiss, R. D., *J. Cell. Comp. Physiol.*, **45**, Suppl. 2, 1 (1955).
26. Hughes-Schrader, S., *Biol. Bull.*, **100**, 178 (1951).
27. LaCour, L. F., Deeley, E. M., and Chayen, J., *Nature*, **177**, 272 (1956).
28. Leuchtenberger, C., Vendrely, R., and Vendrely, C., *Proc. Natl. Acad. Sci. U. S.*, **37**, 33 (1951).
29. Lison, L., *Acta histochem.*, **2**, 47 (1955).
30. McMaster, R. D., *J. Exptl. Zool.*, **130**, 1 (1955).

31. Mechelke, F., *Chromosoma*, **5**, 511 (1953).
32. Miescher, F., *Die histochemischen und physiologischen Arbeiten*, F. C. W. Vogel, Leipzig (1897).
33. Mirsky, A. E., and Ris, H., *J. Gen. Physiol.*, **3**, 7 (1947).
34. Moses, M. J., and Taylor, J. H., *Exptl. Cell Research*, **9**, 474 (1955).
35. Olcott, H. S., and Fraenkel-Conrat, H., *Chem. Revs.*, **41**, 151 (1947).
36. Ornstein, L., *Lab. Invest.*, **1**, 250 (1952).
37. Pasteels, J., and Lison, L., *Compt. rend. Acad. Sci., Paris*, **236**, 236 (1953).
38. Pätau, K., *Chromosoma*, **5**, 341 (1952).
39. Pätau, K., and Swift, H., *Chromosoma*, **6**, 194 (1953).
40. Petrakis, N. L., and Folstad, L. J., *Blood*, **10**, 1204 (1955).
41. Pollister, A. W., and Ris, H., *Cold Spring Harbor Symposia Quant. Biol.*, **12**, 147 (1947).
42. Ris, H., and Mirsky, A. E., *J. Gen. Physiol.*, **33**, 125 (1949).
43. Schrader, F., and Hughes-Schrader, S., *Chromosoma*, **7**, 469 (1956).
44. Schrader, F., and Leuchtenberger, C., *Exptl. Cell Research*, **1**, 421 (1950).
45. Stedman, E., and Stedman, E., *Nature*, **152**, 556 (1943).
46. Swift, H., *Physiol. Zool.*, **23**, 169 (1950).
47. Swift, H., *Intern. Rev. Cytol.*, **2**, 1 (1953).
48. Swift, H., and Kleinfeld, R., *Physiol. Zool.*, **26**, 301 (1953).
49. Taylor, J. H., and McMaster, R. D., *Chromosoma*, **6**, 489 (1954).
50. Vendrely, R., in *The Nucleic Acids*, Vol. II, p. 155, Academic Press, New York (1955).
51. Vendrely, C., Knobloch, A., and Vendrely, R., *Biochim. et Biophys. Acta*, **19**, 472 (1956).
52. Vendrely, R., and Vendrely, C., *Experientia*, **4**, 434 (1948).
53. Walker, P. M. B., and Yates, H. B., *Proc. Roy. Soc. (London)*, B, **140**, 274 (1952).
54. Watson, J. D., and Crick, F. H. C., *Nature*, **171**, 737 (1953).
55. Wilkins, M. H. F., *Cold Spring Harbor Symposia Quant. Biol.*, in press.

DISCUSSION

DR. NASON: Are your spindles free of chromosome material?

DR. MAZIA: No; but the nucleotide impurities on the spindle preparation are of a different order of magnitude.

No, but the DNA content of the chromosomes is known from independent analyses and would account for only a negligible part of the nucleotide recovered from the mitotic apparatus.

DR. McELROY: Has the isolated material been tested for its ability to hydrolyze ATP?

DR. MAZIA: Yes. We haven't found activity. This was the preparation made with detergents. Obviously one should try preparations made with ATP.

DR. GLASS: In many animal cells, according to classical observations, part of the spindle apparatus comes from the nucleus, and we know also that in many protozoa the entire spindle apparatus is inside the nucleus. In your experiments, then, do you have any clue as to what proportion of the spindle is nuclear and what proportion is cytoplasmic in origin?

Dr. Mazia: We can compare the total protein content of one mitotic apparatus at metaphase or anaphase with the total amount of protein that could be contained in one interphase nucleus. It turns out that the interphase nucleus of the sea urchin egg contains only about 2 per cent as much protein as does the mitotic apparatus. Therefore, if the nucleus were merely dumping protein into the system at the time the nuclear membrane disappears, it could be contributing only a small part of the material of the mitotic apparatus. If by "nuclear origin" one means that the protein was ultimately synthesized in the nucleus, that is another matter and one that can't be decided on the basis of what we now know. (See Mazia, D., and Roslansky, J., *Protoplasma*, **44**, 528-534, 1956.)

Dr. Ris: I would like to enlarge on the comment of Dr. Glass. What you call the mitotic apparatus is made up of 3 separate components, the asters which form around the centrosomes, the gel-like spindle body which originates from the nucleus, and chromosomal fibers which originate in connection with the kinetochores. Now these 3 have different origins and different functions. Asters enlarge during the mitotic process; the spindle body elongates in its long axis during anaphase; the chromosomal fibers contract and move the chromosomes to the poles. You mentioned that the mitotic apparatus contains very little beside the material which is cytoplasmic in origin. Therefore, your analysis can perhaps give us only information on the properties of the asters but not on spindle body or chromosomal fibers which make up only a very small fraction of your material.

Dr. Mazia: You speak with some assurance of the nuclear origin of the spindle. I realize that some, but not all, of the cytologists who have worked on mitosis find this a reasonable interpretation of their observations, but is there convincing evidence? In many cases the spindle is quite large, apart from the asters, and again one wonders whether the nucleus could contain the amount of material required. If we succeed in finding evidence of chemical heterogeneity in the isolated mitotic apparatus, we shall probably turn to the hypothesis of the nuclear origin of some parts, the cytoplasmic origin of others. But thus far the protein picture seems remarkably homogeneous. I am aware of the fact that the whole mitotic process takes place within the nucleus in some forms, but am not sure that this is telling us that the spindle is of nuclear origin generally.

Dr. Ris: You say the whole business is inside the nuclear membrane in some organisms: but in these cases it is exactly not the whole business, only part of it—namely the part in which the chromosomes move, the spindle body. The asters are always outside the nucleus. The nuclear membrane may disappear before the spindle is fully formed, or in metaphase, or anaphase and in some cases again it persists all the way through mitosis. The size of the spindle is almost always in direct ratio to the size of the nucleus from which it came. In those cases where we find polysaccharides in the spindle they appear in the nuclear sap during prophase. The film of Michel on cell division in grasshopper spermatocytes shows the nuclear origin of the spindle body in the living cell most beautifully.

DR. BENDICH: I should like to ask Dr. Mazia a question concerning the so-called nucleotide protein. Is the nucleotide protein isolated by the digitonin procedure similar to the nucleotide protein isolated by the ATP procedure? You said it contained purines exclusively.

DR. MAZIA: We haven't tried isolating nucleotide from mitotic apparatus prepared by the ATP procedure. Obviously we would then be worried about how much nucleotide was picked up in the course of the preparation.

DR. HERRIOTT: Did I understand that the precursor protein is later converted into the material with which you then formed these aster formations with cysteine?

DR. MAZIA: Yes. In the model experiments we use solutions containing the cytoplasmic protein that we think may be the precursor to the mitotic apparatus. Thus, while the method of invoking fiber formation is completely artificial, the protein that is used is probably the one that is used by the cell.

DR. OCHOA: What is the mode of action of the ATP in bringing about the solubilization of the cytoplasmic part of the cell? Have you any idea about this? How did you arrive at using ATP there?

DR. MAZIA: In working on the mitotic apparatus, we have kept in mind the experience of others with contractile proteins. We have been particularly curious about some suggestive analogies between the proteins we are dealing with and *actin* from muscle. The possibility that the polymerization and depolymerization of actin involved ATP has been subject of much discussion and experiment. The "plasticizing" action of a high concentration of ATP on muscle is well known and is believed to be related to the relaxation process. These are some of the considerations that led to using ATP as a dispersing agent. We don't know the mode of action, but it may have to do with the fact, stressed by some workers on muscle, that the ATP molecule carries an extraordinary concentration of electric charge.

DR. KAPLAN: Is this a specific agent?

DR. MAZIA: I don't know, but am inclined to predict that it is a nonspecific pyrophosphate effect.

DR. KING: There are some hypotheses that can be raised with regard to the action of kinetochores and the accurate division of the chromosomes. One hypothesis that might be made is that we have two asters that are complementary, in that either they might have different substances diffusing from them or they might have different electrical polarity. There are a number of hypotheses here. Also, the two chromosomes of the same type might have kinetochores that are complementary to each other which will insure their division. You can call one a plus and one a minus—that is, when the chromosomes are reduplicated one is plus and the other is minus. I wanted to ask if there are any results from the cells which have an abnormally large number of asters that would indicate anything with regard to these hypotheses. How are the chromosomes divided?

DR. MAZIA: If there are more than two poles, the chromosomes can't solve the problem and go to the several poles in various numbers.

DR. KING: There is no sign of simple plus or minus connection in the aster?

DR. MAZIA: It seems to me that the most profitable assumption is one for which Pollister has provided an observational basis; namely, that the centrioles and kinetochores are similar structures. We can imagine various ways in which the two facing each other might determine the outgrowth of fibers that join them.

DR. HUXLEY: It may be relevant to what you are saying about the orienting capacities of the centromeres: I was shown the other day by Paul Weiss in New York unpublished electron micrographs of regenerating skin after damage where there seemed clear evidence that the underlying fibroblasts discharged material in the form of ultramicroscopic rodlets which was then oriented by some influence coming from the epidermis. It was really very beautiful to see this organizing influence coming out and arranging these elements in a regular way. There may be something exactly like this in your case with the asters.

DR. MAZIA: We have no real evidence against the idea that these centers are making the fibers, but the hypothesis that they are producing something which aggregates material that is already present seems to be simpler.

DR. SPIEGELMAN: I wanted to ask if you have information about whether the units which go together to make up high polymers pre-exist or if they have to be made fresh.

DR. MAZIA: The evidence I have given favors the pre-existence of the units. I can't say at what point this can be considered to be proved. One attempts to fingerprint the proteins of the mitotic apparatus and to look in the haystack of the cell before division for needles carrying the same fingerprints. We have found a protein meeting the criteria that we have, but the criteria that the protein chemist provides us for what he calls "characterization" are not too sensitive when applied to the job of deciding whether two proteins are the same.

DR. PAPIRMEISTER: What effect would failure of gene replication at interphase have on the mitotic figures or the mitotic apparatus during fission?

DR. MAZIA: I know of no case in which a cell makes the step from interphase into mitosis where chromosome duplication has not taken place. (Meiotic reduction may be an exception to this statement.)

DR. ALFERT: There is one—the supernumerary divisions in pollen grains.

DR. MAZIA: Oh, yes.

DR. BEADLE: But the spindles do form apparently normally. The spindles are formed, but the chromosomes do not divide. The spindles elongate abnormally.

DR. MAZIA: You don't know whether the chromosomes have been replicated.

DR. BEADLE: There are several successive divisions without any chromosome division, so that apparently the chromosomes are not multiplied to the extent of the cell divisions.

DR. ALFERT: I would like to comment on the basophilia of the spindle. This term has been used somewhat loosely at times, because if one looks closely, basophilia is often due to material accumulated among and around the spindle fibers; this is probably due to RNA, which may be lost in the course of the isolation of spindles. If the spindle nucleotide protein itself is basophilic, this constitutes a special situation not comparable to that of muscle nucleotide protein which is noted for its relative lack of basophilia.

DR. MAZIA: In this case one finds that the isolated spindle is basophilic, although analysis thus far shows that it contains nucleotide, not RNA.

DR. HOAGLAND: Do you know anything about the nature of binding of this ATP to the protein? Have you tried to get it off by any mild conditions?

DR. MAZIA: We have looked into that a little. It comes off, as it does in muscle, by heating the protein. It comes off slowly on dialysis, when one dialyzes for days. Heat gets it off. Heating has proved to be the most convenient method.

DR. S. COHEN: I should just like to mention a very few experiments with synchronized bacteria whose extracts produce sedimentation patterns comparable to those observed by Dr. Mazia with his synchronized sea urchin eggs. We synchronized the thymine-requiring bacteria with thymine and observed that, in the period just following doubling of DNA and just prior to division, a unique component of the sedimentation pattern having a sedimentation constant of approximately 25 was specifically reduced to a sedimentation constant of about 12. Then just after the division this material ($S_{20} = 25$) was regenerated. Under no other conditions have we observed a change in this particular component. In other words, there was, under the conditions of division, a change of the polymerization state of a particular component. Whether this was a spindle component or a cell wall component we really don't know.

DR. EPHRUSSI-TAYLOR: I would like to add a remark concerning the question raised by Dr. Spiegelman as to the origin of this protein that

Dr. Mazia is talking about and whether it pre-exists as such long before cell division. It seems to me that the idea, which I think is favored by Dr. Mazia now, is that this protein is present and probably forms a part of some cell structure long prior to cell division. It is rather tempting, because it could—if it were so—provide a basis for the antagonism between the state of cell division and the state of differentiation of the cell. If this protein were shifted from some fixed structure where it played a functional role, and reorganized during division into an inactive protein playing a purely mechanical role, I think this would give a first indication of a chemical basis of the antagonism between cell division and cell function.

THE NUCLEUS AND PROTEIN SYNTHESIS

V. Allfrey and A. E. Mirsky

The Rockefeller Institute for Medical Research, New York

and

S. Osawa

Biological Institute, Nagoya University

In E. B. Wilson's great book, *The Cell in Development and Heredity,* a statement is made which summarizes the results of a great many physiological experiments on living cells. "A cell deprived of its nucleus may for a considerable time live and manifest the power of coordinated movement, but it has lost the power of assimilation, of growth and repair, and sooner or later dies. The operations of destructive metabolism may continue for a considerable time in the absence of a nucleus; those of constructive metabolism quickly cease with its removal." (26)

This picture of a functional, dynamic, synthesizing nucleus is based on studies of nerve fiber regeneration and enucleation studies with amoeba, ciliates, and rhizopods, all of which show that the nucleus is essential for regeneration, for wound healing, for digestion and secretion, for membrane formation, in short for the constructive, synthetic reactions which characterize a living cell. A nucleus in one cell may even make it possible for an adjoining cell without a nucleus to survive and function normally, provided the two are joined by an intercellular bridge. It is this active participation of the nucleus in the life and function of cells which explains how the genetic units within the chromosomes mediate the growth and development of the organisms.

In the experiments about to be described we have attempted to study some of the synthetic reactions within the nucleus—with particular emphasis on the role of deoxyribonucleic acid in protein synthesis.

In earlier work in this laboratory we have been concerned both with the chemistry of the cell nucleus and with the role of the nucleic acids in protein synthesis. Thus it has been shown that nuclei prepared from different somatic cells of the same organism have one main point of similarity, namely, a constant amount of deoxyribonucleic acid (DNA) per nucleus. The germ cells, which contain only one-half the chromosome complement of the somatic cells, contain just one-half as much DNA (16). But although a lymphocyte nucleus and a kidney nucleus or a liver nucleus may be equivalent in DNA content, they are quite distinct chemically in other ways—in their protein composition and in their enzymic constitution (5, 20). These differences in composition suggested that nuclei are engaged in an active metabolic interchange with their cytoplasms.

The activity of the nucleus *in vivo* was then investigated by injecting N^{15}-labeled glycine, and it was shown that the proteins of the nucleus are being synthesized in non-dividing cells, such as those of the liver, kidney, and pancreas of adult animals (3). Furthermore, the rate of nuclear protein synthesis changes when the rate of cytoplasmic protein synthesis is varied. The nucleus therefore is responsive to changes in its immediate environment.

The investigations mentioned depended wholly or in part upon schemes for fractionating cells to yield isolated nuclei. The method of choice in most experiments was a slight modification of a procedure introduced by Martin Behrens (6). This is a scheme which prevents water-soluble materials from moving between nucleus and cytoplasm during the course of the isolation. Its success depends upon the immediate removal of water from the tissue, which is then ground and fractionated in non-aqueous solvents such as cyclohexane and carbon tetrachloride. When the specific gravity of the nucleus differs sufficiently from that of other subcellular components it can be separated from them by centrifugation. This is facilitated by selecting a medium of density lower than the nuclear specific gravity and higher than that of possible cytoplasmic contaminants.

The nuclei of many tissues were prepared in this way and tested for purity. By a variety of chemical, immunological, and enzymatic tests they were shown to be essentially free of cytoplasmic contamination. Such nuclei, prepared in non-aqueous media, constitute a *standard* against which nuclei prepared in aqueous media can be compared. For example, liver or kidney nuclei made in sucrose or citric acid solutions can readily be shown to have lost much of their protein during isolation simply by comparing them with the corresponding Behren's-type nuclei (5, 10).

When such comparisons were made between *thymus* nuclei prepared in sucrose solutions and thymus nuclei isolated in non-aqueous media, it was found that the "sucrose" nuclei were the equivalent of the *standard* in many respects. The DNA analyses for the two preparations were the same (2.5 per cent DNA-P) and so were the overall protein composition and the enzymic constitution (21). Once it was established that thymus nuclei could be prepared in sucrose solutions without extracting their water-soluble components, it was decided to test whether such nuclei can synthesize protein by themselves.

The isolation procedure used is a modification of that introduced by R. M. Schneider and M. L. Petermann (17). Fresh thymus tissue is minced with scissors and then homogenized in a low-speed blendor (4 minutes at 1800 RPM) in 0.25 M sucrose—0.003 M $CaCl_2$ solution. The homogenate is filtered through gauze and through double-napped flannellette to remove clumps of tissue and fiber. The nuclei are then separated by differential centrifugation and washed with sucrose and calcium chloride solution.

Now how good are nuclei prepared in this way? Under the light microscope, stained with crystal violet or unstained, they seem a beautiful preparation—a few whole cells, occasional red cells, some small strands of cytoplasm attached to some of the nuclei. But it is known that some thymocytes contain just a thin halo or crescent of cytoplasm, and it was conceivable that many of the objects considered to be nuclei under the light microscope were cells with scanty or negligible amounts of cytoplasm. To check this possibility two nuclear preparations were examined under the electron microscope. (This was made possible through the generous cooperation of Drs. Watson and Palade of the Rockefeller Institute.) Electron microscopy made it evident that there was some cytoplasmic contamination, but this was also evident in stained preparations under the light microscope. The real advantage of the electron microscope in these studies was the ease of detection of small thymocytes. We counted the number of such small cells in two preparations and observed 45 cells per thousand nuclei in the first preparation and 77 per thousand in the second preparation. The overall extent of cytoplasmic contamination can be estimated chemically, for example by nucleic acid analyses. We consider thymus nuclei prepared in sucrose solutions to be about 90 per cent pure. Even more convincing evidence for the absence of appreciable whole cell contamination was obtained in studying the effect of deoxyribonuclease. These experiments are described in detail below.

AMINO ACID INCORPORATION INTO THE PROTEINS OF ISOLATED NUCLEI

When thymus nuclei are suspended in a buffered sucrose medium and incubated at 37° C. in the presence of isotopically labeled amino acids, there is a rapid and considerable incorporation of the isotope into the proteins of the nucleus (1, 4). Fig. 1 shows the time course of incorporation of alanine-1-C¹⁴ into the mixed proteins of isolated

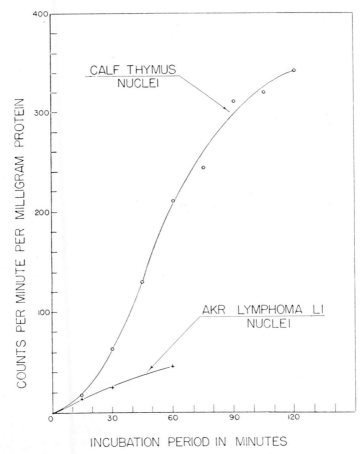

FIG. 1. The time course of alanine-1-C¹⁴ incorporation into the proteins of isolated nuclei. The specific activity of the total, mixed nuclear protein is plotted against the time of incubation of the nuclei. The upper curve shows the incorporation into thymus nuclei. The lower curve shows the rate of alanine-C¹⁴ uptake by nuclei isolated from an AKR lymphoma.

calf thymus nuclei. The lower curve shows the incorporation observed into AKR-lymphoma nuclei isolated by a similar procedure. (The lymphoma tissue was generously supplied by Dr. John Kidd of Cornell University Medical College.) After an initial lag period, the C^{14}-uptake proceeds linearly for about 90 minutes and then begins to taper off.

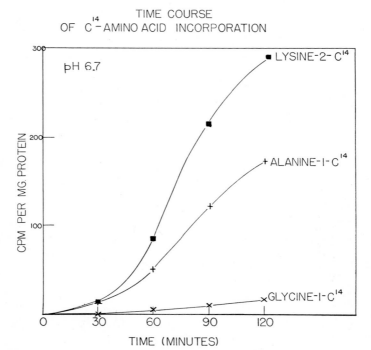

TIME COURSE
OF C^{14} – AMINO ACID INCORPORATION

FIG. 2. The time course of incorporation of alanine-1-C^{14}, glycine-1-C^{14}, and lysine-2-C^{14} into the proteins of isolated thymus nuclei. In this plot the data have been "normalized" to give the relative uptakes for equivalent amounts of the different amino acids where each has the same specific activity in mc. per mM.

Figs. 2 and 3 show the time course of alanine-1-C^{14}, glycine-1-C^{14}, lysine-2-C^{14}, and methionine-S^{35} incorporations. In these, and in most of the experiments to be described below, the uptake was followed by measuring the radioactivity of the total mixed proteins of the nucleus. The results are expressed as counts per minute per mg. protein. The protein was prepared by first extensively washing the

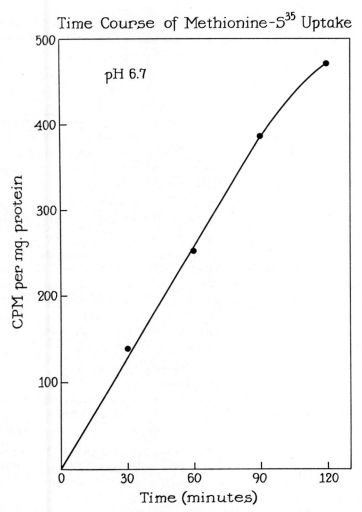

Fɪɢ. 3.   The time course of methionine-S[35] uptake into the proteins of isolated thymus nuclei.

nuclei with trichloroacetic acid (TCA), removing the nucleic acids with hot TCA, and finally removing the lipides with warm ethanol, ethanol-ether-chloroform mixtures, ether and acetone. The protein residue was then homogenized in acetone and filtered off on filter paper planchets. Radioactivity was determined using a G-M tube and scaling circuit, and the measurements were subsequently corrected for self-absorption.

To show that the radioactivity measured was actually in the protein and not merely adsorbed or bound by ester linkages, we treated the protein with alkali and with ninhydrin. In the case of incorporated alanine-1-C^{14} more than 94 per cent of the activity remained after treatment with 0.25 N NaOH for 2 hours, and more than 89 per cent remained after reaction with ninhydrin. Seventy-six per cent of the incorporated methionine-S^{35} was stable to alkali.

A number of experiments next to be described deal with the conditions necessary for amino acid incorporation and with the inhibition of nuclear protein synthesis.

The uptake of amino acids is an aerobic phenomenon, and it is inhibited by a number of substances which are known to block oxidative phosphorylation (Table 1). Cyanide, azide, dinitrophenol, Janus green B, dicumarol, and antimycin A all inhibit alanine uptake. However, methylene blue, a substance which inhibits oxidative phosphorylation in mitochondria, has only a small effect on nuclear isotope incorporation.

Adding metabolites, such as glucose, fructose, or a-ketoglutarate, to the nuclear suspension has little effect on the incorporation of amino acids. Added glucose may at times raise the alanine uptake by about 10 per cent. An attempt to block glycolysis by the addition of fluoride ($10^{-3}M$ NaF) did not result in inhibition of alanine incorporation.

It was shown by Gale and Folkes that chloramphenicol blocks protein synthesis in bacteria (12). This substance had little effect on glycine-1-C^{14} uptake by isolated nuclei. The amino-acid antagonist, p-fluorophenylalanine, also blocks protein synthesis in bacteria (14). We were unable to test this compound at the higher concentrations used in Halvorson and Spiegelman's experiments, but at 5×10^{-3} M it inhibited alanine uptake by only 15 per cent. Similarly, ethionine (1.5×10^{-3} M) had no effect on the incorporation of methionine-S^{35} or lysine-2-C^{14}, and it reduced alanine uptake by only 16 per cent.

TABLE 1

EFFECT OF ANOXIA AND OF SEVERAL INHIBITORS UPON C^{14}-AMINO ACID
INCORPORATION BY ISOLATED CALF THYMUS NUCLEI

Conditions of Experiment	Isotope Administered as	Specific Activity of Nuclear Protein c.p.m. per mg.	Degree of Inhibition per cent
A. Nuclei in O_2	glycine-1-C^{14}	71	—
Nuclei in N_2	"	15	80
B. Nuclei in O_2	DL-alanine-1-C^{14}	72	—
Nuclei in N_2	"	10	85
C. "Control" nuclei	"	72	—
Nuclei in 2×10^{-5} M dinitrophenol	"	11	84
D. "Control" nuclei	"	131	—
Nuclei in 2×10^{-5} M janus green B	"	3	97
E. "Control" nuclei	"	54	—
Nuclei in 1×10^{-3} M NaCN	"	13	76
Nuclei in 1×10^{-3} M NaN$_3$	"	5	91
Nuclei + 0.05 mg. dicumarol per ml.	"	8	85
Nuclei + 1 γ antimycin A per ml.	"	6	89

c.p.m., counts per minute.

TABLE 2

EFFECT OF BENZIMIDAZOLE DERIVATIVES ON ALANINE-1-C^{14} UPTAKE BY
ISOLATED NUCLEI

Derivative Tested		Amount	Specific Activity of Nuclear Protein	Inhibition of Uptake	Relative Inhibition of Virus Multiplication[1]
		mg.	c.p.m. per mg.	per cent	
"Control"		—	50	—	—
5,6-dichloro-benzimidazole	1-β-D-Arabino-pyranoside	0.1	45	10	3.1
" "	1-β-D-Ribo-pyranoside	0.1	36	28	15
" "	1-β-D-Ribo-furanoside	0.1	26	48	92
4,5,6-trichloro-benzimidazole	1-α-D-Ribo-furanoside	0.01	46	8	165
" "	1-β-D-Ribo-furanoside	0.01	36	28	760

[1] Work of Tamm et al. (Refs. 23–25).

The search for antagonists became more fruitful when it was brought to our attention (by Dr. Philip MacMaster) that cortisone injected repeatedly into mice causes involution of the thymus (18). We found that a small amount of cortisone added to the nuclear suspension can reduce alanine uptake by more than 50 per cent.

An inhibitor of considerable interest is 5,6-dichloro-β-D-ribofuranosyl benzimidazole. This structural analog of a purine riboside was found by Tamm and Horsfall to retard influenza virus multiplication in the mouse and in tissue culture (23, 25). It is an effective inhibitor of alanine-1-C^{14} uptake by isolated nuclei. Tests of this and similar compounds (synthesized by C. Shunk and K. Folkers of the Merck Research Laboratories) are summarized in Table 2. It is of interest that the ribosyl benzimidazole inhibits uptake while the corresponding arabinose derivative does not. The data also shows that for effective inhibition, the ribose should exist in the furanose, not the pyranose form, and its linkage to the benzimidazole moiety should have the β-, not the α-configuration.

One of the most striking effects on nuclear amino acid incorporation is that produced by sodium ions. Nuclei isolated in sucrose need a sodium supplement in order to incorporate amino acids actively. Fig. 4 shows the effect of varied sodium concentration on the level of glycine-1-C^{14} uptake. There is a well-defined maximum at about 0.07 M under our test conditions. The sodium requirement seems to be specific. An attempt was made to substitute all or part of the sodium in the medium with an equivalent amount of potassium. In these experiments the total salt concentration was kept constant and the ratio NaCl/KCl was varied. When all the sodium is replaced by potassium, the uptake falls to 15 per cent of the optimal value. Increasing the sodium to potassium ratio gives a corresponding increase in the amount of amino acid incorporated (Fig. 5).

The extreme dependence of the synthetic activity of the nucleus upon sodium ion concentration makes it necessary to control the sodium level of the incubation medium rigorously. This introduces a related problem, namely, the osmotic balance between the nucleus and the suspending medium. It was soon found that nuclei exposed to high sucrose concentrations lost their ability to incorporate amino acid into protein. A more detailed study of this dependence of uptake upon sucrose concentration in the medium is summarized in Fig. 6. The peak of activity occurs at about 0.20 M. The medium also contains

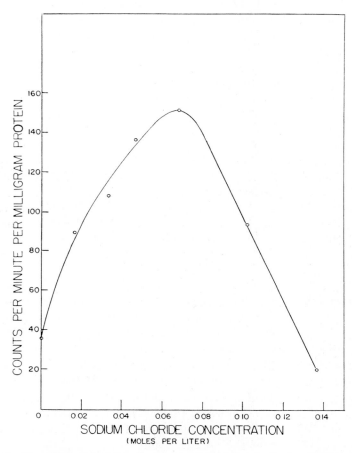

Fɪɢ. 4. The effect of varied sodium ion concentration in the incubation medium upon the ability of thymus nuclei to incorporate glycine-1-C[14]. The specific activity of the nuclear protein after 1 hour incubation of the nuclei in the presence of radioactive glycine is plotted against the sodium concentration of the medium.

sodium phosphate buffer (0.025 M), glucose (0.020 M), and NaCl (0.03 M).

Although it is a simple matter to control the sucrose concentration and sodium level of the medium, there are other factors which influence nuclear amino acid uptake which are not so easy to control. The age of the thymus, the physiological condition of the animal, weather, and feeding, all can vary the synthetic ability of the nucleus in ways that

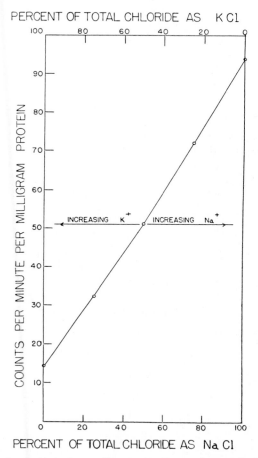

FIG. 5. The effect of varying sodium/potassium ratio on glycine-1-C[14] incorporation by isolated thymus nuclei. The specific activity of the nuclear protein after 60 minutes incubation is plotted against the ratio of sodium to potassium ions in the medium, the total salt concentration being held constant.

cannot be predicted or controlled. The actual amount of amino acid incorporated in a given time varies from one nuclear preparation to another, and it is necessary to run careful "controls" when comparisons are being made.

The synthetic activity of the isolated nucleus can be readily destroyed by heating, by freezing and thawing, or by breaking them in the blendor. Nuclei stored at 2° C. gradually lose their ability to incorporate amino acids. The rate of decline in activity with storage varies considerably in different preparations; but in most cases activity is well retained for 4 to 6 hours and is almost entirely lost after 24 hours at 2° C.

"Synthesis" vs. "Exchange"

Several experiments will now be described which make it clear that the uptake of labeled amino acids into nuclear proteins represents protein synthesis and is not simply a random, non-specific exchange reaction.

The first of these experiments is the demonstration that only the

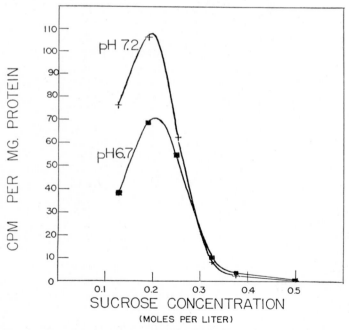

EFFECT OF SUCROSE CONCENTRATION UPON C^{14} - ALANINE
INCORPORATION BY THYMUS NUCLEI

FIG. 6.   The effect of varying sucrose concentration on alanine-1-C^{14} incorporation by isolated nuclei. The specific activity of the nuclear protein after 60 minutes incubation is plotted against the sucrose concentration of the incubation medium.

L-isomer of the administered DL-alanine-1-C^{14} is incorporated into nuclear protein. The ability of the nucleus to distinguish between D and L forms of the amino acid is indicated by the experiments summarized in Fig. 7. In these tests increasing amounts of unlabeled D-alanine or unlabeled L-alanine were added to the incubation medium together with the DL-alanine-1-C^{14}. If both the D and the L forms of the C^{14}-alanine were utilized by the nucleus, then both unlabeled isomers should compete with isotopic molecules for acceptance by the nucleus, and the C^{14} activity of the nuclear protein should be correspondingly lowered. Actually, the addition of unlabeled D-alanine has no such effect; only the L-isomer competes for incorporation. It follows, therefore, that only the L-form of the C^{14}-alanine administered is utilized for protein synthesis by the nucleus.

A second experiment was designed to test whether the incorporated amino acid is in constant exchange with other amino-acid molecules in the medium. If the uptake of amino acids is indeed reversible, then C^{14}-alanine once incorporated into nuclear proteins should be exchanged with unlabeled L-alanine added to the medium after incorporation has occurred. This was tested in the experiments summarized in Fig. 8. Incorporation of C^{14}-alanine was allowed to proceed for 60 minutes. At that time the nuclei were centrifuged down and the isotopic alanine was removed. The nuclei were then resuspended in the presence of a 200-fold excess of unlabeled L-alanine. Samples of the nuclei were removed at 30-minute intervals and the carbon-14 activity of the nuclear protein measured in the usual way. It is evident from the curves that the specific activity of the nuclear protein remains constant for 3 hours even in the presence of a great excess of unlabeled L-alanine. It follows that C^{14}-alanine once incorporated into nuclear protein is not constantly being replaced by unlabeled alanine in the medium. The figure also shows that when additional C^{14}-alanine is added to the nuclei in such experiments, incorporation proceeds in the usual way. Thus the nuclei will continue to incorporate C^{14}-amino acid under conditions where they will not give it up. Similar experiments have been performed using S^{35}-labeled methionine, and the same results were obtained. It follows that the incorporation of amino acids into the proteins of isolated nuclei represents an irreversible, or synthetic, rather than an exchange reaction.

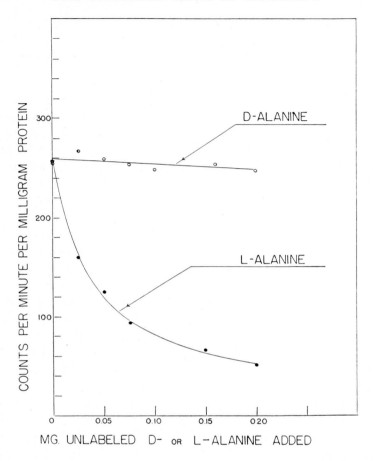

Fig. 7. The effect of unlabeled D- and L-alanines upon incorporation of DL-alanine-1-C14 by isolated thymus nuclei. The specific activity of the nuclear protein after 60 minutes incubation is plotted against the amount of unlabeled D- or L-alanine added to the medium.

It may be of value at this point to clarify our usage of the term "protein synthesis." In the strictest sense this should be applied only when a net synthesis of protein can be demonstrated. When such synthesis occurs in the presence of isotopically labeled amino acids the protein formed will be labeled. However, the incorporation of isotopic amino acids does not in itself constitute a proof that new protein molecules have been synthesized. In our experiments a net synthesis of protein has not been demonstrated directly, but the irreversibility of the amino acid uptake makes it most probable that we are dealing with a very direct aspect of the synthetic mechanism.

From the amount of isotopic alanine incorporated an estimate can be made of the amount of new protein which may be formed. In a typical experiment 30 mg. of nuclei (10^9 nuclei) incorporate 0.6 μg. (2.4 per cent) of the administered C^{14}-alanine in one hour. If the average nuclear protein contains about 7.6 per cent alanine (9), this uptake corresponds to the formation of about 8 μg. of protein per hour, an amount too small to be demonstrated directly by methods now available to us. Nevertheless, the extent of the synthesis can be better appreciated from the calculation that each nucleus synthesizes 22 molecules of protein of average molecular weight 50,000 every second.

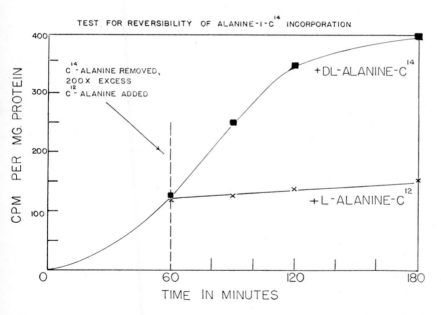

FIG. 8. The retention of incorporated alanine-1-C^{14} following addition of a large excess of unlabeled alanine, after uptake has occurred. [See text.] The specific activity of the nuclear protein at different intervals after adding unlabeled alanine is plotted against time.

Attempts have been made to stimulate the incorporation of isotopic alanine and glycine by the addition of a supplement of mixed L-amino acids to the medium. No stimulation was observed, a result which leads to the conclusion that, if the uptake of isotopic amino acids represents a net synthesis of protein, the other amino acids required must be present in the nuclei. This is indeed the case for thymus nuclei isolated by the Behrens procedure (15).

The Role of Deoxyribonucleic Acid in Protein Synthesis

The notion originally suggested by Brachet and by Caspersson that ribonucleic acids play a role in protein synthesis is now widely accepted as demonstrated. The most direct evidence in its favor stems from the work of Gale and Folkes (13) on amino acid uptake by bacterial cell residues, and from work in our laboratory on amino acid incorporation by a ribonucleoprotein complex of the liver (2). In both cases ribonuclease acts to suppress amino acid incorporation.

The isolated cell nucleus affords a unique opportunity to test the role of the deoxyribonucleic acids in the process of protein synthesis, and the results have a special interest because they ultimately bear on the mode of action of the gene, and on the chemical relationships between the nucleus and the cytoplasm.

A number of experiments which relate deoxyribonucleic acid to the process of protein synthesis in the nucleus will now be described. Several of these experiments deal with the effect of deoxyribonuclease on the uptake of labeled amino acids. When isolated nuclei are treated with crystalline pancreatic deoxyribonuclease before adding isotopic amino acids, the incorporation of the latter is markedly impaired. The degree of impairment becomes more serious as more and more of the deoxyribonucleic acid is removed. Experiments showing the relationship between loss of DNA and inhibition of alanine-1-C^{14} and lysine-2-C^{14} uptakes are summarized in Fig. 9. At the outset there is roughly a 1:1 correspondence between the percentage of DNA removed and the percentage of inhibition of the uptake. The inhibition becomes more marked when 30 to 80 per cent of the DNA is removed. Beyond that point the loss of DNA has little effect on the uptake, which remains constant at about 15 to 20 per cent of that observed in "control" experiments. This sensitivity of the nucleus to treatment with deoxyribonuclease is further evidence for the absence of appreciable whole

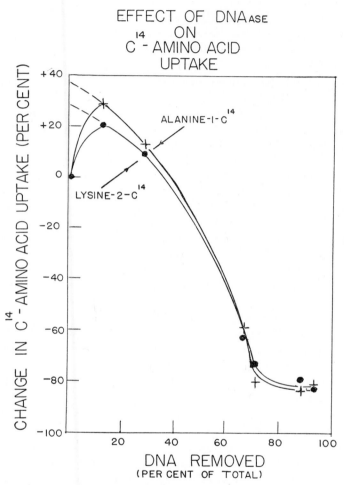

FIG. 9. The effect of removing DNA from thymus nuclei upon the subsequent incorporation of alanine-1-C[14] and lysine-2-C[14]. Nuclei were pretreated with DNAase to remove increasing amounts of their DNA. They were subsequently incubated for 60 minutes in the presence of the isotopic amino acid. The decrease in specific activity of the nuclear protein in treated nuclei, relative to that observed in "control" nuclei, is plotted against the per cent removal of the DNA.

cell contamination, because intact cells are not sensitive to treatment with this enzyme. Thymus tissue slices or minces, for example, show only a very slight inhibition of alanine-1-C^{14} uptake following treatment with deoxyribonuclease, and the inhibition observed could easily be attributed to enzyme attack upon cells which had been damaged mechanically.

The foregoing experiments suggest that deoxyribonucleic acid plays a direct role in nuclear protein synthesis. Additional support for this conclusion arises from experiments which test whether the synthetic activity of nuclei treated with deoxyribonuclease can be restored by the addition of supplementary DNA. In these experiments the nuclei were treated with deoxyribonuclease until 70 per cent or more of the DNA had been released into the medium. The nuclei were then centrifuged down, and the medium containing the products of DNA hydrolysis was removed. The nuclei were then resuspended in the presence of a calf thymus DNA preparation; isotopic amino acid was supplied, and incorporation allowed to proceed for 60 minutes. The specific activity of the protein in nuclei which had received the deoxyribonucleic acid supplement was then compared with the protein "activities" in control nuclei which had been treated with the enzyme in the same way but which had not received any additional deoxyribonucleic acid. The data in Table 3 make it clear that added calf thymus DNA does in fact restore much, and at times, all of the original activity of the nucleus. Pretreatment of the nucleus with deoxyribonuclease affects the uptake of different amino acids to different extents. Methionine-S^{35} incorporation, for example, is reduced only 40 per cent under conditions where alanine-C^{14} uptake is inhibited 75 per cent. However, the addition of supplementary DNA seems to restore the lost activity equally in both cases.

Several experiments were performed to test whether chemically or physically modified DNA could restore the uptake in DNAase-treated nuclei. It was found that DNA denatured by treatment with alkali (pH 12.2 for 16 hours) (11) was just as effective as the original DNA preparation. Apurinic acid, while not as effective as intact DNA, does produce an appreciable stimulation of uptake in the DNAase-treated nuclei. The non-dialyzable DNA "core" which remains after exhaustive digestion of thymus DNA with deoxyribonuclease (27) and the dialyzable split products of the digestion are both able to replace the "whole" DNA in this system.

TABLE 3

Effect of Supplementary Calf Thymus DNA in Restoring C^{14}-Alanine Uptake in DNAase-Treated Nuclei

Supplement tested	Specific Activity of Nuclear Protein			Activity lost c.p.m./mg.	Activity regained c.p.m./mg.	Percentage of lost activity regained
	"Control" nuclei c.p.m./mg.	DNAase-treated nuclei c.p.m./mg.	Treated nuclei + supplement c.p.m./mg.			
A. Thymus DNA	99	15	55	84	40	48
B. Thymus DNA	135	21	93	114	72	64
C. Thymus DNA	99	33	101	66	68	103
", alkali-denatured	99	33	104	66	71	108
D. Thymus DNA	40	10	29	30	19	63
", apurinic acid	40	10	17.4	30	7.4	25
E. Thymus DNA	38	7.5	28	30.5	20.5	67
" "Core" after DNAase digestion	38	7.5	24.5	30.5	17	56
" dialyzable after DNAase digestion	38	7.5	29	30.5	21.5	70

TABLE 5

EFFECT OF RIBONUCLEIC ACID AND RIBONUCLEOTIDES ON C^{14}-ALANINE UPTAKE IN DNAase-TREATED NUCLEI

Supplement tested	Specific Activity of Nuclear Protein			Activity lost c.p.m./mg.	Activity regained c.p.m./mg.	Percentage of lost activity regained
	"Control" nuclei c.p.m./mg.	DNAase-treated nuclei c.p.m./mg.	Treated nuclei + supplement c.p.m./mg.			
A. Calf liver RNA	92	54	80	38	26	68
Calf thymus DNA	92	54	81	38	27	71
B. Thymus DNA	68	23	54	45	31	69
Yeast RNA	68	23	58	45	35	78
" hydrolyzed in 0.3 N NaOH	68	23	23	45	0	0
" dialyzable after RNAase digestion	68	23	36	45	13	29
A,G,C,U mononucleotide mixture	68	23	23	45	0	0
C. Thymus DNA	83	14	46	69	32	46
Yeast RNA	83	14	45	69	31	45
Adenylic-adenylic dinucleotide	83	14	18	69	4	6
Adenylic-guanylic dinucleotide	83	14	18	69	4	6
Adenylic-uridylic dinucleotide	83	14	18	69	4	6
Guanylic-cytidylic dinucleotide	83	14	18	69	4	6

A, adenylic; G, guanylic; C, cytidylic; U, uridylic.

adding C^{14}-amino acids has no effect on the uptake of the latter. However, this result does not permit the conclusion that ribonucleic acid plays no part in nuclear protein synthesis, because in the experiments mentioned only 54 per cent of the nuclear RNA could be released by the action of the enzyme.

It was previously noted that the uptake of isotopic amino acids into the proteins of thymus nuclei is not a readily reversible, exchange-type reaction. This conclusion was obtained from experiments which showed that labeled amino acids once incorporated into nuclear proteins cannot be replaced by non-labeled amino acids in the medium. Similar experiments were performed on DNAase-treated nuclei which were supplemented with either thymus DNA or yeast RNA. These tests are summarized in Fig. 10. In both cases the uptake was irreversible; the nuclei did not lose isotopic amino acid once it was incorporated. The failure to "exchange" cannot be the result of a loss of activity, because such nuclei given C^{14}-alanine show an extensive C^{14} uptake into their proteins.

Since in the intact nucleus, deoxyribonucleic acid is required for protein synthesis, the question naturally arises as to how the DNA participates in amino acid incorporation. Several experiments were performed to test whether the action of deoxyribonucleic acid requires the active participation of its free phosphate groups. The results of these experiments are summarized in Table 6. The procedure used was to add varying amounts of basic compounds which are known to combine with the free phosphoric acid groups of deoxyribonucleic acid. The compounds selected included the basic dye methyl green, and two basic proteins, namely, protamine, and a lysine-rich histone prepared from calf thymus. It is clear that the addition of small amounts of methyl green, protamine or histone to the nuclei before adding the isotopic amino acid has little effect on the uptake. Large amounts lead to a partial impairment of carbon-14 incorporation; but the impairment may reflect osmotic or other damage to the system, since large amounts of added serum albumin also decrease the uptake. The results suggest that some of the free phosphate groups of the DNA can be blocked without affecting the uptake of labeled amino acids.

WHICH NUCLEAR PROTEINS BECOME LABELED?

The answer to this question depends at the outset upon the existence of a dependable and meaningful scheme of fractionating the proteins

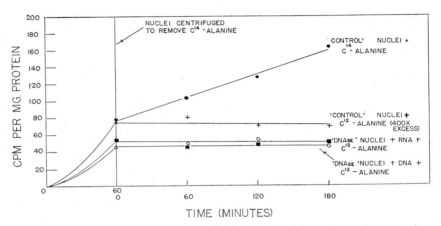

TEST FOR REVERSIBILITY OF ALANINE-I-C^{14} INCORPORATION IN DNA SE-TREATED
NUCLEI 'RESTORED' WITH A NUCLEIC ACID SUPPLEMENT

TIME (MINUTES)

Fig. 10. The retention of alanine-1-C^{14} incorporated into the nuclear proteins of DNAase-treated nuclei "restored" with thymus DNA or yeast RNA. [See text.] The nuclei were treated with DNAase; then given a nucleic acid supplement and incubated in the presence of C^{14}-alanine. They were then centrifuged down and resuspended in the presence of a great excess of unlabeled L-alanine. The specific activity of the nuclear protein at different intervals after adding unlabeled alanine is plotted against time.

of the nucleus. This is a field of endeavor which is now in its earliest stages of development, though it promises to become a major topic of biochemical investigation.

We have developed a *provisional* fractionation procedure which is applicable to the proteins of thymus "sucrose" nuclei, and which permits the separation of several classes of proteins of different properties and considerable biological interest. In its essentials the procedure is as follows (see Flow Sheet, Fig. 11). The nuclei are incubated in buffered sucrose medium in the presence of C^{14}-alanine. After uptake has occurred, the nuclei are centrifuged down, and the protein released into the medium is precipitated with trichloroacetic acid (TCA). The amount of this protein in the medium increases with the time of incubation, but it has a very low specific activity relative to the other proteins of the nucleus. The uptake into this fraction does not seem to be dependent upon DNA, since pretreatment of the nuclei with DNAase does not affect it. The nuclei are next extracted with *p*H 7.1 potassium phosphate buffer. This extract contains some RNA and a

TABLE 6

EFFECT OF METHYL GREEN, PROTAMINE, AND A HISTONE UPON C[14]-AMINO ACID
INCORPORATION BY ISOLATED CALF THYMUS NUCLEI

Conditions of Experiment	Isotope administered as	Specific Activity of Nuclear Protein c.p.m. per mg.	Change in C[14] Uptake per cent
A. "Control" nuclei	DL-alanine-1-C[14]	154	—
Nuclei +0.125 mg. methyl green	" "	167	+8
" +0.25 mg. " "	" "	162	+5
" +0.50 mg. " "	" "	116	−25
B. "Control" nuclei	glycine-1-C[14]	205	—
Nuclei +0.25 mg. methyl green	" "	251	+22
C. "Control" nuclei		89	—
Nuclei +0.50 mg. methyl green		64	−28
D. "Control" nuclei	DL-alanine-1-C[14]	154	—
Nuclei +0.375 mg. protamine	"	168	+9
" +0.75 mg. "	"	159	+3
" +1.50 mg. "	"	164	+6
E. "Control" nuclei	glycine-1-C[14]	79	—
Nuclei +1.5 mg. protamine	"	70	−11
Nuclei +1.5 mg. histone (lysine-rich)	"	76	−4

FRACTIONATION OF THE PROTEINS OF
ISOLATED CALF THYMUS NUCLEI

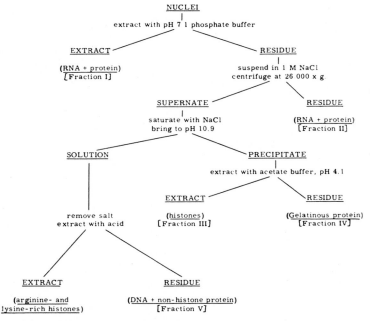

FIG. 11.   Flow-Sheet for the fractionation of the proteins of isolated calf thymus nuclei. [See text.]

small amount of protein, the yield of which seems to diminish as the incubation is prolonged. This protein (Fraction I) has considerable interest because at times it is the most actively labeled fraction of the nucleus. The uptake of isotope into this fraction is almost completely abolished by pretreating the nuclei with DNAase and is not affected by pretreatment with RNAase.

The nuclei are then suspended in 1 M sodium chloride, in which they swell and largely dissolve. The opalescent solution is centrifuged at 26,000 g to sediment the undissolved material. This residue (Fraction II) comprises about 10 per cent of the nuclear mass and contains one-third of the nuclear ribonucleic acid. There is evidence to suggest that this fraction contains the nucleoli (7). The supernatant after high-speed centrifugation contains the bulk of the protein of the nucleus and all of the deoxyribonucleic acid. It can be fractionated to yield different histones, a gelatinous protein, and an unfractionated residue (4). The protein in the latter is firmly attached to the DNA. The distribution of C^{14} activity in these different protein fractions is a matter of some interest (Table 7). (It should be mentioned that the

TABLE 7

ALANINE-1-C^{14} INCORPORATION INTO DIFFERENT PROTEIN FRACTIONS OF THYMUS NUCLEI

Protein Fraction	Specific Activity c.p.m. per mg.
Total nuclear protein	107
Fraction I [protein soluble in pH 7.1 buffer]	179
Fraction II [residue after extraction in M NaCl]	117
Fraction III [histones]	36
Fraction IV [gelatinous protein]	157
Fraction V [non-histone protein associated with DNA]	243

total analine contents of each of the several protein fractions is very similar, so that differences in carbon-14 concentration reflect differences in the metabolic activity of the various proteins.) For example, it was found that the protein most closely associated with the DNA is more active than all other proteins of the nucleus, excepting the small fraction extracted in pH 7.1 buffer. This result lends further support to the conclusion drawn from deoxyribonuclease experiments that the DNA plays a direct role in protein synthesis. A second point of interest is the fact that the level of isotope incorporation into the histone proteins is relatively low. This result agrees with earlier experiments in vivo (8) in which it was noted that the incorporation of glycine-N^{15} into the histones of mouse liver, pancreas, and kidney is much lower than the uptake into the residual proteins of the chromosome.

NUCLEIC ACID SYNTHESIS

The question now arises as to whether the isolated thymus nucleus can synthesize nucleic acid by itself. This was tested by incubating the nuclei in the presence of C^{14}-labeled glycine, a substance known to be a precursor of the purine ring in nucleic acid biosynthesis. Table 8 summarizes some preliminary experiments in which incorporation was demonstrated in three ways. In the first, the total nucleic acid was extracted with hot TCA and prepared by zone electrophoresis. It may contain a trace of adsorbed protein. In the other experiments either

TABLE 8

Incorporation of Glycine-1-C[14] into the Proteins and Nucleic Acids
of Isolated Calf Thymus Nuclei

Nuclear Component	Specific Activity c.p.m. per mg.
Total Nuclear Protein	117
Nucleic Acid prepared by zone electrophoresis	19
Nucleotides prepared on Dowex—1	11
Purines prepared on Dowex—50	57

the nucleotides or the purines were separated on ion-exchange resins. In all cases a detectable amount of isotope appeared in the nucleic acid. Tests are under way to see whether this process, like protein synthesis, is affected by pretreatment of the nuclei with deoxyribonuclease.

Energy-Yielding Mechanisms in Isolated Nuclei

As considerable energy is required for the active synthesis of protein, one would expect the nuclei to contain an energy-generating system, possibly involving energy-rich compounds such as ATP and related nucleotides. It has already been pointed out that the incorporation of C^{14}-amino acids is an aerobic phenomenon which is inhibited by many inhibitors of oxidative phosphorylation.

It has been shown that thymus nuclei isolated by the Behrens procedure have a complete complement of acid-soluble nucleotides, including AMP, ADP, and ATP (4). When similar analyses were performed on thymus nuclei isolated in sucrose solutions it was found that they retained from 60 to 80 per cent of their original acid-soluble nucleotide content. These nucleotides were well retained after repeated washings with cold sucrose and calcium chloride solution. From the analyses of the nucleotides found in thymus nuclei, a surprising observation came to light. During the preparation of "sucrose" nuclei in the cold, the nucleotide monophosphates characteristic of the excised tissue are largely converted back to the energy-rich triphosphate forms which predominate in the living tissue. This was proved to be an intranuclear phenomenon (4), probably the result of extensive aeration of the nuclear suspension during the isolation procedure.

The experiments summarized in Table 9 show that ATP synthesis in the isolated nucleus can be inhibited by a number of substances

TABLE 9

EFFECTS OF METABOLIC INHIBITORS ON PHOSPHORYLATION OF NUCLEOTIDES IN ISOLATED CALF THYMUS SUCROSE NUCLEI

Inhibitor	Concentration	Change in Phosphorylation due to added inhibitor per cent	Inhibitory effect on Nuclear phosphorylation	Mitochondrial phosphorylation
Sodium cyanide	$1 \times 10^{-3}M$	-100	+	+
Carbon monoxide	100 per cent	-100	+	+
2,4-Dinitrophenol	$2 \times 10^{-4}M$	-100	+	+
Sodium azide	$1 \times 10^{-3}M$	-100	+	+
Antimycin A	1 μg./ml.	-61	+	+
Dicumarol	$1 \times 10^{-4}M$	0	−	+
Janus Green B	$2 \times 10^{-5}M$	$+6$	−	+
Methylene Blue	$2 \times 10^{-5}M$	$+30$	−	+
"	$2.5 \times 10^{-4}M$	$+21$	−	+
Calcium ions	$2 \times 10^{-2}M$	0	−	+
" "	$3 \times 10^{-3}M$	0	−	+
" "	$4 \times 10^{-4}M$	0	−	+

which block or uncouple oxidative phosphorylation. The effects obtained resemble those obtained in isolated mitochondria when one considers inhibitors such as cyanide, azide, dinitrophenol, Antimycin A, and carbon monoxide. It differs from any mitochondrial system known to us in its resistance to Janus Green B, Methylene Blue, dicumarol, and calcium ions. [Another point of difference is that thymus nuclei do not appear to contain any cytochrome c oxidase activity (22).]

Other experiments have shown that although the nucleotides are firmly held within the nucleus they can be released (at lower pH values) by adding small amounts of acetate. This permits a correlation to be made between the amount of nucleotide lost and the resulting inhibition of alanine-1-C^{14} uptake. These results will be published elsewhere.

Summary

Nuclei prepared from calf thymus in a sucrose medium actively incorporate labeled amino acids into their proteins. This is an irreversible, synthetic reaction which requires the participation of the deoxyribonucleic acid of the nucleus. Therefore a biochemical function of DNA is to mediate the synthesis of protein in the chromosome.

In the essential mechanism of amino acid uptake, the role of the DNA can be filled by denatured or partially degraded DNA, by DNA from other tissues, and even by RNA. Purine and pyrimidine bases, nucleotides, and certain dinucleotides are unable to substitute for DNA in this system.

When the proteins of the nucleus are fractionated and classified according to their specific activities, one finds the histones to be relatively inert. The protein fraction most closely associated with the DNA has a very high activity. A readily extractable ribonucleoprotein complex is also extremely active. It is tempting to speculate that this may be an intermediary in nucleo-cytoplasmic interaction.

The isolated nucleus can incorporate glycine into its nucleic acids.

Together with earlier observations (e.g., 19) on the incorporation of amino acids by cytoplasmic particulates, these results show that protein synthesis can occur in both nucleus and cytoplasm.

It has been shown that the nucleus can meet the energy requirements of protein synthesis. It is endowed with oxidative systems which generate high-energy phosphate bonds.

REFERENCES

1. Allfrey, V. G., *Proc. Natl. Acad. Sci. U. S.,* **40**, 881 (1954).
2. Allfrey, V. G., Daly, M. M., and Mirsky, A. E., *J. Gen. Physiol.,* **37**, 157 (1953).
3. Allfrey, V. G., Daly, M. M., and Mirsky, A. E., *J. Gen. Physiol.,* **38**, 415 (1955).
4. Allfrey, V. G., Mirsky, A. E., and Osawa, S., *Nature,* **176**, 1042 (1955).
5. Allfrey, V. G., Stern, H., Mirsky, A. E., and Saetren, H., *J. Gen. Physiol.,* **35**, 529 (1952).
6. Behrens, M., in *Handbuch der biologischen Arbeitsmethoden* (E. Abderhalden, ed.), Vol. X, p. 1363, Urban and Schwartzenberg, Berlin and Vienna (1938).
7. Bessis, M. C., in *Traité de Cytologie Sanguine,* p. 83, Masson & Cie., Paris (1954).
8. Daly, M. M., Allfrey, V. G., and Mirsky, A. E., *J. Gen. Physiol.,* **36**, 173 (1952).
9. Daly, M. M., and Mirsky, A. E., *J. Gen. Physiol.,* **38**, 405 (1955).
10. Dounce, A. L., Tischkoff, G. H., Barnett, S. R., and Freer, R. M., *J. Gen. Physiol.,* **33**, 629 (1949).
11. Ehrlich, P., and Doty, P., *J. Am. Chem. Soc.,* in press.
12. Gale, E. F., and Folkes, J. P., *Biochem. J.,* **53**, 493 (1953).
13. Gale, E. F., and Folkes, J. P., *Biochem. J.,* **55**, xi (1953).
14. Halvorson, H. O., and Spiegelman, S., *J. Bacteriol.,* **64**, 207 (1952).
15. Kay, E. R. M., *Federation Proc.,* **15**, 107 (1956).
16. Mirsky, A. E., and Ris, H., *Nature,* **163**, 666 (1949).
17. Schneider, R. M., and Peterman, M. L., *Cancer Research,* **10**, 751 (1950).
18. Santisteban, G. A., and Dougherty, T. F., *Endocrinology,* **54**, 130 (1954).
19. Siekevitz, P., *J. Biol. Chem.,* **195**, 549 (1952).
20. Stern, H., Allfrey, V. G., Mirsky, A. E., and Saetren, H., *J. Gen. Physiol.,* **35**, 559 (1952).
21. Stern, H., and Mirsky, A. E., *J. Gen. Physiol.,* **37**, 177 (1953).
22. Stern, H., and Timonen, S., *J. Gen. Physiol.,* **38**, 41 (1954).
23. Tamm, I., *Science,* **120**, 847 (1954).
24. Tamm, I., Folkers, K., and Shunk, C. H., *J. Bacteriol.,* in press.
25. Tamm, I., Folkers, K., Shunk, C. H., and Horsfall, F. L., Jr., *J. Exptl. Med.,* **99**, 227 (1954).
26. Wilson, E. B., *The Cell in Development and Heredity,* 3rd ed., p. 25, Macmillan, New York (1925).
27. Zamenhof, S., and Chargaff, E., *J. Biol. Chem.,* **187**, 1 (1950).

NUCLEIC ACIDS AND THE SYNTHESIS OF PROTEINS[1, 2]

S. SPIEGELMAN

Department of Bacteriology,
University of Illinois,
Urbana, Illinois

INTRODUCTION

THE PAST DECADE has witnessed the universal acceptance of a doctrine which may be phrased as follows: The key to the resolution of the basic issues of biologically specific syntheses is to be found in the interrelations existing within the triad of macromolecules RNA, DNA, and protein.

Data emerging from rather diverse disciplines have tended to support such concepts. While no one group of results can be taken as conclusive, the cumulative effect has served to elevate the "doctrine of the triad" to a central tenet of present-day biological thinking.

The present paper will attempt to inquire into the following questions:

(1) How well do the data on protein synthesis conform to the dogma so acceptable to our times?

(2) Where do we go from here?

In surveying knowledge relevant to the first question, we begin with the data on precursors and intermediates in protein synthesis and the implications of these for a template mechanism. The theoretical and experimental information pertinent to a decision on the chemical nature of the template are then examined. As a result we come to the somewhat reluctant conclusion that the time has come to take our faith

[1] The original investigations stemming from the author's laboratory were aided by grants from the National Cancer Institute of the U. S. Public Health Service and from the Office of Naval Research.

[2] The following abbreviations have been used: ribonucleic acid (RNA), deoxyribonucleic acid (DNA), ribonuclease (RNAase), deoxyribonuclease (DNAase), adenosinetriphosphate (ATP).

seriously and subject it to an experimental test which could hope to disprove it. This brings us naturally to the second question posed and to a consideration of the subcellular fractions developed in recent years by investigators who are seeking systems permitting a more direct dissective analysis of the protein-synthesizing mechanism.

THE TEMPLATE QUESTION

Two principal processes have been proposed as mechanisms for the formation of protein molecules. One envisages a step-wise synthesis of polypeptides of increasing length and complexity, ending ultimately in the finished product. It is implicitly assumed in such hypotheses that the individual steps are mediated by a series of specific enzymes. The alternative essentially denies this possibility and adopts the view that a single template is responsible for and guides the fabrication of a particular protein molecule.

The crucial difference between the two models lies in what may be referred to as the "geometrical sensing" inherent in each model. Aside from the initial reactions, the first mechanism implies that at each step contact between the appropriate catalyst and the molecule being formed is limited to relatively small proportions of the molecular structure of either. Consequently, each of the many catalysts can have but limited information of what has gone before. In the template mechanism, on the other hand, contact between the molecule being synthesized and the single guiding catalyst is comprehensive. The template can therefore in principle possess complete knowledge of geometrical detail at all stages in the synthesis of the protein molecule.

For simplicity, we will refer to these two alternatives as the "poly-enzyme" and "template" models. The question of which of these to adopt as a point of departure in the further analysis of the protein-synthesizing mechanism has been the subject of intensive (and repetitive) discussion in the published accounts of the multitude of symposia held within the past few years. The question is not definitively settled, and opinion, although favoring the template model, is not unanimous in the minds of those competent to form judgments (cf. Synge, 89). A justification is as yet therefore required of reasons for preferring the template hypothesis.

From the theoretical point of view, the poly-enzyme mechanism runs quickly into a dilemma which, if not insurmountable, is at least unpleasant. I refer to the question of the mechanism involved in the synthesis of the proteins which are presumed to serve as the individual catalysts in the formation of the other proteins.

Another difficulty is encountered in the face of the mounting evidence that the amino acid sequence of protein molecules is specified with considerable accuracy. The very fact that a unique sequence could have emerged from the ingenious experiments of Sanger (75) on the structure of insulin already argues forcibly for the relative rigidity of the specification. There is in addition the evidence (31) stemming from analysis of end and subterminal groups to support the same contention.

It is difficult to see how a multitude of sequentially cooperating individual enzymes could provide a mechanism for ordering amino acids in a previously specified sequence. Enzymes which are known to be capable of peptide bond formation do not have the requisite degree of specificity. There is the further problem of geometrical sensing. Consider the situation in which 50 out of 100 residues of a particular protein molecule have been put together. To make the proper choice, the catalyst presumed by the poly-enzyme mechanism to mediate the addition of the 51st amino acid would have to possess detailed information on the succession of the existing 50 amino acids. The difficulty of transmitting the required information would appear to pyramid for the stepwise mechanism as the synthesis progresses. It is evident that the theoretical difficulties just noted pose no problem for the template mechanism.

The available experimental data are equally discouraging for the poly-enzyme mechanism. Briefly noted are the following relevant findings.

(a) Preventing the utilization of any one amino acid by an effective analogue concomitantly suppresses the incorporation of all others into peptide linkages (45, 48).

(b) Experiments on the induced synthesis of specific proteins, such as enzymes and antibodies, lead to the conclusion that amino acids, or their activated derivatives, are the immediate precursors of finished protein molecules (20, 40, 46, 47, 52, 60, 62, 68, 71, 72, 77, 93). These experiments have used amino acid analogues, amino-acid–deficient organisms, tracers, and subsequent isolation of protein formed. All are in agreement.

(c) Nutritional experiments with whole animals, as well as cell and tissue cultures, lead to the same conclusions (26, 38, 39, 79).

(d) No convincing evidence for the existence of peptide intermediates has been found even under conditions where they might reasonably be expected to accumulate (45, 48, 19).

Labeling experiments in whole animals have, for the most part, supported the template mechanism (6, 7, 9, 11, 22, 49, 80). The only data which can be taken as even remotely supporting the existence of peptide intermediates are those of Anfinsen and his colleagues (4, 85, 94), who found evidence of unequal labeling in the synthesis of ovalbumen, insulin, and ribonuclease. However, a unique interpretation of unequal labeling is made impossible by a number of potential complications. Gale (33) and his colleagues have shown by the use of analogues and single amino acid supplementation that it is possible to dissociate incorporation from protein synthesis. One must therefore raise the question whether incorporation experiments exhibiting unequal labeling may not be telling us something about the geometry of the protein molecule, in terms of differential ease of exchange at localized points, rather than about the mechanism employed in putting this molecule together. It is important to emphasize that we do not maintain that the incorporation reaction is not part of the synthetic mechanism. It may, for example, occur only on the template. The point is that it need not involve the entire molecule, since Gale's evidence shows that incorporation can occur without being accompanied by the synthesis of a complete molecule. Unless an estimate of the extent of this "nonsynthetic" incorporation can be made, an unambiguous interpretation of the data is difficult. The possibilities that some tissues or proteins may be more prone to this type of reaction may explain the difference between the results obtained with Anfinsen's material and others.

Some General Considerations on the Nature of the Template

Those who adopt the template model of protein synthesis are mandatorily forced to accept as a more or less immediate task the identification of its chemical nature. There are two features one would ascribe a priori to a mold which is to serve as a guide in the construction of a protein molecule. One is that it must be at least as large as the compound being synthesized, and the other that it contain in its structure the information prescribing the residue sequence.

Disregarding the physical and concentrating only on the purely logical aspects of the situation, any macromolecule composed of two or more distinguishable elements could serve the purpose. That two are sufficient follows immediately from the existence of Boolean algebra. It should be noted that the term "element" possesses in the present context a rather broad significance. Thus, a macromolecule composed of identical residues could still in principle satisfy the requirement if it possessed two types of linkages between the residues. Such limitations of logic would admit many sorts of molecules as suitable candidates for our template, including lipids and polysaccharides. In point of fact, of course, relatively few are given serious consideration in the literature, and many possibilities have never even been mentioned as such. This raises an interesting question of omission which has received but little explicit attention and which we may pause here briefly to discuss. Aside from the question of faith in the triad concept, a number of rational arguments can in fact be invoked to narrow down considerably the number of macromolecules worthy of careful examination.

On the assumption that the template structure functions physically in imposing a restriction of sequence, plausible grounds can be offered for eliminating certain types of macromolecules as possible candidates for a template. Thus, despite the logical sufficiency, it seems unlikely that macromolecules composed of only two elements could serve in determining protein structure. The reasons are essentially geometrical in nature and involve questions of molecular distances. Selection must be made from amongst 20 different amino acids. Consequently, a two-element template would have to employ a minimum of five elements in the choice of a given amino acid at a particular point of a sequence. For compounds like polysaccharides this would involve distances of about 25Å. Similarly, one would tend to disregard macromolecules composed of three or even more elements in which all but two were present in relatively small proportions.

Another factor influencing our search amongst the macromolecules for a suitable template stems from our belief in the basic similarity and unity of biosynthetic systems. Unless forced to do so by incontrovertible evidence, we are not likely to entertain the premise that such a centrally necessary mechanism as protein synthesis would be mediated in some forms by one type of chemical template, and by a completely different sort in others. This point of view necessarily leads to the immediate elimination of many macromolecules which are unique to particular cell types. Attention is thereby focused on a small class which is known to be universally distributed throughout the living kingdom.

One other point may be made, related to the very probable assumption that the amino acid sequence of a protein molecule is rigidly determined. It follows that the sequence of template elements must be ordered with an equivalent accuracy. If this be accepted, we must discard all macromolecules which are synthesized by a mechanism which does not inherently contain a plausible device for specifying element sequence. Thus, the very reasons that led us earlier to adopt a template model for protein synthesis force us to eliminate as templates macromolecules which are synthesized stepwise by one or more cooperating enzymes.

It is important to emphasize explicitly that we are not categorically denying the involvement of enzymes in the formation of templates. We are proposing that if enzymes do play a role they cannot be the determinants of the sequence of elements in a template.

In summary, then, the general analysis of the protein template problem leads us to postulate a macromolecule which is universally distributed, composed in large part of at least three elements in roughly equivalent proportions, and synthesized by a mechanism insuring accurate ordering.

There are only three candidates which one can at the present time offer as suitable, and we are thus returned to members of our triad, RNA, DNA, and protein. Here we must admit we are making a virtue out of our ignorance, particularly with regard to the third property noted. Many macromolecules are eliminated by virtue of the fact that we know enough of the details of their synthesis to be certain that ordering does not emerge as a consequence of the mechanism. Our uncertainty as to the synthetic details of our three candidates is sufficient to permit retention of the hope that an ordering device exists.

The analysis can be pushed one step further under the rather naive assumption that only one of the three serves as the template and that it is functionally and generically independent of the other two. Thus, consider the proposition that protein is the template for making more protein. One is immediately faced with a dilemma we have already encountered—what makes the protein templates? There are two ways out, both, however, equally unpalatable biologically. One could suppose that all proteins are capable of self-duplication. The other would assume that only certain proteins can serve as templates for the synthesis of other proteins, but that these templates possess, in addition to this heterocatalytic capacity, the ability to catalyze their own synthesis. Either hypothesis would confer a degree of biological autonomy on proteins that few would agree to and for which there exists no supporting experimental evidence.

It should be noted that this line of reasoning argues only against protein alone being the template. It does not make unlikely the possibility that protein may function as a component of the template in consort with one or the other of the nucleic acids.

We should now like to turn our attention to data which could help in deciding between the two nucleic acids as components of the protein-synthesizing mechanism. We shall first consider data derived from experiments with intact cells and tissues.

Experiments with Intact Cells Relevant to the Chemical Nature of the Template

Evidence from work with the transformation principles offers convincing evidence that genetic information can be stored in and transmitted through DNA. The potentiality, therefore, of forming any specific kind of protein molecule must ultimately be referable to the DNA of the cell. However, the question being entertained at the present moment is whether DNA is directly and *personally* involved in the synthesis of protein or whether it effects its influence *via* an intermediary differing from itself and which is the actual template. Evidence leading to a decisive conclusion with intact cells is at present not available and, by the very nature of the question, probably not attainable. With such material the best that can be offered is a series of experiments inquiring whether a correlation can be established between the metabolic activity or state of DNA and the act of the synthesis of new protein molecules.

There exists a variety of experiments which demonstrate a complete dissociation of DNA metabolism from the synthesis of protein. DNA formation is known (1) to be far more sensitive to inhibition by radiation with x-rays than is protein formation. Baron, Spiegelman, and Quastler (8) have shown that x-ray dosages far exceeding those expected to stop the formation of DNA completely permit, nevertheless, normal enzyme synthesis in yeasts. Kelner's studies (56) on photoreactivation of *Escherichia coli* following exposure to ultraviolet have provided an elegant method for a virtually complete separation of RNA and protein formation from net DNA synthesis. Halvorson and Jackson (44), employing yeasts, have repeated and confirmed these findings.

Cohen and Barner (27) have reported the ability of a thymine-less mutant of *E. coli* which can synthesize xylose isomerase in the absence of an added supply of thymine. This important finding was confirmed in our own laboratory (42), using the same mutant but examining the formation of β-galactosidase. It was found that cells of this strain synthesized considerable amounts of the enzyme when suspended in a synthetic medium lacking thymine. The use of C^{14}-glycine in the same investigation provided convincing evidence that the DNA was metabolically inert. The behavior of the thymine-less strain is in striking contrast to that observed with mutants possessing other metabolic deficiencies. Thus, in our own experience and in that of others (68, 70), mutants deficient for adenine, uracil, or amino acids synthesize little or no enzyme in the absence of the required metabolite.

An interesting apparent exception to the data just cited is that of Allfrey's observation (2) with isolated nuclei of thymocytes. He found that treatment with DNAase suppressed the ability of his preparations to incorporate labeled amino acids. The fact that DNA from a variety of sources, as well as degraded DNA, can restore incorporating ability (3) makes it difficult to interpret these findings at present.

The data cited above demonstrate that drastic interference with DNA synthesis is often not accompanied by very striking effects on the formation of protein. They would appear to make unlikely the possibility that DNA is actively participating in the fabrication of new protein molecules. The credence and weight assignable to such negative conclusions with respect to DNA gain further weight from similar experiments which have studied the relation between protein synthesis and RNA metabolism and which yielded strikingly different results.

Ever since the suggestions of Caspersson (23) and Brachet (13), many have postulated RNA as a key substance in protein synthesis. Chantrenne (24) and Brachet (15) have recently summarized such speculations and examined the nature of the supporting evidence.

Much of the earlier data is essentially correlative and need not be detailed here. It may be said at the outset that the relationship between RNA and protein synthesis is not reciprocal since RNA formation can occur unaccompanied by protein synthesis. The recent remarkable findings being summarized in the present symposium by Ochoa represent a dramatic example of such dissociation.

Certain suggestive interrelations between RNA and protein synthesis emerged from the earlier studies of Gale and Folkes (34, 34a) and from some more recent investigations which we should like to note. They reveal an intriguing dependence of nucleic acid synthesis on amino acid availability which is also strikingly exhibited in experiments with osmotically-ruptured preparations of protoplasts to be described in subsequent sections.

Using washed suspensions of *Staphylococcus aureus*, Gale and Folkes (34a) found that the formation of nucleic acid in the presence of an added supply of purine and pyrimidine bases was greatly stimulated by including an amino acid mixture.

The interesting thing about this augmentation is that it also occurs (34) in the presence of sufficient chloramphenicol to prevent protein synthesis. This shows that nucleic acid formation can be dissociated from protein synthesis, a possibility subsequently confirmed by Wisseman and his colleagues (98a). Of greater immediate interest is the elimination of protein synthesis in attempts to explain the stimulation of nucleic acid formation by amino acids. The data suggest the necessity of looking for the answer in terms of the amino acids themselves or small molecular weight derivatives of them.

Pardee and Prestidge (70a) recently reexamined this question with the aid of amino acid auxotrophic mutants. They found that the synthesis of RNA was virtually eliminated in arginineless, valineless, tryptophanless, and threonineless mutants when the required amino acid was omitted from the incubation mixture. The amount of RNA formed when these mutants were supplemented with the relevant amino acid was proportional to the amount of the amino acid added. This strong dependence on the presence of the required metabolite was not exhibited, however, in the case of methionineless mutants. The peculiarity with respect to the methionine requirement is referable to the amino acid deficiency rather than to the strain, since in the case of a double mutant, which was methionineless and leucineless, RNA synthesis was possible in the absence of methionine but not when leucine was omitted.

The effect of chloramphenicol on these systems was revealing. In the presence of limiting amounts of the required amino acids, chloramphenicol stimulated the synthesis of RNA, whereas in the absence of these trace amounts the presence of the antibiotic did not lead to RNA formation.

These data support rather strongly the conclusion derivable from the Gale and Folkes experiments. The experiments of Pardee and Prestidge permit a further analysis of this intriguing situation. In view of the number and kinds of amino acids they tested and found necessary, it seems unlikely that we are dealing here with a supply of precursors of the nucleic acid building blocks. Their findings imply rather that the amino acids are serving in some sort of catalytic role. Again, the fact that chloramphenicol stimulates this catalytic activity precisely when the supply of a necessary amino acid is limited would appear to make unlikely the possibility that the catalytic effect is mediated through the formation of some necessary protein.

Pardee and Prestidge are inclined to reject the hypothesis that the amino acids stimulate RNA synthesis by serving as "low molecular weight cofactors." I am, however, inclined to retain this possibility in at least one particular form. The experiments we have just summarized suggest the possible existence of a common precursor for both protein and RNA. The work of Hoagland (51) and DeMoss and Novelli (29) already implicates nucleotide–amino acid complexes as the immediate precursors of protein. Why could they not also serve as the immediate precursor for nucleic acid? Such a complex is a sort of double-headed substrate which could provide either active nucleotide for nucleic acid synthesis or activated amino acid for protein synthesis.

A mechanism of this sort would explain many features of the data we have described, as well as others. The need for an available supply of amino acids for its functioning is obvious. One might perhaps find certain amino acids not required for nucleic acid synthesis, since all 80 possible complexes are theoretically not needed. Further, it is evident that when one or more of the amino acids is limited, suppression of their relatively irreversible incorporation into protein would conserve their use in nucleic acid formation. One can thereby explain the chloramphenicol effect and the need for a trace supply of amino acids to exhibit this sort of stimulation.

Any agent which prevented the formation of one of these necessary complexes would simultaneously inhibit the synthesis of both protein and nucleic acid. This may well explain the results of Schmidt et al. (75a), who find that in sulfur-starved yeast ethionine, which does not interfere with purine synthesis, nevertheless prevents the synthesis of both protein and polymerized nucleic acid.

There are other more or less obvious implications of a mechanism of this sort but we need not detail them here.

While RNA formation is evidently possible in the absence of protein synthesis, the majority of the available data suggests that the opposite situation does not obtain. There are certain apparent exceptions and since these provide the most rigorous test of the central concept of RNA as the template, we may briefly consider a few such instances here. For example, Abrams (1) found that x-rays inhibited the synthesis of RNA and DNA, as measured by incorporation of C^{14}-labeled glycine, but had little effect on the incorporation into protein. It is interesting to note that McQuillen (63), using uranyl chloride as the inhibitory agent, made a very analogous finding with protoplasts of *Bacillus megaterium*. However, is the incorporation of glycine necessarily an adequate measure of the ability of RNA to function actively as a protein-synthesizing machine?

The pertinence of this question is emphasized by the experiments of Hokin and Hokin (53), who used P^{32}-incorporation as the indicator of activity and obtained results at variance with those of Abrams. It is possible, and even probable, that P^{32} may be superior to glycine as an indicator of RNA functional activity for the same reason that it obviously would be a more informative tool in estimating the metabolic activity of ATP.

Another interesting case is that of virus protein synthesis in the coli-phage system. This was taken for some time as an instance of rapid protein synthesis in the absence of RNA metabolism. However, as pointed out by Hershey (50), if 5 per cent of the total RNA were undergoing moderately rapid turnover, the RNA synthesis could easily keep pace with the other synthetic processes without having been detected. That this is indeed the case has been revealed by the recent experiments of Volkin (95), who showed that a specific RNA fraction found in the supernatant RNA actively incorporated P^{32} in virus-infected cells.

The coil-phage system illustrates in an experimentally subtle manner that not all the RNA need be functional. This complication to a simple interpretation of correlative experiments is more obviously displayed by the mature rabbit erythrocyte, which contains 40 mg. per cent of RNA and yet exhibits no ability to synthesize protein (43). In accord with this is the failure to uncover any stoichiometrical relationship between the over-all synthesis of RNA and specific proteins (58).

In designing experiments which could hope to establish a dissociation between RNA metabolism and protein synthesis, recognition must be given to the possibility that a simple and invariant relation between the two may not exist. Such a relation would hold only if a significant proportion of the RNA molecules were participating *via* a chemical mechanism detectable by the test employed.

The ultimate proof of a specific relation between RNA and protein is more likely to come from experiments examining the formation of individual proteins. As a consequence, the tendency in recent years has been to concentrate on the synthesis of specific proteins identifiable by their serological or enzymatic properties. We may briefly summarize some of the recent findings along these lines.

Swenson and Giese (88) demonstrated that exposure to ultraviolet dosages far exceeding those required to stop DNA formation were necessary to result in the inhibition of induced enzyme synthesis in yeasts. An examination (87) of the action spectrum revealed that it coincided with the absorption spectrum of nucleic acid. Halvorson and Jackson (44) extended these interesting observations. They examined the effects of various dosages on the synthesis of α-glucosidase, the ability to use free amino acid pool components, and the incorporation of P^{32} into the nucleotides of RNA. Their data established an excellent parallelism between the loss in the capacity to utilize the free amino acids and the ability to synthesize enzyme. Ultraviolet dosages resulting in a 22 per cent inhibition of RNA metabolism suppressed enzyme formation by 95 per cent. Experiments such as these indicate that relatively slight damage to the RNA molecules can have serious consequences and suggest that RNA has an active role in the process of protein synthesis.

Further evidence along these lines comes from the use of metabolic analogues and various deficient mutants. One of the most effective compounds tested was 5-OH-uridine, which is able to prevent (81) the utilization of uracil for the synthesis of RNA. The present of as little as 5 μg./ml. of this compound results in a virtual cessation of β-galactosidase formation in *E. coli*. Furthermore, this inhibition can be achieved even if the OH-uridine is introduced subsequent to the addition of inducer, at a time when a maximal rate of enzyme formation has already been attained (83).

Several illuminating facts emerged from these experiments. One was that the OH-uridine could effect a complete inhibition of β-galactosidase formation at concentrations which had no effect on over-all protein synthesis. The apparently greater sensitivity of the β-galactosidase-forming system suggests that it requires a larger effective supply of RNA precursors than other protein-synthesizing systems. A second fact of interest is the ability of the OH-uridine to prevent enzyme formation even after its onset. This would suggest that continued synthesis of RNA is required for the uninterrupted production of new enzyme. The same conclusion was derived by Pardee (70) from the observation that uracil-less mutants cease making enzyme immediately upon the exhaustion of externally supplied uracil.

The dependence of new enzyme formation on nucleic acid synthesis was also exhibited by Spiegelman, Halvorson, and Ben-Ishai (83) in the case of α-glucosidase formation in *Saccharomyces cerevisiae*. In addition to their free amino acid pools, yeast cells also possess a considable internal supply of nucleotides and their polyphosphate derivatives (76). It was found possible to deplete the nucleotide pool specifically by incubation in the presence of an external supply of amino acids and energy. This treatment leads to a loss of enzyme-forming capacity but leaves the free amino acid pool intact. If cells are first partially induced and their nucleotide pool then depleted, they fail to form enzyme on being re-exposed to inducer. If their nucleotide pool is replenished, however, enzyme synthesis proceeds normally. These experiments illustrate in a different manner and with another system the apparent requirement that RNA synthesis be possible if induced enzyme formation is to continue.

It should be noted that the requirement for active RNA synthesis may turn out to be a property unique to induced protein formation. Creaser (28) studied the effect of azaguanine on the synthesis of catalase and β-galactosidase in two strains of *S. aureus*. The β-galactosidase was inducible in both strains, whereas the catalase was inducible in one and constitutive in the other. Azaguanine inhibited the synthesis of the inducible enzymes at all growth stages. Further, it was equally effective subsequent to the onset of enzyme synthesis. Its presence, however, had no influence on the synthesis of the constitutively formed catalase and glucozymase. The results obtained could imply that the synthesis of constitutive enzymes may not demand the concomitant formation of RNA. Creaser suggests that the difference may lie in the relative instability of the RNA template in instances of inducible enzymes.

Should these results be generalized by confirmation with other enzyme systems, a significant difference between induced and constitutive protein formation will have been uncovered. There exists, however, one apparent disagreement with this conclusion. Thus, Gros and Spiegelman (41) found that the formation of β-galactosidase in constitutive mutants of *E. coli* was as sensitive to inhibition by 5-OH-uridine as in their inducible counterparts. However, the possibility remains that this contradiction is more apparent than real. The formation of β-galactosidase in the constitutive mutants of *E. coli* may be due to the endogenous formation of an inducer rather than to any modification in the stability of the template.

The data described thus far, relating the synthesis of specific proteins and RNA metabolism, are still essentially only correlative. Two recent reports, although only of a preliminary nature, carry the analysis one step further. One is that of Volkin (95), who provides evidence that the RNA synthesized subsequent to infection by bacterial virus possesses a base ratio which differs from that normally found in the uninfected *E. coli* cell. The other is the report of Chantrenne (25), who finds that the induced synthesis of catalase in yeast is accompanied by an increased incorporation of labeled purines and pyrimidines into RNA. Ammonium sulfate fractionation of the RNA yielded several fractions differing considerably in specific activities. These results are interpreted to indicate that the effect of enzyme induction in modifying RNA metabolism is not a generalized one but rather is referable to one or more specific fractions. Aside from the obvious instances of certain of the RNA plant and animal viruses, these two investigations provide the first suggestive leads to a possible specificity in the function and structure of RNA.

EXPERIMENTS WITH SUBCELLULAR FRACTIONS

The data surveyed in the previous section leave little doubt that RNA is implicated in some way with the synthesis of new protein molecules. They do not, however, constitute proof that the RNA is serving as *the* specific template. The same results would have been obtained were RNA to constitute a nonspecific source of energy required, for example, for the activation of the individual amino acids as a preliminary to their insertion into peptide linkages. One need only imagine the excellent sort of correlative data which would have been obtained had attention been focused on the relation between the metabolism of ATP and protein synthesis.

There is no doubt that interesting and even ingenious experiments have been, and will continue to be, performed with intact cells. Nevertheless, it has been painfully obvious for some time that the distance between the data and the deductions derived from the analyses of intact cells is far too great for certainty. As between the two, many of us would, I suspect, prefer to be ingenious rather than courageous. It is therefore with reluctance that one accepts the conclusion that ingenuity alone will no longer suffice and that the age of courage and the direct approach has arrived. As pointed out in the introduction, the analysis of the problem has reached the stage in which the working hypothesis must be taken seriously and subjected to direct tests. Those who accept the RNA template dogma can no longer delay the search for and the design of experimental systems which will ultimately permit an unequivocal demonstration that *a specific RNA functions as a guide in the formation of a specific protein*. The possibility must not be overlooked that the same experimental systems may prove with equal certainty that RNA is not the template.

It must not be imagined that one must arrive in a single leap at the ideal situation of the isolated template operating in pristine purity and fabricating protein molecules from an appropriate mixture of synthetic amino acids. There is little doubt but that the presence of unknown numbers of cooperating factors, both large and small, are necessary for the final synthesis. A more realistic and realizable immediate goal would be the attainment of a subcellular preparation sufficiently organized to provide the as yet unspecified components, and sufficiently disorganized to permit the selective removal and insertion of macromolecules of interest. A gradual simplification should emerge as a natural consequence of the increasing understanding which will attend the study of such systems.

In the past few years a number of laboratories have reported the successful preparation of various subcellular fractions exhibiting in one form or another protein-synthesizing capacity. We should like to summarize the results obtained to date with such systems.

A. *Anucleate Systems.*

One of the most direct ways of deciding whether the physical presence of DNA is necessary to the formation of new protein molecules is to examine the consequences of nuclear absence. There are biological systems, for example, reticulocytes, which suggest themselves as natural experimental material for such purposes, since their maturation is paralleled by the loss of their nuclei as microscopically defined structures. It has been shown (12) that reticulocytes incorporate labeled amino acids into their protein and glycine into their DNA (58) long after the nucleus has disappeared. The possibility of specific protein synthesis has also been exhibited with the same material (69, 57).

Anucleate fragments of eggs obtained by centrifugation (66) or ligation (90) can incorporate radioactive precursors into RNA and protein. Indeed, the incorporation of labeled glycine into RNA is notably more rapid in the anucleate fraction.

The most extensive investigations along these lines have emerged from the laboratories of Brachet and Mazia. In both investigations, organisms were used permitting micromanipulative removal of nuclei. In the case of *Amoeba proteus*, the results obtained in the two laboratories are in essential agreement (14, 54, 67). Enucleation results in a considerable loss of RNA and a corresponding decrease, but not a complete loss, in the ability to incorporate labeled methionine or phenylalanine into protein.

Interpretation of these results is complicated, however, by the fact that the anucleate fragment is unable to feed. Hence these experiments are carried out under starvation conditions in which the synthesis of protein and nucleic acid would be at a minimum. This may well explain the very different results obtained by Brachet and his collaborators (16) when they employed the alga *Acetabularia mediterranea* in analogous experiments. Here, the enucleated halves retain their photosynthetic capacity and hence possess the energy and material requisite for macromolecular synthesis. Removal of the nucleus in these organisms leads to a stimulation in the net synthesis of protein and RNA which lasts for about 15 hours for protein and 5 hours for RNA. Subsequently, a slower synthetic rate sets in which can continue for periods extending over several months.

The enucleation experiments provide some of the strongest evidence available against the supposition that DNA must serve as a physical template for protein synthesis. We shall consider comparable data in subsequent sections which describe experiments with bacterial protoplasts performed in our own laboratory.

We have already referred to the complementary experiments with isolated nuclei free of cytoplasm. The results obtained with them are fully detailed elsewhere in this symposium by Allfrey.

B. *Experiments with Cytoplasmic Particulates*

A continuing investigation by Zamecnik and his collaborators over the past few years has provided valuable information on the properties of a subcellular system derived from animal tissue. The work started with observations by Siekevitz and Zamecnik (78), who demonstrated that a crude rat liver homogenate could incorporate amino acids under conditions where oxidative phosphorylation was possible. Zamecnik and Keller (99) succeeded in preparing a microsome fraction which actively incorporated amino acids when supplemented with some component of the supernatant fraction and an ATP-generating system. Subsequent work (55, 100) on the supernatant fraction indicated the presence therein of an enzyme which generated guanosine triphosphate, a derivative of which functions in the insertion of the amino acids into peptide linkages. Hoagland (51) studied the nature of the activating enzyme from the supernate and the role of ATP in the process in some further detail. The addition of a complete complement of *L*-amino acids to the supernatant fraction enhanced the rate of exchange of inorganic pyrophosphate into ATP, and α-aminohydroxamic acids are produced if hydroxylamine is included as a trapping agent. The data suggested a collection of separate enzymes which function in a carboxyl activation of the individual amino acids as an initial step to their incorporation into the microsomes. The data of DeMoss and Novelli (29) also suggest involvement of polyphosphate derivatives of nucleotides as activators of amino acids.

While no net synthesis has been observed with this microsomal fraction, the evidence supports the contention that a step relevant to protein synthesis is being studied. Most important was the demonstration (100) that hydrolysis of the protein isolated from the microsomes after incubation with C^{14}-leucine led to the isolation of a peptide containing the radioactive amino acid linked to isoleucine and valine in an α-peptide bond. Further, the incorporation of the labeled amino acid into the microsomes is irreversible, a fact which argues against any nonspecific absorption phenomenon or easily exchangeable reaction of some other sort. The incorporation occurs most readily into a protein which is not separated from the RNA by exposure to 0.5 per cent Na-desoxycholate.

Webster and Johnson (96) have reported the preparation of a particulate fraction from pea roots which incorporates labeled amino acids. The activity is destroyed some 50 per cent by treatment with RNAase or by extraction with 1 M sodium chloride. Restoration of incorporation can be achieved by the addition of RNA from a variety of sources, as well as by RNAase or mild KOH digests of RNA. This system also responds to mixtures of nucleotides and nucleosides, as well as the bases.

Extremely provocative preliminary reports have emerged from Straub's laboratory to suggest that net protein synthesis has been achieved in a cell-free system. Ullman and Straub (92) reported the formation of amylase in homogenates of pigeon pancreas. Synthesis required supplementation with a complete amino acid mixture and ATP at .02 M. In the original report the amylase-synthesizing activity was found to be associated with a fraction sedimentable from 0.3 M sucrose solutions at speeds corresponding to between "1,000 and 20,000 g" in 30 minutes. In a subsequent report, they announce (86) a solubilized preparation derived by homogenizing the fresh organ in cold acetone and drying the residue in vacuo. A water extract of the acetone powder is brought to pH 5.0, and the resulting precipitate is centrifuged and resuspended in a buffered incubation medium. The synthesis of amylase in this system corresponds in the best case to about a 50 per cent increase and more usually is in the neighborhood of about 20 per cent. ATP is required and enzyme formation is stopped by treatment with ribonuclease or by inclusion of p-fluoro-phenylalanine. The inhibition of the latter is reversed by the addition of the normal homologue.

C. Experiments with Ruptured Cells.

The work of Gale and Folkes (35, 36) on sonically ruptured cells has justifiably attracted wide interest. The findings have been extensively summarized in recent discussions, and we need note here only certain interesting features of the system as reported in the original publications. Suspensions are disrupted by sonic disintegration to yield preparations low in viable cells (between 0.015 and 0.3% of the original suspension) and retaining the ability to incorporate amino acids and synthesize specific enzymes.

One of the most useful features of these preparations resides in the fact that they can be selectively resolved with respect to their nucleic acid content by the use of the corresponding nuclease or by extraction with 1 M sodium chloride. The extent of the resolution with respect to the two nucleic acids is a function of the degree of disintegration to which the original preparation was exposed. By varying this factor, fractions have been obtained and studied with differing RNA and DNA contents.

The extent of the resolution for RNA extends between 87 per cent for what is called stage "B" to about 96 per cent for stage "D". For DNA, the corresponding numbers are 82 per cent and 92 per cent. Striking restorations of synthetic activity upon supplementation with nucleic acids are obtained only with preparations in which the percentage of removal has been extensive.

The incorporation of C^{14}-glutamic acid requires the presence of an energy supply, which can be provided by ATP and hexose diphosphate (HDP). If glutamic acid is the only amino acid present, the incorporation ceases when only a fraction of the added amino acid is incorporated, and the kinetics behave as if the system were equilibrating. The reversible nature of the incorporation is easily demonstrated by allowing the C^{14}-glutamic acid to be incorporated and then adding unlabeled glutamic acid. The labeled amino acid then emerges. If a complete amino acid mixture is present, the kinetics of incorporation behave differently, proceeding linearly and showing no sign of leveling off within the period of the experiment.

When the preparation is depleted of nucleic acid, a marked decrease in the rate and extent of incorporation results. Restoration of the incorporating ability can be achieved by the addition of *staphylococcal* nucleic acid of either kind, DNA however being more active than RNA on a dry weight basis.

Nucleic acid preparations from other sources *(Pseudomonas aeruginosa, Clostridium welchii,* thymus, wheat germ, herring roe, *Saccharomyces cerevisiae,* and ox liver) were found to be ineffective. On the other hand, nucleic acid from another strain of *S. aureus* possessed essentially the same activity as that derived from the strain being employed.

The incorporation studies quickly ran into some puzzling properties. If *staphylococcal* RNA was digested with the corresponding nuclease and the residual nucleic acid was reprecipitated and dialyzed, the subsequent preparations possessed no activity. However, if the complete digest was added to the disrupted cells, the stimulating effect on incorporation remained and was, in some cases, enhanced. Furthermore, inactive RNA from unrelated species could be made active by similar digestions. This suggested that at least part of the incorporating activity was referable to small components, and in a subsequent study (37) such indeed appeared to be the case.

The apparent specificity of the intact nucleic acids is paradoxical in the light of these findings. One possibility is to ascribe the specificity to endogenous nucleases capable of hydrolyzing with ease only *staphylococcal* nucleic acids to active fragments. The problem remains, however, unresolved.

Several other peculiarities emerged upon comparison of the incorporation of a number of amino acids into such preparations. It was found that the addition of nucleic acid to resolved preparations did not restore incorporating ability equally, the extent varying with the amino acid tested. Thus, for example, activation by nucleic acid of a salt-resolved preparation influenced incorporation as follows: glycine, 550%; aspartic acid, 210%; glutamic acid, 150%; lysine, 20%; and alanine, 0%. These differing responses were observed independently of the method of resolution for nucleic acid. No procedure was found which resulted in any effect of nucleic acid on the incorporation of alanine.

It had been hoped that incorporation could be used as a measure of protein synthesis if it were carried out in the presence of all the amino acids. However, the same differential effects on individual amino acids are observed whether the complete mixture or only a single amino acid is supplied.

Gale (32) comes to the conclusion that either incorporation is not suitable for the study of protein synthesis as such, or the effects of nucleic acids on protein synthesis are related to specific amino acids rather than to specific proteins. The formation of "glucozymase," catalase, and β-galactosidase was adopted as a more certain criterion of protein synthesis. The conclusion that the observed increases in activity were reflections of protein synthesis was based on the requirement for a complete amino acid mixture and inhibition with chloramphenicol.

The behavior of the three enzymes differed from each other and also varied with the degree of resolution with respect to nucleic acids. Preparations in which 85 per cent of the nucleic acids of both types have been removed are able to synthesize all three enzymes when incubated with a complete mixture of amino acids. Supplementation with nucleic acids has little or no effect. When, however, 93 per cent of the RNA and approximately 90 per cent of the DNA have been removed, little enzyme-forming ability is observed unless the preparations are supplemented either with nucleic acid or its derivatives. Catalase formation is strongly stimulated by RNA and does not respond to a mixture of purine and pyrimidine bases. The synthesis of β-galactosidase, on the other hand, is stimulated by the latter but not by RNA. DNA possesses little or no activating effect in these preparations. If the resolution is carried one step further, leading to the removal of 92 per cent of the DNA and approximately 96 per cent of the RNA, one obtains preparations which respond less markedly to either RNA or to the purines and pyrimidines, and are stimulated markedly by DNA.

The properties of enzyme synthesis in the highly resolved preparations are consistent with the generally accepted view of the interrelations between RNA, DNA, and protein, which assumes that DNA makes RNA and that the latter in turn synthesizes protein. The fact that DNA becomes mandatory for the synthesis of the constitutive enzymes in the most highly resolved preparations may simply be a reflection of a greater stability of DNA to the isolation procedures employed. The inability of RNA to stimulate the β-galactosidase formation at any stage of resolution can be interpreted in terms of a greater instability of RNA templates associated with inducible enzymes.

It is clear that this system possesses great potentiality. The crucial and decisive experiments relative to the specificity of the nucleic acids remain to be performed.

D. Experiments with Bacterial Protoplasts.

Work on protoplasts began with Weibull's observation (97) that exposure of *Bacillus megaterium* to lysozyme under hypertonic conditions leads to the formation of structures he labeled "protoplasts." Usually, each rod-like cell yields two or three of the spherical protoplasts. Osmotically stabilized suspensions of the protoplasts were found to be metabolically active, possessing a high endogenous respiration and capable of oxidizing glucose at constant rates for extended periods of time (98). It was generally recognized that a subcellular system of potential usefulness in the analysis of cellular syntheses had been uncovered.

A number of laboratories undertook a study of the synthetic capacities of these protoplasts. It was shown independently by Brenner and Stent (18), as well as by Salton and McQuillen (74), that bacteriophage multiplication can occur in protoplasts of *B. megaterium* if the bacteria are infected or induced prior to the removal of the cell wall. Virus yields were in the neighborhood of 30 per cent of those obtainable with intact cells. Single burst experiments demonstrated that virus synthesis was occurring in a major proportion of the infected protoplasts.

It became quickly evident that protoplasts retained a major proportion of the synthetic potentiality of the cells from which they are derived, as is dramatically exhibited by Salton's experiments on spore formation (73). Approximately 1 per cent of the protoplasts were convertible to spores. Thus far, no one has achieved direct conversion of *B. megaterium* protoplasts to viable cells by resynthesis of the cell wall. McQuillen (64) has, however, provided evidence indicating a limited residual capacity for division. When properly supplemented and incubated with aeration for periods extending between 4 and 6 hours, protoplasts take on dumb-bell shapes which are highly suggestive of incipient division.

Attempts to study protein synthesis by tracer procedures were actually made prior to the appearance of Weibull's publication, and while it was not realized that under certain conditions the treatment of sensitive cells with lysozyme results in the appearance of microscopically visible structural elements. Lester (61) exposed *Micrococcus lysodeikticus* to lysozyme in the presence of sucrose and found that such "lysates" could still incorporate C^{14}-labeled leucine into the protein fraction. The addition of desoxyribonuclease enhanced the incorporation, whereas ribonuclease abolished it. Similar findings were reported by Beljanski (10), who used labeled glycine. Here again, stimulation with DNAase and inhibition with RNAase were observed.

The first extensive investigation of incorporation in defined protoplast preparations was reported by McQuillen (63). A variety of C^{14}-labeled compounds was used and a comparison of protoplasts and intact cells made. The results obtained in the two were qualitatively similar. C^{14}-carboxyl-labeled glycine made its way into protein as glycine and also into the adenine and guanine of the nucleic acids. The rate of incorporation in the protoplasts was between 50 and 100 per cent of that observed with intact cells.

The synthesis of enzymatically active proteins in suspensions of protoplasts was achieved simultaneously in several laboratories. Wiame and his collaborators (98) showed that arabinokinase was formed in protoplasts prepared from *Bacillus subtilis* when they were incubated aerobically in the presence of arabinose, yeast extract, and ammonium sulfate, with 0.5 M sodium chloride as a stabilizing agent. McQuillen (65) and Landman and Spiegelman (59) demonstrated that protoplasts of *Bacillus megaterium*, strain KM, can be induced to synthesize β-galactosidase. As with other synthetic functions, the properties of enzyme formation in protoplasts and intact cells were markedly similar, providing the comparisons are carried out under hypertonic conditions.

The interest in the protoplasts as possible tools in the further analysis of enzyme synthesis stems, of course, from the possibility that they might be more amenable to specific enzymatic resolution than the intact cells from which they are derived. Fortunately this possibility is potentially obtainable, for it is when one examines responses to various enzymes that striking differences between cells and protoplasts begin to emerge. It was found (59) that the ability to synthesize enzymes could be abolished in protoplasts by treatment with either lipase or trypsin. Intact cells are completely insensitive to these enzymes.

These results illustrate a point worthy of the attention of those concerned with performing and interpreting experiments with subcellular fractions of any sort. Based simply on the observation recorded with lipase, one might be led to conjecture that a lipid is a key component to the enzyme-forming mechanism. However, the fact is that the loss of enzyme-synthesizing ability is a simple consequence of the physical dissolution of protoplasts. After incubation with either lipase or trypsin at the levels indicated, few protoplasts can be recovered. It is thus important in any given case to demonstrate that an inhibition of synthetic activity which follows a particular treatment is not the result of a generalized destruction. This caution is also relevant to experiments involving other enzymes such as ribonuclease and desoxyribonuclease. Lysis of protoplasts by RNAase has been observed by Brenner (17), as well as in our own laboratory, under certain conditions. To be interpretable, experiments of this nature must be accompanied by evidence that enzymatic, or any other, treatment has resulted in the selective removal of the relevant compounds.

An extensive examination has been made of the effects of both RNAase and DNAase on the chemistry and the synthesis of β-galactosidase in both intact cells and protoplasts. No effects were observed with intact cells under any conditions. Striking modifications were, however, obtained with protoplasts (82).

A few words may perhaps be interposed on the conditions necessary for consistent results. The earlier phases of this investigation were plagued by extremely poor reproducibility. As a result of purely empirical efforts, a procedure was finally devised which yielded protoplast preparations giving comfortably concordant results in repetitive experiments. The major difficulty was finally located at the stage of cell preparation. Customarily, cells for an experiment were obtained by inoculation into 2% peptone, followed by incubation with shaking overnight at 30° C. By morning, the cultures were in the stationary phase and were then put through a "rejuvenation" prior to use. Rejuvenation consisted of diluting the cultures five-fold with fresh medium and reincubating until they had entered the logarithmic growth phase, as determined by periodic examinations of the optical density. Extreme care had to be exercised in controlling the time allowed for rejuvenation, if protoplast preparations were to be obtained exhibiting uniform behavior with respect to enzyme-forming ability and response to resolution.

The precision which had to be exercised was puzzling. Consequently an investigation (Spiegelman, unpub.) was made of the cells during the course of their rejuvenation, and this disclosed that our procedure had inadvertently led to a marked phasing of DNA synthesis. Total RNA formation showed only slight evidence of cycling. However, enzyme-forming ability varied twenty-fold during the course of one cycle. The details of the interrelations are still being unraveled. The studies did make possible the preparation of protoplasts capable of extensive enzyme synthesis and which responded homogeneously to the action of enzymes. The observations on accessibility to enzymes may perhaps be related to the recently published experiments of Thomas (91), who noted a periodic variation in the permeability of pneumococci to large molecules such as DNA and DNAase.

Even with the rejuvenation aspect of the system under control, a consistent removal of RNA and DNA by the corresponding nuclease was not achieved until the age of protoplasts at the time of treatment was carefully standardized. Protoplasts incubated in the stabilizing medium became progressively more impervious to enzymatic resolution. Eventually it was found most convenient to treat the protoplasts with the nuclease enzymes during their formation.

The procedure finally employed for resolution may be outlined as follows. The rejuvenated cells are suspended in the hypertonic medium supplemented with 1% casein hydrolysate, lysozyme at a level of 200 μg. per ml., and the enzyme to be tested for ability to resolve the protoplasts. The incubation is carried out for a period of 45 minutes at 30° C. with constant shaking, by which time the cells have been converted into protoplasts and the resolution will have been accomplished. The protoplasts are then recovered by centrifugation, an aliquot removed for test of enzyme-forming ability, and the remainder retained for chemical analysis. Residual capacity to synthesize enzyme was examined by suspending the treated protoplasts in hypertonic medium containing amino acids and hexose diphosphate and lactose as the inducer. The resultant suspension was then incubated on a roller-type device for 2 to 3 hours with periodic sampling for enzyme assay. The latter was performed with the aid of the chromogenic substrate, ortho-nitrophenyl-β-D-galactoside. Untreated controls were always run in parallel.

The first series of experiments performed was designed to provide an answer to the question of whether the physical presence of intact DNA and RNA was necessary for the induced synthesis of β-galactosidase. Table 1 summarizes a typical series of experiments in which the effect of DNAase on protoplasts was examined in terms of the percentage of removal of DNA, RNA, and the residual enzyme-forming capacity. The results with respect to enzyme-forming abilities are clear-cut. It is quite evident from the data that considerable amounts of DNA can be removed, up to 99 per cent, without loss of enzyme-forming ability. Indeed, rather considerable stimulations of enzyme synthesis are consistently observed. However, it will be noted that in those cases where 30 per cent or more of the RNA is lost serious inhibitions of enzyme-forming ability resulted.

Table 2 summarizes a comparable series of experiments in which the protoplasts were treated with RNAase, and here the picture is also clear. In most cases, there is relatively little concomitant loss in DNA. Again, one can observe that, wherever the removal of RNA exceeds 35 per cent, drastic inhibitions of enzyme-forming capacity result.

TABLE 1

THE EFFECT OF DNAASE ON ENZYME SYNTHESIS AND DNA AND RNA CONTENT

DNAase (400 μg./ml.) was present in the experimental flasks during protoplast formation (45 minutes). Protoplasts were then recovered by centrifugation and washed. An aliquot was used for determination of DNA, RNA, and protein. The extent of removal of each nucleic acid is determined in terms of ratio of protein in the protoplast pellet and comparison with untreated control. This corrects for loss due to lysis during treatment. Enzyme-forming ability is examined with another aliquot of the protoplasts which is resuspended in an induction mixture (0.5 M K_2HPO_4, pH 7.8; 2% amino acids; 0.6% hexose diphosphate; and 0.06 M lactose). Samples are removed periodically for enzyme assay. Enzyme activity is determined in terms of the millimicromoles of o-nitrophenyl-β-D-galactoside hydrolyzed per milligram of protein per minute. The rate of enzyme formation is obtained as the number of enzyme activity units synthesized per milligram of protein per hour.

| | Per cent removal | | Enzyme formed (in % of |
Experiment	DNA	RNA	untreated controls)
$1020C_1$	87	0	400
$1020C_2$	94	0	420
$1020C_3$	97	0	540
$1019D_2$	41	4	104
$1019C_2$	43	17	120
$1019C_3$	99	13	100
718	65	31	13
715	65	32	15
719	59	46	0
712	39	42	12

It would appear that enzymatic resolution of protoplasts provides information consistent with the thesis that the physical integrity of RNA, rather than that of DNA, is the principal requisite for the retention of enzyme-forming ability. However, one cannot from such experiments categorically deny an immediate role of DNA in the process of enzyme formation. Uncertainty stems essentially from the fact that treatment of protoplasts with DNAase, while leading to the disappearance of acid-precipitable DNA, does not lead to the complete removal of the acid-soluble fragments to which the DNA is degraded. Analysis of the acid-soluble fraction following DNAase treatment indicates that 60 per cent of the degraded DNA remains in the protoplasts. It could be argued that these fragments are either themselves functional or convertible to active elements. To obviate objections of this nature, it would be necessary to get protoplasts to the state in which removal of acid-soluble fragments could be achieved. Presumably then an unequivocal experimental decision would be attainable.

TABLE 2

THE EFFECT OF RNAASE ON ENZYME SYNTHESIS AND DNA AND RNA CONTENT

RNAase (500 μg./ml.) was present in the experimental flasks during protoplast formation (45 minutes). Protoplasts were then recovered by centrifugation and washed. An aliquot was used for determination of DNA, RNA, and protein. The extent of removal of each nucleic acid is determined in terms of ratio to protein in the protoplast pellet and comparison with untreated control. This corrects for loss due to lysis during treatment. Enzyme-forming ability is examined with another aliquot of the protoplasts which is resuspended in an induction mixture (0.5 M K_2HPO_4, pH 7.8; 2% amino acids; 0.6% hexose diphosphate; and 0.06 M lactose). Samples are removed periodically for enzyme assay. Enzyme activity is determined in terms of the millimicromoles of o-nitrophenyl-β-D-galactoside hydrolyzed per milligram protein per minute. The rate of enzyme formation is obtained as the number of enzyme activity units synthesized per milligram protein per hour.

Experiment	Per cent removal		Enzyme synthesized (in % of untreated controls)
	DNA	RNA	
1013	21	33	30
930B	0	34	0
926B	0	36	21
1004D	14	39	38
1004C	16	52	14
1020B	0	54	16
1004F	0	72	10
1014B	0	72	0
1020B2	13	75	1
1020B3	58	78	0

There were other reasons which impelled us to abandon the study of intact protoplasts. It is obvious that a loss of enzyme-forming ability paralleling the destruction of a particular macromolecule is not adequate evidence for concluding that the macromolecule in question is serving in a specific manner in the synthesis of the protein being studied. To complete the evidence and make the conclusion inescapable, it is necessary to restore the enzyme-forming ability in such a resolved preparation by the addition of the macromolecule which has been removed or destroyed. As a result of accumulating experience with protoplasts, it became evident that reconstitution would be extremely difficult to achieve. Once made, there is a period of 30 to 45 minutes during which the removal and replacement of large molecules appears possible. This period is not long enough to permit performance of all the necessary operations. We therefore turned our attention to the search for procedures which would yield preparations still capable of enzyme formation and yet more or less permanently accessible to the activity of large molecules. The next section summarizes the results obtained.

E. Experiments with Osmotically Shocked Protoplasts.

The direction taken was conditioned by the experience we had gained in the course of the search for a suitable stabilizing medium for enzyme synthesis. It was noted that certain procedures, while leading to considerable lysis, nevertheless on a number of occasions yielded pellets containing a surprising amount of enzyme-synthesizing ability. A systematic investigation was therefore undertaken of the chemical composition and synthetic capacities of protoplasts subjected to controlled lysis in a variety of media.

We need not here detail the various procedures tried and which led to inactive preparations. It was ultimately found (84) that consistent results could be obtained if 0.5 M succinate was used as the stabilizing medium and if lysis was achieved by osmotic shocking through the sudden addition of water followed by immediate centrifugation. The resulting pellet was then resuspended in stabilizing medium.

The extent of the osmotic shocking must be carefully controlled. There exists a rather narrow range within which the procedure yields pellets relatively free of protoplasts and retaining enzyme-forming ability. The chemical composition and enzyme-forming ability of variously shocked preparations are compared with protoplasts in Table 3. It will be noted that 1:3 and 1:4 shockates possess somewhat better enzyme-forming ability on a per mg. nitrogen basis than the control protoplasts. Both of these shockates lose RNA and protein.

TABLE 3

Composition and Enzyme Forming Ability of Pellets from
Osmotically Shocked Protoplasts

Enzyme formation (EF) is expressed as increase in enzyme units per mg. of protein per hour. The three components are given in terms of mg. per ml. Centrifugation at 8,000 r.p.m. for 5 minutes was begun immediately after addition of H_2O to protoplasts suspended in 0.5 M succinate medium, as described in the text.

Material	DNA	DNA/prot.	RNA	RNA/prot.	Prot.	EF
Protoplasts	29	.032	341	.31	880	900
1:3 Shockate	30	.088	123	.36	340	1120
1:4 Shockate	23	.114	70	.35	200	1300
1:5 Shockate	18	.100	4	.02	179	0

However, there is no drastic change in the RNA/protein ratio. On the other hand, diluting 1:5 yields a pellet possessing no enzyme-forming ability and a RNA/protein ratio which has been reduced by a factor of 15.

It will be noted that the pellets from all the shockates exhibit a rather surprising ability to retain the DNA originally present in the protoplasts. This is related to the fact that the DNA is associated with a nucleus-like structure (5) which does not burst immediately unless the osmotic shocking is much more extensive. These nuclear structures and the DNA associated with them sediment at the speeds employed (8,000 r.p.m. for 5 minutes). On resuspension of the pellet by repeated blowing through a pipette, most of the DNA goes into solution as acid-precipitable material but no longer sedimentable at the speeds employed. This property is illustrated by the first number in column 4 of Table 4.

Microscopically, shockates of 1:4 and above consist primarily of membranous bodies of the same size and shape of protoplasts but of lower optical density. The most striking difference between protoplasts and the osmotically shocked preparations is the modification in chemical composition which follows various treatments. This difference is exhibited in Table 4. It will be noted that protoplasts respond neither quantitatively nor qualitatively to resuspension, treatment with the two nucleases, or extraction with molar sodium chloride and resolving mixture (RM). Shockates, on the other hand, are markedly modified by any of these treatments. As noted previously, resuspension of the pellet from a shockate and subsequent spinning yields a pellet in

TABLE 4

RESOLVABILITY OF PROTOPLASTS AND SHOCKATES

Resuspension was done in 0.5 M succinate. Enzyme treatment and extractions carried out for 30 minutes at 30° C. with proper ionic supplements. Pellets recovered for analysis by centrifugation at 8,000 r.p.m. for 5 minutes. RM, Resolving mixture—see text. Figures are percentages of untreated control pellets.

Treatment	Protoplasts			Shockate (1:4.2)		
	DNA	RNA*	PROT.	DNA	RNA	PROT.
Resuspension	95	97	95	15	83	80
RNAase (400μg./ml.)	91	89	105	18	30	66
DNAase (400μg./ml.)	100	98	102	3	84	85
1M NaCl	87	81	80	9	58	68
RM	100	100	100	2	86	67

which 85 per cent of the DNA has been lost to the supernate. There is a small loss in both RNA and protein but not preferentially for either. Exposure to RNAase results in a marked drop of RNA, and similarly DNAase is capable of removing about 80 per cent of the DNA which remains sedimentable after a simple resuspension. Extraction with 1 M sodium chloride removes both RNA and DNA and some protein.

A word may be said here about the resolving mixture (RM). It was found empirically that if shockate pellets are resuspended in 0.5 M succinate as a stabilizing medium, containing in addition 0.1 M phosphate and a complete mixture of amino acids, a highly selective and efficient removal of DNA results. The reasons for this removal are under investigation. We have, however, used this empirical method as an extremely convenient device for the selective removal of DNA. It will be noted in Table 2 that this treatment has little effect on either RNA or protein.

We next undertook to examine the effect of these various procedures on the enzyme-forming ability. The results of a typical experiment are summarized in Table 5. The DNA analyses of the acid-soluble and

TABLE 5

Nucleic Acid Resolution and Enzyme Formation in Shockates

Treatments carried out as in Table 4, but extended to 50 minutes at 30° C. Cold 0.2 N perchloric used to separate acid-soluble and acid-insoluble fractions. Enzyme formation (EF) measured as in Tables 1 and 3.

				Distribution of DNA of resolved shockate in mg./10 ml.			
	In percentages of controls			Pellet		Supernate	
Treatment	DNA	RNA	EF	Acid-Insol.	Acid-sol.	Acid-insol.	Acid-sol.
RM	<1	100	150	<2	<2	190	95
RM DNAase	<1	89	130	<2	<2	8	305
DNAase	<1	92	140	<2	<2	2	302
(1 M NaCl)	5	49	14	—	—	—	—
RNAase	74	42	10	—	—	—	—

insoluble fractions are given for the first three pellets along with the corresponding figures for the supernatants. The procedures for removing DNA used singly and in combination were clearly effective, there being no detectable DNA left in the pellet either as small or large fragments. Nevertheless, no inhibition of enzyme synthesis resulted.

On the other hand, treatment with RNAase or extraction with 1 *M* sodium chloride, both of which lead to removal of RNA, resulted in a corresponding decrease in enzyme-forming capacity.

We would appear to have here a completely convincing experiment demonstrating the possibility of the formation of new enzyme molecules in the absence of DNA. There remained, however, one unlikely possibility that the preparations could resynthesize the DNA during the subsequent incubation required for the test of enzyme-forming ability. Samples were therefore taken at the end of three hours' incubation and analyzed for DNA. To our complete astonishment, extensive resynthesis of DNA had occurred. Needless to say, this observation modified temporarily the direction of our investigations.

Table 6 summarizes a representative set of experiments with various

TABLE 6

Resynthesis of DNA in Pellets from Osmotically Shocked Protoplasts

Incubation carried out at 30° C. with shaking. Medium is as described in text. In all cases pellets washed once prior to incubation. Some were subjected to resolution for DNA. Figures represent μg./10 ml. as determined by Burton's modification of the Dische reaction on the acid-precipitable fraction.

Shockate Preparation	Zero Time	3 Hours
1:4	4	118
1:4	11	130
1:4.2	4	76
1:4.2	40	273
1:4.7	18	153
1:4.7	—	44

types of shockates resolved initially to various extents and then subjected to a three-hour incubation. It is to be seen that the amounts of DNA synthesized are considerable. That the material being synthesized is DNA was established by a number of criteria. First, it is converted to acid-soluble form by treatment with deoxyribonuclease. Secondly, on removal of RNA by alkaline digestion, and hydrolysis with hot 0.5 *N* perchloric acid, the ultraviolet absorptions at 260 and 290 mμ were in quantitative agreement with the values expected on the basis of the Dische (30) and Burton (21) reactions of the same material.

It is, of course, needless to emphasize that a shockate is hardly an enzyme preparation, and much remains to be done to analyze the nature of the system further. There are certain features which we might note. The principal components of the incubation medium are succinate (0.5 *M*), KCl (0.1 *M*), amino acids (1% enzymatic hydrolysate of casein), hexose diphosphate (.6%), magnesium chloride (0.02 *M*), and manganese chloride (0.001 *M*). The omission of the amino acids abolishes DNA formation. These can, however, be partially replaced by the four deoxynucleotides and ATP. The kinetics of the resynthesis is of interest. Following a lag period of 40 to 90 minutes, synthesis begins and proceeds linearly for a period exceeding five hours. The rate achieved is not dependent upon the initial amount of DNA left in the preparation. Noteworthy is the fact that the rate of DNA synthesis (μg. per mg. protein per hour) in these shockates can exceed by a factor of 10 the maximal rate attained by a culture growing logarithmically in 2 per cent peptone. The relation of this DNA synthesis to the system described by Kornberg in the present symposium cannot be specified as yet.

In view of this remarkable capacity to synthesize one of the important macromolecules, an examination was naturally made for net formation of RNA and protein. The results are summarized in Table 7,

TABLE 7

RESYNTHESIS OF NUCLEIC ACIDS IN SHOCKATES AND PROTOPLASTS

Conditions are as described in previous tables. Figures represent percentages after 3 hours of amounts at zero time. Analysis carried out on acid-insoluble fraction.

Preparation and Treatment		DNA	RNA	Protein
1:4 Shockate	RM	3000	410	350
	RM	1200	520	460
	RM	720	210	140
	RM	420	120	80
	1 M NaCl	0	130	102
	RNAase	40	80	64
Protoplasts	RM	510	600	550

in which synthesis in protoplasts and 1:4 shockates subjected to various treatments are recorded. One finds that protoplasts can synthesize all three components, but in a manner which always leads to an equal proportionate increase in all three components. Shockates, on the other hand, in general display an unbalanced synthetic ability. Finally, it will be noted that shockate preparations treated with either molar sodium chloride or RNAase lose their ability to synthesize all three components. This loss has thus far been an invariable consequence of the removal or damage of RNA. The implications of this for the hierarchichal relationships amongst the three macromolecules are suggestive but at the present time hardly conclusive.

An extensive attempt has been made to restore the enzyme-forming ability of resolved preparations. Restoration has been achieved by ATP in some cases and by a mixture of the nucleoside diphosphates in others. These substances are active providing the resolution with respect to RNA has not been too severe. The effect of supplementing with purified Ochoa enzyme, derived from *E. coli*, was also examined. The puzzling result was obtained that the enzyme abolished the stimulating effects of the diphosphates. Obviously, other enzyme preparations must be tested, particularly a purified preparation from *B. megaterium*. Until these experiments are performed, no certain conclusions can be drawn.

Many questions are raised by the results we have thus far reported with the osmotically shocked protoplasts of *B. megaterium*. Principal interest in our minds centers on the biological competence of the macromolecules which these preparations can synthesize. There is no doubt but what they can fabricate enzymatically active protein. It remains, however, to be established whether the DNA and RNA formed are nonsensical or possess biologically meaningful content. It will be a tedious task to attempt a resolution of this question with *B. megaterium*. Little genetic work has been done with this organism and the necessary mutant collection is not available.

Fortunately, protoplast formation with *E. coli* has been recently achieved by a number of investigators, including Lederberg, Zinder, and Mahler and Frazer. All were kind enough to communicate their methods prior to publication. We have used Lederberg's procedure, which involves growth in the presence of penicillin in a sucrose-stabilized medium. Our preliminary results have demonstrated that active shockates can be prepared as easily from *E. coli* protoplasts as from *B. megaterium*. The wealth of genetically defined material available with *E. coli* makes it the obvious choice for future investigations of certain basic problems.

Conclusion

The problem of protein synthesis has been brought to the point where further questions must be posed in terms of the chemical structures and reactive interrelationships amongst RNA, DNA, and protein. The work with the subcellular systems reviewed in the last sections of this paper makes it evident that the era of the direct attack has arrived. The crucial experiments have not yet been executed. However, the systems required for their performance are with us, or close at hand. The outlook is depressingly bright for the quick resolution of many interesting problems.

REFERENCES

1. Abrams, R., *Arch. Biochem.*, **30**, 90 (1951).
2. Allfrey, V. G., *Proc. Natl. Acad. Sci. U. S.*, **40**, 881 (1954).
3. Allfrey, V. G., present symposium.
4. Anfinsen, C. B., and Steinberg, D., *J. Biol. Chem.*, **189**, 739 (1951).
5. Aronson, A., and Spiegelman, S., unpub.
6. Askonas, B. A., Campbell, P. N., and Work, T. S., *Biochem. J. (London)*, **56**, *Proc. Biochem. Soc.*, p. iv. (1954).
7. Askonas, B. A., Campbell, P. N., and Work, T. S., *Biochem. J. (London)*, **58**, 326 (1954).
8. Baron, L. S., Spiegelman, S., and Quastler, H. J., *J. Gen. Physiol.*, **36**, 631 (1953).
9. Barry, J. M., *J. Biol. Chem.*, **195**, 795 (1952).
10. Beljanski, M., *Biochem. et Biophys. Acta*, **15**, 425 (1954).
11. Borsook, H., *J. Cell. Comp. Physiol.*, **47** (Suppl. 1), 35 (1956).
12. Borsook, H., Deasy, C. C., Haager-Smit, A., J., Keighley, D., and Lowy, P. H., *J. Biol. Chem.*, **196**, 669 (1952).
13. Brachet, J., *Arch. Biol. (Liége)*, **53**, 207 (1941).
14. Brachet, J., *Biochim. et Biophys. Acta*, **18**, 247 (1955).
15. Brachet, J., in *The Nucleic Acids* (J. N. Davidson and Erwin Chargaff, eds.), Academic Press, New York (1955).
16. Brachet, J., Chantrenne, H., and Vanderhaeghe, F., *Biochim. et Biophys. Acta*, **18**, 544 (1955).
17. Brenner, S., *Biochem. et Biophys. Acta*, **18**, 531 (1955).
18. Brenner, S., and Stent, G. S., *Biochem. et Biophys. Acta*, **17**, 473 (1955).
19. Britten, R. J., Roberts, R. B., and French, E. F., *Proc. Natl. Acad. Sci. U. S.*, **41**, 863 (1955).
20. Bulman, N., and Campbell, D. H., *Federation Proc.*, **10**, 404 (1951).
21. Burton, K., *Biochem. J. (London)*, **62**, 315 (1956).
22. Campbell, P. N., and Work, T. S., *Biochem. J. (London)*, **52**, 217 (1952).
23. Caspersson, T., *Symposia Soc. Exptl. Biol.*, **1**, 127 (1947).
24. Chantrenne, H., *Symposia Soc. Gen. Microbiol.*, Nature of Virus Multiplication, pp. 1-15, Cambridge University Press (1953).
25. Chantrenne, H., *Nature*, **177**, 579 (1956).
26. Christensen, H. N., *J. Nutrition*, **42**, 189 (1950).
27. Cohen, S. S., and Barner, H. D., *Proc. Natl. Acad. Sci. U. S.*, **40**, 885 (1954).
28. Creaser, E. H., *Nature*, **176**, 556 (1955).
29. DeMoss, J. A., and Novelli, D., *Bacteriol. Proc.*, p. 125 (1955).
30. Dische, Z., *Mikrochemie*, **8**, 4 (1930).
31. Fraenkel-Conrat, H., *J. Cell. Comp. Physiol.*, **47** (Suppl. 1), 133 (1956).
32. Gale, E. F., *Proc. 3rd Intern. Congr. Biochem., Brussels*, p. 345 (1955).

33. Gale, E. F., in *Symposium on Amino Acid Metabolism* (W. D. McElroy and B. Glass, eds.), Johns Hopkins Press, Baltimore (1955).
34. Gale, E. F., and Folkes, J. P., *Biochem. J. (London)*, **53**, 493 (1955).
34a. Gale, E. F., and Folkes, J. P., *Biochem. J. (London)*, **53**, 483 (1953).
35. Gale, E. F., and Folkes, J. P., *Biochem. J. (London)*, **59**, 661 (1955).
36. Gale, E. F., and Folkes, J. P., *Biochem. J. (London)*, **59**, 675 (1955).
37. Gale, E. F., and Folkes, J. P., *Nature,* **175**, 592 (1955).
38. Geiger, E., *Science,* **111**, 594 (1950).
39. Gerarde, H. W., Jones, M., and Winnick, T., *J. Biol. Chem.*, **196**, 51 (1952).
40. Green, H., and Anker, H. S., *Biochim. et Biophys. Acta.*, **13**, 365 (1954).
41. Gros, F., and Spiegelman, S., unpub.
42. Gros, F., Spiegelman, S., and Gros-Doulcat, F., *Proc. 3rd Intern. Congr. Biochem. (Brussels),* 74 (1955).
43. Halloway, B. J., and Ripley, S. H., *J. Biol. Chem.*, **196**, 695 (1952).
44. Halvorson, H. O., and Jackson, L., *Bacteriol. Proc.*, p. 117 (1954).
45. Halvorson, H. O., and Spiegelman, S., *J. Bacteriol.*, **64**, 207 (1952).
46. Halvorson, H. O., and Spiegelman, S., *J. Bacteriol.*, **65**, 496 (1953a).
47. Halvorson, H. O., and Spiegelman, S., *J. Bacteriol.*, **65**, 601 (1953).
48. Halvorson, H. O., Spiegelman, S., and Hinman, R., *Arch. Biochem. and Biophys.*, **55**, 512 (1955).
49. Heimberg, M., and Velick, S. F., *J. Biol. Chem.*, **208**, 725 (1954).
50. Hershey, A. D., *J. Gen. Physiol.*, **37**, 1 (1953).
51. Hoagland, M. B., *Biochim. et Biophys. Acta,* **16**, 288 (1955).
52. Hogness, D. S., Cohn, M., and Monod, J., *Biochim. et Biophys. Acta,* **16**, 99 (1955).
53. Hokin, M. R., and Holzin, L. E., *J. Biol. Chem.*, **219**, 85 (1956).
54. James, T. W., *Biochim. et Biophys. Acta,* **15**, 367 (1954).
55. Keller, E. B., and Zamecnik, P. C., *Federation Proc.*, **14**, 234 (1955).
56. Kelner, A., *J. Bacteriol.*, **65**, 252 (1953).
57. Koritz, S. B., and Chantrenne, H., *Biochim. et Biophys. Acta,* **13**, 209 (1954).
58. Kruh, J., and Borsook, H., *Nature,* **175**, 386 (1955).
59. Landman, O. E., and Spiegelman, S., *Proc. Natl. Acad. Sci. U. S.,* **41**, 698 (1955).
60. Lee, N. D., and Williams, R. H., *Biochim. et Biophys. Acta,* **9**, 698 (1952).
61. Lester, R. L., *J. Am. Chem. Soc.*, **75**, 5448 (1953).
62. Loftfield, Robert B., and Harris, Anne, *J. Biol. Chem.*, **219**, 151 (1956).
63. McQuillen, K., *Biochem. et Biophys. Acta*, **17**, 382 (1955).
64. McQuillen, K., *Biochem. et Biophys. Acta*, **18**, 458 (1955).
65. McQuillen, K., in *Bacterial Anatomy* (E. T. C. Spooner and B. A. D. Stocker, eds.), Cambridge Univ. Press (1956).
66. Malkin, H. M., *J. Cell. Comp. Physiol.*, **44**, 105 (1954).
67. Mazia, D., and Prescott, D. M., *Biochim. et Biophys. Acta*, **17**, 23 (1955).
68. Monod, J., Pappenheimer, A. M., Jr., and Cohen-Bazire, G., *Biochim. et Biophys. Acta*, **9**, 648 (1952).
69. Nizet, A., and Lamburt, S., *Bull. soc. chim. biol.*, **35**, 771 (1953).
70. Pardee, A. B., *Proc. Natl. Acad. Sci. U. S.,* **40**, 263 (1954).
70a. Pardee, A. B., and Prestidge, L. S., *J. Bacteriol.*, **71**, 677 (1956).
71. Ranney, H. M., and London, I. M., *Federation Proc.*, **10**, 562 (1951).
72. Rotman, B., and Spiegelman, S., *J. Bacteriol.*, **68**, 419 (1954).
73. Salton, M. R. J., *J. Gen. Microbiol.*, **13**, iv (1955).
74. Salton, M. R. J., and McQuillen, K., *Biochem. et Biophys. Acta,* **17**, 465 (1955).

75. Sanger, F., in *Currents in Biochemical Research* (D. E. Green, ed.), Interscience Publishers, New York (1956).
75a. Schmidt, G., et al., *Biochim. et Biophys. Acta,* **20**, 135 (1956).
76. Schmitz, H., *Biochem. Z.,* **325**, 555 (1954).
77. Schucher, Rueben, Hokin, Lowell E., *J. Biol. Chem.,* **210**, 551 (1954).
78. Siekevitz, P., and Zamecnik, P., *Federation Proc.,* **10**, 246 (1951).
79. Silber, R. H., and Porter, C. C., *J. Nutrition,* **38**, 155 (1949).
80. Simpson, M. V., and Velick, S. F., *J. Biol. Chem.,* **208**, 61 (1954).
81. Slotnick, C. J., Visser, D. W., and Rittenberg, S. C., *J. Biol. Chem.,* **203**, 647 (1953).
82. Spiegelman, S., in *Enzymes: Units of Biological Structure and Function* (O. H. Gaebler, ed.), Academic Press, New York (1956).
83. Spiegelman, S., Halvorson, H. O., and Ben-Ishai, R., in *Symposium on Amino Acid Metabolism* (W. D. McElroy and B. Glass, eds.), Johns Hopkins Press, Baltimore (1955).
84. Spiegelman, S., Wolin, E., and Liu, G. B., unpub.
85. Steinberg, D., and Anfinsen, C. B., *J. Biol. Chem.,* **199**, 25 (1952).
86. Straub, F. B., Ullmann, A., and Hos, G., *Biochim. et Biophys. Acta,* **18**, 439 (1955).
87. Swenson, P. A., *Proc. Natl. Acad. Sci. U. S.,* **36**, 699 (1950).
88. Swenson, P. A., and Giese, A. G., *J. Cell. Comp. Physiol.,* **36**, 369 (1950).
89. Synge, R. L. M., in *The Chemical Structure of Proteins* (G. E. W. Wostenholme and M. P. Cameron, eds.), Little Brown and Company, Boston (1952).
90. Tiedemann, H., and Tiedemann, H., *Naturwissenschaften,* **41**, 535 (1954).
91. Thomas, R., *Biochim. et Biophys. Acta,* **18**, 467 (1955).
92. Ullmann, A., and Straub, F. B., *Acta Physiol. Acad. Sci. Hung.,* **6**, 377 (1954).
93. Ushiba, D., and Magasanik, B., *Proc. Soc. Exptl. Biol. Med.,* **80**, 626 (1952).
94. Vaughn, M., and Anfinsen, C. B., *J. Biol. Chem.,* **211**, 367 (1954).
95. Volkin, Elliott, present symposium.
96. Webster, G. C., and Johnson, M. P., *J. Biol. Chem.,* **217**, 641 (1955).
97. Weibull, C., *J. Bacteriol.,* **66**, 688 (1953).
98. Wiame, J. M., Storck, R., and Vanderwinckel, E., *Biochim. et Biophys. Acta,* **18**, 353 (1955).
98a. Wisseman, C. L., et al., *J. Bacteriol.,* **67**, 662 (1954).
99. Zamecnik, P. C., and Keller, E. B., *J. Biol. Chem.,* **209**, 337 (1954).
100. Zamecnik, P. C., Keller, E. B., Littlefield, J. W., Hoagland, M. B., and Loftfield, R. B., *J. Cell. Comp. Physiol.,* **47**, 81 (1955).

EFFECTS OF NUCLEOTIDES ON THE INCORPORATION OF AMINO ACIDS INTO PROTEIN*

GEORGE C. WEBSTER

*Department of Agricultural Biochemistry,
The Ohio State University,
Columbus 10, Ohio*

MICROSOME-LIKE particles derived from pea seedlings have the ability to incorporate a variety of amino acids into their protein. Incorporation of any single amino acid is enhanced by a mixture of seventeen other amino acids, magnesium and potassium ions, and low concentrations of adenosine triphosphate (11, 12). Incorporation is inhibited by adenosine diphosphate, by rubidium ions, and by various amino acid analogues (11, 12). The particles are unstable after removal from their cellular environment, and steadily disintegrate during incubation at 38° C., with the liberation of ribonucleotides. This disintegration process severely limits the time during which amino acid incorporation into protein can occur. Extensive investigations of optimal environmental conditions for the preparation and incubation of the particles have extended their useful stability to 90-120 minutes, and have resulted in greatly increased amounts of amino acid being incorporated into protein.

Ribonucleic acid is essential for amino acid incorporation into particulate protein. Pretreatment of the particles with ribonuclease results in the release of dialyzable nucleotides and the coincident inhibition of incorporating activity. Furthermore, both 4-aminofolic acid, an inhibitor of nucleic acid synthesis (5, 9), and various purine and pyrimidine analogues are inhibitors of amino acid incorporation into protein.

Gale and Folkes (3) have made the significant observation that the amino-acid-incorporating ability of bacterial extracts, previously inhibited by ribonuclease treatment, is restored by the addition of bacterial ribonucleic acid. Similar results have been observed with the

* This work was aided by a grant from the Charles F. Kettering Foundation.

268

present system, but, unexpectedly, the effect is not dependent on an intact ribonucleic acid molecule. Instead, a mixture of the four nucleosides derived from ribonucleic acid is considerably more effective in promoting amino acid incorporation than is ribonucleic acid itself (14). These findings raise a number of questions concerning the functions of both ribonucleic acid and its constituents in the incorporation of amino acids into protein. In order to learn more about the relationships of nucleosides and amino acid incorporation, our previous studies (14) have been extended to include considerations of the specificity of the nucleoside effect on incorporation, the possible functions of nucleosides and nucleotides in the amino acid incorporation system, and their relationship to actual protein synthesis.

SPECIFICITY OF THE NUCLEOSIDE EFFECT

In view of the striking effect of a mixture of the four nucleosides derived from ribonucleic acid on amino acid incorporation into protein (14), it was of considerable interest to determine the chemical structures of the nucleoside molecules necessary for promoting incorporation. It has already been shown (14) that removal of the ribose moiety results in a decreased ability of the nucleoside to enhance amino acid incorporation. Fig. 1 shows the effect of substitution of deoxyribose for ribose. It can be seen that deoxyribonucleosides, both singly and together, are without effect on the incorporation of glutamate-C^{14} into protein. Likewise, substitution of inosine, xanthosine, or purine riboside for guanosine or adenosine results in a diminution of the promoting effect of these nucleosides. Kinetin (6-furfurylaminopurine), a potent cell-division factor for certain plant tissue cultures (7), is also without effect on amino acid incorporation. The promoting effect, therefore, is seemingly specific for the nucleosides derived from ribonucleic acid.

In contrast to nucleosides, where alteration of the molecular structure results in loss of promoting ability, nucleotides exhibit variable effects depending on the position of the phosphate group in the molecule. As is evident from Fig. 2, nucleoside-3'-phosphates are less capable of promoting amino acid incorporation than free nucleosides. As the cytoplasmic particles are able to remove the phosphate group from nucleoside-3'-phosphates, it is entirely possible that the promotion observed with nucleoside-3'-phosphates is a reflection of their conversion to free nucleosides. In contrast, a mixture of nucleoside-

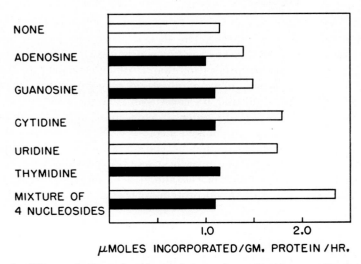

Fig. 1. Effects of ribonucleosides and deoxyribonucleosides on glutamate-C[14] incorporation into protein. Open bars, ribonucleosides; solid bars. deoxyribonucleosides. Complete system containing glutamate-C[14], amino acid mixture, adenosine triphosphate, phosphoenolpyruvate, $MgCl_2$, KCl, and the nucleosides was incubated for 60 minutes at 38° C.

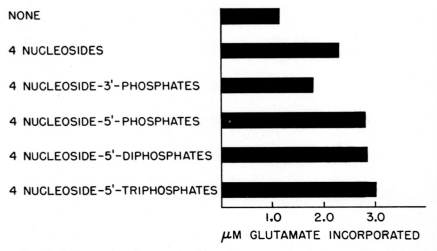

Fig. 2. Effects of various nucleotide mixtures on the incorporation of glutamate-C[14] into protein. The nucleoside moieties in each case were adenosine, guanosine, cytidine, and uridine. Reaction conditions were the same as described with Fig. 1.

5′-phosphates is more effective in augmenting incorporation than free nucleosides. Nucleoside-5′-diphosphates are only slightly more effective than the monophosphates, but a mixture of nucleoside-5′-triphosphates elicits the greatest enhancement of incorporation thus far obtained.

Gale and Folkes (4) have reported that, under certain conditions, the incorporation of a particular amino acid into bacterial protein is promoted by specific di- and tri-nucleotides obtained from ribonuclease digests of ribonucleic acid. Similar polynucleotide fractions have been isolated from a ribonuclease digest of yeast ribonucleic acid and purified by chromatography on Dowex-1 (1). When these polynucleotides are incubated with the particular preparation, amino acid mixture, Mg^{++}, K^+, and adenosine triphosphate, they fail to enhance the incorporation of any of the following amino acids into protein: alanine, arginine, aspartic acid, cysteine, glutamic acid, glycine, histidine, leucine, lysine, methionine, phenylalanine, and valine. In a few cases, in fact, 20-30 per cent inhibitions of amino acid incorporation result from the presence of the polynucleotides. Promotion of incorporation is obtained only when a concentrate of the crude ribonuclease digest (after removal of the nondialyzable polynucleotide) is incubated with the incorporating system. Although it is suspected that this promoting effect is due to the presence of mononucleotides in the digest, the possibility cannot be ruled out as yet that some unidentified promoting factor is present in such preparations.

Effects of nucleosides on the protein content of cytoplasmic particles. In addition to promoting the incorporation of amino acids into protein, nucleoside-5′-triphosphates effect an apparent increase in the protein content of the cytoplasmic particles (13). This increase requires the presence of a mixture of 18 amino acids, and magnesium and potassium ions (Table 1). However, the maximum protein increase that has been obtained thus far is disappointingly small and amounts to only 8 per cent of the particulate protein. Whether this increase represents a general synthesis of particulate protein, or whether it is due to the formation of a specific polypeptide is not yet clear. The fact that the protein increase is dependent on nucleotides and amino acids, in the same manner as amino acid incorporation into protein, suggests, however, that C^{14}-amino-acid incorporation into the particulate protein (14) is probably the result of this protein increase. Unfortunately, despite considerable effort, it has not been possible to elicit greater

TABLE 1

CHARACTERISTICS OF THE INCREASE IN PARTICULATE PROTEIN

System	Micrograms protein formed per milligram particulate protein per hour
Complete	58.
minus amino acid mixture	0.
minus magnesium ions	25.
minus potassium ions	38.
minus adenosine triphosphate	15.
minus nucleoside triphosphate mixture	30.
plus p-fluorophenylalanine	23.
plus ribonuclease	0.
plus hydroxylamine	0.

increases in protein. The most obvious difficulty in obtaining greater increases is due to the steady disintegration of the particulate nucleic acid during incubation. Further alterations of environmental conditions during the preparation and incubation of the particles, or the addition of a variety of possible stabilizing materials have failed to decrease further the rate of particle inactivation.

FUNCTION OF NUCLEOTIDES IN THE INCORPORATION OF AMINO ACIDS INTO PROTEIN

In view of the above results showing that ribonucleotides specifically increase both the rate of amino acid incorporation into protein and the protein content of the particles, the manner in which nucleotides function in both of these processes is of primary interest. Although they may exert several different influences, one attractive possibility is that nucleoside-5'-phosphates are efficient precursors of ribonucleic acid. The results of recent investigations with purine- or pyrimidine-requiring mutants of bacteria (8, 10), as well as with purine analogues (2), have indicated that protein formation depends upon the simultaneous formation of nucleic acid. In the present system, the effectiveness of nucleoside-5'-phosphates in promoting amino acid incorporation into protein could be due to their providing an abundant supply of nucleic acid precursors. That this may indeed be the case is shown by the data of Table 2, in which the rates of incorporation into ribonucleic acid of a series of precursors are compared. As is evident, the carbons of C^{14}-adenosine-5'-phosphates are incorporated considerably faster into ribonucleic acid adenine than are the carbons of any other precursors examined. The rates of incorporation, in fact, roughly

TABLE 2

Incorporation of Various C^{14}-Labeled Compounds into the Adenine of Ribonucleic Acid

Substrate	Micromoles incorporated per hour
Glycine	0.03
Adenine	0.15
Adenosine	0.23
Adenosine-3'-phosphate	0.17
Adenosine-5'-phosphate	0.29
Adenosine-5'-diphosphate	0.30
Adenosine-5'-triphosphate	0.33

parallel the extent to which the various substances enhance the incorporation of amino acids into protein. Nucleoside-5'-phosphates, therefore, may be promoting amino acid incorporation into protein by promoting the concurrently necessary formation of ribonucleic acid.

In order to ascertain whether protein and nucleic acid syntheses are interdependent in the cytoplasmic particles, the effects of selective inhibitors on each process have been examined. Table 3 presents the

TABLE 3

Effects of Selective Inhibitors on the Incorporation of Metabolites into Protein and Ribonucleic Acid

Inhibitor	Per cent inhibition of incorporation of	
	C^{14}-glutamate into protein	C^{14}-adenosine triphosphate into ribonucleic acid adenine
p-Fluorophenylalanine	41.	50.
β-Thienylalanine	45.	38.
Ethionine	18.	21.
Hydroxylamine	100.	100.
Chloramphenicol	100.	100.
Purine	83.	71.
6-Mercaptopurine	25.	19.
Benzimidazole	41.	33.

results of these studies. In every case, inhibitors of nucleic acid synthesis inhibit amino acid incorporation into protein, while inhibitors of protein synthesis inhibit the incorporation of C^{14}-adenosine-5'-triphosphate into the adenine of ribonucleic acid. Extensive studies have as yet failed to provide an inhibitor that will "uncouple" the two processes.

At least two other possible functions of nucleotides in promoting amino acid incorporation should be mentioned. The possibility that nucleotides promote incorporation by inhibiting decomposition of particulate ribonucleic acid has been tested experimentally. No evidence for the function of nucleotides in the inhibition of ribonucleic acid decomposition has been obtained. Of greater potential interest is the possibility that nucleotides act as (or are converted to) cofactors for protein synthesis. The observation of Keller and Zamecnik (6) that leucine incorporation into the protein of liver microsomes is specifically enhanced by guanosine diphosphate may be an example of such a cofactor function. Similar effects of guanosine diphosphate have not been observed with the present system, but it is possible that the nucleotide is already firmly bound to the particles.

DISCUSSION

Experiments with the present system have demonstrated two noteworthy facts. First, they have shown that the requirements for the incorporation of amino acids into protein at maximal rates are complex and involve (in addition to amino acid mixtures, adenosine triphosphate, Mg^{++}, and K^+) both intact ribonucleic acid molecules and certain mononucleotides. Secondly, if close attention is paid to the above requirements for maximal incorporation, as well as to optimal environmental conditions for the preparation and incubation of the particles, then indications of net protein synthesis can be obtained. These findings, together with those of other investigators (3, 15), demonstrate conclusively the value of cell-free preparations in elucidating the nature of the process of amino acid incorporation.

It would seem, however, that intact particles are of only limited value in elucidating the exact manner in which amino acids are incorporated into protein, and the manner in which ribonucleic acid or ribonucleotides participate in this process. The difficulties encountered in the study of both amino acid incorporation and net protein synthesis due to the activities of various degradative enzymes in the particles have already been mentioned. In order to overcome these difficulties, a systematic investigation has been undertaken of amino acid incorporation into protein by the nucleoprotein fractions liberated by sonic disruption of the microsome-like particles. Although only preliminary results are available, they indicate amino-acid incorporating systems of less complexity than the cytoplasmic particles can be prepared, and that these systems can provide additional information on the chemical steps involved in the incorporation of amino acids into protein.

REFERENCES

1. Cohn, W. E., Doherty, D. G., and Volkin, E., in *Phosphorus Metabolism* (W. D. McElroy and B. Glass, eds.), Vol. II, p. 339, Johns Hopkins Press, Baltimore (1952).
2. Creaser, E. H., *Nature*, **176**, 556 (1955).
3. Gale, E. F., and Folkes, J. P., *Biochem. J. (London)*, **59**, 661 (1955).
4. Gale, E. F., and Folkes, J. P., *Nature*, **175**, 592 (1955).
5. Goldthwaite, D. A., and Bendich, A., *J. Biol. Chem.*, **196**, 841 (1952).
6. Keller, E. B., and Zamecnik, P. C., *Federation Proc.*, **14**, 234 (1955).
7. Miller, C. O., Skoog, F., VonSalza, M., and Strong, F., *J. Am. Chem. Soc.*, **77**, 1392 (1955).
8. Pardee, A. B., *Proc. Natl. Acad. Sci. U. S.*, **40**, 263 (1954).
9. Skipper, H. E., Mitchell, J. H., Jr., and Bennett, L. L., Jr., *Cancer Research*, **10**, 510 (1950).
10. Spiegelman, S., Halvorson, H. O., and Ben-Ishai, R., in *Amino Acid Metabolism* (W. D. McElroy and B. Glass, eds.), p. 124, Johns Hopkins Press, Baltimore (1955).
11. Webster, G. C., *Plant Physiol.*, **30**, 351 (1955).
12. Webster, G. C., *Biochim. et Biophys. Acta*, **20**, 565 (1956).
13. Webster, G. C., *Federation Proc.*, **15**, 380 (1956).
14. Webster, G. C., and Johnson, M. P., *J. Biol. Chem.*, **217**, 641 (1955).
15. Zamecnik, P. C., and Keller, E. B., *J. Biol. Chem.*, **209**, 337 (1954).

REPRESSION AND INDUCTION AS CONTROL MECHANISMS OF ENZYME BIOGENESIS: THE "ADAPTIVE" FORMATION OF ACETYLORNITHINASE*

HENRY J. VOGEL

Department of Microbiology,
Yale University,
New Haven, Connecticut

THE INTIMATE connection that exists between the genetic apparatus of cells and the formation of enzymes (and other proteins) has been brought into sharp focus by the researches in microbial genetics (5, 11, 19, 28). For a full understanding of gene physiology and its chemical basis it would, therefore, seem essential to gain insight into the mechanics of protein synthesis. Undoubtedly, a clarification in detail of gene function as related to protein biogenesis is one of the central issues of contemporary "molecular biology."

Much of our knowledge of protein synthesis has come from several beautiful and incisive studies of enzymatic adaptation or induced enzyme formation (10, 14, 15, 17, 18). The important consequences of this work have riveted attention on the induction process, the inducer, and the latter's supposed locale of action, the enzyme-forming site.

IS INDUCTION A SINE QUA NON OF ENZYME FORMATION?

The present article is concerned, among other things, with the question whether or not induction is a necessary characteristic of all enzyme formation. Certain aspects of this question have been critically discussed by Cohn and Monod (7). They have cited the frequently expressed "unitary" view that there are no serious grounds for a fundamental distinction between inducible and constitutive enzymes. It follows, then, either that (i) induction is universal but masked in the

* Previously unpublished results obtained at Yale University were aided by a contract between the Office of Naval Research, Department of the Navy, and Yale University.

276

case of constitutive systems (generalized induction hypothesis), or that (ii) induction is a secondary and contingent phenomenon that is not a necessary characteristic of enzyme syntheses (secondary induction hypothesis) (7).

Cohn and Monod have made it clear that the problem of generalized versus secondary induction is as yet unresolved, but did propose that constitutive enzymes are formed through the agency of endogenous (internal) inducers (7). As an argument against the "secondary" hypothesis, these authors held that, if the said hypothesis is correct, the observed specific structural relationship of enzyme to inducer can be accounted for only on the assumption (which appears to be unwarranted) that induced enzyme synthesis somehow results from a specific combination of preexisting enzyme and inducer (7). It seems to the writer, however, that another assumption would be in accord with a "secondary" hypothesis, namely, that induced enzyme formation depends in part on an entity that is neither the enzyme nor the inducer, but has elements of structural complementariness to the inducer.

In connection with the generalized induction hypothesis, Cohn and Monod (7) considered the concept of the organizer (16) in induced enzyme formation. They pointed out that this concept implies that the characteristic pattern of an enzyme's "dynamic" site is imposed on it by a prosthetic group or co-organizer, which in turn is derived from the corresponding inducer. In other words, the inducer would carry at least part of the information for the structure of the enzymatically active portion of the protein. However, there is a good basis for the belief that the cell has this kind of information prior to induction, in view of certain specific inhibition effects observed (7), and for other reasons. It would thus seem that the inducer is dispensable with respect to the structural information required for enzyme synthesis.

Accordingly, there would appear to be no valid theoretical objections to a secondary induction hypothesis. On such a hypothesis, the nature of enzyme induction would be primarily that of a control mechanism. This view has been maintained from time to time and has been advocated in a recent paper by Lederberg (12). Indeed, the picture of induced enzyme formation as a regulatory device is consistent with the available results, including the following: enzymes of indistinguishable specificity are evoked by different inducers; there is no necessary relationship between the properties of a given substance as inducer, substrate, or complexant; and inducible enzymes usually show a "basal level" in the absence of added inducers. Moreover, on the basis of a "secondary" hypothesis one need not postulate (generally undemonstrable) endogenous inducers to account for the synthesis of constitutive enzymes (or for the basal levels of inducible enzymes).

The findings with acetylornithinase are in harmony with the notion that an induction process is not a *sine qua non* in the formation of this enzyme. Although an adaptive phenomenon has been encountered in the biosynthesis of this enzyme (22), it has not been possible to demonstrate an induction effect, nor indeed has it been necessary to postulate one.

The Case of Acetylornithinase

The adaptive phenomenon observed with acetylornithinase seemed of particular interest because it initially suggested the possibility of induced enzyme formation involving a constitutive, biosynthetic enzyme (22, 29; cf. 7).

The biosynthetic pathway with which this phenomenon was associated is the one leading to ornithine, citrulline, and eventually to arginine in *Escherichia coli*. In this organism, ornithine has been found to arise via a series of acetylated intermediates (20, 23-25). The last step in the formation of ornithine is the hydrolytic deacetylation of N^α-acetylornithine to ornithine. This step is mediated by the enzyme acetylornithinase (21, 23, 27). The activity of acetylornithinase is enhanced by the cobaltous ion and is stimulated and preserved by glutathione; the enzyme has no demonstrable requirements for any other organic factor (23, 27). Various other properties of the enzyme have also been recorded (27).

The adaptive phenomenon. For the adaptation experiments, a mutant (39A-23R1) of *E. coli*[1] was used that is blocked in the formation of acetylornithine; it gives a growth response either to acetylornithine or to ornithine or citrulline or arginine. Since the mutant is blocked in the arginine pathway at a step prior to that catalyzed by acetyl-

---

[1] Strain 39A-23R1 is a single-colony isolate from a culture of strain 39A-23 (cf. 22), which in turn is derived from *E. coli*, ATCC 9637. Results with different isolates were qualitatively similar, but quantitatively somewhat variable. In terms of the ultimate growth level attained by strain 39A-23R1, acetylornithine (on a molar basis) is at least as effective a growth factor as arginine. The L-isomers of acetylornithine (20, 24) and of arginine were used throughout.

ornithinase, this organism could be employed in experiments designed to exhibit a possible inducing effect of the *exogenously* supplied substrate on acetylornithinase formation (without interference from *endogenously* produced substrate). It thus seemed feasible to test for an induction effect that might be masked in the corresponding wild-type organism due to the continuous presence of the substrate of the constitutive enzyme involved.

An adaptive response could indeed be shown in growth experiments (Fig. 1). When an arginine-grown inoculum is cultivated under anaerobic conditions at 37° C. in a glucose-salt medium supplemented with arginine, exponential growth at wild-type rate results (see the straight line ABC in Fig. 1). However, if the arginine-grown inoculum is cultivated in the presence of a supplement of acetylornithine (under otherwise unchanged conditions), the adaptive response represented by the curve AD is obtained. Acetylornithine-grown inocula, when again cultivated on acetylornithine, fail to give the pronounced lag shown in Fig. 1 (cf. **22, 29**).

The adaptation observed suggested that the enzyme utilizing acetylornithine was being elicited through the agency of its substrate. In this connection, it should be noted that no growth of the mutant is obtained unless either acetylornithine or arginine (or the latter's functional equivalent) is provided. Hence, what appeared to be an enzyme induction by acetylornithine might have reflected the resumption of spontaneous (non-induced) enzyme formation after a possible prior depression by arginine (during the growth of the inoculum).

An indication of such an antagonistic effect on acetylornithinase formation presented itself in growth experiments with mixed supplements of arginine and acetylornithine.

Diphasic growth. When the mutant strain is cultivated, in the general manner described, on a mixed supplement of a limiting amount of arginine and an excess (in terms of growth requirement) of acetylornithine, diphasic growth results, as represented by ABE in Fig. 1 (cf. **22**). During the first phase, the growth proceeds exponentially at wild-type rate with virtually exclusive utilization of the arginine supplied.[2] At the point of exhaustion of the arginine, a relatively

---

[2] The preferential utilization of arginine would seem to be due either to an inhibition of acetylornithine utilization at the level of enzyme *function* (rather than of enzyme formation) or to an interference with the access of acetylornithine to acetylornithinase (cf. footnote 4).

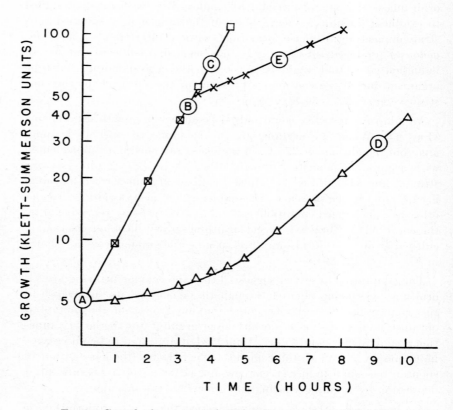

Fɪɢ. 1.   *Growth of mutant strain 39A-23R1 on various supplements*

The organism was grown anaerobically (nitrogen atmosphere) at 37° C. on a glucose-salt medium supplemented either with arginine alone (squares), or with acetylornithine alone (triangles), or with a mixture of 0.06 millimolar arginine and 0.30 millimolar acetylornithine (crosses).

The inoculum used was cultivated on the glucose-salt medium supplemented with 0.05 millimolar arginine; the inoculations were performed shortly after growth of the inoculum had ceased.

Growth of the cultures was followed turbidimetrically. A Klett-Summerson instrument (No. 66 filter) was employed; Klett-Summerson units are proportional to optical density.

See text and Table 1 in reference to the circled letters in this figure.

sharp "break" occurs; the organisms then enter a second phase, during which they grow at a reduced exponential rate. In general, no appreciable lag intervenes between the two phases. During the second phase, the organisms grow at the expense of the acetylornithine that was included in the medium. That the reduced second-phase growth rates observed reflect a restrictive rate of conversion of acetylornithine to ornithine is readily shown by the immediate acceleration of growth produced upon addition of ornithine to second-phase cultures.

An antagonistic effect of arginine seemed to be revealed, when it was noted that the longer the duration of the first phase (i.e., the more arginine there was in the mixed supplement), the slower was the resulting second-phase growth rate (22).

As a working hypothesis to account for the diphasic growth behavior, the possibility has been considered that the second phases correspond to an arginine-regulated capacity of the organisms to synthesize acetylornithinase. Other interpretations, however, have not been excluded. For instance, the second-phase growth rates could reflect the amount (controlled by arginine) of enzyme present in the cells at the "break"; and the constancy of these rates could be due to a physiological adjustment of the organisms (under the prevailing cultural conditions) to the initial pace set, even if relatively increased quantities of acetylornithinase should become available. Either hypothesis would be consonant with an antagonistic action of arginine (or a derivative thereof) on acetylornithinase formation.

Enzyme studies with mutant strain 39A-23R1. When the relative specific activity (see Table 1) of acetylornithinase extracted from acetylornithine-grown cells was compared with that from arginine-grown cells, the former was found to be substantially higher than the latter. The enzyme from acetylornithine-grown organisms and that from arginine-grown organisms were indistinguishable on the basis of their behavior toward cobalt and glutathione and of their substrate affinity; mixture experiments with enzyme from the two sources gave additive results.[3] It was therefore inferred that the adaptive phenomenon observed actually reflects the formation of acetylornithinase.

When a culture was sampled during second-phase growth at a point corresponding to E in Fig. 1, a relative specific activity smaller than

---

[3] The enzyme from the two sources is also indistinguishable from the acetylornithinase of wild-type *E. coli*, ATCC 9637.

TABLE 1

EFFECT OF CULTIVATION CONDITIONS ON THE RELATIVE SPECIFIC ACETYLORNITHINASE
ACTIVITY OF STRAIN 39A-23R1

The organisms were cultivated in the general manner described (see Fig. 1) in the presence of the supplements shown. Cultures were sampled for enzyme assay, as indicated, at points corresponding to A, B, C, D, and E in Fig. 1. The samples taken were chilled in ice and centrifuged at 0° C., and the resulting supernatant liquids were discarded. The sedimented bacteria from each sample were suspended in ice-cold 0.125 *M* phosphate buffer (*p*H 7) containing 1.0 m*M* glutathione and were then disrupted by sonic vibration. The sonicates produced were assayed for acetylornithinase activity, essentially as previously reported (27). The relative specific activity of the enzyme was computed as units of acetylornithinase activity per unit weight of total protein relative to the value (taken as 1.0) obtained for the arginine-grown inoculum.

Inoculum	Supplement, concentration (m*M*)	Point of sampling*	Relative specific activity
Arginine-grown	None	A	1.0**
Arginine-grown	Acetylornithine, 0.30	D	8.3
Arginine-grown	Arginine, 0.10	C	0.6
Arginine-grown	Arginine, 0.06	B	0.7
Arginine-grown	Arginine, 0.06, plus Acetylornithine, 6.00	B	0.7
Arginine-grown	Arginine, 0.06, plus Acetylornithine, 0.30	E	3.7
Acetylornithine-grown	Arginine, 0.06	B	1.2
Acetylornithine-grown	Arginine, 0.06, plus Acetylornithine, 6.00	B	1.2

* The acetylornithine-grown (like the arginine-grown) inoculum, when cultivated on the supplement of arginine shown, gave a growth rate corresponding to the line AB in Fig. 1. The same growth rate (at least up to the point of sampling) was observed for the two cultures that grew on the mixed supplement of 0.06 m*M* arginine plus 6.00 m*M* acetylornithine.

** Value for the arginine-grown inoculum used.

the "adapted" value, corresponding to D, was found (see Table 1). This result is in harmony with the conclusion, previously drawn from growth experiments, that arginine (or a derivative) appears to exert an antagonistic effect on acetylornithinase synthesis while the organisms are growing in the first phase.

In view of the apparent antagonism of arginine, the question arose whether this amino acid produces its effect through interference with a possible inducing function of acetylornithine in the synthesis of acetylornithinase. It was endeavored to obtain an answer to this question by examining, under various cultural conditions, the effect on the formation of acetylornithinase of the simultaneous presence of relatively large amounts of acetylornithine and relatively small amounts of arginine. Under these circumstances, an antagonism, possibly of a competitive nature, between acetylornithine and arginine might have been anticipated. However, this anticipation was not fulfilled, and in fact, no evidence for an inducing action of acetylornithine on acetylornithinase formation could be obtained from the experiments described below.

(i) An arginine-grown inoculum was cultivated, under the general conditions outlined above, on a quantity of arginine sufficient to permit growth up to the optical density of the "break," as represented in Fig. 1. The culture was sampled at a point corresponding to B shortly prior to attainment of this optical density. The enzyme level obtained is included in Table 1. An arginine-grown inoculum was then cultivated analogously on a mixed supplement of arginine and acetylornithine, the quantity of arginine again being sufficient to permit growth up to the point of the "break" and the molar ratio of acetylornithine to arginine being 100 to 1. When the resulting culture was sampled at an optical density corresponding to B, precisely the same specific activity of extracted acetylornithinase was found as that obtained when the organisms were grown in the absence of acetylornithine. Since the arginine, but not the acetylornithine, supplied is used up during the growth of the culture, the ratio of acetylornithine to arginine becomes progressively larger; at the point of sampling, nearly all the added arginine has been exhausted, and this ratio is seen to be very greatly in excess of the initial one of 100 to 1. Mixed supplements containing less acetylornithine likewise led to the same enzyme level as that obtained with arginine as sole supplement.

(ii) A similar experiment was performed with an acetylornithine-grown inoculum. During cultivation on arginine or on arginine plus acetylornithine, as in (1), the specific activity fell, in both cases, from the "adapted" value of the inoculum to that shown in Table 1.

(iii) An arginine-grown inoculum was permitted to undergo diphasic growth on a mixed supplement of 0.05 mM arginine and 0.3 mM acetylornithine. In a parallel procedure, a culture was grown on a mixed supplement of 0.05 mM arginine and 15 mM acetylornithine. On sampling both cultures at corresponding points during second-phase growth, identical acetylornithinase levels were found.

Enzyme studies with wild-type E. coli. The wild-type organism, from which mutant 39A-23R1 was derived, was also examined as to a possible elicitation of acetylornithinase by its substrate. It was discovered that wild-type cells grown on minimal medium and such cells grown on minimal medium in the presence of 1.0 mM acetylornithine gave identical acetylornithinase levels. In contrast, when the cells were cultivated in minimal medium containing 1.0 mM arginine, the specific gravity of acetylornithinase was reduced by 70 per cent. (In these experiments, the general cultural conditions employed were the same as those described for the mutant strain; the wild-type cultures were harvested at Klett-Summerson readings of about 90.)

The pronounced depressing action of arginine on acetylornithinase synthesis in the wild-type strain has a measure of specificity, since various other amino acids (not directly related to arginine) tested exhibited no such effect.

REPRESSION AND INDUCTION IN THE REGULATION OF ENZYME BIOGENESIS

Comments on the experiments with the acetylornithinase system. That the arginine supplied to the organisms (or a metabolic transformation product of arginine) antagonizes acetylornithinase formation was clearly indicated in the experiments cited. Moreover, no inducing function of acetylornithine in acetylornithinase synthesis could be demonstrated, nor any reversal of the antagonistic effect of arginine. In these experiments, first- and second-phase cultivation of arginine-grown and acetylornithine-grown inocula of the mutant strain and cultivation of the parental wild-type strain were employed. In first-phase growth, the inclusion of various proportions of acetylornithine in the culture medium failed to exert any detectable effect on the system studied, not even when relatively massive amounts of acetylornithine were supplied. In second-phase growth (i.e., after the added arginine had been consumed), the level of acetylornithinase produced was again independent of acetylornithine concentration over a wide range. In the experiments with the wild-type organisms, added acetylornithine and arginine could be tested under conditions when neither was required for growth. In this case too, acetylornithine was entirely inert, whereas arginine depressed acetylornithinase formation.

These findings do not *prove* that acetylornithinase is *not* induced by its substrate. For example, one can imagine that, when the mutant strain is grown in the presence of a mixed supplement of arginine and acetylornithine, the (low) acetylornithinase level obtained (prior to the exhaustion of arginine) is, after all, induced by the acetylornithine supplied. When the mutant strain is grown on a supplement of arginine only, the hypothesis that the acetylornithinase formed under these conditions arises through substrate-induction may be maintained only on the assumption that the cells can somehow produce an amount of acetylornithine sufficient to give the same enzyme level as that obtained with the mixed supplement. Any such assumed formation of acetylornithine is not likely to occur from the added arginine by reversal of the normal synthetic pathway (24), since the cleavage of acetylornithine to yield ornithine is, for practical purposes, irreversible (27). However, it is *unnecessary* to postulate that acetylornithinase is induced by its substrate, nor indeed, by any other substance. The results under discussion can be explained on the hypothesis that acetylornithinase synthesis is spontaneous (non-induced) and antagonizable by arginine (or a chemical relative of arginine), and that, following the disappearance of added arginine, the rate of enzyme synthesis accelerates through *release* from the antagonistic influence.

As mentioned above, wild-type cells growing on a minimal medium, although producing arginine, synthesize acetylornithinase at levels that can be depressed by cultivation in the presence of exogenous arginine. It would seem to follow that endogenous arginine either is formed in quantities insufficient to give the reduction in enzyme level obtained with the exogenous arginine, or can be distinguished by the cells from exogenous arginine. Such distinctions between endogenous and exogenous metabolites are known: for instance, endogenous ornithine is metabolized differently from exogenous ornithine by *Neurospora crassa* (2, 26) and *Torulopsis utilis* (2). The arginine produced by mutant strain 39A-23R1, when the latter is cultivated on a supplement of acetylornithine, presumably resembles, in the respect mentioned, the arginine formed by the wild-type strain.

Repression of enzyme formation. The action of arginine on acetylornithinase formation may be regarded as a rather specific antagonistic effect on enzyme synthesis of a substance following in biosynthetic sequence the substrate of the enzyme; in this case, the substance is the "end-product" of the biosynthetic sequence involved. It is readily seen that this action of arginine constitutes a control mechanism that presumably is of great value to the organism: for example, an *E. coli* (wild-type) cell, in an environment that supplies arginine, will utilize this exogenous arginine [4] and at the same time will conserve its resources by sharply curtailing the now unnecessary synthesis of acetylornithinase.

The regulation of acetylornithinase formation by arginine by no means appears to be an isolated occurrence of its kind. For instance, enzymes concerned with the synthesis of methionine (8, 30), tryptophan (13), valine (3), and pyrimidine compounds (4) probably are subject to similar regulation. This type of control may thus be quite a general phenomenon.

In order to facilitate further discussion, the following terminology [5] will be used hereafter: a relative decrease, resulting from the exposure of cells to a given substance, in the rate of synthesis of a particular apoenzyme is termed "enzyme repression"; the substance thus decelerating enzyme synthesis is a "represser" ("repressor"); an enzyme-forming system that can be antagonized by a represser is "repressible"; and, under conditions of repression, the formation of the enzyme is "repressed." [6]

Repression and induction. It is evident that the repression of the formation of a "constitutive" enzyme in response to the corresponding "end-product" represents a control mechanism that is complementary to the induction of an "adaptive" enzyme in response to a suitable inducer. In either case, the cell tends to form enzymes when they are needed, and tends not to form enzymes when they are not needed.

The following "small-molecule" control situations with respect to enzyme formation are conceivable:

[4] The preferential utilization of exogenous arginine (to the virtual exclusion of endogenous arginine) for protein synthesis in *E. coli* has been demonstrated with isotopic competition experiments (1); under conditions of such preferential utilization, the synthesis of arginine by the cells is inhibited (6). This inhibition reflects an interference with the functioning of one or more enzymes already present in the cells. The inhibition of enzyme *function* operates in addition to the antagonism to enzyme *formation,* thus providing the organisms with two coacting mechanisms for conserving their resources.

[5] This terminology is modeled after that proposed for induced enzyme formation by Cohn et al. (9). These authors define enzyme induction as "a relative increase in the rate of synthesis of a specific apoenzyme resulting from exposure to a chemical substance."

[6] "Repression" would seem preferable to such terms as "inhibition" or "suppression," which have well-established connotations in enzyme chemistry and in genetics, respectively. It will be noted that enzyme repression, as defined here, includes interference of a substance with induced enzyme formation.

(i) indifferent enzyme synthesis (no control);

(ii) induced enzyme synthesis;

(iii) repressed enzyme synthesis.

One and the same enzyme-forming system could be both inducible and repressible, or could be neither. Again, a given enzyme-forming system could be inducible, but not repressible, or repressible but not inducible. The latter category includes the case of acetylornithinase, as far as the available evidence goes. The adaptive effect obtained with the mutant strain used could then be termed a "repression-release" phenomenon.

A possible mechanism of repression. It would seem reasonable to assume that repression of enzyme formation reflects an interference with the functioning of the enzyme-forming system.

The question then arises as to the mechanism by which a represser (or a represser derivative), presumably of small molecular weight compared to that of a protein, can hamper the performance of an enzyme-forming system. One conceivable mechanism would seem to consist in the binding of a newly synthesized enzyme molecule to the site of its formation through the agency of the represser (or its "active" derivative). Such binding might block the further production of enzyme molecules until the enzyme-forming site affected is freed again. Whether or not this type of binding, mediated by a repressing substance, would involve the "dynamic" site of the enzyme (which may have affinity for the "active" represser) is, at present, unknown.

In line with such a picture of repression, the induction process could be regarded, at least in some instances, as comprising a promotion of the removal of an enzyme molecule from its site of synthesis. In indifferent enzyme synthesis, the newly produced enzyme would vacate its forming-site with neither assistance nor hindrance from specific small molecules.

General biological implications of enzyme repression. In view of the above-mentioned utility to the cell of repression mechanisms, it seems warranted to assume that an organism that developed a repressible enzyme in the course of evolution thereby gained an asset, which under conditions of competition would have a positive selective value. Presumably, therefore, the selection for repressibility mechanisms constitutes a factor in evolution, and it would thus appear to be no accident that instances of enzyme repression can be readily discovered.

It seems quite probable that enzyme repression, like enzyme induction, occurs in the higher forms of life. If so, the arguments advanced by a number of authors in support of a possible role of enzyme induction in development, or even in differentiation, apply with equal force to a possible role of enzyme repression in these important biological phenomena.

As discussed above, the notion that induction is not a sine qua non of enzyme synthesis has led to the inference that, in general, the cell possesses all the information required for the structure of its enzymes. One might imagine that much, if not all, of this information is contained in, and preserved by, the nuclear genes of the organism, no matter how fuzzy at the edges they turn out to be. At any rate, in consideration of the subject matter of this Symposium, it seems appropriate to end this article with a tribute to the genetic, rather than to the non-genetic, powers of the cell!

Summary

An adaptive phenomenon, which superficially seemed to reflect a substrate-induced formation of the biosynthetic enzyme acetylornithinase, has been analyzed.

The adaptive effect is attributed to the *removal* of an antagonistic influence of arginine on the synthesis of acetylornithinase, rather than to an induced formation of this enzyme. Thus, in a variety of experiments with an acetylornithine-requiring mutant strain (which permits the testing of the substrate as a possible exogenous inducer) of *Escherichia coli* and with a wild-type strain of this species, an antagonistic effect of arginine, but no inducing action of acetylornithine, could be demonstrated.

This general type of antagonism is referred to as "enzyme repression," in analogy with "enzyme induction."

Induction probably is not a sine qua non of enzyme synthesis; hence, the information required for the structure of enzymes and presumably contained in genetic material, does not appear to be supplemented through the agency of inducers.

Both repression and induction are viewed as control mechanisms of enzyme biogenesis.

Arginine, the represser studied, is the "end-product" of the biosynthetic pathway in which acetylornithinase participates. Repressibility of an enzyme, by a substance following in biosynthetic sequence the substrate of this enzyme, is thought to be of value to the cell involved and presumably is positively selected in the course of evolution.

REFERENCES

1. Abelson, P. H., *J. Biol. Chem.*, **206**, 335 (1954).
2. Abelson, P. H., and Vogel, H. J., *J. Biol. Chem.*, **213**, 355 (1955).
3. Adelberg, E. A., and Umbarger, H. E., *J. Biol. Chem.*, **205**, 475 (1953).
4. Back, K. J. C., and Woods, D. D., *Biochem. J. (London)*, **55**, xii (1953).
5. Beadle, G. W., in *Genetics in the 20th Century* (L. C. Dunn, ed.), p. 221. Macmillan Co., New York (1951).
6. Britten, R., *Science*, **119**, 578 (1954).
7. Cohn, M., and Monod, J., *Symposium Soc. Gen. Microbiol. (Adaptation in Micro-organisms)*, **3**, 132 (1953).
8. Cohn, M., Cohen, G. N., and Monod, J., *Compt. rend. Acad. Sci. Paris*, **236**, 746 (1953).
9. Cohn, M., Monod, J., Pollock, M. R., Spiegelman, S., and Stanier, R. Y., *Nature*, **172**, 1096 (1953).
10. Gale, E. F., in *Enzymes: Units of Biological Structure and Function* (O. H. Gaebler, ed.), p. 49. Academic Press, New York (1956).
11. Horowitz, N. H., and Fling, M., in *Enzymes: Units of Biological Structure and Function* (O. H. Gaebler, ed.), p. 139. Academic Press, New York (1956).
12. Lederberg, J., in *Enzymes: Units of Biological Structure and Function* (O. H. Gaebler, ed.), p. 161. Academic Press, New York (1956).
13. Monod, J., and Cohen-Bazire, G., *Compt. rend Acad. Sci. Paris*, **236**, 530 (1953).
14. Monod, J., and Cohn, M., *Advances in Enzymol.*, **13**, 67 (1952).
15. Pollock, M. R., *2nd Intern. Congr. Biochem., Paris (Symposium sur la biogenèse des protéines)*, p. 67 (1952).
16. Pollock, M. R., *Symposium Soc. Gen. Microbiol. (Adaptation in Micro-organisms)*, p. 150 (1953).
17. Spiegelman, S., in *Enzymes: Units of Biological Structure and Function* (O. H. Gaebler, ed.), p. 67. Academic Press, New York (1956).
18. Stanier, R. Y., *Ann. Rev. Microbiol.*, **5**, 35 (1951).
19. Tatum, E. L., in *Enzymes: Units of Biological Structure and Function* (O. H. Gaebler, ed.), p. 107. Academic Press, New York (1956).
20. Vogel, H. J., *Abstr. Am. Chem. Soc. (Atlantic City)*, 43C (1952).
21. Vogel, H. J., *Proc. 6th Intern. Congr. Microbiol. (Rome)*, **1**, 267 (1953).
22. Vogel, H. J., *Proc. 6th Intern. Congr. Microbiol. (Rome)*, **1**, 269 (1953).
23. Vogel, H. J., *Proc. Natl. Acad. Sci. U. S.*, **39**, 578 (1953).
24. Vogel, H. J., in *Amino Acid Metabolism* (W. D. McElroy and B. Glass, eds.), p. 335. The Johns Hopkins Press, Baltimore (1955).
25. Vogel, H. J., Abelson, P. H., and Bolton, E. T., *Biochim. et Biophys. Acta*, **11**, 584 (1953).
26. Vogel, H. J., and Bonner, D. M., *Proc. Natl. Acad. Sci. U. S.*, **40**, 688 (1954).
27. Vogel, H. J., and Bonner, D. M., *J. Biol. Chem.*, **218**, 97 (1956).
28. Vogel, H. J., and Bonner, D. M., in *Handbuch der Pflanzenphysiologie* (W. Ruhland, ed.), Vol. 11, Chapter II. Springer-Verlag, Heidelberg (in press).
29. Vogel, H. J., and Davis, B. D., *Federation Proc.*, **11**, 485 (1952).
30. Wijesundera, S., and Woods, D. D., *Biochem. J. (London)*, **55**, viii (1953).

DISCUSSION

DR. P. BERG: I would just like to ask Dr. Spiegelman what the shockate preparation is. Is it the pellet that you spin down after dilution of the protoplasts?

DR. SPIEGELMAN: Yes.

DR. BERG: In other words, the acid-soluble nucleotide fraction is now removed after treatment with the so-called RM mixture.

DR. SPIEGELMAN: No.

DR. BERG: The supernatant is removed?

DR. SPIEGELMAN: Yes. The supernatant is always removed.

DR. BERG: What constitutes the induction mixture for the synthesis of DNA?

DR. SPIEGELMAN: We need a complete mixture of amino acids, HDP, potassium ion, manganese and magnesium ions. In the presence of this they will make everything that I have indicated: protein, RNA, and DNA.

DR. BERG: What then is the source of the nucleotides for RNA and DNA synthesis since you show that most of the nucleotides remain in the supernatant after this treatment?

DR. SPIEGELMAN: Well, they are making them.

DR. KORNBERG: How can they make more DNA?

DR. SPIEGELMAN: I don't understand.

DR. KORNBERG: What is the source of the deoxynucleotides?

DR. SPIEGELMAN: They are presumably synthesizing them from material they have or what we are supplying. I should like to note that a supply of amino acids is essential for extensive DNA synthesis. However, in the absence of amino acids, some DNA formation occurs if desoxynucleotides are provided. I should like to emphasize again that we don't have here an isolated enzyme. Our preparation is hardly in a state to suit the needs of the biochemist seeking to unravel the intermediate details of DNA synthesis.

DR. CHARGAFF: I have one question for Dr. Spiegelman and one for Dr. Allfrey. I refuse to use the shocking word shockate, and would prefer to use the word micromush. When you get DNA synthesis or RNA synthesis, do you look at the sugar reactions, or do you look at the spectrum? Do you have enough bases in your preparation to put them back into the nucleic acid, or do you simply get a polyribose derivative?

DR. SPIEGELMAN: I mentioned the fact, I think, that we measure the absorption spectrum of the material synthesized after hydrolysis. Let me describe it. We do an acid precipitation after the synthesis is over. A 30° C. alkaline hydrolysis is then performed and the DNA precipitated from this digest. The precipitate is then hydrolyzed with hot

0.5N perchloric acid and UV absorption performed at 260 and 290 mμ. The values are then compared with analysis of the same material, using Burton's modification of the Dische reaction.

Dr. CHARGAFF: You see, there are some very characteristic spectroscopic changes when you go from a mixture of nucleotides to a polynucleotide. For instance, there is a very marked decrease in the extinction. This will be, in a way, the test of polymerization. Altogether there are very marked spectroscopic shifts. One can't really speak of synthesis unless one has this kind of information.

Dr. SPIEGELMAN: We can't have this information on this system. There is too much interfering material. However, we make milligrams of this material and isolate and analyze the product made. It seems to me that this provides much more direct evidence of its nature.

Dr. CHARGAFF: I would like to ask Dr. Allfrey a simpler question. You had a slide on the effects of ordinary alanine compared with C^{14} alanine showing that the nuclei after centrifugation could still go on and incorporate it. I was wondering, if you have C^{14} alanine and get an increase in incorporation (increasing counts), shouldn't we expect that if you have the unlabeled alanine you will get a decrease in incorporation, because presumably the nuclei cannot differentiate between the isotopic and the non-isotopic amino acids? I noticed that, after labeling, in one case the C^{14} went up in the continued presence of isotope, but, in the presence of C^{12} alanine, the label was almost stationary, instead of going down in a symmetric fashion.

Dr. ALLFREY: The reason is this: In the operation of that experiment the technique will allow the uptake to proceed for 60 minutes; then we remove the C^{14} alanine or other amino acids which may have been used. At that point we add an excess of C^{12} alanine, so that in the usual experiment there is no further chance for incorporation. You can show that these nuclei can still take up isotopes, so to do that at 60 minutes you give this group a fresh dose of the C^{14} isotope, and so uptake proceeds again in this case. As I understand it, you are asking if in the case where you add C^{14} after 60 minutes it goes up, why in the case where you add the unlabeled amino acid it does not go down. The reason is that, for one thing, it is a tracer experiment and you take up minute amounts of unlabeled isotope, which isn't going to change the level of the isotope in the protein. The other thing is, of course, that it is not a reversible system, which is the main point of the experiment.

Dr. OCHOA: I would like to ask a question. Dr. Spiegelman's shockates have shocked me more than they shocked him. I can't help being shocked when I hear that the Ochoa mixture and the Ochoa enzyme nullify themselves. Now, Sol, the question is: Did you use resolved cell fragments in that experiment where you showed increase of all of the components—DNA, RNA, and protein on addition of the polynucleotide phosphorylase digest of RNA? Were they resolved by the RM treatments?

DR. OCHOA: Your synthesizing medium contains no added bases?

DR. SPIEGELMAN: No.

DR. OCHOA: You think the system may be synthesizing the bases from scratch?

DR. SPIEGELMAN: Yes, to a certain extent.

DR. BERG: I would like to make one comment on Dr. Allfrey's talk concerning the amino acid incorporation into nuclei proteins. It seems to me that one of the points we should discuss concerns the criteria of alkali lability and a ninhydrin reaction which are being used to establish whether this is an incorporation into a peptide structure. I don't know how valid these two criteria are for actually establishing whether this is incorporation into a protein. One could argue from the data that have been presented that this is linkage of amino acid with DNA —not that this would be uninteresting by itself. However, the point is that one of the criteria which must be used is to actually isolate polypeptide structures, dipeptides or tripeptides showing that the amino acid is incorporated in such a linkage rather than just using the criteria of alkali lability and reactivity with ninhydrin.

DR. ALLFREY: I thought I had made the answer to that in the course of the talk. You see, they were introduced as criteria for incorporation into the total protein, but subsequently to that we isolated these proteins, such as the lysine-rich histones and the arginine-rich histones. In those cases, we found that the amino acid present, like lysine, was actually in the protein. Now, there is another point. Could it be absorbed on the DNA? Even when we were making the total protein from the nucleus we were sure to get rid of all of the nucleic acid.

DR. LEVINTHAL: I have a question for Dr. Spiegelman. Do you have any evidence or any data for the kinetics of the increase of total absorption at 260 mμ in your incubation mixture?

DR. SPIEGELMAN: Yes. I do. I have separate figures for DNA, RNA, and protein. I can sum them. I have never done that. It seems to me that a chemical analysis is superior to a UV absorption at 260 mμ.

DR. NASON: I have a question for Dr. Allfrey concerning the possibility of incorporation vs. protein synthesis. Is it possible, in view of the extremely small amount of incorporation of C^{14} compared to the very high endogenous protein in your nuclei, that now after you removed C^{14} and provide the C^{12} you don't detect any appearance of C^{14} in the medium as a result of further change because of the great dilution effect in the nucleus itself? The second question is to Dr. Spiegelman. On the first slide on which you used the term shockate, the fourth shockate showed a loss of about 80% of its RNA, and yet your enzyme formation had gone up continually. Did I read that correctly?

DR. SPIEGELMAN: Did you look at the ratio between RNA and protein? You always have to look at ratios here, not at absolute numbers.

DR. NASON: But in your control you go from an absolute number of 314 to 70 with respect to RNA.

DR. SPIEGELMAN: You are talking about comparison of various shockates. You see, in that 1 to 4 shockate I have 200 gammas of protein and 70 gammas of RNA. In the 1:3 shockate I have 340 gammas of protein and 123 gammas of RNA, so that the relative content of RNA does not differ very much between a 1 to 3 and a 1 to 4. The big difference comes in the 1 to 5 shockate, where you have only 4 gammas of RNA and 179 gammas of protein.

DR. ALLFREY: In answer to your question about exchange, I don't think that the objection that you raised fits into this argument, because we did not measure the release of isotope into the medium after the uptake had occurred, but rather what we did was to measure the retention of isotope in the insoluble protein.

DR. HOAGLAND: I would like to say a word about the microsomes. The group at Massachusetts General Hospital has described a liver system containing microsomes, supernatant, ATP, GTP, and labeled amino acids which produces incorporation of the labeled amino acids into the microsome protein. This incorporation into the microsomes is very rapid and is initially more rapid than in any other fraction, including the nuclei. Littlefield and Keller in our laboratory have recently shown that ribonucleoprotein particles received from the microsomes of mouse ascites tumor cells have the capacity for incorporating amino acids at a rapid rate into their protein structure, and these particles, as they prepare them, have about 50% RNA and 50% protein. Furthermore, in relation to the importance of the supernatant fraction in this process, we have recently been studying the activation enzymes of which, as Dr. Spiegelman pointed out, there may be one in number for each amino acid activated prior to incorporation. These enzymes are separate from the microsome fraction. It looks as if there is a nucleotide associated with these activating enzymes and we are trying to identify it. Dr. Lipman, who has recently prepared in high purity a tryptophan-activating enzyme, has also found a firmly bound nucleotide associated with the enzyme. I mention these matters because I think there is much to be said for a system in which one can make such progress in more clearly defining the actual nucleotide and enzyme requirements for irreversible incorporation of labeled amino acids into ribonucleoprotein particles, a process which we now feel safe in calling protein synthesis.

DR. KAPLAN: Dr. Allfrey, you say that with your particle the incorporation of amino acids is abolished by dinitrophenol and other factors. Do you think that the nucleus itself is carrying out oxidative phosphorylation?

DR. ALLFREY: I didn't have time to go into that, but we have very good evidence indeed that the nucleus is carrying out oxidative phosphorylation. We have shown that you do get ATP synthesis in isolated nuclei, and it is not inhibited by a number of inhibitors which do block ATP synthesis in mitochondria.

Dr. R. Williams: What is the relative magnitude of the amount of incorporation of amino acids in the case of isolated nuclei, compared with what these nuclei would have assimilated in the same length of time in the intact cell? Have you done the experiment the same way with intact cells? The same question, I think, applies to the protoplast compared with the intact *megaterium*.

Dr. Allfrey: In our experiments comparing nuclei with tissue slices or minces the nucleus is either just as active as the whole cell or perhaps half as active.

Dr. Hotchkiss: I would like to ask Dr. Spiegelman to clarify one point. The synthesizing medium sounds so much like the resolution medium that I would like to know what turns on the synthesis.

Dr. Spiegelman: We substituted chloride for phosphate and added HDP in the synthesizing medium.

Dr. Potter: I would like to comment on the iconoclastic position of Dr. Spiegelman. I think that it detracts somewhat from the extreme scientific interest of your presentation. I think when a fellow is iconoclastic he should state which particular prophets he is counter-manding. I found nothing particularly novel in the concepts that were presented, but I thought the data were extremely interesting.

Dr. Spiegelman: Dr. Potter, at the present time I see no point in following any other prophets than the data.

Dr. Berg: I would like Dr. Allfrey to state explicitly the experimental operation involved in showing the leakage or non-leakage from the protein that had already incorporated label—that is, what did you do to show that the label remained in protein? Did you make an acid precipitation, or did you spin down the nuclei, wash them, measure, and so on?

Dr. Allfrey: Oh, no. Nothing of the kind. After the uptake had occurred, the nuclei are spun down and washed exhaustively with trichloroacetic acid. Then the nucleic acid is removed with hot TCA; then the lipids are removed; then we wash again; and then finally we have a protein residue that we assay.

Dr. M. Green: Dr. Allfrey, you said that your criterion for protein synthesis was that you isolated labeled protein from the nuclei. Did you employ this criterion in your experiments with reconstituted nuclei —that is, where you added either DNA or degraded DNA or RNA, and got an increase in the incorporation of isotopic amino acid?

Dr. Allfrey: In those experiments we did not isolate proteins after uptake had occurred; but we did see whether isotope, once incorporated, did exchange; and it did not.

Dr. Berg: There is one comment about the degradation of *E. coli* RNA and yeast RNA which Dr. Spiegelman used to prepare the diphosphates. A purified preparation of polynucleotide phosphorylase from *E. coli* prepared by DiHaver and Kornberg does not appreciably degrade purified RNA. It appears to degrade only the polymers which it makes. In this particular case you have used a similar *E. coli* enzyme to generate and manufacture the nucleoside diphosphates.

DR. SPIEGELMAN: We used an enzyme prepared according to a procedure devised by Razell of Illinois and a highly purified preparation kindly supplied by Dr. Uri Littauer of Kornberg's laboratory. Our substrate was commercial yeast RNA which was not highly polymerized.

DR. BERG: As I understand it, the *E. coli* and the *Azotobacter* polynucleotide phosphorylases enzymes do not significantly degrade yeast RNA or their own natural RNA.

DR. OCHOA: Dr. Heppel has rather recent data indicating that the *Azotobacter* enzyme can bring about the phosphorolysis of one of the virus RNA's—I think it was the turnip yellow mosaic virus—and also very recently the phosphorolysis of Allen's preparation of yeast RNA, so it does seem to act on some RNA's fairly well.

DR. SPIEGELMAN: I might add that we did isolate the diphosphates— the 7-minute material—and it goes up after the digestion with enzyme.

DR. BERG: I didn't question that. I think it's an important point, because it may provide a way for producing nucleoside diphosphates enzymatically from a readily available source.

DR. HOGNESS: I would like to ask Dr. Spiegelman a question. In cases where you regenerated activity of the shockate by the addition of ribonucleoside diphosphates, what was the percentage of regeneration?

DR. SPIEGELMAN: It was 100% where it worked, but if the shockate is too highly resolved for RNA, diphosphates won't work and we don't know why. At present the implications are that the systems have to have some intact RNA to respond.

DR. SMITH: I was wondering whether the DNA synthesized in your system has the composition of that of the normal bacteria.

DR. SPIEGELMAN: I don't know.

DR. VOLKIN: I would like to ask Dr. Allfrey whether this incorporation represents a *de novo* synthesis of intact protein or if the labeled amino acid might be attached just as an end group on preformed protein.

DR. ALLFREY: I can't give you a positive answer either way on it. The only way to prove it would be to show that new protein is synthesized, and we haven't done it. All that we have shown is that the label goes in and stays there.

DR. HOAGLAND: In the microsome system, the label is incorporated into the protein molecule and can be demonstrated to occur in peptide fragments obtained by partial acid hydrolysis (*J. Cell. and Comp. Physiol.*, **47**, supplement 1, May 1956). The labeled amino acid is not just terminal, but substantially exists within the protein structure.

DR. LOOMIS: I would like to ask Dr. Allfrey what the highest P/O ratio is that he has obtained with nuclei.

DR. ALLFREY: I can't answer that. All of that work was done by Dr. Osawa in our laboratory, and he is much better qualified than I to answer that question.

DR. DOUNCE: I would like to ask Dr. Spiegelman whether his results have not effectively ruled out the use of RNA and DNA as information carriers. If you take out both the RNA and the DNA and then replace with the Ochoa digest you have no information carrier left.

DR. SPIEGELMAN: In none of our preparations have we ever removed all of the RNA. As soon as 50% removal is reached, you lose the ability to synthesize DNA and protein. I might add that obviously the DNA that is synthesized in these preparations can, of course, be nonsense DNA. What we need, then, is a test for the biological specificity of the DNA. The base ratios will certainly be important, but obviously not decisive. To test for the biological specificity is going to be a rather difficult job, because genetic recombinations of any type are virtually unknown in *B. megaterium*. It was for this reason that we were very happy to learn by personal communication from Dr. Lederberg and Dr. Zinder that protoplasts can be made from *E. coli*. We have employed Dr. Lederberg's procedure to prepare protoplasts of *E. coli* and derived shockates from them which retain considerable enzyme synthesizing ability. We hope that with them, or with the very closely related *Salmonella* system, we will be in a position to test whether genetically competent DNA is being synthesized.

Part III

NUCLEIC ACIDS AS TRANSFORMING AGENTS

X-RAY INACTIVATION STUDIES ON SOLUTIONS OF TRANSFORMING DNA OF PNEUMOCOCCUS

HARRIETT EPHRUSSI-TAYLOR

Laboratory of Genetics,
University of Paris,
Paris, France

INVESTIGATIONS OF THE action of ionizing radiations on transforming factors of pneumococcus have been undertaken with the hope of determining the dimensions of the biologically active particle (1, 2, 3). At the outset, the method would seem particularly suitable in view of the fact that with small viruses, the radiation-sensitive volume is observed to be in close agreement with particle size, as estimated from sedimentation and electron microscope studies (4). This is to say that an ionization occurring anywhere within the particle has a high probability of destroying its biological activity. DNA particles are of the same order of size as small viruses, and would seem, from the point of view of size, to be as favorable a material for the application of radiation methods.

However, investigations pursued in my laboratory during the past few years with the assistance and collaboration of several colleagues have led to the conclusion that the target theory in any simple form is inapplicable, in so far as the inactivation of the streptomycin-resistance transforming factor of pneumococcus is concerned. It is concluded that the transforming factor is a complex target, and that this accounts for its complex inactivation behavior. Because of the special role which DNA is generally believed to occupy in genetic structures, it seems worthwhile to summarize the principal results obtained.

The validity of inactivation experiments resides first of all in the validity of the methods employed for titration of activity. Consequently, problems of quantitation of transforming activity will be discussed in some detail before turning to the results of the inactivation experiments.

299

I. Quantitation of Transforming Activity

Schematically, two reactants are involved: reactive, or competent, bacteria, and DNA particles endowed with transforming activity. One of the reactants, the competent bacteria, is highly unstable, the competent state lasting, on the average, about 15 minutes per bacterium (5, 6). The other reactant, the transforming DNA, presents the complication of being impure, in that along with molecules bearing the selective marker there is an unknown number of molecules which lack the selected marker, but which bear, presumably, other kinds of specific transforming functions. The development of effective titration methods requires that these special features be taken into consideration.

It is now evident that the pattern by which competence develops is a function of the species of bacterium, and of culture conditions (5, 6, 7). The conditions employed in the experiments to be described lead to an almost synchronous development of competence by a large but indeterminate proportion of the population, during exponential growth of the culture. Since competence lasts only 15 minutes, one observes, as a function of time, a tremendous fluctuation in the numbers of cells which can be transformed for a particular marker. In the space of a single generation (30 minutes), the number may pass from zero to 10^5 and drop back to ten or a hundred, in a culture containing 5×10^6 bacteria. A second wave of competent cells usually appears on the heels of the first.

In such synchronized cultures, the reaction between bacteria and DNA can be performed in two ways:

(1) At a moment when a growing culture contains many competent bacteria, the culture may be chilled and samples transferred rapidly to a medium containing measured amounts of the DNA to be assayed.

(2) Bacteria and the DNA to be assayed can be mixed in the culture medium at the outset, and the cultures incubated long enough to go through one or more cycles of competence. In each instance, time is then allowed for phenotypic expression, and the reaction mixtures are assayed on selective media. However the reaction is carried out, replicates give results as accurate as the plating method itself. The second method gives higher numbers of transformed cells per unit weight of DNA, since the number of competent cells involved is always greater than in the first method. With either titration technique, low concentrations of transforming DNA yield transformed cells in proportion to the amount of DNA added.

curves observed vary, but their similarity is always apparent. It is possible that this complex situation is a result of special conditions prevailing in my own laboratory, but it may be noted that curves published by others (9, 2) definitely suggest that a similar behavior is to be observed under the conditions employed by them. Almost none of the titration curves published thus far have a form compatible with the simple saturation of competent bacteria by transforming agent. Thomas, on the other hand, who observed a simple plateau in experiments done in my laboratory (4), was working under conditions in which rate of transformation was very low, and this might explain why he failed to detect the complex nature of the titration curve.

It is most desirable to understand the reasons for the complexity of titration curves, in order to perform quantitative experiments in security. The most likely cause of complex behavior was suspected to be the heterogeneity of the transforming DNA, and accordingly experiments were devised in which this heterogeneity was deliberately increased in a known fashion. This was done by adding to the DNA extracted from the streptomycin-resistant strain, known amounts of DNA prepared from a pneumococcal strain which lacked the marker. Fig. 2 shows the results of such an experiment. The following points can be noted:

(1) The numbers of transformed cells observed at both the first and second plateaus are decreased roughly in proportion to the increased numbers of unmarked DNA particles present.

(2) The first plateau sets in at lower concentrations of the S_r transforming factor; that is, it sets in as a function of the total amount of DNA in the system.

These results suggest the following interpretation of the titration curves:

That the first break in the curve occurs when bacteria are beginning to react with more than one unit of DNA, and is due to a marked inhibition of transformation in bacteria which have so reacted.

That as multiplicity augments, inhibition is reversed in those bacteria which have reacted with a great enough number (or perhaps variety) of DNA units.

Finally, that a second break occurs because either the number of units of DNA a bacterium can absorb is limited, or the probability of acquiring the right varieties is low. This being granted, the actual titration curves observed for a particular marker are only a reduced

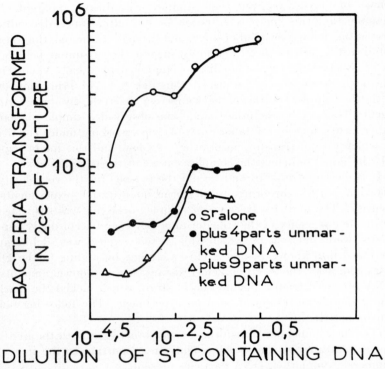

Fig. 2. Curves relating transformations induced to DNA concentration, at high DNA levels, and in the presence of competing DNA. Experimental details as in Fig. 1.

image of the total events. Absolute values will be limited in the linear portion of the curve by the proportion of DNA units bearing the marker and by the total number of competent cells, and in the non-linear portion by the intensity of interference and the number of DNA units a bacterium can absorb.

Justification of this interpretation can be found in the work of Hotchkiss (5) and Hotchkiss and Marmur (10), who have established beyond doubt the reality of interference. Further supporting evidence has been obtained by myself and Dr. Furness, in experiments employing a DNA containing two markers: resistance to streptomycin and to canavanine (8). In this instance, the numbers of bacteria acquiring one or both markers are determined. From the curve for single transformations, the position of the plateaus can be determined. Assuming that the two markers are unlinked, doubly transformed bacteria should appear when the probability of two effective hits becomes high. Experiments show that in practice doubly transformed bacteria cannot be found until DNA concentrations are reached which yield the first plateau for singles. This, then, strongly supports the idea that the first plateau sets in when the probability of two hits becomes high. There is, however, one difficulty. Can one be sure that the two markers are unlinked? Interestingly enough, when doubly transformed cells make their appearance, their numbers appear to increase almost proportionally with DNA concentration. A linear increase would be expected from two factors linked on a single particle, but not for two independent factors. However, it is precisely at these concentrations of DNA that inhibition of transformation has been invoked to explain the existence of the plateau for single transformations. A linear increase in doubles would be compatible with location of the markers on two separate particles if the inhibition is sufficient to change an exponential increase into a linear one. A definite proof was needed as to whether or not two particles were involved.

This proof may be obtained in the following way. It has been shown that in the region of the first plateau the effect of competing DNA is to decrease transformations approximately in proportion to the increased heterogeneity of the DNA. Where two particles are involved, doubles should be decreased in proportion to the square of the decrease in singles. Too few experiments have been performed to say whether the reduction is exactly proportional to the square, but results definitely show that the reduction is near this level. The figures shown in Table 1 can be cited in evidence.

It seems most likely that the two factors are located on separate particles, and consequently, that the interpretation proposed to explain the titration curves is a valid one. It may be added incidentally that interference experiments would seem to provide the most direct test for linkage of two factors, involving the fewest assumptions and the least work.

In any event, it is clear that the non-linear region of the titration curve cannot be considered to follow the behavior of a typical bimolecular reaction. Nor can the mechanisms operating involve a simple competition for a site in the bacterium. In view of the importance of multiplicity in determining lysogeny and transduction in *Salmonella*,

TABLE 1

The effect of competing DNA on single transformations to streptomycin resistance and doubles to canavanine and streptomycin resistance, induced by a transforming DNA prepared from a doubly marked strain. Control: the transforming DNA acting alone. Experimental: the transforming DNA in the presence of competing DNA which lacks the markers.

Dilution of Transforming DNA	Singles to S^r		Doubles	
	Control	Experimental	Control	Experimental
10^{-1}	1.4×10^5	1.38×10^4	345	8
$10^{-1.5}$	6×10^4	7×10^3	226	2
10^{-2}	3.9×10^4	3.75×10^3	157	3
$10^{-2.5}$	2.5×10^4	6.8×10^3	62	0
10^{-3}	9×10^3	8.5×10^3	25	2

it is worthwhile to speculate briefly on the possible nature of interference between transforming factors. The explanation which *a priori* seems most intelligible is that the observed kinetic behavior is an expression of the well-known phenomenon of genic imbalance: that when a bacterium has acquired one molecule of DNA, genic disequilibrium is relatively slight, but as second, third, and fourth molecules enter the cell, such a disturbance is created that the transformed cell fails to transform, or even dies. Genic balance would be restored in those cells which pick up enough different molecules so that something approaching a complete set of genetically distinct molecules is attained. Such an hypothesis implies that whether or not a molecule is integrated into the genome, it exerts a physiological action in the cell. This is not difficult to admit in view of the experiments of Stocker on abortive transductions (11). Integration into the genome may express only an attachment to a centromore-like structure, and be quite beside the point in so far as physiological action or even DNA duplication is concerned. The hypothesis further leaves open the possibility that differently marked DNA molecules may unfavorably affect the cell to different extents. Data with canavanine resistance as a marker suggest, in fact, that the first break in the titration curve occurs at slightly higher DNA concentrations than for streptomycin resistance. This could best be explained by assuming that the imbalance is in part a function of the qualities of the molecules absorbed. Finally, according to this hypothesis, the degree of multiplicity required for interference to disappear would be a function of the number of different types of DNA molecules present in the pneumococcal cell. This multiplicity is of the order of ten. But it would not be fruitful at present to try to calculate the number of different molecules involved on the basis of this figure, for too many assumptions are involved.

In connection with this hypothesis that imbalance can be created by excess DNA, it is interesting that several lines of evidence lead to the idea that bacterial viruses contain more DNA than is required to transmit the genetic information needed for virus synthesis. This has been suggested by Levinthal, for phage T2 (12); by Luria, for those phages in which host-induced variations are found (13); and by Zinder, for transducing phage (14). Were the uptake of a certain quantity of DNA to lead to genic imbalance, the "extra" DNA of phages could be ascribed a very important function, namely, that of creating a disturbance of the host cell which would be favorable to the infective process. On the other hand, the amount of "extra" DNA may play a decisive role in determining the establishment of lysogeny. Those phages which have either very little or very much "extra" DNA along with their virus DNA will tend to be lysogenic rather than lytic, owing to the slightness of the genic imbalance they created. That this "extra" DNA need be of the right specificity would account for the non-genetic host-induced modifications described by Luria. It is the utility of this hypothesis which has made it attractive enough to present here in this symposium, in spite of the lack of direct evidence to support it.

Turning now to the problem of the quantitative estimation of the inactivation of transforming agents by diverse treatments, we see clearly that inactivation, whatever its nature, results in an increased heterogeneity of the DNA solution. In addition to the inherent heterogeneity, there are inactivated molecules, and in some instances fragments of molecules, which will be exerting their effects. The active particles will thus comprise much less of the total mass of DNA, and, what may be more critical, may be reduced to a very small proportion of the total number of particles. It is necessary to determine whether interference sets in as a function of the mass of DNA absorbed by the bacterium, or as a function of the particles of DNA absorbed, more or less irrespective of the mass of each individual particle.

To test this point for the irradiation experiments to be described, a highly irradiated sample of transforming DNA was prepared, and a curve established relating transformations induced to DNA concentration. This curve is compared with a simultaneous titration of

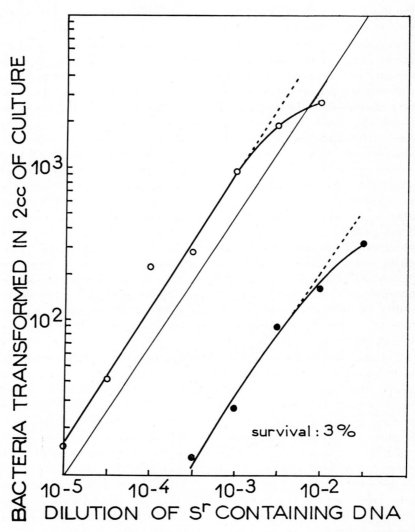

F_IG. 3. Comparison of titration curves obtained with x-ray inactivated and control samples of DNA containing the streptomycin-resistance factor. The fine line gives the slope expected from a linear relationship between amount of DNA and numbers of transformations. White circles: control; black circles: irradiated.

unirradiated DNA. The results of an experiment are shown in Fig. 3. Although the DNA has received a very strong irradiation, so that only 3 to 4 per cent of activity remains, linear results are obtained at low DNA concentrations, and the first plateau sets in approximately as in the control. If there is a difference, it is in the direction of a less sharp break in the curve on the irradiated material.

These results are compatible with three interpretations. Either the plateau sets in as a function of the total mass of DNA in the titration, or no fragments are formed by the x-rays, or the fragments formed do not contribute to the interference phenomenon. Since in all likelihood fragments are formed, it can be concluded that either inhibition is predominantly a matter of the mass of DNA absorbed, or that the fragments formed are inactive. It is clear that in x-ray inactivation work, titrations can be set up taking into account that it is the mass of DNA added which determines whether the results will be linear or not. This has been done in the experiments now to be reported by establishing in each experiment that the scale of concentrations of DNA employed does not exceed the limiting concentration, as determined on the control DNA. In addition, in the most heavily irradiated samples, titrations were performed at two levels of DNA, in order to be certain of the linearity of the titration of the most irradiated samples.

II. Quantitative Radiation Studies on the Streptomycin-Resistance Factor

One of the striking properties of the streptomycin-resistance transforming factor is its extreme sensitivity to the free radicals formed in water during irradiation (3). This sensitivity is revealed by the fact that the addition of organic matter to the solution of transforming DNA gives only a partial protection from indirect effects. It is necessary, for the determination of the radiation-sensitive volume, to exclude inactivation due to indirect effects, but it is extremely difficult to know when this has been completely accomplished. In the experiments to be described, irradiation in the frozen state has been employed in order to eliminate, in so far as possible, the action of free radicals. When the DNA solutions are frozen during irradiation, inactivation curves are identical irrespective of the amount of protective substances added, and yield the smallest radiation-sensitive volume (15). At worst, this volume is in error by being still too large, to the extent that free radicals are still causing some inactivation. The extreme sensitivity of the transforming factor to indirect effects is doubtless a consequence of the enormous surface which the DNA molecule offers for chemical reactions with the solvent phase.

In the experiments to be described, irradiations were performed under two conditions. The S^r-containing DNA is diluted in 1 per cent Yeast Extract (Difco) and irradiated (a) in the liquid state, where 90 per cent of inactivation is due to secondary effects; or (b) in the frozen state, where most if not all inactivation is due to direct hits.

Irradiation in the frozen state is used where the radiation-sensitive volume is to be determined, and in the liquid state where regions of low survival are to be examined. The latter expedient is chosen in order to avoid the very long exposures which would otherwise be necessary were all irradiation done on frozen material, for in unfrozen material inactivation is ten times faster than in frozen.

An example of the first kind of curve is seen in Fig. 4; of the second in Fig. 6, A.

When the disappearance of transforming activity is studied as a function of radiation dose, one observes first an exponential drop in activity, followed by a break in the curve which sets in when between 5 and 10 per cent activity remains (see Fig. 4). The break in the curve is due to the presence of highly resistant residual activity. It is difficult to determine precisely the sensitivity of this resistant residual activity, owing to the limitations of the titration system, and owing to the complication of using such high doses of x-rays. This activity seems to be about ten times more resistant to the radiation than that which disappears in the first, exponential part of the curve (15). Curves of this type have been observed both for ionizing radiations (2, 3) and for ultraviolet light (16). A similar curve may also be obtained with succinic peroxide, a substance having a radiomimetic action, as an inactivating agent (17). The bulk of all of this work has been performed on the streptomycin-resistance factor, but Marmur and Fluke (3) have investigated the mannitol-utilization, the penicillin-resistance, and the sulfanilamide-resistance factors as well.

Confining interest first to the exponential portion of the curve, it must be stated at the outset that considerable difference exists in the rates of inactivation observed in different investigations (1, 2, 3). Inactivation doses have been found which are compatible with molecular weights ranging from 7×10^5 to $2\text{-}6 \times 10^6$. Owing to the extreme sensitivity of the transforming agent to indirect effects, it is likely

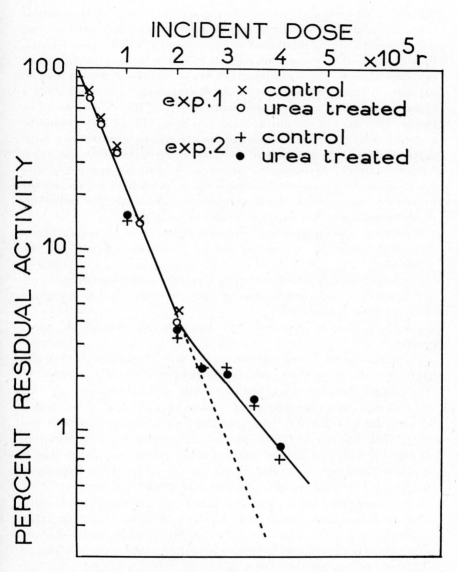

Fig. 4. Treatment of transforming DNA with 5 *M* urea. No change is observed in inactivation characteristics. Irradiation is performed under conditions in which about 90 per cent of the inactivation is due to indirect effects.

that the smaller value is more nearly correct. Accepting for the moment the smaller value, it should be noted that it is ten times smaller than the molecular weight attributed to pneumococcal DNA (Doty, 1955). If we assume that every ionization is effective we must also assume two sizes of units in transforming DNA, viz., molecules having a mean molecular weight of 7×10^6, and the S^r-transforming factor having a radiation-sensitive volume of not more than 7×10^5. There would be two obvious ways of visualizing these two units. The S^r factor could be a smaller particle than the average, or it could be located on a large particle, most of the structure of which is not concerned with the transforming activity. According to the second hypothesis, any potentially inactivating event occurring outside of a particular region of the molecule would cause no inactivation, and consequently, the radiation-sensitive volume would be smaller than particle size.

Turning now to the resistant residual activity, there are several situations that might be responsible for it. The more obvious are the following:

(a) owing to indirect effects, when a certain percentage of inactivation is reached, the already inactive particles may exert a protecting effect on those remaining active;

(b) there may be a genetically distinct x-ray-resistant S^r factor present;

(c) activity may be associated with two sorts of particles, having different sensitivities to x-rays, ultraviolet light, and succinic peroxide; or

(d) aggregates, requiring very many hits, are present.

The first explanation is excluded by the fact that irradiations performed on very dilute DNA solutions give these broken curves (0.0001 per cent). The amount of DNA present in such cases is so small in comparison with the amount of protecting substances added that it cannot be the DNA which determines the curve. Also, this hypothesis could not explain the results obtained with ultraviolet light.

The second explanation was eliminated by preparing transforming DNA from bacterial clones derived from cells transformed by DNA subjected to heavy irradiation. The DNA "clones" derived from activity surviving irradiation have inactivation characteristics identical with those of the "parent" DNA (2).

There remain the last two hypotheses.

Hypothesis c. Were the residual resistant activity associated with a distinctive particle, it might be supposed that fractionation of transforming DNA by the method of Brown and Watson (18) would yield materials having different x-ray inactivation properties. This possibility has been examined by irradiating two fractions obtained from an experiment performed by Dr. G. L. Brown of King's College. One fraction had a high guanine content and a high specific activity, while the second had a lower guanine content and a low specific activity. The results of an experiment (Table 2) indicate no significant difference

TABLE 2

Destruction of transforming activity in two fractions of pneumococcal DNA prepared by Dr. G. L. Brown. Fraction 9 is rich in guanine and has a high specific activity. Fraction 30 is guanine-poor, and has a low activity. X-ray inactivation is under conditions of indirect effect.

Irradiation dose $r \times 10^3$	Per cent residual transforming activity		
	Unfractionated	Fraction 9	Fraction 30
25	46	36.4	40.6
50	21	13.4	24.3
75	13.8	9.4	14.6
100	10.2	6.61	5.4
150	—	3.9	3.4
200	1.9	1.7	1.7
300	0.6	0.5	—

between the two samples with respect to their x-ray inactivation. The result is particularly interesting in view of the finding that macromolecular weight is greatest in those DNA's having a high guanine content (19). However, there is no correlation between x-ray sensitivity and guanine content. Furthermore, and much more important, if two different sorts of S^r particles exist, they must be supposed to remain in essentially the same proportions in the two widely separated fractions which were examined. This result is not in favor of the hypothesis that two sorts of particles are involved.

Hypothesis d. Were formation of aggregates responsible for the residual resistant activity, strong urea might be expected to make it disappear, in view of the well-known effects of urea in diminishing intermolecular attractions. Accordingly, samples of transforming DNA were treated with 5 M urea for a number of hours, and the x-ray inactivation of the treated material was then compared with that of controls. Urea has no effect upon biological activity, nor does it alter the inactivation characteristics of the DNA. The latter fact is demonstrated in Fig. 4.

Thus, it has not been possible to obtain evidence in favor of any one of the four above hypotheses. However, it is difficult to obtain evidence categorically against several of them. It has nonetheless proven possible to amplify the evidence against a formation of aggregates as the cause of the resistance.

The occasion arose in examining pneumococcal DNA, prepared by Dr. N. S. Simmons, which proved to be very difficult to dissolve, and which, after hours of shaking, gave an opalescent solution of low viscosity. The S^r-transforming activity of the solution was from 10 to 20 per cent that of a normal DNA preparation. The activity showed, however, a remarkable resistance to irradiation with x-rays, as may be seen in Fig. 5. This curve is typical of an active unit which requires

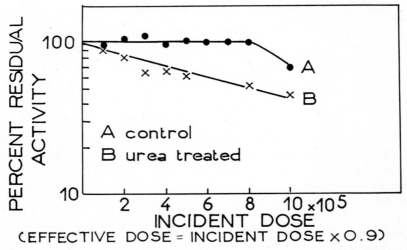

Fig. 5. Irradiation of highly aggregated transforming DNA, under conditions of direct effect. A, aggregated sample. B, the same, after treatment with 5 M urea. (From ref. 15).

several hits in order for activity to disappear. The number of hits lies somewhere between 3 and 10. This fact immediately suggested that the DNA was aggregated and that the particles comprised from 3 to 10 transforming units. Here, then, was a material upon which to test the action of urea. Treatment with 5 M urea resulted in the appearance of viscosity, and in a threefold increase in activity. Urea-treated samples showed, finally, a normal inactivation curve, when subjected to irradiation with x-rays. A curve obtained after urea treatment is shown in Fig. 5. There can be no doubt that in the original solution large aggregates were present, and that they have been dispersed by urea. Doubtless these aggregates are composed not only of several S^r particles, but of other kinds of DNA molecules as well, unless specific attraction is to be invoked. The aggregates may be presumed to be very large indeed, and it is interesting to have another form of evidence indicating that bacterial cells can react with a large mass of DNA. The fact that in this instance urea can dissociate DNA aggregates strengthens the argument that the residual resistant activity is not a consequence of the formation of aggregates, but is caused by some other peculiarity of structure.

Since the purpose of these experiments was to try to superimpose the image of the active transforming site upon the image of the molecule as depicted by the physical chemists, it seemed highly desirable to prepare a transforming DNA by a method currently employed in obtaining DNA for physical-chemical study, and to perform on the DNA both x-ray inactivation studies and physical-chemical measurements. Thanks to the interest and assistance of Dr. N. S. Simmons and Professor P. Doty, one such experiment has been realized. Dr. Simmons prepared the DNA by his method, and the material was subjected to physical-chemical study in Professor Doty's laboratory. As a preliminary, the relatively dilute solution was subjected to centrifugation in order to eliminate undispersed DNA. Two fractions were thus obtained. Fraction 1 comprised the upper supernatant liquid, while Fraction 2 included a small pellet plus the lower supernatant liquid.

Fraction 1 contains molecules of the size and configuration typical of calf thymus DNA prepared in identical fashion (Doty, 1955). The S^r transforming factor in the solution behaves, however, as though it were a particle having a molecular weight of not more than 7×10^5, until 10 per cent survival is reached, at which point one observes the break in the curve that demonstrates the presence of resistant residual activity. The same discrepancy exists, therefore, between the x-ray-sensitive volume and the molecular weight, as had been noted with our preparations of transforming DNA. Furthermore, the resistant residual activity has not been eliminated.

Fraction 2 reserved a surprise. Here, in the material normally rejected in light-scattering work, was found activity which was three to four times more sensitive than usual. This can be seen in Fig. 6, in

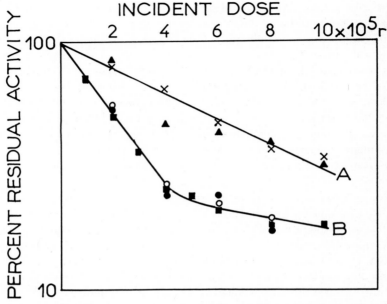

Fig. 6. Irradiation of Fraction 1 (curve A) and Fraction 2 (curve B) under conditions of direct effect. Fraction 1 gives a curve typical of most transforming DNA preparations, with an inactivation dose in the neighborhood of 7×10^5 r. Fraction 2 contains x-ray-sensitive material having an inactivation dose in the neighborhood of 2.5×10^5. (From ref. 15).

which the inactivation curves of Fractions 1 and 2 are shown. The problem which arises more persistently than ever is this: with how many kinds of targets is S^r activity associated? Already three sorts have been described: the activity associated with a unit having a mass of the order of 7×10^5, the resistant residual activity, and the x-ray-resistant unit requiring multiple hits for its inactivation. Since the last-mentioned unit is unstable to urea treatment, and is converted into the first, there remain basically two varieties of S^r activity. It was decided to see whether the fourth kind of unit, the x-ray-sensitive one, was also stable to urea treatment. In fact, it is not (15). Treatment with urea renders samples of Fraction 2 essentially like Fraction 1 in the vast majority of transforming DNA solutions examined. It seems, therefore, most probable that the x-ray-sensitive particle is also a product of aggregation, and is not a basic constituent of transforming DNA.

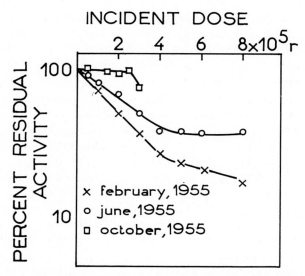

F IG. 7. Progressive change in the inactivation behavior of Fraction 2. Evolution is toward aggregation. Irradiation is under conditions of direct effect. (From ref. 15).

How is it possible that aggregation can give rise to two units differing so radically in their inactivation characteristics? Part of the answer is demonstrated by Fig. 7. Here are shown inactivation curves performed on Fraction 2, allowed to stand for ten months with only very little stirring. A progressive change in inactivation behavior is evident, and evolution is toward the formation of x-ray-resistant units requiring multiple hits. Apparently, the x-ray-sensitive, urea-unstable unit is found during the initial phase of aggregation. It remains to be explained why a small aggregate should be more sensitive to x-rays than the basic unit of which it is composed. This question will be considered shortly.

D ISCUSSION

It is customary to find the properties of DNA highly complex. In the described x-ray inactivation work, complexity has taken the form of a plethora of units having different sensitive volumes, all endowed with streptomycin-resistance transforming activity. In addition to two urea-stable units differing in x-ray sensitivity by a factor of ten-fold, two other kinds of units are described which are unstable to urea treatment. Both of the latter are presumably aggregated forms of the urea-stable units. One of these aggregates is highly resistant to x-rays, and requires many hits for inactivation to occur, while the other is more sensitive to x-rays than the basic units of which it is composed, and is inactivated by a single hit.

Restricting attention first to the urea-stable units, the following remarks may be made about them. They may be considered to be fundamental units of transforming DNA, because they are stable to urea, and because they are consistently found in DNA prepared by two different methods. Experiments thus far performed which might have proven that these two units are physically discrete have failed to do so. The units may of course be discrete and the methods thus far employed to separate them inadequate. However, if we suppose that they are not discrete, but are functional aspects of a single entity, what needs to be postulated to explain the inactivation curves obtained? It need only be supposed that the target offered by the S^r transforming factor is complex: that S^r activity is due to the properties of only a very small region of the DNA molecule, but that the probability of this region becoming incorporated by the bacterium is very greatly increased if a large region around it is intact. Accordingly, the dimensions of the S^r region would be those of the resistant residual activity, while those of the sensitive region around it would be of the order of 7×10^5. The larger target is ten times smaller than the average DNA molecule, but the causes of this cannot be stated with certainty. It may be that the larger sensitive region is itself only part of the molecule involved, or, as has been mentioned above, it may represent the entire molecule, but be measured as smaller owing to errors in the radiation method. The dimensions of the smaller target are of the order of 7×10^4. If one takes these figures at face value, the larger target contains one-tenth of the nucleotides of the total molecule, i.e., 2×10^3, and the smaller target contains one-hundredth, or about 2×10^2. The calculation cannot be taken too seriously, however, owing to the uncertainty already discussed, and owing to the possibility that the projectile used may be too big for the smaller target.

It is interesting to note that the notion of a complex target, essentially like that invoked above, has been put forward by Garen and Zinder (20) in radiation studies on transducing phage, and that in this latter instance, too, DNA may be presumed to be the site of action of the radiation.

Turning finally to the behavior of aggregates toward irradiation with x-rays, the following problem arises. How can it be that during the initial phases of aggregation S^r particles are inactivated more readily than unaggregated material, and by a single hit, while in later stages, many hits are required? The DNA in the solutions containing the aggregates shows a high degree of orientation, as evidenced by its crystallinity (21). It may be supposed that the molecule-fibers are packed in parallel and orderly array. The fact that the smaller aggregates offer a larger target than unaggregated DNA can only be explained by supposing that a hit in an aggregate has effects which spread beyond the limits of a single molecule. This may result as a consequence of energy transfer, but is more likely to be the result of the formation of stable cross-links between adjacent molecules. Cross-links might very well block the integration by bacteria of S^r-bearing molecules. X-ray inactivation probably occurs in the same fashion in both small and large aggregates, but since the spreading effect would tend to be limited, an aggregate would show multi-hit behavior as soon as two S^r particles were associated in a particle whose dimensions exceeded the radius of spread. It has not been possible to test this point, owing to the variable results observed with the inhomogeneous suspensions of the large aggregates.

Radiation studies unfortunately yield data which can be interpreted only with the aid of a fair number of assumptions. However, the use of urea in the present investigation has been of enormous help in unsnarling the complexities encountered, and has enabled a more direct testing of several hypotheses than is customarily possible in x-ray work. It is quite clear that, in certain types of pneumococcal DNA preparations, aggregation occurs giving rise to particles having properties different from those manifested by the basic elements of the solution. Stability toward urea might profitably be used in defining a large variety of properties of DNA particles.

REFERENCES

1. Brown, G. L., M'Ewen, M. B., and Pratt, M. I., *Nature,* **176**, 161 (1955).
2. Brown, G. L., and Watson, M., *Nature,* **172**, 339 (1953).
3. Ephrussi-Taylor, H., and Latarjet, R., *Biochim. et Biophys. Acta,* **16**, 183 (1955).
4. Fluke, D. J., Drew, R., and Pollard, E., *Proc. Natl. Acad. Sci. U. S.,* **38**, 180 (1952).
5. Garen, A., and Zinder, N., *Virology,* **1**, 335 (1956).
6. Hotchkiss, R. D., *Proc. Natl. Acad. Sci. U. S.,* **40**, 49 (1954).

7. Hotchkiss, R. D., and Marmur, J., *Proc. Natl. Acad. Sci. U. S.*, **40**, 55 (1954).
8. Latarjet, R., in *Ionizing Radiations and Cell Metabolism*, J. A. Churchill Ltd., London (1956).
9. Lea, D. E., *Actions of Radiations on Living Cells*, Cambridge, England (1946).
10. Levinthal, C., *Proc. Natl. Acad. Sci. U. S.*, **42**, 394 (1956).
11. Luria, S. E., *Cold Spring Harbor Symposia Quant. Biol.*, **18**, 237 (1953).
12. Marmur, J., and Fluke, D. J., *Arch. Biochem. and Biophys.*, **57**, 506 (1955).
13. Marmur, J., and Hotchkiss, R. D., *J. Biol. Chem.*, **214**, 383 (1955).
14. Schaeffer, P., *Ann. inst. Pasteur* (in press).
15. Stocker, B. A. D., *J. Gen. Microbiol.*, in press (1956).
16. Thomas, R., *Biochim. et Biophys. Acta*, **18**, 467 (1955).
17. Zinder, N., *Cold Spring Harbor Symposia Quant. Biol.*, **18**, 261 (1953).

CRITERIA FOR QUANTITATIVE GENETIC
TRANSFORMATION OF BACTERIA

ROLLIN D. HOTCHKISS

Rockefeller Institute for Medical Research, New York, N. Y.

GRIFFITH, WHO discovered the transformation of bacteria, and Avery, who did so much to define it, amply demonstrated the heritable and specific nature of the changes brought about. Although the process was always by implication genetic, it was by no means obvious that it is closely related to the nuclear genetic processes of higher plants and animals. Now, however, many homologies have been indicated, and it will not be useful to dwell upon them here. Rather, after briefly indicating the genetic nature of transformations, we shall turn to the discussion of what seem to be their unique features, their nature as physico-chemically definable interactions between cells and cell parts.

It has been pointed out elsewhere that transformations are step-by-step transfers of unit portions of the genetic potentialities of the donor cells (12, 14). The cell properties transferred reflect accurately the unitary nature, great or little, simple or complex in effect, of the donor strain as inferred from a known mutational history. Transforming agents from pneumococci were shown to transmit a genetic potentiality (the ability adaptively to dehydrogenate mannitol) without reflecting the attained enzymatic state, adapted or unadapted, of the cells from which the agents were extracted (22). Such findings led to the deliberate conclusion that the transforming deoxyribonucleates (DNA) contained biologically specific entities operationally equivalent to bacterial genes.

With the help of a system of linked genes in pneumococcal DNA, it was possible to derive evidence that the effective units introduced in transformation are not only smaller than the total bacterial genome, but are variable fragments of individual DNA particles themselves (17). It is important to distinguish the type of genetic recombination involved in transformation from those which seem to be involved in such higher order processes as crossing over. Formally, at least, the latter result from reciprocal exchanges between homologous intact

321

strands, across distances of several thousand Å. We believe the evidence indicates that bacterial transformation results from an extraneous DNA fragment acting at short range, and in a non-reciprocal manner modifying, or substituting in, the DNA of the cell during replication (17). Other bacterial or phage genetic recombinations, and transduction, appear to be similar non-reciprocal short-range processes.

LIMITATIONS OF THE CLASSICAL SYSTEM

The capsule transformations were detected by Avery, MacLeod, and McCarty (4) by exposing the DNA-treated culture to an antibody broth in which the unencapsulated organism would grow, be agglutinated, and fall to the bottom of the tube, leaving transformants to grow in the upper levels. As we gained some experience with this system, it became clear that many pitfalls awaited the newborn transformant before it would have a chance to be detected. In the first place, many capsulated transformants would be found among the sedimented organisms at the bottom of the tube, and not duplicating successfully. This was so serious a matter that if the sedimentation were speeded up by using an inoculum as little as three or four times too heavy, or by lightly centrifuging the culture at an early time, transformation would be recorded as negative. Furthermore, delaying the sedimentation (Table 1) by such means as remixing the upper and

TABLE 1

THE EFFECT OF VARIOUS KINDS OF INTERVENTION ON THE RECOVERY OF CAPSULE TRANSFORMANTS

Transformants not recovered in supernatant culture as a result of
1. Too early sedimentation, carrying down the transformants
   a. Inoculum 4× too large; clumps settle 1 hour early
   b. Light centrifugation
   c. Growth more rapid than usual
2. Too late sedimentation, inhibiting development
   a. Inoculum too small; clumps form late
   b. Antibody concentration too low; cells do not sediment, or overgrowth of untransformed cells in upper layer
   c. Culture mixed up after being partly sedimented
Standard system, giving transformants in upper layer
1. Sedimentation carries down some potential transformants while leaving others in upper layer to develop
2. One transformant in upper layer, if free to express itself, can give same maximal expression as many thousands; yet many thousands may be carried down in sediment and never be detected
3. Higher yield obtained by deliberately mixing up after full expression period, then speeding up removal of untransformed cells by centrifuging lightly after antibody has reagglutinated them

lower layers, would also have the same effect. Thus, if the sedimentation occurred early enough to reduce competition for the transformants in the upper layer, it was inevitably carrying down a large proportion of the unexpressed transformants into a highly competitive, concentrated, bottom layer. Taking advantage of these properties of the system, it was easier to observe more nearly the true yield and also to show that antibody played only a selective role. A culture is grown in the absence of antibody, DNA is added, and the excess is destroyed shortly thereafter. Using antiserum medium for detecting the transformants, it is easily demonstrated that they are produced in essentially equal amounts with or without antibody in the initial phases. Since the recovery of capsule transformants is disturbed when sedimentation is disturbed, it becomes clear that the role of antibody is essentially a selective one.

It was evident that there is a vulnerability of the capsule transformants while in the nascent state, a vulnerability so great that in this classical selection system the outcome might easily seem to indicate that no transformation was occurring. These and other experiments indicated that transformants only slowly develop their new capsule character, and even more slowly become effectively able to survive in growth competition with the excess of untransformed cells present.

These observations, furthermore, made it seem unlikely that the frequency of capsule transformation could be determined with quantitative precision. Even when the number of encapsulated cells is reasonably precisely determined (12, 26), the uncontrolled adverse selection to which they have been exposed before plating makes the result in all probability unreliable. When they are not enumerated (1, 3, 4, 6, 23, 24, 29, 30), the "determination" can be at best only a statistically uncertain end-point dilution, in terms of DNA concentration. The uncertainties of selection more or less ensure likewise that end-point dilutions for determining encapsulated transformants (12, 26) will give only a semiquantitative idea of the number of cells transformed.

QUANTITATIVE DETERMINATION OF TRANSFORMANTS

To improve the basis of selection, we turned some years ago to drug-resistance transformations (12). In numerous public and private discussions further developments have been described and made available, but no written publication contains a record of the basic quantitative concepts involved. Such a presentation seems timely at this point, inasmuch as the procedures and principles outlined in our laboratory have become variously involved in the literature of the subject, including that of this symposium.

In principle, it is merely necessary to add DNA from a drug-resistant strain, and then after an appropriate interval to dilute the culture into drug medium which kills or prevents growth of all except the transformants. With accurate control of the time of interaction by adding DNA at precisely known times and following it shortly thereafter with crystalline DNAase, well-defined kinetic quantitative experiments can be done. In all such experiments, drug-resistant transformants appear in a two-step pattern. The first step is an extremely rapid one, beginning about one division period after the DNA exposure. It is followed by a clearly perceptible one- to two-hour period during which no increase occurs. After this interval, the duration of which depends upon population density and nutritional factors, there is a slower and exponential rise in the number of transformants. Typical complete kinetic curves essentially as described were reported for streptomycin-resistance transformation in pneumococcus (14, 16) (Fig. 1), and show that the total culture was still growing when the lag plateau in transformants appeared. Such a course had already been suspected, as I have mentioned, in the capsule transformation, and it was indicated in the data reported with the initial description of drug-resistance transformation (12). In the experiments published then, it appeared that more than 90 minutes of growth were required before penicillin resistance was fully developed. Subsequent replication obviously occurred, since colonies were eventually obtained, but precise data were not available at that time concerning late events in the undiluted culture. The streptomycin-resistance transformation in *Hemophilus* (2) showed a similar rapid, followed by a negligible, rise of streptomycin-resistant transformants under conditions (seeded on fresh agar medium, incubated in an air-bath incubator) in which the total cells were unquestionably dividing, but for an imprecisely known incubation time. Thomas has recently presented a partial curve showing again, for pneumococci, the first step and a subsequent plateau of transformants (27); but he had no actual data on the total culture growth to show that it was still growing during the plateau period.

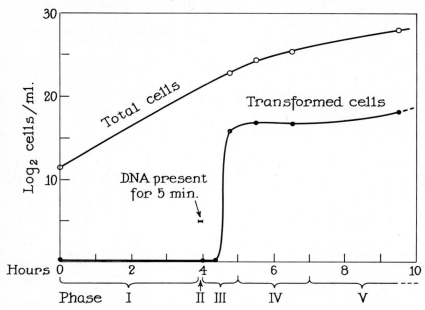

FIG. 1. Kinetics of streptomycin-resistance transformation in pneumococci at 37° C.

SIGNIFICANCE OF A TRANSFORMANT AS A UNIQUELY DETERMINED ENTITY

Taking advantage of the growth of pneumococci as single clone-clusters settling to the bottom of the culture tube after small numbers are inoculated into antiserum broth (15), we have devised a simplified individual growth-rate determination. Single viable units, distributed with suitable statistical precautions in single tubes of antibody broth, will grow to produce single colonies. If disturbed, however, by vigorous shaking, after one (or two) divisions, the microclusters are separated into two (or four) units, and after further undisturbed incubation, two (or four) colonies will be formed. By simply shaking different sets of diluted cultures after suitable periods of incubation, both the individual and the average number of divisions can be directly indicated. If a transformed culture is so diluted, and treated with streptomycin as well as shaken, the rate of division of individual transformants can be similarly determined. In the experiment indicated

TABLE 2

DIVISIONS AMONG TRANSFORMANTS AND AVERAGE CELLS IN TRANSFORMED CULTURE

Tube #	Expected distribution of 19 cells in 20 tubes	Transformed colonies found in twenty replicate dilution tubes at			
		60 min.	120 min.	180 min.	240 min.
1	4 cells in	3	6	15	42
2	0.3 tubes	2	5	12	38
3		2	4	12	36
4	3 in 1.1	2	4	11	27
5		2	3	10	23
6	2 in 3.5	1	3	8	20
7		1	1	8	17
8	1 in 7.3	1	1	6	14
9		1	1	4	14
10		1	1	3	13
11	0 in 7.8	1	0	1	13
12		1	0	0	8
13		1	0	0	7
14		0	0	0	0
15-20 incl.		0	0	0	0
Unoccupied tubes	8	7	10	9	7
Mean transformants per tube	(0.95)	0.95	1.45	4.5	13.6
Factor of increase		1.0	1.5	4.7	14
Variance	0.91	0.75	3.5	26	183

	Total cells in average replicate tubes of same dilution				
	0 min.	60 min.	120 min.	180 min.	240 min.
Total cells	135	190	1200	7100	43,000
Factor of increase	0.67	(1.0)	6.3	37	225
Ratio, total cells to transformants	(142)	200	825	1600	3150

in Table 2, a culture was diluted immediately after treatment with DNA, and 20 identical sets of dilution tubes were thus examined for the number of streptomycin-resistant transformants at a series of times. At the first time, 60 minutes, expression was complete, and the expected 19 transformants had shown a distribution among the twenty tubes close indeed to that predicted from the Poisson distribution calculated for this expectancy. It may be noted that variance is within the value of the mean, for this set, and that the expected 7 to 8 unoccupied tubes were found. The first significant finding in this experiment is that, as incubation before the addition of streptomycin is prolonged and greater numbers of colonies are recovered, each set of 20 tubes still continues to give its share of about 8 unoccupied tubes. In other words, the second portion of transformants now beginning to appear *are not coming from new occurrences,* but are coming from a replication of the rapidly appearing first group. The same indication is obtained from the greatly increased variance from all of the tubes as soon as time has allowed some factor other than sampling distribution to influence the numbers of colonies present. Thirdly, the numbers of colonies found show clearly that there is *a delayed onset of division among the average transformants.* This delay can be compared to the rate of division of average untransformed cells *in the same culture dilutions,* shown at the bottom of Table 2. It will be seen that the latter were dividing regularly and rapidly as a result of the dilution into a large volume of fresh medium, giving about a six-fold increase per hour. Finally, *the onset of this replication for individual cells is irregular,* coming within the second hour for perhaps half of them and not until the fourth hour for some last few, even in the fresh medium. This particular aspect has been seen repeatedly and best in many experiments in which the number of cells per tube is held at a lower level.

The delayed onset of divisions in the transformant class has been in part explained as a segregation lag during which untransformed parental types are separating at the early divisions (14, 17). The genetics of this process will not be considered here. The irregular delay in onset of individual divisions, by whatever cause, brings us another lesson of caution. Bacteria, of which large populations seem to offer an easy route to statistically significant observations, can unobtrusively obscure the true ratios of different transformant types in case there is *temporarily* delayed division in part of the group. It is easy to see that the slowest transformants to replicate in the experiment of Table 2 drifted from a position as 1/19 of the transformants to 1/90, and from 1/140 of the whole population to 1/1600 merely by means of this delay. It has been shown by Witkin that similar division delays supervene, at least in agar microcolonies, after transduction or ultraviolet irradiation (28).

For the present purpose, emphasis is placed on the fact that at last we have a direct demonstration that the appearance of a transformant clone is an event uniquely determined by brief contact of an individual cell with intact DNA. Immediately after this contact and thereafter, this cell behaves as a unit with a predetermined potentiality. The rapid rise of a new cell type is simply the expression of this potentiality and takes place without distortion or influence if the culture is diluted into fresh medium at a suitably early time. The rate of transformation of the culture is therefore the number of such modified cells divided by the number of total cells present at the time DNA is used. The number of transformants can, however, only be judged when these modified cells are placed in a colony-forming situation before replication of the new property has begun, and only if they are not exposed to the selective agent (e.g., streptomycin) before the selective property is fully developed. These criteria have been established in several systems in our laboratory, and empirical details have been provided to a number of coworkers and colleagues. A number of investigations based upon these procedures have been published (5, 9, 12, 15, 16, 17, 19, 21, 22, 25); parts of the procedures have been adopted in others (2, 3, 7, 8, 10, 20, 27).

Time of Exposure to DNA

Several factors make it important to limit the time of exposure of sensitive cells to specific DNA, by adding it at a known time and terminating its action five to ten minutes later with DNAase. One of these is the changing state of the culture, since *physiological sensitivity* develops gradually during late exponential growth and then decays slowly. This period of receptivity is rather broad (at least 2 hours or 4 to 5 division periods) in our complex media, but it can be shortened and made steeper in rise and fall either (a) by diluting the medium, or using a less adequate medium, or (b) by using a larger inoculum with any medium. It seems probable that the brief, steep period of sensitivity reported by Thomas (27) and by Ephrussi-Taylor (7) comes from such shortening of the physiological sensitivity, and in any case it is not reasonable to speak of the cultures as "synchronized". Phasing of cultures by temperature change shortly before DNA addition has superimposed peaks of *cumulative sensitivity* (10 to 17% of the cells being transformed after 5 min. exposure) upon a broad physiological sensitivity level of 2 to 5 per cent, and there is some suggestive evidence that synchronization of cell division may be responsible (15). The transformability "peaks" described by Thomas rise to about 0.1 per cent of the population with the same pneumococcal strain and marker, and they might well reflect only a small part of what is happening when the yield is 20 to 100 times higher. In any case, it is not clear that they can be used to explain our own results.

All of those who have occupied themselves with this question, however, agree that both populations and individual cells seem to pass through rather cyclical rises and falls of sensitivity. Therefore the timing of DNA addition and duration of exposure may enormously influence, and interfere with, the quantitation of the number of cells transformed. We have employed a 5-minute exposure in the main, begun at a time when the culture is expected to be at a relatively flat portion of the physiological sensitivity curve. Others have used a similar short 5 to 10 min. period (2, 20, 21, 25), or 15 minutes (3), which is about the indicated duration of cell sensitivity; a time of 30 minutes (7, 12, 26, 27) would seem dangerously long in our own system. A number of workers keep the DNA present throughout the culture growth (4, 7, 8, 23, 24, 30) and do not terminate its action; it is usually unstable in this environment, so that a rising population is reacting to a falling DNA concentration. These choices undoubtedly make quantitation less precise and perhaps render some of the conclusions incorrect.

Another reason prolonged DNA exposure may be destructive to quantitative work lies in the very nature of the expression process. Fox has shown in this laboratory (9) that the expression times for individuals in a population treated briefly with DNA distribute normally over a series of times (approximately 20 to 80 min. after DNA administration). From this it would seem that for a 30-min. exposure the late-reacting group of cells would not be finished expressing their transformation when the first reacting ones might be beginning to replicate.

RELATION BETWEEN THE NUMBER OF TRANSFORMANTS AND DNA CONCENTRATION

Even when working with the qualitative capsule transformations, it was recognized that higher concentrations of DNA gave more transformants, and the agent has often been assayed by dilution end-points (3, 4, 6, 11, 23). In these one observes the *number of test populations* containing transformants when limiting dilutions of DNA are used, rather than the number of *cells* induced to become transformed. The uncertainties of selection already mentioned are combined with statistical ones when approximately five replicate cultures (1, 3, 4, 6, 11, 23) are used at the end-point. Ravin has employed an elegant variation of this procedure in which approximately 50 microcolonies are grown in soft agar in a known initial concentration of DNA, and in this case the number of test populations containing transformants can clearly be made a significant measure of the transforming activity (24). Unfortunately, the activity measured is that of a prolonged exposure to a falling (through decay in the medium at 37° C.) concentration of DNA.

The studies by Zamenhof (29, 30) present data of considerable potential interest obtained by methods that at best can be semi-quantitative, and may conceivably be qualitatively deceptive. The method he has used almost exclusively has been end-point dilutions of DNA acting upon only two test populations of *Hemophilus* for each concentration, the significant dilution being considered to be that at which neither duplicate can be shown to contain transformants after overnight growth. Even if there were no selective forces inimical to the transformants, the statistical scatter at the end-points (for both DNA and cells) should render quantitation hazardous. Even the easily measurable drug-resistant transformants are measured only in test-population units in the same way. The dangers of this method may be thought to be even more grave here than elsewhere, since Zamenhof has undertaken to compare activities of DNA preparations inactivated by a variety of chemical and physical agents. In effect, the attempt is to measure the ability of a DNA preparation to be diluted. If a preparation is rendered inhomogeneous by these treatments, and the components have different affinity, rate, or adsorption constants of interaction with receptive cells, it might well be that the activity estimated will be only that of the most highly dilutable component.

Concentration response data were obtained for the capsule system by end-point dilutions to determine transformants created at intermediate (not limiting) concentrations of DNA (12, 26). The first data from an essentially quantitative system were those presented for penicillin-resistant transformation (12). A crude saturation type of curve is indicated from the data, and the relation has often been described; but the only curves published have been those for the marker mannitol (22), as well as those of Marmur and Fluke with other markers used in this laboratory (21). Alexander, Leidy, and Hahn published in 1954 a concentration-response curve showing the typical linear region over a 1000-fold concentration range in which number of transformants was proportional to the first power of concentration (log-log slope = 1) for streptomycin resistance in *Hemo-*

philus (2). Ravin gave linear curves with the same general relationship for number of colonies containing capsule transformants versus DNA concentration (24).

Meaning of Concentration-Response Relationships

It might be well to discuss some typical concentration-response curves as a basis for measuring DNA transforming activity. The curves in Fig. 2 show the response to several known mixtures of pneumococcal transforming preparations. When the activity being scored, S (streptomycin-resistance), is plotted against the concentration, the linear relation is followed over 3 logarithmic decades. When a "foreign" DNA not bearing S activity (F, sulfanilamide-resistance) is being added along with the S-DNA, the curve follows the same linear path. In other words, there is no detectable competition between different DNA's in the linear, low-concentration range.

The yield of transformants at saturation shows a very different thing, however. Under the conditions of our experiments, the capacity of the cells to respond is saturated when about 0.1 μg. total DNA/ml. is present, and although Fig. 2 does not show it, the plateaus are horizontal ($\pm$ 10%) for 50-fold concentration ranges of DNA. It will be noted that each of the mixtures levels off at a yield of transformants approximately proportional to its S-DNA content, *and this yield cannot be increased by adding more of the same mixture.* Here then, we see that the saturation yield of transformants is a measure of the *quality* of a DNA preparation, its ability to supply active DNA bearing a certain marker relative to its total DNA content.

Confirmation of these relations has been obtained for a large number of different artificial mixtures. It is not known whether the pure-strain standard DNA contains undetected DNA particles which do not carry the particular marker being measured and are instead inhibitory, as would be the case if the various known linkage groups are in different particles. Since calf thymus DNA, for example, is similarly inhibitory on a weight-for-weight basis at plateau concentrations, it may be assumed that the unmarked pneumococcal DNA would also be competitive. If this is the case, the maximal or 100 per cent plateau yield is merely that of the best preparation so far available, and the yield at saturation becomes the most significant test for quality of any new fraction or preparation of transforming DNA.

Competition between Intact DNA's

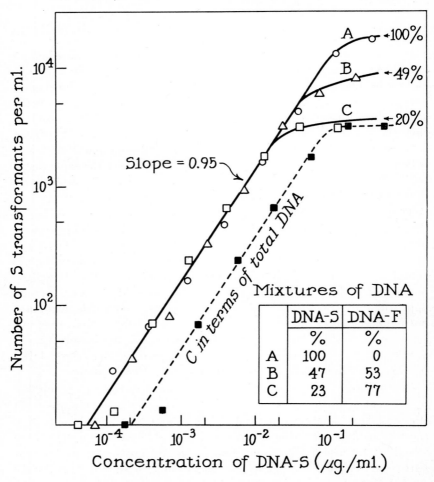

Fig. 2. Concentration-response curve of streptomycin-resistant transformants plotted against concentration of high-molecular DNA bearing S marker, both logarithmic. The indicated mixtures with other pneumococcus DNA (F-marker, not bearing S) were made and added, in increasing quantities, to aliquots of the same culture. Time of exposure, 5 minutes at 37° C.

The actual absolute yield at saturation is of course dependent upon individual factors of number, sensitivity, and duration of exposure of the cultures used for assay, as already indicated. We have found that the logarithm of (1 minus the fraction transformed) is linear with DNA concentration for all of our quantitative systems. This concentration rate of attack upon untransformed cells becomes reproducible from experiment to experiment and independent of absolute yield or culture conditions, since the fraction transformed is taken as the number transformed divided by the number transformed at saturation. Most suggestive is the observation that this attack rate of a DNA preparation on transformable cells (with respect to its own marker) appears to be exactly the same as its attack rate upon cells being transformed by another DNA (where it competitively *reduces* the number transformed to another marker). These studies will be extended and reported elsewhere, partly in collaboration with Dr. F. Gros.

It should be noted that when one does not know the degree of admixture with an "inert" DNA, or is seeking information about this, one will then be plotting a concentration curve as shown in the dotted line in Fig. 2, which represents the data of curve C on a total DNA basis. In this case the activity level of mixture C can be judged at a glance from the plateau reached, but its activity can also be compared on a weight basis with that of any standard DNA in the linear region. What is most important to stress is that the relative activities at saturation can be judged without accurate information about DNA concentration. For assay in the linear region, it is necessary to know accurately the amount of DNA; for this, absorption at 260 mμ is not adequately specific, and colorimetric measurements may require large amounts of material. We have employed for some years a method based upon the increase in optical density (hyperchromic effect) when the preparation is treated with purified DNAase (18).

Finally, when working with irradiated, degraded, or fractionated transforming DNA, and attempting to judge the relative activity of such preparations, it seems advisable to establish the approximate form and reliability of the concentration-response relation for each significant treated preparation or fraction. If non-linear or multistep curves are obtained, the explanation may first be sought in the difficulty of meeting experimentally some of the requirements for quantitation outlined above. In any case, the multiple-inflection curves presented at this symposium (7) suggest great discontinuities difficult to explain rationally, and ones which we have never observed. In general, it might be said that new or modified DNA whose nature is not fully understood should be compared with standard preparations at each of several concentration levels.

Transforming DNA very slightly degraded by careful exposure to DNAase by Dr. F. Gros in this laboratory shows typical linear response saturation curves, and its competitive ability in inhibiting an intact DNA bearing other markers is in the early stages markedly increased. This work will be the basis of another communication.

Conclusions and Summary

Genetic transformation is a unique response of bacteria to appropriate specific DNA, and the outcome for each individual cell is essentially predetermined at the time of contact with DNA. Subsequent stages include a discrete expression period, distributed in time about a mean, and a period during which replication as transformant does not occur, followed by normal division. Quantitation is accomplished by maintaining potential transformants in a growth environment which is not adversely selective until genetic expression has occurred, distributing them into a selective medium favorable for the transformant type during the period of no replication, and then observing the number of colonies formed after replication has proceeded.

Quantitative data will have maximum validity if some attempt is made to show that the following conditions are satisfied:

1. The culture is at a known and not rapidly changing level of transformability.
2. DNA is used at concentrations above the limiting end-point, and preferably at several concentrations.
3. DNA content is based upon analysis for high-molecular DNA.
4. Exposure to DNA is controlled and of brief duration (less than 15 min.).
5. Transformants are freed from disadvantageous competition with an untransformed background population.
6. The culture is diluted into selective medium at a time when the transformants have not yet replicated.
7. The yield of transformants is related both to the total number of cells present at the time of DNA treatment and to the yield from standard DNA on same population.

8. If relative activity is judged from the yield at the saturation region, it should be known that saturation yield has been obtained.

9. If the activity of a modified or fractionated preparation is observed at a low concentration region, evidence should be provided of the nature of the concentration-response behavior of the preparation, as well as that of the standard.

REFERENCES

1. Alexander, H. E., and Leidy, G., *J. Exptl. Med.,* **93**, 345 (1951).
2. Alexander, H. E., and Leidy, G., *J. Exptl. Med.,* **97**, 17 (1953).
3. Alexander, H. E., Leidy, G., and Hahn, E., *J. Exptl. Med.,* **99**, 505 (1954).
4. Avery, O. T., MacLeod, C. M., and McCarty, M., *J. Exptl. Med.,* **79**, 137 (1944).
5. Bendich, A., Pohl, H., and Beiser, S., *Cold Spring Harbor Symposia Quant. Biol.,* **21**, in press.
6. Ephrussi-Taylor, H., *Exptl. Cell Research,* **2**, 589 (1951).
7. Ephrussi-Taylor, H., this symposium.
8. Ephrussi-Taylor, H., and Latarjet, R. *Biochim. et Biophys. Acta,* **16**, 183 (1955).
9. Fox, M. S., and Hotchkiss, R. D., *Abstr. 3. Intern. Congr. Biochem.,* 74 (1955).
10. Goodgal, S. H., and Herriott, R. M., *Federation Proc.,* **15**, 590 (1956).
11. Hotchkiss, R. D., *Colloq. intern. centre natl. recherche sci. (Paris),* **8** [*Unités biol. douées contin. génét.*], 57 (1949).
12. Hotchkiss, R. D., *Cold Spring Harbor Symposia Quant. Biol.,* **16**, 457 (1951).
13. Hotchkiss, R. D., in *Phosphorus Metabolism* (W. D. McElroy and B. Glass, eds.), Vol. 2, p. 426. The Johns Hopkins Press, Baltimore (1952).
14. Hotchkiss, R. D., *Harvey Lectures,* **49**, 124 (1953-54).
15. Hotchkiss, R. D., *Proc. Natl. Acad. Sci. U.S.,* **40**, 49 (1954).
16. Hotchkiss, R. D., in *Dynamics of Virus and Rickettsial Infections,* (F. W. Hartman, F. L. Horsfall, J. G. Kidd, eds.), p. 405, Blakiston, New York (1954).
17. Hotchkiss, R. D., in *Enzymes: Units of Structure and Function* (O. H. Gaebler, ed.), p. 119, Academic Press, New York (1956).
18. Hotchkiss, R. D., in *Methods in Enzymology* (S. P. Colowick and N. O. Kaplan, eds.), Vol. 2, p. 708. Academic Press, New York (1956).
19. Hotchkiss, R. D., and Marmur, J., *Proc. Natl. Acad. Sci. U.S.,* **40**, 55 (1954).
20. Lerman, L. S., *Biochim. et Biophys. Acta,* **18**, 132 (1955).
21. Marmur, J., and Fluke, D. J., *Arch. Biochem. and Biophys.,* **57**, 506 (1955).
22. Marmur, J., and Hotchkiss, R. D., *J. Biol. Chem.,* **214**, 383 (1955).
23. McCarty, M., *J. Exptl. Med.,* **81**, 501 (1945).
24. Ravin, A. W., *Exptl. Cell Research,* **7**, 58 (1954).
25. Schaeffer, P., in press.
26. Stocker, B. A. D., Krauss, M. R., and MacLeod, C. M, *J. Pathol. Bacteriol.,*
27. Thomas, R., *Biochim, et Biophys. Acta,* **18**, 467 (1955). **66**, 330 (1953).
28. Witkin, E. M., and Thomas, C., *Bacteriol. Proc.,* 54 (1955).
29. Zamenhof, S., this symposium.
30. Zamenhof, S., Alexander, H. E., and Leidy, G., *J. Exptl. Med.,* **98**, 373 (1953).

STUDIES ON TRANSFORMATION OF
HEMOPHILUS INFLUENZAE *

Sol H. Goodgal and Roger M. Herriott

Department of Biochemistry, Johns Hopkins University,
School of Hygiene and Public Health,
Baltimore, Maryland

BACTERIAL TRANSFORMATIONS have been demonstrated to occur as a result of the addition of DNA derived from a variant population to a susceptible host population (3). The mechanism by which this process takes place is unknown. In the following preliminary report of studies on the transforming DNA of *Hemophilus influenzae*, it is shown that the number of transformations is directly related to the amount of transforming DNA taken up irreversibly by the cell population, and this DNA may be considered to have penetrated the cell. In addition, an analysis of the molecular weight of the transforming factors (TP) by sedimentation and diffusion methods and a sedimentation analysis of the total DNA have been made with the object of defining transformations in quantitative terms, i.e., in terms of interacting units, molecules of DNA, and numbers of cells.

Uptake of Transforming DNA by Susceptible Cells.

DNA labelled with P^{32} is taken up by hemophilus cells in two forms, a reversible form, which is sensitive to DNAase or which may be washed off by saline, and an irreversible form, which is insensitive to DNAase and cannot be removed by washing. The irreversibly absorbed DNA is maintained by the cell population as DNA and is not lost to any other fraction during subsequent growth.

Hemophilus influenzae cells which transform do so as a result of the uptake of transforming DNA. In dilute solutions of transforming DNA (10^{-6} to 10^{-3} μg./ml.) the number of sensitive *Hemophilus*

* Carried out under a grant (Contract No. AT(30–1)–1371) from the U. S Atomic Energy Commission.

influenzae cells that transform to cells with streptomycin resistance is directly related to the concentration of DNA applied. This result is to be expected if a single unit or molecule is the cause of the transformation. At concentrations above 1 to 10 molecules of DNA per cell the number of transformations is less than expected, so as to suggest that competition or an interference by DNA molecules other than the specific factor being measured is responsible for the observed deviation. The number of cells transforming is directly proportional to the DNA taken up irreversibly, regardless of the relative concentration of cells or of DNA.

Using a value of 15,000,000 for the molecular weight of DNA, determination of which is discussed later, the number of molecules taken up irreversibly by the cell population for each cell transformed was found to be 120. This is shown in Table 1, where values of the reciprocal ratio are given, i.e., the number of transformations per 1000 molecules absorbed irreversibly. This figure is remarkably constant over a wide range of transforming factor concentration and at different stages of cell growth.

Evidence for Cell Penetration by Transforming DNA.

Transforming DNA taken up irreversibly by a cell population can be liberated from the cell within 10 minutes after absorption by lysing the cells with lysozyme. The liberated transforming factor is then demonstrated (by titrating against a standard titration curve) and gives a value corresponding to the expected amount of transforming factor. The liberated transforming factor is sensitive to DNAase; however, whether or not it has been physically or chemically altered has not yet been determined.

Evidence that the Uptake of Transforming DNA is Not Selective for Specific Factors.

The following evidence suggests that there is no fractional uptake of transforming factor by the cell: (1) Transforming factor and DNA have a constant relationship where the amounts of transforming factor and DNA taken up by the cells vary over a considerable range from 0–90 per cent. This also applies to the reversibly bound DNA which is washed off and analyzed. (2) Hemophilus cells will take up their own or homologous DNA (but do not transform) to the same extent as they take up transforming DNA.

TABLE 1

Relationship between the Quantity of TP–DNA and the Transformation of Cells

Sample	No. of host cells/ml.	DNA added μg./ml.	DNA added No. molecules per cell**	DNA taken up by cells* μg./ml.	DNA taken up by cells* Molecules per cell**	DNA taken up by cells* % of added†	Cells transformed Per 1000 cells exposed	Cells transformed Per 1000 molecules DNA taken up
9-19-9-20	4×10^9	.002		.00032				8.0
10-21	4×10^9	.014	.14	.0012	.012	9	.10	8.2
10-21	3.6×10^9	.028	.28	.0019	.02	7	.16	8.0
10-19	3.7×10^9	.07	.76	.012	.13	16	1.3	8.2
11-7	3.6×10^9	.10	1.2	.0045	.05	4.5	0.3	8.2
		1.5	16.	.022	.24	1.5	2.1	8.7
2-29, 3-1	1.6×10^9	.017	.4	.0068	.16	40	1.4	9.0
	1.6×10^9	.025	.64	.011	.28	44	1.8	6.5
	1.6×10^9	.033	.84	.013	.32	38	2.5	7.8
	1.6×10^9	.05	1.24	.013	.32	26	2.6	8.2
	1.6×10^9	.1	2.5	.015	.38	15	2.8	7.5

* This refers to the DNA in an irreversible form only, i.e., resistant to DNAase.

** Using a value of 15×10^6 for the molecular weight of the TP–DNA, 1 μg. $= 4 \times 10^{10}$ molecules.

† These experiments were not carried out under the conditions of maximal uptake, i.e., where the cell concentration is very for such results are too variable, for reasons that are not clear.

Diverse Nature of the Donor DNA.

Inasmuch as no fractionation of transforming DNA was observed and there was only one transformation for every 120 molecules of DNA taken up, only one in every 120 molecules of DNA may be assumed to carry the factor for streptomycin resistance. Since a donor cell contains approximately 100-120 molecules of DNA, it is possible that each donor cell contains only a single molecule of the streptomycin-resistance factor. The above data do not exclude the possibility that every DNA molecule carries the streptomycin-resistance factor and that the over-all efficiency of the transformation is merely 1 in 120. This possibility, however, seems unlikely in view of the constancy of the results obtained under the varied experimental conditions that might be expected to alter the efficiency of transformation.

This value of one transforming factor for streptomycin resistance per cell is independent of the molecular weight.

The Molecular Weight of the Transforming Factor for Streptomycin Resistance.

It was reported in the symposium meetings that preliminary data on the molecular size of the streptomycin-resistance factor calculated from sedimentation and diffusion measurements indicated its weight to be in the neighborhood of 6,000,000. This is close to the value reported for thymus DNA (2, 4, 7). Since then more complete data, especially diffusion measurements, have led to a higher value. The sedimentation data obtained (see Table 2), using dilute DNA solutions of 0.1 μg. to 10 μg./ml., show that DNA, as measured by P^{32}, and the transforming factor are sedimented together, and that a large fraction (90 per cent or more) of the DNA consists of material of high molecular weight and of a fairly uniform rate of sedimentation. The sedimentation constants for DNA and the transforming activity shown in Table 2 have not been corrected for any blank or low molecular weight values.

The diffusion data obtained by using the Northrop-Anson porous disc method (1, 6) show a decrease in the diffusion constant during the first forty days. In this period about 8 per cent of the total material diffused out. During the period of forty to one hundred twenty days determinations of transforming activity from 3 diffusion cells have led to a value of 1×10^{-8} for D_{20}. Using this D_{20} and a figure of 27 for

TABLE 2

SEDIMENTATION CONSTANT (S_{20}) OF TP AND DNA*

Expt. No.	Concentration of DNA μg./ml.	Upper cell concentration as a fraction of initial concentration**		$S_{(20°C.)}$†	
		DNA (P^{32})	TP	DNA (P^{32})	TP
1	10	.16	.11	21	22.4
2	1	.18	.13	20.3	21.8
3	0.1	.20	.16	23	24.2
4	1	.45	.38	28	31.9
5	1	.15	.09	27.6	29.8
6	1	.10	.06	23.3	24.6
7	10	.57	.61	29.6	26.6
8	10	.26	.23	30.1	31.9

* Solvent = 0.3 M NaCl + .014 M citrate buffer, pH 7.
** Uncorrected.
† Calculated from formula derived by Sher and Mallette (8).

S_{20} in the usual formula (5), a value of 15,000,000 for the molecular weight of the unlinked transforming factors for streptomycin resistance and for erythromycin resistance was obtained.

REFERENCES

1. Anson, M. L., and Northrop, J. H., *J. Gen. Physiol.*, **20**, 575 (1937).
2. Doty, P., and Bunce, B., *J. Am. Chem. Soc.*, **74**, 5029 (1952).
3. Hotchkiss, R. D., in *Phosphorus Metabolism* (W. D. McElroy and B. Glass, eds.), Vol. II, p. 426. Johns Hopkins Press, Baltimore (1952); also, this volume.
4. For review see Jordan, D. O., in *The Nucleic Acids* (E. Chargaff and J. D. Davidson, eds.), Vol. I, p. 447. Academic Press, New York (1955).
5. Lundgren, H. P., and Ward, W. H., in *Amino Acids and Proteins* (D. M. Greenberg, ed.), p. 391. Charles C Thomas, Springfield, Ill. (1951).
6. Northrop, J. H., and Anson, M. L., *J. Gen. Physiol.*, **4**, 543 (1929).
7. Peacocke, A. R., and Schachman, H. K., *Biochim. et Biophys. Acta*, **15**, 198 (1954).
8. Sher, I. H., and Mallette, M. F., *Arch. Biochem. and Biophys.*, **53**, 370 (1954).

PHOTOREACTIVATION OF *HEMOPHILUS INFLUENZAE* TRANSFORMING FACTOR FOR STREPTOMYCIN RESISTANCE BY AN EXTRACT OF *ESCHERICHIA COLI* B

Sol H. Goodgal, Claud S. Rupert, and Roger M. Herriott

The Departments of Biochemistry and Biophysics,
The Johns Hopkins University,
Baltimore, Maryland

The phenomenon of photoreactivation originally described by Kelner (5) has been demonstrated for a wide variety of organisms and tissues (3), but very little is known of the nature of the process. Kelner has shown that DNA synthesis is inhibited by relatively low doses of ultraviolet light and that this inhibition can be reversed by using photoreactivating light (6). In addition, the photoreactivation process is known to be temperature-dependent, with a temperature coefficient (near 2 in the region of 37° C. for bacteria and bacteriophage (3, 5)) and an activation energy (approximately 17,000 calories for *Neurospora* microconidia (4)) that suggest an enzymatically controlled biological reaction. Dulbecco's studies on phage photoreactivation likewise indicate that the process is dependent on the cell's enzymatic apparatus (2).

Some recent studies of photoreactivation have indicated that the nucleus is the site of photoreversal and that cytoplasmic effects of ultraviolet radiation are not subject to photoreactivation (1, 7).

In our hands attempts to photoreactivate *Hemophilus influenzae* and *Diplococcus pneumoniae* for growth proved to be unsuccessful, although *Escherichia coli* under similar conditions underwent photoreactivation, consistent with previous reports (6). The photoreactivation of ultraviolet-inactivated transforming factor after the uptake of transforming DNA by *Hemophilus influenzae* also proved to be unsuccessful. Therefore, an attempt was made to transform ultraviolet-inactivated transforming factor for streptomycin resistance by the use of extracts of *E. coli* and *Hemophilus influenzae*. The hemophilus extract in conjunction with visible light failed to produce any increase in the frequency of transformation. The results of the two experiments with *E. coli* extracts are given in Table 1.

341

TABLE 1

Experiment I

PHOTOREACTIVATION OF ULTRAVIOLET-INACTIVATED *H. influenzae* TRANSFORMING
FACTOR (TP) FOR STREPTOMYCIN RESISTANCE BY AN EXTRACT OF *E. coli* B

Tube No.	Mixture incubated 20 minutes at 37°C. with Mg^{++} and ATP*	Condition	Titer of TP
1	TP + buffer (citrate .014 M + .15 saline)	Dark	1.5×10^4
2	UVTP† + buffer	Dark	6.6×10^2
3	UVTP + *E. coli* extract**	Light	4.4×10^3
4	UVTP + *E. coli* extract	Dark	4.6×10^2
5	UVTP + heated *E. coli* extract	Light	4.4×10^1
6	UVTP + heated *E. coli* extract	Dark	5.2×10^1
7	TP + *E. coli* extract	Light or Dark	1.9×10^4
8	TP + heated *E. coli* extract	Dark	2.6×10^3
	Streptomycin-resistant viable cell count of *E. coli* extract		0
	Streptomycin-resistant viable cell count of TP		0

* The Mg++ concentration in the reaction mixture was 0.014 M. The ATP
concentration in the same mixture was 0.003 M.

† UVTP, ultraviolet-irradiated transforming factor.

** The extract in the reaction mixture represented material from 10^{11} *E. coli*/ml.

Experiment II

Tube No.	Mixture incubated at 37°C. with Mg^{++} and ATP	Conditions	Titer of TP	
			0 min.	20 min.
1	TP + *E. coli* extract	Dark	1.7×10^4	$2.5 \times 10^{4*}$
2	UVTP + *E. coli* extract	Dark	3.8×10^2	4.6×10^2
3	UVTP + *E. coli* extract	Light	3.6×10^2	4.8×10^3

* 60 minutes in dark.

A comparison of the light-treated and dark-treated tubes after incubation with *E. coli* extract shows a 10-fold increase in the frequency
of transformation of the light-treated tubes. A small but perhaps significant increase is also shown in the incubation mixture of purified
transforming factor (not inactivated by ultraviolet) and *E. coli* extract
when compared with the same mixture at time zero or containing
buffer in place of cell extract. The difference is quite marked when
comparisons are made between transforming factor incubated with
heat-treated extract and transforming factor with unheated extract, the
latter being far higher in titer.

A detailed discussion of the interpretation of these results must await further experimentation, but there is an increase of activity of ultra-violet-inactivated *Hemophilus influenzae* transforming factor when both visible light and an extract of *E. coli* B are present.

REFERENCES

1. Brandt, C. L., and Giese, A. C., *J. Gen. Physiol.,* **39**, 735 (1956).
2. Dulbecco, R., *J. Bacteriol.,* **59**, 329 (1950).
3. Dulbecco, R., in *Radiation Biology* (A. Hollaender, ed.), Vol. II, p. 455. McGraw-Hill Book Co., New York (1955).
4. Goodgal, S. H., "The Effect of Photoreactivating Light on the Survival and Frequency of Mutations in Ultraviolet Irradiated Microconidia of *Neurospora crassa.*" Doctoral dissertation, The Johns Hopkins University, Baltimore, 1950.
5. Kelner, A., *Proc. Natl. Acad. Sci. U. S.,* **35**, 73 (1949).
6. Kelner, A., *J. Bacteriol.,* **65**, 252 (1953).
7. Von Borstel, R. C., and Wolff, S., *Proc. Natl. Acad. Sci. U. S.,* **41**, 1004 (1955).

DISCUSSION

DR. RAVIN: I would just like to ask whether the number of doubles that you find there is the number that you would expect if you thought that SR and CR were unlinked, as you assumed.

DR. EPHRUSSI-TAYLOR: The number is much too low. However, the calculation is not of great value since in making it, it is necessary to assume that the totality of the population is competent. The advantage of the interference method for the study of linkage lies just in the fact that it is not necessary to suppose that all of the population is competent.

DR. GOODGAL: Does the expected column refer to DNA plus interference?

DR. EPHRUSSI-TAYLOR: There is no "expected" column. The figures in Table 1 are experimental values, obtained in the absence and in the presence of competing DNA.

DR. GOODGAL: I wonder if you might have analyzed your data by assuming a certain fraction of your cells are competent and determining the frequency of doubles as a random function of the number of singles. In *Hemophilus influenzae,* if we assume that the frequency of transformations for singles is based on the competency of the whole population, we obtain far too many doubles for unlinked markers. However, if we make a correction for the number of competent cells available, assuming any frequency of transformation above 1/300 is due to the presence of cells which are not competent, we obtain the expected frequency of double transformations.

DR. EPHRUSSI-TAYLOR: We have not done experiments of that particular sort. The point to be made in connection with the complex titration curves is that the DNA may be acting as a selecting agent. In the regions of the titration curve where response is no longer linear, the bacteria which transform may be just those which have reacted with the largest numbers of DNA molecules. This could give an entirely distorted picture of the relative frequencies of single and double transformations.

DR. GOODGAL: If one interferes with the frequency of transformation of *Hemophilus influenzae* by adding homologous DNA, the interference is directly proportional to the amount of DNA added, and the frequency of doubles obtained is merely what one would expect on the basis of competency and the number of single transformations. There does not seem to bè any complication in this respect.

DR. LURIA: If I understand the point correctly, you suggest that there is a fraction of competent cells, whereas Dr. Ephrussi-Taylor is making the very interesting point that the proportion of competent cells may in itself be determined by the amount of DNA to which they have been exposed.

DR. EPHRUSSI-TAYLOR: Error would obviously be introduced by only a fraction of the cells being competent, and this fraction has never been determined in any experiment I know of. What I am saying in connection with my data is that when one employs a concentration of DNA at which multiple hits are frequent, it is just those cells which have reacted with a large number (5-10) of molecules which will appear preferentially as transformed cells. These cells would also be expected to give double transformations.

DR. LURIA: In a numerical sense that amounts to the same conclusion.

DR. BENDICH: It may be appropriate at this point to mention some of our work (carried out jointly with Drs. S. M. Beiser and H. B. Pahl) on the determination of transforming activity in fractions of pneumococcal DNA which have been obtained by a fractionation procedure using a substituted cellulose anion exchanger known as ECTEOLA (cf. A. Bendich, J. R. Fresco, H. S. Rosenkranz, S. M. Beiser, *J. Amer. Chem. Soc., 77,* 3671 (1955)). Except for the fact that it was possible with this pneumococcal DNA preparation to demonstrate a particular biological activity (transformation to streptomycin-resistance), it was like the DNA from a wide variety of other sources in that it too appeared to consist of a mixture of polynucleotides. The chromatographic pattern of the pneumococcal DNA is shown in Figure 1. The DNA was placed on a column of the cellulose exchanger and fractions of DNA were obtained by passing through solutions of increasing sodium chloride concentration followed by sodium chloride solutions of increasing *p*H. A number of fractions were obtained and certain of these were tested for their ability to transform pneumococci to streptomycin-resistant cells. The relative specific transforming activity of these fractions is given in Table 1 which lists the composition

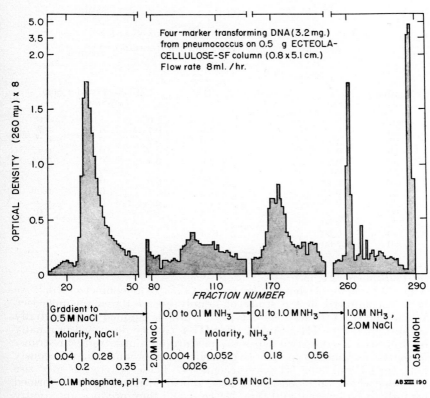

Fig. 1. Profile obtained by chromatography of pneumococcal transforming DNA on the substituted cellulose anion exchanger ECTEOLA (cf. E. A. Peterson and H. A. Sober, *J. Amer. Chem. Soc.*, **78**, 751 (1956).

of the eluent in terms of sodium chloride molarity and *p*H. In the last three columns are given the results of three sets of transforming activity measurements. Streptomycin-resistance activity was found in many different fractions and relative transforming activity varied some fifty-fold from fraction to fraction. It is of considerable interest that some fractions were five times more active than the original. It would appear that the DNA of these pneumococci consists of different molecules of greater or lesser streptomycin transforming activity, as well as molecules which do not show this property. There was no evidence that the fractionation procedure caused loss of biological activity. A discussion of the possible significance of the heterogeneity of the DNA from pneumococcus and other sources is given in A. Bendich, H. B. Pahl and S. M. Beiser, *Cold Spring Harbor Symposia for Quanti-*

TABLE 1

Chromatographic Fractions of Pneumococcal DNA
(Transformation to Streptomycin Resistance)

Fraction Number	Composition of Eluent		pH	Relative Transforming Activity		
	Molarity, NaCl	Molarity, NH₃				
original			7.0	1.0	1.0	1.0
25	0.17		7.0	0.7	0.8	0.7
27	0.19		7.0	0.2	0.4	0.2
29	0.21		7.0	0.5	0.6	0.4
32	0.25		7.0	0.4	0.1	0.04
35	0.28		7.0	1.2	0.8	1.9
40	0.32		7.0	0.9	0.7	1.2
67	0.45		7.0	0	0.1	0.06
78	0.47		7.0	0	0.1	0.03
99	0.50	0.02	8.4	1.9	1.8	2.0
173	0.50	0.22	9.5		5.1	4.2
190	0.50	0.56	10.4	1.1	1.0	
260	2.00	1.0	11.0		5.1	4.8

tative Biology, **21**, in press.

Dr. Austrian: I should like to mention two phenomena which we have encountered in the study of doubly encapsulated pneumococci. When the DNA from a wild type I strain is applied to a partially encapsulated type III strain of the SIII-1 variety described originally by Ephrussi Taylor, two types of cells are obtained from this transformation: ordinary type I cells and cells which produce simultaneously both type I and type III polysaccharides. These latter cells give rise to clones which, on blood agar plates, appear identical to those formed by fully encapsulated wild type III cells and they produce apparently normal amounts of type III polysaccharide. When such doubly encapsulated cells are analyzed by the Ouchterlony agar precipitin technique, they are found to produce two distinct capsular components which give reactions of identity with either the type I or the type III capsular polysaccharide obtained from wild-type singly encapsulated cells. When DNA from a doubly encapsulated strain is applied to a non-encapsulated strain of pneumococcus, three types of clones are obtained: the SIII-1 variant which produces negligible amounts of type III polysaccharide, the wild type I variant (SI) and a few doubly encapsulated variants (SI-III). The interesting fact revealed by this experiment is that the presence of the type I genetic unit in association with the SIII-1 unit leads apparently to restoration of the normal synthesis of type III polysaccharide by the cell without any alteration of the SIII-1 unit itself. When DNA is extracted from the doubly encapsulated SI-III cell, it behaves as if the two genetic units controlling capsule formation have been unmodified and not as if the DNA from the SI cell had contributed something to the reconstitution of a normal SIII unit by alteration of the mutant SIII-1 factor.

As noted above, when the DNA of an SI strain is applied to cells of an SIII-1 strain, two capsular variants are obtained with regularity: SI and SI-III. The reaction may be represented schematically in the following fashion:

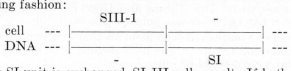

If only the SI unit is exchanged, SI-III cells result. If both units from the SI cell "cross over," SI cells are the product of the transformation. When the DNA from SI-III cells is applied to the parent SIII-1 strain, the results of transformation are different, as SI-III cells predominate overwhelmingly following this reaction and SI cells are found extremely rarely in contradistinction to the result obtained by applying SI DNA to the same SIII-1 variant. If the reaction of SI-III DNA with SIII-1 cells is diagrammed in a fashion analogous to the scheme employed above, a reasonable hypothesis to explain the observed results may be developed:

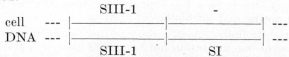

If only the SI unit is exchanged, SI-III cells result. If both capsular genetic units from the SI-III strain are exchanged, however, SI-III cells are again the product of the reaction. Thus, by modifying the genome of the cell supplying the SI unit so that it now contains the SIII-1 unit, one can alter significantly the products of the transformation.

Dr. KAPLAN: I was wondering, Dr. Ephrussi-Taylor, if you have made any chemical or physical measurements of your x-ray-treated or succinic-peroxide–treated material. Did you see any spectral changes or other changes after treatment?

Dr. EPHRUSSI-TAYLOR: That work is just really getting under way.

Dr. DOTY: From a little work that Dr. Ephrussi-Taylor and I have been doing together on the physical changes undergone by DNA upon x-radiation, we find practically no optical density changes in the ultra-violet over the range of radiation required for major inactivation.

Dr. LURIA: I would like to ask Dr. Ephrussi-Taylor a question. How much trust do you put in this factor 10 in molecular weight, or a factor 10 in volume based on the assumptions of target theory—that is, one ionization, ion distribution, and so on? Generally one assumes that a factor of 10 of uncertainty is about as good as you can get in this kind of calculation.

Dr. EPHRUSSI-TAYLOR: We consider the volume obtained to be an upper limit. It is, of course, difficult to know how the ionizations occur and act. I am not responsible for that calculation, nor competent to defend it to any extent. The assumptions made were checked by using phage S 13 as a control material. Its choice was determined by the fact that it is small—believed to be of the order of size of the DNA molecule. Subsequently, doubt has been thrown on the identity of the granules measured by Drs. Elford and Hotchin, which they believed to be phage S 13. Dr. Stent has pointed this out to me.

DR. WATSON: Your calculation assumes that every ionization within the DNA molecule results in loss of biological activity. If this is not so, molecular weight could be much larger.

DR. LURIA: There are two types of corrections we can make in such types of measurements: one would make this the maximal estimate, but assuming that there still may be some residual indirect effect. The other correction would make the estimate minimal since it is assumed that every ionization is effective. Especially in a molecule of the type of DNA you may find that only a few ion clusters are completely effective. You don't know how much damage you need to destroy the biological activity.

DR. EPHRUSSI-TAYLOR: When one speaks of the efficiency of ionization, this may simply be a less explicit way of saying that part of the molecule is not needed for biological activity.

DR. LURIA: Radiobiologically you can distinguish in this way. It is not a matter of one ionization not being effective. It's the fact of the ionization not being distributed completely at random. You have a waste effect. For all we know, in the material described it may be a factor of 10.

DR. EPHRUSSI-TAYLOR: You feel, then, that the, radiobiological data fit fairly well with the physical-chemical data?

DR. LURIA: I have long given up trying to find any too good fit in radiobiological data.

DR. STENT: In the case of bacteriophage T1, some experiments of Adams and Pollard show that, under the conditions of irradiation employed by you, actually less than one-tenth of the ionizations are effective. Adams and Pollard found that the x-ray sensitivity of dried T1, where the indirect effect is excluded, increases by a factor of ten when the temperature of irradiation is raised to 100° C. Thus, at low temperatures many ionizations are wasted which could have become effective during irradiation at higher temperatures.

DR. LEDERBERG: I have a very elementary question. I want if possible to get on the record some simple numbers—for example, the amount of DNA there is per cell, the amount of DNA that is required in these cases for transformation, and so on.

DR. EPHRUSSI-TAYLOR: I have not determined the amount of DNA per cell, but in connection with the question of the minimal amount of DNA per transformation, it should be pointed out that it is impossible to calculate it from kinetic data, for at all DNA concentrations at which one obtains transformations there are vastly more molecules present than are taken up. From the dose-response curves, one ends up with a figure of the order of 103 per transformation, but this only means that transformation is an inefficient process.

DR. LEDERBERG: Then how can you do an assay of activity at all if you don't exhaust a measurable part of the material you are assaying for?

DR. EPHRUSSI-TAYLOR: One assays the numbers of transformations induced at a series of concentrations of DNA.

DR. HOTCHKISS: You can measure the effect of something without exhausting it from the medium. A good example is the glass electrode, which exhausts a very negligible amount of hydrogen ions but records the chemical potential or concentration of these ions very accurately. In one experiment we attempted to show exhaustion when two cultures were successively exposed to the same DNA. Penicillin-resistant cells were added after penicillin-sensitive cells, to varying amounts of DNA to see how many could be transformed by the remaining DNA. We found the same number, whether or not other cells had been present and transformed, so with a biological marker there was no detectable exhaustion of DNA from the solution. There are now at least three groups—Dr. Fox in our laboratory, Drs. Goodgal and Herriott here, and Dr. Lerman in Colorado—studying the behavior of a chemical marker, P^{32}, in this kind of material. When you measure P^{32} you can detect the absorbed DNA, and I believe all of these people are getting the impression that only a small number of particles are being taken up per transformation. Dr. Fox's experiments suggest that this number may be around 3 per recorded transformation of a particular marker.

DR. LEDERBERG: What does an assay curve mean, then?

DR. HOTCHKISS: You are measuring the rate of supply, in other words the effective concentration, of biologically active DNA.

DR. LURIA: You are measuring this in the same way as you can measure the amount of antibodies in large excess, by measuring the number of, let's say, bacteriophage particles that can be inactivated in the presence of excess antibodies. A change of the concentration of antibodies will change the rate of inactivation.

DR. LEDERBERG: Does this mean that by putting in twice as many cells you will get twice as many transformants?

DR. LURIA: That's what Dr. Ephrussi-Taylor said at the beginning.

DR. GOODGAL: First of all, I want to mention that in *Hemophilus* one can readily measure the amount of DNA taken up from solution, either by measuring the uptake of DNA directly by means of P^{32}-labeled DNA or by determining the amount of DNA taken out of solution by transforming cells. Cells and DNA are mixed and incubated; then the cells are removed by centrifugation. A transformation titration experiment will determine the amount of transforming factor left in solution or taken out by the cells. One can remove practically all of the DNA with a suitable number of cells and a suitable amount of DNA. Or, one can remove a very small amount of DNA, then add more cells, and find about the same number of cells transformed. The experiments that Dr. Hotchkiss and Dr. Ephrussi-Taylor report probably result, as they have indicated, from having removed only a small fraction of the DNA which they add.

PROPERTIES OF THE TRANSFORMING PRINCIPLES [1]

STEPHEN ZAMENHOF

Department of Biochemistry,
College of Physicians and Surgeons,
Columbia University, New York

THIS DISCUSSION will deal with only one type of those biological substances known as transforming principles or transforming agents. It is proper to explain first why the study of these substances should be of particular interest. The evidence presented in preceding contributions to this Symposium and to be added in those which are to follow clearly points to nucleic acids as being determinants of heredity. The evidence in the field of virus research seems even to indicate that the nucleic acids are the *sole* determinants of heredity in these simple living entities. As to cellular organisms, the evidence is still insufficient, in my own opinion, to determine that the nucleic acids are the sole heredity determinants of *all* the hereditary characters. In other words, there is still no proof that all cellular substances other than nucleic acids are entirely devoid of the master properties of self-determination and self-reproduction. Nevertheless, the studies on the transforming phenomena leave little doubt that some of the (mutable) hereditary characters are determined solely by deoxyribonucleic acids (DNA) and that any help received by DNA from other substances is not of the determining ("master") kind.

A biochemist is naturally interested in studying such biologically active substances in vitro and in vivo. The DNA of bacterial viruses or of metazoa can be obtained in vitro but thus far cannot be reintroduced into the living system to see whether they are still active. The situation in the field of crystalline plant viruses may be more promising, as will be shown by Dr. Fraenkel-Conrat later on in this symposium. However, in those small and simple living entities the nucleic acid is of the ribose type and is therefore of less interest for the study of bacterial viruses and of all the cellular organisms where the heredity determinants seem to be nucleic acids of the deoxyribose type. Thus,

[1] The author's investigations reported in this paper were supported by research grants from the National Institutes of Health, Public Health Service and from the American Cancer Society.

for the study of biologically active DNA we have at present only one tool, the transforming principles.

The transforming principles indeed offer some unique possibilities: they can be extracted from the cell, purified, chemically identified, and analyzed; they can be chemically changed in vitro, reintroduced into the cell, and studied to establish the relationship between the change in structure and the change in function. In short, this mode of attack offers possibilities of applying to the problem of heredity the same rational approach which yielded elucidations in so many fields of biochemistry and biophysics.

While the foregoing reasons for an interest in the transforming principle appear personally to be the most important ones, the biophysicist's interest may often come from the study of DNA itself. In early chemical approaches the DNA was subjected to degradation, with complete disregard of the macromolecular nature of the substance. This error was compensated for in the last decade by extensive biophysical studies of the giant molecule of DNA; but biophysicists soon faced a dilemma: whether their substance was indeed "native" or was actually degraded. The discovery that certain purified highly polymerized DNA's have transforming activity but lose it on the slightest degradation, provided the desired yardstick of "intactness"; for although no one can say whether this DNA preparation is in the same state as the DNA that exists in the cell, the "functionally intact" unit seems important enough to warrant study, and constant enough to serve as a standard.

Another reason for interest in the transforming principle is a practical one. Subtle reactions of certain agents, notably mutagenic, carcinogenic, and carcinostatic ones, with DNA can often be demonstrated by studying the loss of transforming activity, long before these reactions can be apprehended by any chemical or physical method. On the other hand, several carcinogenic and carcinostatic agents have no effect on the transforming activity. This may indicate that the primary action of these substances is through cell components other than DNA.

The above points will be discussed below. To avoid repetition, the transforming phenomenon itself will not be discussed here and will be considered merely as a detector of activity of the transforming principle. However, the transforming phenomenon involves several steps, and at present it is not possible to decide which is (are) responsible for inactivation in any particular case: thus, if a transforming principle loses its ability to transform, it might be due to any of the following (hypothetical) failures: the inability to penetrate into the cell, to reach the genetical locus, to displace the previous occupant (DNA) of the locus, to attach itself to the protein of the locus, to reproduce itself (even though established in the locus) or to exert its phenotypical action (even though reproduced), etc.

The chemistry and physics of DNA itself have been the subject of many reviews (cf. 59). I will therefore discuss only these subjects with reference to the transforming principle.

The Chemical Nature of the Transforming Principles

In 1944, Avery, MacLeod, and McCarty (5) found that the purified transforming principle has all the properties of a highly polymerized DNA. Their conclusion that the transforming principle *is* DNA was based on the following observations: (1) elementary analysis of the transforming principle shows it to correspond to that of DNA; (2) chemical tests reveal the presence of DNA in the transforming principle; no other substance could be detected in it by either chemical or physical (ultracentrifuge, electrophoresis) methods; (3) serological tests fail to detect the presence in it of any immunologically active substances (such as polysaccharides); (4) of several enzymes tested, only (crude) deoxyribonuclease (DNAase) was able to destroy the transforming activity. At the same time, physical studies (viscosity, ultracentrifugation) revealed that the substance is in a highly polymerized state. These findings, especially that of destruction by DNAase, were amplified by further studies of McCarty and Avery (41).

In subsequent years, there was some criticism of the identification of the transforming principle with DNA (45). The main points of criticism were the following: (1) the chemical methods were not sensitive enough to exclude the presence of some impurity (such as protein) which might be responsible for the activity; (2) even accepting the evidence that the destruction of DNA by DNAase destroys the activity of the transforming principle, it could still be that DNA is not active alone, but merely in combination with some such hypothetical protein, so that the destruction of either moiety would result in inactivation; indeed, for a long time the genes were believed to be nucleoproteins in which various proteins were carriers of specificity, whereas the undiversified DNA was merely an unspecific prosthetic group; and (3) the failure by a few proteolytic enzymes to destroy the transforming activity does not by itself prove the non-protein nature of the transforming principle, because proteins are known which resist many proteolytic enzymes.

To answer the first point of criticism, attempts were made in recent years to improve the methods of purification and analysis. Zamenhof et al. (69, 62) purified the transforming principle of *Hemophilus influenzae* to the point where it contained less than 0.4 per cent (referred to DNA) of each of the following impurities: proteins, immunologically active substances, and ribonucleic acids. No loss of biological activity occurred during the gradual removal of impurities (cf. also 28). Hotchkiss (30) found less than 0.02 per cent of protein in his purified transforming principle of pneumococcus. According to a recent estimate (62), the amount of DNA sufficient to transform one cell of *H. influenzae* is of the order of 10^{-8} μg.; an impurity of 0.01 per cent would correspond to about 6 molecules of a molecular weight of 10^5, or less than one of a molecular weight of 10^6. Thus, one has approached the situation where the protein nature of the transforming principle can be excluded on purely analytical grounds.

Besides the above studies, some recent ones offer more suggestions (but no absolute proof) that the transforming principle is DNA. Crystalline pancreatic DNAase in concentrations lower than 10^{-4} μg./ml. produces a 10-fold decrease of activity within 28 minutes (62). The temperature at which the transforming principle begins to lose its activity (81° C., 1 hr.) is the same as the temperature at which the viscosity of the bulk of the preparation begins to decrease. The pH values (on both the acid and alkaline sides) at which the activity begins to decrease are again the same as the pH values at which the viscosity begins to decrease (62). Thus, the active molecule of the transforming principle seems to behave like the average molecule of DNA. Two hours at pH 14.0 (30° C.) or 1 hr. at 98° C. (pH 7) fail to destroy completely the activity of some transforming principles (70). Few, if any, other biologically active substances would be that stable.

In summary, extensive evidence favors the view that the transforming principle is DNA; no evidence to the contrary has ever been presented.

COMPOSITION

As already mentioned, the chemical analysis of the purified transforming principles reveals only the presence of normal components of DNA: nitrogenous bases, deoxy sugar, and orthophosphate, all in usual proportions (5, 28, 69, 62). Of these, only the proportions of individual purines and pyrimidines may be of more than routine interest, in view of the observation that these proportions (for the whole DNA) are characteristic for the species from which they have been derived (14) (for a review, see 59). Such analyses have as yet been made only for the transforming principles of pneumococcus (28, 15), *H. influenzae* (60, 63), and the hypothetical transforming principle (DNA) of *Escherichia coli* (25). The molar ratios of individual purines and pyrimidines for the DNA of pneumococcus and of *H. influenzae*, although characteristic of their respective species, are not far from the values of human DNA, that is, the DNA of their host (14). On the other hand, the values for DNA of *E. coli* are strikingly different; in fact, this is the only analyzed DNA in which the molar ratios of individual purines and pyrimidines are close to unity. No satisfactory explanation of this peculiarity can be offered at present.

The principle that the composition of the whole DNA is characteristic of the species from which it was derived does not necessarily imply that this composition is unchangeable; the alteration of DNA composition by a change in the nutrient medium has indeed been demonstrated (56, 18, 67, 66, 74). When *E. coli* was grown in the presence of 5-bromouracil, 5-iodouracil, or 5-chlorouracil, a considerable part of the thymine in the DNA (up to 48 molar per cent in case of 5-bromouracil) became replaced by these "unnatural" analogs of thymine. The change is readily reversible. It has recently been demonstrated that the change occurs also without DNA synthesis de novo and that the composition of DNA at any particular moment is merely a function of the environment (74, 75).

Space will not permit a detailed discussion of these findings. One might add, however, that the presence of unnatural bases in the medium is not a prerequisite for a change in the DNA composition: as reported recently by Dunn and Smith (19), the content of 6-methylaminopurine, which occurs naturally in the DNA of *E. coli*, can be changed more than 10-fold merely by changing the thymine content of the medium.

The effect of these changes in composition on the transforming activities in pneumococcus or in *H. influenzae* has not yet been studied, because of the difficulties in introducing the "unnatural" bases into the DNA of those species. However, the transformation of *E. coli* has also been reported (7-9, 33), and in another approach a study has been made of the effects of the replacement of half of the thymine in DNA by 5-bromouracil on the phenotype and the genotype of that species (66).

HETEROGENEITY

The data reported in the literature for the composition of the DNA of any species refer to the whole DNA preparation from many, presumably identical, cells. A chemist will, of course, be interested to know whether the preparation really represents a single chemical species or a mixture of many. If one performs a transformation experiment using the principle from a donor carrying several transformable characters ("markers"), each of the resulting transformed cells carries, as a rule, only a single marker (4, 29, 2) ; thus, the preparation behaves like a mixture of independent transforming particles. The doubly transformed cells occur as rarely as predictable from the probability of two independent particles hitting the same cell (29, 32) (an interesting exception will be discussed later on). On this basis one usually assumes that the DNA of each cell consists of many *different* molecules (different chemical species) that determine different hereditary characters.

The nature of the difference could be manifold. The molecules could differ in sequence of nucleotides or in steric pattern or in pattern of bonds, such as hydrogen bonds, or in some other unknown features of this kind. If these were the only differences, the analysis of the mixture could still represent the actual analysis of each molecule. If, on the other hand, the molecules differ in proportions of individual purines and pyrimidines, then the analysis refers merely to the average composition. This difference in proportion could be due to an actual difference in pattern, or merely to the difference in length of the molecule: since the distribution of individual bases is dyssymetrical (64), the difference in length might result in a difference in proportion.

At present no method exists to test the possibility that the differences between various DNA molecules of the same species are merely differences in nucleotide sequence or bond pattern. On the other hand, the detection of the heterogeneity in length might be within the sensitivity of the present methods. Stern and Atlas (54) found that the DNA preparations from calf thymus, upon ultracentrifugation, show polydispersity, which suggests the existence of such an heterogeneity in length of the molecule. The solutions used for this study were rather dilute (0.04 per cent), as otherwise meaningless hyper-sharp boundaries are obtained. It might be stressed that such results are only as good as the preparation studied. Many steps in preparation, and especially failure to exclude the action of DNAase, may result in a depolymerized and therefore polydisperse artifact; indeed, the DNA prepared by an early Hammarsten method (DNAase action not excluded) were polydisperse (54) even at concentrations (0.9 per cent) at which carefully prepared DNA gives hyper-sharp boundaries.

That the DNA molecules of one species can actually exhibit demonstrable differences in their proportions of individual purines and pyrimidines has been shown by the important discovery of DNA fractionation (13; see also 12, 6, 38, 11). In these experiments it has been shown that the DNA preparations from calf thymus or from *E. coli* are non-homogeneous in so far as their dissociation from basic proteins or from ion exchangers is concerned. This phenomenon has been used as a basis for the separation of DNA into several fractions. Such results would be explicable if the size or the acidic characters of the molecules were different. The analysis of the fractions obtained in some procedures revealed that they differ in proportions of individual purines and pyrimidines. The compositions of the whole DNA preparations recorded in the literature are therefore not the compositions of individual molecules but of the averages of compositions.

It would be of obvious interest to study whether the transforming principle preparation carrying several "markers" can be separated into fractions, each containing one marker only. Attempts in this direction are under way in several laboratories, but to date only preliminary results have been published (22, 6, 37). One difficulty is that some preparation and fractionation procedures result in a considerable inactivation of the transforming principle, so that the "fractionation" achieved may actually represent merely a separation of injured molecules or a "fractional inactivation": as will be shown further on, the individual markers in the same preparation of the transforming principle vary indeed greatly in so far as their resistance to inactivating agents is concerned.

Add that it has never been demonstrated that the differences in composition or length of individual molecules have any relation to differences in the determinants of heredity carried by these molecules: it is still possible that a molecule on reproduction changes somewhat its composition or length (see also last chapter), while still retaining its heredity determinants functionally unchanged.

The "Native State" of DNA

The study of the chemical nature and composition of DNA may eventually be undertaken even with degraded preparations of the transforming principle (provided that no fragments are lost). On the other hand, the physical study of the size and shape of the molecule demands that the subject of study be as "native" as possible.

At present, it is not known whether even a most carefully isolated DNA preparation can be identical in all respects with the DNA as it existed in the living cell (65): the DNA is found in the cell not as such but merely as part of a nucleoprotein, which, in turn, may have bonds to still other substances. The term "native" when applied to the preparation of DNA in vitro is therefore rather misleading. What this usually means is that such a preparation exhibits certain features which it must have had when it was in the living cell. The most obvious and the most important of these features is the proper biological activity. It is indeed a feature of which one can safely say that it could not have been created artificially by the process of isolation. Such an active DNA preparation may be called *"functionally intact"* and can serve as a yardstick. Obviously, its properties are more constant and are of more interest than the properties of the products of some undetermined degree of "denaturation"; in particular, the studies of the functionally intact DNA preparation may disclose a correlation between the function and the structure.

As discussed before, the transforming activity is such a proper biological activity, which can be demonstrated in certain bacterial DNA preparations; these DNA preparations can therefore be called functionally intact. The studies of DNA preparations other than these are open to the criticism that the starting material was a product of degradation. While a completely satisfactory study of such functionally intact DNA preparations cannot be offered at present, advantage can be taken of the fact that the DNA of different species exhibits similarities in resistance to various agents (68); thus, a DNA isolated under conditions which would not inactivate another DNA having transforming activity may lead to a "functionally intact" product. Another possibility is to add small amounts of active transforming principle during the isolation of any DNA (68). This transforming principle is to signalize the absence of denaturation. The recovery of the activity in the final preparation of a DNA is an indication that the latter has not been mistreated.

Physical Properties of the Transforming Principles

Avery, MacLeod, and McCarty (5) have made some qualitative studies of the behavior of the transforming principle during ultra-centrifugation and electrophoresis, and concluded that in these respects the transforming principle resembles calf thymus DNA. The ultra-violet absorption spectrum was also similar to that of calf thymus DNA.

Zamenhof et al. (69) determined the electrophoretic mobility of the DNA of *H. influenzae* possessing transforming activity: the ascending mobility was —17 $\times$ 10^{-5} sq. cm./v./sec., in 0.15 M aqueous sodium chloride which was 0.02 M with respect to sodium phosphate (final pH 7.2). The entire transforming activity was associated with this DNA fraction. A quantitative study of the viscosity of a similar preparation has also been made (62); the specific viscosity, when measured under similar conditions, was again similar to that of calf thymus DNA or human spleen DNA (68). From an x-ray diffraction study of pneumococcal transforming principle (57), the crystalline structure was found to be similar to that of calf thymus DNA.

An attempt to determine the molecular weight of the pneumococcal transforming principle by electron and deuteron bombardment has been made by Fluke, Drew, and Pollard (24); the molecular weight so estimated was 6 $\times$ 10^6, which is similar to values obtained by the light-scattering method for calf thymus DNA (16, 52, 50, 10).

The measurement of the sensitive volume inactivated by x-rays yielded values from 7 $\times$ 10^5 to 5 $\times$ 10^6 (44, 23). The discrepancy may be apparent rather than real, since the method may actually measure the size of the vulnerable region of the molecule and not the molecule as a whole. As will be shown further on, even small injuries to the molecule of DNA produce its complete inactivation; thus far, an integral molecule seems to be necessary if there is to be any activity at all. This does not preclude the possibility that the actual active center (or centers) is (are) smaller than the entire molecule (see below).

The discontinuity in the curve of inactivation by x-rays (44, 23) has been interpreted as signifying that the active particles fall into two classes differing in size (44). In the author's opinion such a conclusion may be questioned, since many factors other than the size may account for differences in stabilities (compare last section). It should also be noted that the x-ray irradiation method, which involves drying of the transforming principle prior to irradiation (44), is open to objection inasmuch as drying is known to injure the transforming principle (62). In general, caution should be exerted when using pneumococcus for quantitative studies because pneumococcal cultures contain deoxyribonuclease, which may have a chance to injure the transforming principle both during the isolation and during the testing of the activity. As will be shown further on, injured DNA molecules are artifacts which behave differently from the intact product.

The Molecule of the Transforming Principle

In the foregoing sections each transforming principle has been chiefly discussed as if a single substance; yet in the section on heterogeneity it was shown that a preparation of the transforming principle of a single species may actually be a mixture. In this section the emphasis will be mainly on a single molecule of the transforming principle.

One of the first questions in such an approach is to ask: how many molecules of transforming principle are necessary to transform one cell?

The lowest concentration of transforming principle which will still accomplish transformation in pneumococcus has been estimated by Avery, MacLeod, and McCarty (5), by McCarty and Avery (41), and by Hotchkiss (28) to be of the order of 2×10^{-3} to 10^{-2} μg./ml. These weights refer either to the weights of a purified preparation, or to the weights of DNA, which for all practical purposes are equivalent. Although seemingly low, these concentrations still represent 2×10^8 to 10^9 molecules of DNA (of a molecular weight of the order of 5×10^6) per ml. In these studies the number of the transformed cells was not counted, and therefore the amount of DNA per single transformed cell could not be estimated. As mentioned above, for a study involving very small amounts of DNA, the pneumococcus is not best suited because of the presence of DNAase in the culture.

A quantitative study has been recently made with the transforming principle of *H. influenzae* (62). In one type of experiment a small total volume (0.02 ml.) was used, and the minimal total amount of DNA necessary to transform at least one cell was determined; the value so obtained was 3×10^{-7} μg. In another type of experiment the number of transformed cells was counted; the minimal amount of DNA per transformed cell was found to be 10^{-8} μg. Assuming the molecular weight of DNA to be of the order of 5×10^6, one can calculate that the number of molecules of transforming principle (computed as molecules of DNA) necessary to transform one cell in this system is of the order of 10^3.

It is of interest to compare this minimal effective amount of DNA with the total amount of DNA in one cell of *H. influenzae*. This latter amount has been found to be 2×10^{-9} μg. (62); thus the minimal amount of DNA necessary to transform one cell is only five times higher than the total amount of DNA in the cell. (This estimate is, of course, independent of the actual molecular weight of DNA).

The section on the heterogeneity of DNA contains a discussion of the premise that each DNA molecule of the cell is different because each determines a different hereditary character. If such an assumption is made here,[2] then the number of molecules of DNA of *one kind* necessary for transformation would be of the order of five. If this number can further be reduced, support will be gained for the hypothesis that practically all molecules of one kind are active. If, in addition, every DNA molecule in the cell is assumed to be a potential transforming principle, then the physical and chemical behavior of the bulk of the DNA preparation represents the physical and chemical behavior of the active molecules. Obviously, more evidence is needed before such a view can be fully accepted, but even at the present status of the matter the "infectivity" (31, 48) of DNA particles is comparable to that of bacterial viruses.

If one assumes the molecular weight of DNA to be of the order of 5×10^6, then the above figure of 2×10^{-9} μg. DNA per cell corresponds to 200 molecules. Even if one assumes that all the molecules of DNA in the cell are functional, there still appear to be too few of them to serve as determinants of *all* the hereditary characters of the cell. One is tempted to speculate that not *all* the characters are determined by DNA or else that one molecule of DNA determines several characters. That the latter may be true is indeed suggested by the discovery of multiple transformation in *H. influenzae* (36) and subsequently in pneumococcus (32, 49, 3). In *H. influenzae* a new strain *ab* has been obtained by exposing cells of type *b* to the transforming principle from cells of type *a* (TP$_a$). The new type produces *two* capsular substances *(a* and *b)* at once and yields a new transforming principle TP$_{ab}$ capable of producing *ab* cells from competent receptor

---

[2] Obviously, this study is not meant to contribute to the problem of heterogeneity as such; if several DNA molecules in the cell carry the same marker, then more than five molecules are necessary to transform one cell (22).

cells. These results cannot be obtained by simply mixing TP_a and TP_b in vitro.

In the pneumococcus, the exposure of sensitive cells to the transforming principle from cells bearing two genetic markers produces more cells bearing two markers than would be expected from randomly distributed, *independent* transformations. Again, this result cannot be obtained by simply mixing the two transforming principles in vitro.

Several explanations of these interesting phenomena appear possible at present. (1) It might be that each of the two markers is carried by a separate DNA molecule, but these molecules are linked by some such device as a protein bridge. The experimental evidence speaks against this explanation: the protein content of the preparation can be reduced to less than 0.02 per cent (30); the usual deproteinization (involving protein denaturation) (36, 32) and autolytic proteolysis (32) did not abolish the "linkage." (2) Perhaps a linkage between the two independent DNA molecules is caused by some direct bond which resists rupture in the preparative methods. This explanation (purely speculative) would mean that the aggregate would have a double molecular weight, and this might result in some fractionation during the purification; no evidence of such fractionation has been obtained. (3) If no evidence for either explanation (1) or (2) is forthcoming, then the most likely explanation may be that, indeed, one molecule of DNA can determine more than one genetical marker. Just how one molecule of DNA can reproduce faultily in the presence of another one (in the same locus?) remains entirely in the domain of speculation. It is to be noted that the idea that a faulty reproduction of DNA (mutation?) is *always* an extremely rare phenomenon may not be correct.

THE RESISTANCE TO PHYSICAL AND CHEMICAL AGENTS

The literature on the effects of physical and chemical factors on DNA is rather voluminous; however, the starting material for these studies was in many cases prepared by the methods which are now known to give denatured and therefore less resistant DNA. Here the discussion will be limited to studies in which the starting material had full transforming activity. Most of the studies have been done on the transforming principle of *Hemophilus influenzae* because the cultures of this organism do not contain detectable amounts of deoxyribonuclease (62).

1. Heat

Avery, MacLeod, and McCarty (5) reported that the crude (but not the purified) transforming principle of pneumococcus withstands heating for 30 to 60 min. at 65° C. Zamenhof, Alexander, and Leidy (62) made a quantitative study of the resistance to heat of the purified transforming principle of *H. influenzae.* This study revealed that both viscosity and activity of the transforming principle are indeed rather stable to heat. In citrate buffer a decrease (in both properties) occurs only after 1 hour of heating to temperatures higher than 81° C. The change in concentration of DNA does not affect the stability. These stabilities are much greater than those stated above for the activity of the purified transforming principle of pneumococcus and for the viscosity of DNA of calf thymus (26, 46). That this discrepancy is not due to the species difference is shown by the fact that when human DNA and calf thymus DNA were prepared and tested under conditions similar to those used for the transforming principle, they exhibited a similar stability, as demonstrated by viscosity measurements (68). This high stability is undoubtedly partly due to the avoidance of unstabilizing steps (initial enzyme action, dialysis, drying).

The temperature coefficients of the (biological) inactivation rates between 85 and 95° C. are very large, and suggestive of large energies of activation. If the phenomenon for DNA is similar to thermal denaturation of protein, the above finding may mean that in order to produce comparable denaturation more bonds (H-bonds?) or stronger bonds must be broken in the case of DNA than in the case of most proteins.

It is interesting to note that those molecules of the transforming principle which remained active after a sub-lethal treatment with heat lose their stability to heating at 76° C. or even to storage in the cold (71, 72). This subject will be fully discussed further on.

2. H+ and OH− ions

Avery, MacLeod, and McCarty (5) reported that the inactivation of pneumococcal transforming principle occurs more rapidly at pH 5 and below. A quantitative study of the resistance to acid and alkali of purified transforming principle of *H. influenzae* (62) revealed that both the viscosity and the activity are completely stable over a wide range on either side of pH 7.4 (the normal pH of the human blood). This stability may be species-specific. It has been shown (65) that in yeast cells, whose cytoplasm has a much lower pH, the region of the stability of its DNA is extended towards a lower pH.

As in the case of heating, those molecules of the transforming principle which remained active after a sub-lethal treatment with acid lose their stability to heating at 76° C. (pH 7) or even to storage in the cold (71, 72).

Beyond the stability range, a rapid drop of activity occurs accompanied by a loss of viscosity. At pH 5 (the threshold of stability for *H. influenzae* DNA), less than one primary phosphate group per 10^4 is undissociated; thus, one might conclude that in order to be active, the transforming principle must be in the form of a salt (deoxyribonucleate). However, at the low pH the inactivation might also be a result of the removal of purines (and/or hypothetical hydrogen bonds to these purines). A study (62) of the amount of such a "depurination" of the transforming principle reveals that a 100-fold inactivation concurs with the removal of less than two purines per thousand; thus, practically every purine may be necessary for the activity.[3]

3. Deoxyribonuclease

Avery, MacLeod, and McCarty (5) observed that crude DNAases from dog intestinal mucosa, pneumococcus autolysates, or normal sera inactivate the pneumococcal transforming principle. McCarty and Avery (41) studied inactivation by purified pancreatic DNAase, and Hotchkiss (28) that produced by streptococcal DNAase and by crystalline pancreatic DNAase; 2.5×10^{-4} μg. of the latter per ml. were sufficient to decrease the activity.

Zamenhof, Alexander, and Leidy (62) made a quantitative study of the effects of crystalline pancreatic DNAase on the viscosity and activity of the transforming principle of *H. influenzae*. Less than 10^{-4} μg. of this enzyme per ml. was sufficient to cause a ten-fold decrease in activity within 28 minutes, and a complete inactivation within 140 minutes (30° C.; 300 μg. DNA/ml.). On the other hand, the drop of viscosity at the beginning of inactivation is insignificant. A similar lag period in the depolymerizing action of the enzyme could be demonstrated when calf thymus DNA and human spleen DNA were used as substrates (68). Despite this lag in depolymerization, the enzyme

---

[3] This may be the case only on the assumption that the active molecule behaves like an average molecule of DNA.

does exert some action in this period, as evidenced by a marked decrease in activity (62) and by the loss of stability to heat (68, 71, 72) of the DNA preparations exposed to such initial action of the enzyme. The nature of the initial changes is still not clear. They may involve the breaking of a few phosphate bonds insufficient in number to cause any decrease of size of the molecule which is still held together by the hydrogen bonds.

4. Ionic strength

Avery, MacLeod, and McCarty (5) observed that the *purified* pneumococcal transforming principle rapidly loses activity if dissolved in distilled water. A quantitative study of the effects of exposure to various ionic strengths on activity and viscosity has been made for the transforming principle of *H. influenzae* (62). Previous exposure to lower or higher ionic strengths did not affect the viscosities (as measured in a standard buffer). On the other hand, the activities were reduced by the exposure to lower ionic strength but not by one to higher ionic strength. The previous exposure to lower ionic strength was also found to decrease the stability to heat (68) (as measured under standard conditions). The damage could be due to the breakage of a few vital bonds, such as hydrogen bonds, during the stretching caused by repulsion of anions in the DNA molecule in the absence of salts (62, 55).

5. Dehydration

Avery, MacLeod, and McCarty (5) observed that drying of the purified pneumococcal transforming principle from the frozen state in the lyophilizing apparatus results in a loss of activity. Such a procedure usually involves dialysis prior to drying, and the reported inactivation may represent the combined effect of both these processes. Lyophilization has also been found to degrade calf thymus DNA (68).

A quantitative study of the effect of various conditions of dehydration and storage on activity has been made for the transforming principle of *H. influenzae* (62). None of the commonly used drying methods was harmless; the popular method of drying the DNA fibers with ethanol and ether resulted in an almost complete inactivation. Parallel studies on other DNA (68) revealed that the dried DNA loses its stability to heat (when tested in solution, under standard conditions); again, the most damaging method was drying with ethanol and ether.

The over-all effect of drying and of storage in the dried state may actually be due to several causes: instantaneous injury; slow injury by thermal oscillations in a molecule rendered more vulnerable; or slow injury by progressive dehydration. The exact nature of the injuries is not known.

6. Deamination

A quantitative study of the effects of various chemical agents on activity was made only for the transforming principle of *H. influenzae* (62).

Incubation of the transforming principle with 2 *M* or 1 *M* NaNO$_2$ at *p*H 5.3 resulted in a rapid inactivation of the transforming principle. However, the viscosity remained constant, showing that the average DNA molecule was but slightly altered. An estimate was made of the extent of deamination corresponding to a 1000-fold decrease of activity: this extent was found to be of the order of 0.1 per cent. Thus it seems that practically all the primary amino groups must be intact for activity to remain.[3]

7. Mutagenic agents

The agents in this very heterogeneous class will be grouped together here, although the mechanism of their action may be entirely different.

McElroy (42) suggested that the processes leading to mutation and death are essentially the same, with the exception that the latter are accompanied by more extensive molecular changes. If mutation indeed occurs through a direct action of the mutagenic agents on DNA, then the *inactivation* of the transforming principle by these agents could be a demonstration of such a "too strong mutation."

It is to be emphasized that the transforming principle (DNA) can be harmlessly subjected in vitro to the action of a greater variety of (and more concentrated) mutagenic agents than can the DNA in a living cell. In the case of the transforming principle, the excess of such strong agents can be removed prior to the reintroduction of the transforming principle into the cell. In the case of the living cell, these strong agents may never reach the nuclear DNA, or they may cause death of the cell for reasons other than a reaction with DNA.

Of particular interest is the phenomenon of the unstabilization of the *active* transforming principle, for this may be the first step of the mutational process; this subject will be discussed further on.

Ultraviolet irradiation. The effect of ultraviolet radiation on the activity of the transforming principle of *H. influenzae* has been studied quantitatively (73, 72). The curve for the inactivation of the transforming principle for capsule b formation is shown in Fig. 1. The results suggest a "multi-hit" inactivation. A dose of 500 ergs per sq. mm. was sufficient to cause 1000-fold inactivation. This dose is of the same order of magnitude as that necessary to inactivate the bacterial viruses (for review, see 39). It is important to note that this dose is about 500 times lower than the lowest dose necessary to produce any demonstrable decrease of viscosity of DNA by ultraviolet irradiation (72). Attempts at photoreactivation were not successful.

Ultraviolet irradiation also destroys the stability of the transforming principle to heat (71, 72)—see below.

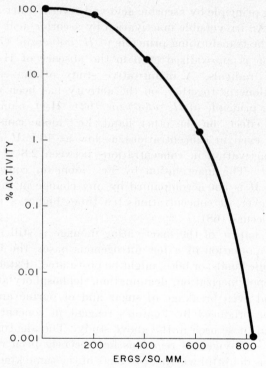

Fig. 1. Inactivation of the transforming principle (capsule b formation) by ultraviolet irradiation. The ordinate indicates the surviving transforming activity as percentage of the original activity on a logarithmic scale; the abscissa indicates the ultraviolet dose. DNA concentration, 227 μg./ml.

Other types of radiation. The inactivation of pneumococcal transforming principle by electron and deuteron bombardment (24) and by x-rays (44, 23) has already been discussed. Drew (17) subjected pneumococcal transforming principle to γ-irradiation; cysteine was found to exert some protective action against this. It is interesting to note that pneumococcal cells injured by γ-irradiation still yielded fully active transforming principle.

Ferrous ion and hydrogen peroxide. The action of ultraviolet irradiation is now believed to be due to free radicals, H$\cdot$ and OH$\cdot$, and to peroxides formed during the irradiation of organic molecules. Similar free radicals are believed to be produced by Fenton's reagent (Fe^{++} + H$_2$O$_2$).

McCarty (40) observed reversible inactivation of pneumococcal transforming principle by ascorbic acid and several other autoxidizable substances. An irreversible inactivation by ascorbic acid has also been studied for the transforming principle of *H. influenzae* (72).

Ferrous ion is autoxidized even in the absence of H$_2$O$_2$ and may produce free radicals. A quantitative study of the effects of Fe^{++} and H$_2$O$_2$, alone or together, on the activity has been made for the transforming principle of *H. influenzae* (62). H$_2$O$_2$ alone had a mild inactivating effect; on the other hand, Fe^{++} alone caused a 10-fold inactivation even in concentrations as low as 10^{-5} M and produced complete inactivation in concentrations between 2.8×10^{-5} M and 2×10^{-4} M. The inactivation by Fe^{++} alone in concentrations up to 2×10^{-4} M is not accompanied by any change in the viscosity of DNA. However, at concentrations ten times higher a rapid depolymerization occurs (68).

The exact nature of the inactivating damage is still unknown. An oxidative deamination of a few nitrogenous bases, the breaking of a few vital labile bonds, or both, might be postulated. Extensive damage, including depolymerization, deamination, dephosphorylation, splitting of bases, and even breakage of sugar and of purine and pyrimidine rings, can be produced by Fenton's reagent in concentrations much stronger than those used in the above study. The identification of the products of such vigorous reactions has recently been reported (53). However, it is doubtful whether products of the same kind are involved in the mild reactions which cause inactivation of the transforming principle or which occur during sublethal mutagenic treatment by free radicals.

Formaldehyde, reported to be a mutagenic agent (47, 20), in strong concentrations (4 M) causes both inactivation and a decrease in the viscosity of the transforming principle of *H. influenzae* (62). A probable interpretation is that formaldehyde reacts slowly with the primary amino groups of adenine, guanine, and/or cytosine, and that in this reaction enough labile bonds (hydrogen bonds?) are broken to cause a decrease in the asymmetry of the molecule as well as inactivation. The latter may again be indicative of the importance of free amino groups for the activity of the transforming principle.

Mustards. Herriott (27) studied inactivation of pneumococcal transforming principle by di(2-chloroethyl) sulfide (mustard gas). This mustard in a concentration as low as 6×10^{-5} M was able to cause complete inactivation in 2 hours. The inactivation of the transforming principle of *H. influenzae* by various nitrogen mustards was studied by Zamenhof et al. (73, 72). Di(2-chloroethyl)-methylamine (HN2) causes a complete inactivation at a mustard concentration of 10^{-4} M. A 10-fold decrease of activity (of capsule b formation) is observed at a mustard concentration of 10^{-5} M (6 hrs., 23° C.), which is 300 times lower than the lowest concentration producing any detectable decrease in the viscosity of DNA (72). The inactivating power of this and other nitrogen mustards for the transforming principle seems to be of the same order of magnitude as the carcinostatic power of these compounds, and suggests some correlation between these phenomena (73, 72). Such results cannot be predicted from the chemical reactivities nor from the DNA-depolymerizing power of the compounds. The transforming principle which survives the mustard treatment also undergoes a change; it becomes unstable to heat (71, 72).

Other alkylating agents. The mutagenic agents dimethyl sulfate, diethyl sulfate, methyl iodide, and β-propiolactone have been quantitatively tested for their ability to inactivate the transforming principle of *H. influenzae* (72). In general, they were comparable in this respect to the monofunctional nitrogen mustard (HN1).

The main reactions of compounds of this kind with DNA are: (1) alkylation of amino groups (especially primary amino groups) of nitrogenous bases; and (2) esterification of the phosphate groups. Recently, a study has been made (51) of these reactions at the low concentrations of these compounds sufficient for inactivation or unstabilization.

The study included a monofunctional nitrogen mustard N,N-diethyl-β-chloroethylamine (HN1) as well as dimethyl sulfate and diethyl sulfate. The study revealed first that the purine bases were much more reactive than the pyrimidines. At the lowest concentrations of dimethyl sulfate which still cause inactivation, only one derivative of bases could be demonstrated in the DNA so treated. The derivative was tentatively identified as 7-methyl guanine. Esterification of the phosphate groups was also detectable with some reagents. Thus, as far as this study is concerned, both alkylation and esterification might be responsible for inactivation or unstabilization.

Non-inactivating agents. The study of agents which even in high concentrations do not inactivate the transforming principle may be of interest from both the theoretical and the practical points of view. Such a quantitative study has been made for the transforming principle of *H. influenzae* (62, 73, 72). For convenience only, these agents have been divided into groups:

(1) *Protein denaturing and sterilizing agents,* in many cases do not cause any inactivation of the transforming principle. Urea ($4M$) can serve as one example (72). This finding may be regarded as a further indication that the transforming principle is not a protein or a virus; and that to produce denaturation more bonds (H-bonds?) or stronger bonds must be broken in the case of DNA than in the case of most proteins (see also section on "Heat"). From the practical point of view, such a study helps to devise deproteinization methods harmless for DNA.

(2) *Agents reported to have mutagenic action* in general, strongly inactivate the transforming principle. However, a few were found (manganous ions, urethane, acriflavine, etc.) to have no inactivating effect at all. The nature of this discrepancy is not clear. One of many possible explanations is that such agents need the presence of the cell to show any action on DNA, either mutagenic or lethal.

(3) *Carcinogenic and carcinostatic agents* are of two classes (73, 72), (a) those (as discussed before) which even in minute doses completely inactivate the transforming principle (U.V., mustards); (b) and those which have no inactivating effect at all (methylcholanthrene, urethane, carcinogenic azo dyes). The mechanism of action of some of these agents (such as azo dyes) may not involve DNA at all. Others may again need the presence of the cell to show any action.

Summary. The effects of strong mutagenic agents on the transforming principle of *H. influenzae* have been summarized in Table 1. This table also includes agents (H^+, DNAase, HNO_2) for which mutagenic action has not yet been demonstrated; this may be due to the inability of these agents to reach DNA in the cell.

In general, the transforming principle is sensitive to all strong mutagens. This fact may suggest that the DNA is indeed the site of their mutagenic action. Obviously, more direct evidence is needed before such a view can be fully accepted.

The Unstable Transforming Principle

As mentioned above, the sublethal treatment of the transforming principle of *H. influenzae* by heat, acids, mustards, deoxyribonuclease, or ultraviolet irradiation results in a product which is unstable to heat or even to storage in the cold (71, 72). The kinetics of inactivation by heat reveal that more than one reaction is involved (such as unstabilization followed by inactivation). When the transforming principle, rendered very unstable by a sublethal heat, ultraviolet, or mustard treatment, was used for transformation experiments, the transformed cells yielded transforming principle which was completely stable: thus, the change (unstabilization) in vitro was not retained on reproduction and therefore was not a "mutation in vitro."

The chemical nature of a true mutation is, of course, still unknown. If it concerns DNA at all, it may involve any of the changes mentioned in the discussion of differences between individual DNA molecules

TABLE 1

Inactivation of the Transforming Principle of *H. influenzae*
by Mutagenic Agents

(Character transferred: capsule b formation.
DNA 200 μg./ml.; 23° C., 6 hrs., except as noted).

Agent	Mutagenicity	Conc. or Dose for 10-Fold Inactivation
H^+	?	$10^{-4}M$
DNAase	?	$<8 \times 10^{-5}$ μg./ml. $\begin{cases} \sim 10^{-12}M \\ 25 \text{ min. } 30°\text{C.} \end{cases}$
HNO_2	?	$<5 \times 10^{-3}M$
Fe^{++}	+	$10^{-5}M$
Ultraviolet	+	200 ergs/sq.mm.
β-Propiolactone	+	$<10^{-3}M$
Nitrogen mustard HN_2	+	$10^{-5}M$
Dimethyl sulfate	+	$3 \times 10^{-4}M$
Diaminobiuret	+	$4 \times 10^{-4}M$
Urea	−	$4 M$—no inactivation

(sequence of nucleotides, proportions, etc.), see section on Heterogeneity. At present, any such change could be visualized as a (rare) fault occurring during DNA reproduction. However, the probability and the location of the fault along the DNA molecule may be determined by a preceding process, the gene unstabilization (61).

It has repeatedly been suggested (1, 58, 43, 35) that the first action of the mutagenic agents is to bring the gene into an unstable state from which it can either return to the previous state or change into a stable mutant gene; this secondary change may not require the presence of the mutagenic agent any more. The phenomenon of delayed mutations may point in this direction. It is conceivable that such unstabilization is also possible in vitro and that the unstabilization of the transforming principle is indeed a demonstration of such a change.

DIFFERENTIAL STABILITIES OF INDIVIDUAL HEREDITARY DETERMINANTS

The study of the loss of viscosity in DNA preparations as a whole has revealed that the *average* stability of DNA molecules towards various agents is similar in different species (*H. influenzae*, 62; human and ox, 68). However, in some species the stability may be extended to meet special environmental conditions (such as low pH in yeast, 65).

It is of interest to study whether *individual* heredity determinants differ in their stabilities. Such a study, in vitro, can be done only on transforming principles. Marmur and Fluke (44) were unable to demonstrate any difference in the stability of several pneumococcal transforming factors towards ionizing radiation. The stability towards other agents has been quantitatively studied in the transforming principle of *H. influenzae* (70) and is reported below.

Purified transforming principle was prepared as described before, using as donors streptomycin-resistant encapsulated strains of types b, c, or d. Each preparation thus carried two "markers"; as receptors, streptomycin-sensitive non-encapsulated strains R_b or R_d served. The transforming principle was exposed to various agents as described previously (62, 72). The results are represented in Figs. 2 and 3.

It will first be seen that several transforming activities differ in stability: In the case of ultraviolet irradiation a dose up to 60 times higher is required to produce the same amount of destruction in activity for streptomycin resistance (from type b) as for activity for production of capsules b or c. Such a study also reveals (Fig. 3) that the activity for streptomycin resistance from type b is not identical with that from type d. Possibly they depend on different heredity determinants.

The differences in stability of the activities for capsule b formation and for streptomycin resistance are most pronounced in the case of ultraviolet irradiation. However, these differences can easily be demonstrated also for other agents, such as nitrogen mustards (Fig. 3), heat, H^+, or Fe^{++}. As already discussed, the processes leading to inactivation by these agents are probably different; however, the present results suggest that some feature or features of stability may be common to all these agents (though, as shown here, different for different heredity determinants). The inactivation by OH^- seems to be an exception: no differences could be detected in that case, a fact which suggests an entirely different mechanism of inactivation.

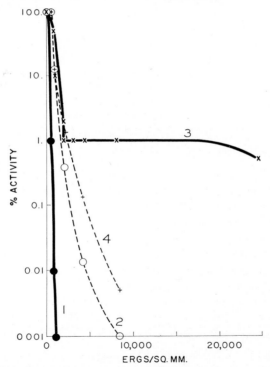

FIG. 2. Stability to ultraviolet irradiation of the following transforming activities: for capsule b or c formation (curve 1), capsule d formation (curve 2), streptomycin resistance in type b (curve 3) and streptomycin resistance in type d (curve 4). The ordinate, abscissa, and DNA concentration as in Fig. 1.

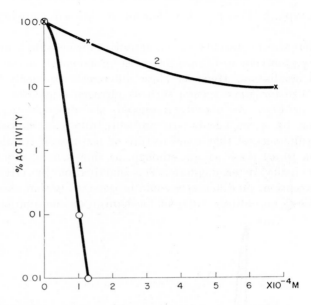

Fɪɢ. 3. Stability of the transforming activity for capsule b formation (curve 1) and the transforming activity for streptomycin resistance in type b (curve 2) to the action of the nitrogen mustard p-di-(2-chloroethyl)-amino-phenylalanine (DL) (6 hrs., 23° C.). The ordinate and the DNA concentration as in Fig. 1; the abscissa indicates the concentration of mustard.

The study also indicates that it is possible to "separate" the mixture of heredity determinants by completely destroying some of them but not completely destroying the others.[4]

In several cases the above properties did not seem to be substantially affected by the choice of receptor (homologous or heterologous) nor by the passage (reproduction) of a transforming principle through a homologous or heterologous receptor (i.e., there was no significant "host modification" caused by the passage).

It is also of interest that even the more resistant activities *begin* to decrease at a temperature or a pH value at which the viscosity of the bulk of the preparation begins to decrease. The stability of the activity

[4] The finding that some heredity determinants show higher resistance to mutagenic agents than others may have a bearing on the phenomenon of induction of phage development (intact DNA?) in lysogenic bacteria (for review, see 34). It is also of interest to note that this development is not induced by those reported mutagens which in the present work have been found not to inactivate the transforming principle.

for streptomycin resistance (in type b) is not *uniformly* high. The curves of this stability to ultraviolet irradiation (Fig. 2) and to the action of nitrogen mustard (Fig. 3) first drop more rapidly, but eventually reach a very distinct plateau. This fact suggests that some of the molecules may be much more stable than others. Thus it appears that not only individual heredity determinants as wholes, but also individual molecules within (presumably) a single kind of heredity determinant differ widely in stability. A break in the exponential inactivation curve was also observed by Ephrussi-Taylor and Latarjet (23) in their study of the inactivation of pneumococcal transforming principle by x-rays. In order to test whether such diverse stabilities are due to the presence of several heredity determinants or to heterogeneous stabilities of what is essentially a single heredity determinant, those authors repeated the transformation but using the more resistant fraction of the transforming principle remaining after sublethal irradiation. The transformed cells yielded a transforming principle which again showed heterogeneous stabilities. This result suggested that here a single heredity determinant, which on reproduction assumes heterogeneous stabilities, may be involved.

Essentially similar results were obtained in the present study with the transforming principle of *Hemophilus influenzae*. A transformation experiment was performed using irradiated transforming principle (streptomycin resistance, type b) which had 1 to 2 per cent of residual activity completely resistant to a total dose of at least 16,000 ergs/sq.mm. (plateau in Fig. 2). R_b or R_d served as receptor cells. The transformed cells yielded a transforming principle whose activity could again be destroyed (in 80 to 90 per cent) by less than 900 ergs/sq.mm. All these experiments suggest that the transforming principle does not breed true, at least in so far as a uniform stability is concerned. Several "special" cases where the transforming principle does not breed true have been reported in recent years (21, 36, 32, 49, 3).

As already discussed, the heterogeneity in resistance towards irradiation may mean heterogeneity in size, heterogeneity in some other factors contributing to bond stability, or both. The parallel heterogeneity in resistance towards other agents (mustards, heat, H^+, Fe^{++}) may also be related to size. It follows that some heterogeneity in size of the active molecules of the transforming principle, either carrying the same or different markers, cannot be excluded at present.

REFERENCES

1. Auerbach, C., Robson, J. M., and Carr, J. G., *Science,* **105**, 243 (1947).
2. Austrian, R., *J. Exptl. Med.,* **98**, 21, 35 (1953).
3. Austrian, R., and Bernheimer, H. P., *J. Clin. Invest.,* **34**, 920 (1955).
4. Austrian, R., and MacLeod, C. M., *J. Exptl. Med.,* **89**, 439, 451 (1949).
5. Avery, O. T., MacLeod, C. M., and McCarty, M., *J. Exptl. Med.,* **79**, 137 (1944).
6. Bendich, A., Fresco, J. R., Rosenkranz, H. S., and Beiser, S. M., *J. Am. Chem. Soc.,* **77**, 3671 (1955).
7. Boivin, A., *Cold Spring Harbor Symposia Quant. Biol.,* **12**, 7 (1947).
8. Boivin, A., Vandrely, R., and Lehoult, Y., *Compt. rend. Acad. Sci., Paris,* **221**, 646 (1945).
9. Boivin, A., Tulasne, R., and Vendrely, R., *Compt. rend. Acad. Sci., Paris,* **225**, 703 (1947).
10. Brown, G. L., M'Ewen, M. B., and Pratt, M. I., *Nature,* **176**, 161 (1955).
11. Brown, G. L., and Martin, A. V., *Nature,* **176**, 971 (1955).
12. Brown, G. L., and Watson, M., *Nature,* **172**, 339 (1953).
13. Chargaff, E., Crampton, C. F., and Lipshitz, R., *Nature,* **172**, 289 (1953).
14. Chargaff, E., Zamenhof, S., and Green, C., *Nature,* **165**, 756 (1950).
15. Daly, M. M., Allfrey, V. G., and Mirsky, A. E., *J. Gen. Physiol.,* **33**, 497 (1949).
16. Doty, P., and Bunce, B. H., *J. Am. Chem. Soc.,* **74**, 5029 (1952).
17. Drew, R. M., *Radiation Research,* **3**, 116 (1955).
18. Dunn, D. B., and Smith, J. D., *Nature,* **174**, 305 (1954).
19. Dunn, D. B., and Smith, J. D., *Nature,* **175**, 336 (1955).
20. Englesberg, E., *J. Bacteriol.,* **63**, 1 (1952).
21. Ephrussi-Taylor, H., *Exptl. Cell Research,* **2**, 589 (1951).
22. Ephrussi-Taylor, H., *Advances in Virus Research,* **3**, 275 (1955).
23. Ephrussi-Taylor, H., and Latarjet, R., *Biochim. et Biophys. Acta,* **16**, 183 (1955).
24. Fluke, D., Drew, R., and Pollard, E., *Proc. Natl. Acad. Sci. U.S.,* **38**, 180 (1952).
25. Gandelman, B., Zamenhof, S., and Chargaff, E., *Biochim. et Biophys. Acta,* **9**, 399 (1952).
26. Goldstein, G., and Stern, K. G., *J. Polymer Sci.,* **5**, 687 (1950).
27. Herriott, R. M., *J. Gen. Physiol.,* **32**, 221 (1948).
28. Hotchkiss, R. D., *Colloq. intern. centre. natl. recherche Sci. (Paris),* **8** [Unités biologiques douées de continuité génétique], 57 (1949).
29. Hotchkiss, R., *Cold Spring Harbor Symposia Quant. Biol.,* **16**, 457 (1951); Symposium sur le mode d'action des antibiotiques, *2. Congr. intern. Biochim. (Paris),* 40 (1952).
30. Hotchkiss, R. D., in *Phosphorus Metabolism* (W. D. McElroy and B. Glass, ed.), Vol. II, p. 426, Johns Hopkins Press, Baltimore (1952).
31. Hotchkiss, R., in *The Dynamics of Virus and Rickettsial Infections* (F. W. Hartman et al., eds.), p. 405. Blakiston, New York (1954).
32. Hotchkiss, R. D., and Marmur, J., *Proc. Natl. Acad. Sci. U.S.,* **40**, 55 (1954).
33. Ishii, O., *J. Osaka City Med. Center,* **3**, 238 (1954); [*Chem. Abstr.,* **49**, 7051 (1955)].
34. Jacob, F., and Wollman, E. L., *Cold Spring Harbor Symposia Quant. Biol.,* **18**, 101 (1953).
35. Kaplan, R. W., *Z. Naturforsch.,* **7b**, 291 (1952).

36. Leidy, G., Hahn, E., and Alexander, H. E., *J. Exptl. Med.,* **97**, 467 (1953).
37. Lerman, L. S., *Biochim. et Biophys. Acta,* **18**, 132 (1955).
38. Lucy, J. A., and Butler, J. A. V., *Nature,* **174**, 32 (1954).
39. Luria, S. E., *General Virology,* John Wiley & Sons, New York (1953).
40. McCarty, M., *J. Exptl. Med.,* **81**, 501 (1945).
41. McCarty, M., and Avery, O. T., *J. Exptl. Med.,* **83**, 89, 97 (1946).
42. McElroy, W. D., *Science,* **115**, 623 (1952).
43. McElroy, W. D., and Swanson, C. P., *Quart. Rev. Biol.,* **26**, 348 (1951).
44. Marmur, J., and Fluke, D. J., *Arch. Biochem. and Biophys.,* **57**, 506 (1955).
45. Mirsky, A. E., *Cold Spring Harbor Symposia Quant. Biol.,* **12**, 15 (1947).
46. Miyaji, T., and Price, V. E., *Proc. Soc. Exptl. Biol. Med.,* **75**, 311 (1950).
47. Rapoport, I. A., *Compt. rend. acad. sci. U.R.S.S.,* **54**, 65 (1946).
48. Ravin, A. W., *Am. Scientist,* **43**, 468 (1955).
49. Ravin, A. W., *Records Genet. Soc. Am.,* **24**, 591 (1955); *Brookhaven Symposia Biol.,* **8**, 33 (1955).
50. Reichmann, M. E., Rice, S. A., Thomas, C. A., and Doty, P., *J. Am. Chem. Soc.,* **76**, 3047 (1954).
51. Reiner, B. D., and Zamenhof, S., unpub.
52. Rowen, J. W., *Biochim. et Biophys. Acta,* **10**, 391 (1953).
53. Scholes, G., and Weiss, J., *Biochem. J.,* **53**, 567 (1953).
54. Stern, K. G., and Atlas, S. M., *J. Biol. Chem.,* **203**, 795 (1953).
55. Thomas, R., *Biochim. et Biophys. Acta,* **14**, 231 (1954).
56. Weygand, F., Wacker, A., and Dellweg, H., *Z. Naturforsch.,* **7b**, 19 (1952).
57. Wilkins, M. H. F., Stokes, A. R., and Wilson, H. R., *Nature,* **171**, 738 (1953).
58. Witkin, E. M., *Cold Spring Harbor Symposia Quant. Biol.,* **16**, 357 (1951).
59. Zamenhof, S., in *Phosphorus Metabolism* (W. D. McElroy and B. Glass, eds.), Vol. II, p. 301. Johns Hopkins Press, Baltimore (1952).
60. Zamenhof, S., *Bull. N.Y. Acad. Med.,* **28**, 349 (1952).
61. Zamenhof, S., *Science,* **120**, 791 (1954).
62. Zamenhof, S., Alexander, H. E., and Leidy, G., *J. Exptl. Med.,* **98**, 373 (1953).
63. Zamenhof, S., Brawerman, G., and Chargaff, E., *Biochim. et Biophys. Acta,* **9**, 402 (1952).
64. Zamenhof, S., and Chargaff, E., *J. Biol. Chem.,* **178**, 531 (1949); **187**, 1 (1950).
65. Zamenhof, S., and Chargaff, E., *J. Biol. Chem.,* **186**, 207 (1950).
66. Zamenhof, S., De Giovanni, R., and Rich, K., *J. Bacteriol.,* **71**, 60 (1956).
67. Zamenhof, S., and Griboff, G., *Nature,* **174**, 306, 307 (1954).
68. Zamenhof, S., Griboff, G., and Marullo, S., *Biochim. et Biophys. Acta,* **13**, 459 (1954).
69. Zamenhof, S., Leidy, G., Alexander, H. E., FitzGerald, P. L., and Chargaff, E., *Arch. Biochem. and Biophys.,* **40**, 50 (1952).
70. Zamenhof, S., Leidy, G., and Greer, S., unpub.
71. Zamenhof, S., Leidy, G., and Hahn, E., *Records Genet. Soc. Am.,* **23**, 75 (1954).
72. Zamenhof, S. Leidy, G., Hahn, E., and Alexander, H. E., *J. Bacteriol.,* **72**, 1 (1956).
73. Zamenhof, S., Leidy, G., and Reiner, B., *Proc. Am. Assoc. Cancer Research,* **1**, 53 (1954).
74. Zamenhof, S., Reiner, B., De Giovanni, R., and Rich, K., *J. Biol. Chem.,* **219**, 165 (1956).
75. Zamenhof, S., Rich, K., and De Giovanni, R., *Federation Proc.,* **15**, 390 (1956).

CHROMATOGRAPHIC FRACTIONATION OF *E. COLI* DNA CONTAINING 5-BROMOURACIL-2-C^{14} *

AARON BENDICH, HERBERT B. PAHL** AND GEORGE BOSWORTH BROWN

The Sloan-Kettering Division of Cornell University
Medical College, New York, N. Y.

INTRODUCTION

EVIDENCE HAS BEEN obtained by a variety of independent procedures which clearly indicates that the total DNA of the cell consists of a complex mixture of different macromolecules (2-8, 10-12, 17, 18, 22). It is not known at present whether all these molecules are concerned with genetic function, or whether some are involved in other biological phenomena. Certain column chromatography procedures (4-6, 14, 16) have been used to advantage in the study of the transforming DNA of pneumococcus, because the DNA fractions which are obtained possess a demonstrable biological property. However, biological properties for the DNA's from other sources have not yet been observed, and therefore additional approaches by which such properties may be revealed have been sought.

The demonstration by Weygand, Wacker, and Dellweg (24) of the uptake of radioactivity by the nucleic acid fraction of *Streptococcus faecalis* when grown in the presence of bromine-labeled 5-bromouracil led to the definitive experiments of Dunn and Smith (13) and of Zamenhof and Griboff (25), in which it was shown that the halogenated pyrimidine replaced the thymine of both *Escherichia coli* and bacteriophage DNA on an equimolar basis. In *E. coli,* nearly 50 per cent of the thymine can be replaced. Both Zamenhof (25) and Wacker et al. (23) have expressed the thought that there may be among the DNA molecules within the cell a fraction which does not incorporate 5-bromouracil to the same degree as do the majority of DNA molecules.

* This investigation was supported by funds from the National Cancer Institute, National Institutes of Health, Public Health Service (Grant #C-471), and from the Atomic Energy Commission (Contract #AT(30–1)–910).

** Fellow of the National Cancer Institute of the Public Health Service.

The amount of bromouracil incorporated could conceivably depend upon the extent to which the particular DNA molecule acts as a genetic determinant.

Because of the availability of methods for the possible selective labeling (incorporation of 5-bromouracil) of the DNA's of a cell and for the fractionation of DNA into many components, by means of chromatography on the substituted-cellulose derivative ECTEOLA (4-6), it appeared reasonable to test the hypotheses of Zamenhof and of Wacker mentioned above. The present study is concerned with the demonstration that the DNA of *E. coli* is heterogeneous with respect to incorporation of bromouracil.

EXPERIMENTAL PROCEDURE

A thymineless mutant of *E. coli*, Strain I[1], was grown in either proteose-peptone or synthetic media supplemented with 5-bromouracil. When synthetic medium was employed, a supplement of thymine was added. The organisms were grown for 18-24 hours at 37° C. with aeration, and at the end of this period the cells were harvested, washed, and the DNA isolated after lysis with detergent[1]. Deproteinization was carried out either with detergent (15) or by shaking with chloroform-pentanol (21). Ribonucleic acid was degraded with ribonuclease, and the products of hydrolysis were removed by dialysis against 2 M NaCl (19). The final product was white and fibrous, and yielded a clear, viscous solution. It assayed for 94-100 per cent of DNA by the Ceriotti test (9) when calf thymus DNA prepared by the method of Schwander and Signer (20) was used as a standard, and for 0-6 per cent of DNA by the orcinol procedure (1).

Radioactive 5-bromouracil was synthesized by direct bromination of uracil-2-C[14]. The 5-bromouracil was freed of uracil either by repeated recrystallizations or by fractionation of the mixture on a Dowex-1 (hydroxyl form) column.

For the chromatographic fractionation of the DNA the procedure of Bendich et al. (4-6) was employed. Gradient elution was used, first with NaCl solutions of increasing concentration at constant but neutral pH, then with increasing pH but constant salt concentration. The amount of DNA in each fraction was determined by spectrophotometric

[1] The strain of *E. coli* and details for isolating the DNA were kindly provided by Dr. S. Zamenhof.

measurement. Each fraction was dialyzed exhaustively, and the radio-activity of aliquots was determined to within ±10 per cent error. In each experiment 100 ± 5 per cent of the DNA was recovered from the column on a spectrophotometric basis, and 74-86 per cent on the basis of radioactivity (from an added radioactivity of the order of 600,000 c.p.m.).

The DNA was isolated from appropriate column fractions for base analysis. The bases were determined by spectrophotometric methods after paper chromatographic separation from perchloric acid hydrolysates.

RESULTS AND DISCUSSION

In a preliminary study (Experiment 1) the DNA isolated from *E. coli* grown in the presence of 5-bromouracil-2-C-[14] was fractionated on ECTEOLA. Determinations of thymine/5-bromouracil ratios on DNA's isolated from a few major pooled fractions revealed no significant differences between chromatographic peaks.

Since the chromatographic pattern given by the DNA containing 5-bromouracil might be expected to be different from that of normal DNA, the absence of significant differences in the thymine/bromouracil ratio between peaks was ambiguous. This result might mean either that (a) there was a uniformity in uptake of bromouracil by all the DNA's in the cell, and therefore all column fractions had the same amount of bromouracil per unit of DNA, or (b) the population of DNA's within the cell was heterogeneous with respect to bromouracil content, but the cellulose exchanger, or the method of sampling used, did not permit discrimination between a DNA containing 5-bromouracil and one from which this base is absent.

Since the latter interpretation was subject to test by experimentation, the following was carried out (Experiment 2): two separate cultures of *E. coli* were grown simultaneously under the same conditions except that one culture was supplemented with 5-bromouracil-2-C[14]. Each culture was harvested and washed separately and the wet weight determined. The moist cells from both cultures were then mixed in such proportions that approximately one-third of the final weight was due to those cells which had been grown in the presence of bromouracil. The intimately mixed cells were lysed and the DNA isolated. This DNA, when fractionated on a column of ECTEOLA, gave the information shown in Fig. 1 and Table 1. It is to be seen in Fig. 1 that some

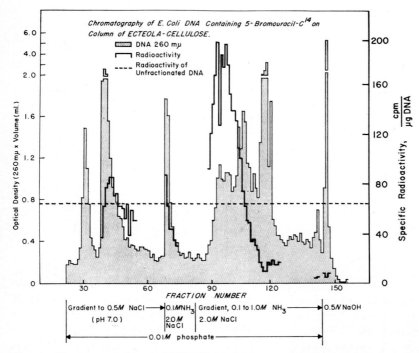

Fɪɢ. 1. Chromatography on ECTEOLA of 3.9 mg. of DNA isolated from an *E. coli* mixture composed of two parts (by wet weight) of cells grown in the absence of 5-bromouracil-2-C14 and one part of cells grown in the presence of this pyrimidine. Of the total radioactivity added to the column (252,000 c.p.m.), 76 per cent was recovered in the 58 per cent of the fractions which were dialyzed and assayed for C14 content. The stippled area represents the DNA content of a fraction (left-hand ordinate), and the heavy black line the specific radioactivity of the fraction (right-hand ordinate). The horizontal dashed line shows the specific radioactivity of the starting, unfractionated DNA. The ECTEOLA column was 5.0 × 1.15 cm. See Table 1 for the calculated relative specific activities of selected column fractions. (This figure refers to Experiment 2.)

fractions, especially those in the high alkaline range, have a considerable amount of DNA, but only very little radioactivity. This indicates that the chromatographic profile of the DNA which lacks 5-bromouracil is not identical with that of the DNA which contains this pyrimidine. Whether some of the DNA in these particular peaks (those with a low specific activity) comes from those cells which were grown in the presence of bromouracil-C14 cannot be ascertained from these data. It is highly probable that the DNA in that chromatographic

TABLE 1

SPECIFIC ACTIVITY OF COLUMN FRACTIONS

(*E. coli* DNA Containing 5-Bromouracil-2-C^{14})

The data in this table are calculated from the results of Experiment 2 (Fig. 1).

Composition of Eluent	Fraction Number	cpm / µg.DNA	Sp. Act. of Fraction / Sp. Act. of Original
	Original	66	1.0
From 0.0 to 0.5 *M* NaCl	39	38	0.6
	43	88	1.3
	55	51	0.8
From 0.0 to 0.1 *M* NH$_3$ in 2.0 *M* NaCl	69	90	1.4
	74	31	0.5
	89	93	1.4
	93	198	3.0
From 0.1 to 1.0 *M* NH$_3$ in 2.0 *M* NaCl	94	129	2.0
	97	197	3.0
	118	11	0.2
	142	4	0.1
0.5 *M* NaOH	147	4	0.1

peak which shows the highest specific activity (fractions 90-115) was derived almost entirely from the bromouracil-grown cells, for the maximum specific activity attained (Table 1) is three-fold that of the unfractionated DNA (the proportion of labeled cells to total cells was 1:3). A further point of interest, which will be discussed later, concerns the shape of the specific activity curve within any one chromatographic peak. These results (Experiment 2) indicate that the cellulose exchanger does discriminate decisively between DNA's which contain bromouracil and those which do not. The extent to which the content of bromouracil in two DNA's can be different and still not show chromatographic differences is not yet known. In this experiment the one DNA had no bromouracil, while in the other approximately 47 per cent of the thymine had been replaced. It can be seen from the shape of the specific activity curve of Experiment 2 (Fig. 1) that the pooling of fractions in any peak would smooth out both those differences which are present in the individual fractions of each peak, and those which exist between separate peaks. Since this possibility might explain the apparent lack of differences in the ratios of thymine to 5-bromouracil in Experiment 1, it was considered necessary to assay individual column fractions of DNA obtained from a single culture grown in the presence of 5-bromouracil. An appropriate isotope tracer study (Experiment 3) was therefore carried out.

In this experiment (Experiment 3) a culture of *E. coli* was grown in synthetic medium in the presence of 5-bromouracil-2-C^{14}, and the DNA isolated and chromatographed as before (Fig. 2). A comparison of Fig. 2 with Fig. 1 shows that, in general, the chromatographic profile is similar, the main differences existing in the region of high *p*H. This region is, however, where the DNA from non-labeled cells is eluted (see Fig. 1), and this provides further evidence for the essential reproducibility of the chromatographic pattern even when separate DNA samples prepared at different times are used (6).

It is to be seen in Fig. 2 that, in general, the shape of the specific activity curve follows the shape of the optical density curve, although the two curves are not superimposable. The same correlation is seen in Fig. 1. Thus it may be concluded that the shape of the specific activity curve shown in Fig. 1 is not due entirely to the fact that a mixture of DNA's was used, since the same kind of result is obtained (Fig. 2) when the DNA from a single culture is fractionated. Although the physicochemical basis for the particular shape of the specific activity curve is not as yet known, the observed differences in specific activity are significant, and are interpreted as providing evidence in support of the idea that the DNA population is heterogeneous within the cell.

Although the nature of the experimental technique used does not point out the type of heterogeneity being studied here, the DNA's with the lower concentration of bromouracil may have come from young cells, while DNA's with the higher specific activities could have been derived from older cells. This idea is intriguing in view of the recent report by Zamenhof et al. (26, 27) of an exchange of 5-bromouracil for thymine in cells which are no longer dividing. In the present investigation the cells grown in the presence of bromouracil were harvested after 18-24 hours. Thus the final content of bromouracil in the DNA could represent both that amount which was incorporated during synthesis of the DNA as well as that which replaced thymine by exchange after cell division had stopped. It would be of interest to repeat the present chromatographic experiments with bromouracil-labeled DNA isolated after various times of bacterial growth in the presence of that pyrimidine, since the distribution of 5-bromouracil along the polynucleotide chain may depend upon the mode of incorporation, i.e., either by total synthesis or by "exchange." A difference in the distribution of bromouracil residues might be expected to modify

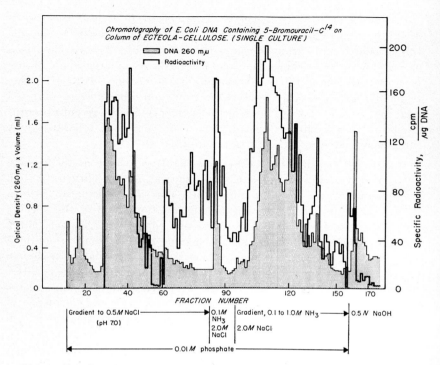

Fig. 2. Fractionation on ECTEOLA of 3.0 mg. of DNA isolated from *E. coli* grown in the presence of 5-bromouracil-2-C[14]. 86 per cent of the radioactivity added to the column (613,000 cpm.) was recovered. For each fraction, the stippled area shows the DNA content (left-hand ordinate) and the heavy black line the specific radioactivity (right-hand ordinate). 0.75 g. of ECTEOLA exchanger were used for the chromatography. (This figure refers to Experiment 3.)

the specific configuration of the DNA molecule and possibly its chromatographic behavior. The DNA peaks which were eluted with NaOH in both Experiments 2 and 3 (Figs. 1 and 2) had relatively low specific activities, and it is therefore possible that a portion of the DNA eluted in this *p*H region in Experiment 2 came from the bromouracil-grown cells.

It has been reported that the specific transforming activity (streptomycin resistance) of pneumococcal DNA, after fractionation on ECTEOLA, is highest in those column fractions which are eluted in the alkaline region (6). In addition, it has been found (6) that the ratios of adenine to thymine and guanine to cytosine approach unity in fractions obtained in this region. The specific activity of the alkaline column fractions of DNA isolated from bromouracil-C^{14}-grown cells is low, and indicates that these molecules do not incorporate bromouracil to a great extent. Taken together, these three findings may indicate that the DNA which is eluted from the column in the later stages of the chromatography is related to the essential "genetic" DNA mentioned by Zamenhof (25) and by Wacker et al. (23), although other column fractions may also have biological significance.

SUMMARY

The application of the procedure for the chromatographic fractionation of DNA to a study of the DNA isolated from *E. coli* grown in the presence of 5-bromouracil indicates that the DNA population is heterogeneous with respect to the incorporation of this pyrimidine. These results have been discussed in terms of the recent findings of Zamenhof that bromouracil can be incorporated into *E. coli* DNA by two routes: total synthesis, and exchange with thymine residues after cell division has ceased.

It is postulated that the DNA eluted from the column in the region of high alkalinity may be more closely related to the "native" DNA.

REFERENCES

1. Albaum, H. G., and Umbreit, W. W., *J. Biol. Chem.,* **167**, 369 (1947).
2. Bendich, A., *Exptl. Cell. Research* **3** (suppl. 2), 181 (1952).
3. Bendich, A., Russell, P. J., Jr., and Brown, G. B., *J. Biol. Chem.,* **203**, 305 (1953).
4. Bendich, A., Fresco, J. R., Rosenkranz, H. S., and Beiser, S. M., *J. Am. Chem. Soc.,* **77**, 3671 (1955).
5. Bendich, A., in *Essays in Biochemistry* (S. Graff, ed.), p. 14. Johns Wiley & Sons, New York (1956).
6 Bendich, A., Pahl, H. B., and Beiser, S. M., *Cold Spring Harbor Symposia Quant. Biol.,* **21** (in press).
7. Brown, G. L., and Martin, A. V., *Nature,* **176**, 971 (1955).
8. Brown, G. L., and Watson, M., *Nature,* **172**, 339 (1953).
9. Ceriotti, G., *J. Biol. Chem.,* **214**, 59 (1955).
10. Chargaff, E., in *The Nucleic Acids* (E. Chargaff and J. N. Davidson, eds.), Vol. I, p. 307. Academic Press, New York (1955).
11. Chargaff, E., Crampton, C. F., and Lipshitz, R., *Nature,* **172**, 289 (1953).
12. Crampton, C. F., Lipshitz, R., and Chargaff, E., *J. Biol. Chem.,* **211**, 125 (1954).
13. Dunn, D. B., and Smith, J. D., *Nature,* **174**, 305 (1954).
14. Ephrussi-Taylor, H., in *Advances in Virus Research* (K. M. Smith and M. A. Lauffer, eds.), Vol. III, p. 275. Academic Press, New York (1955).

15. Kay, E. R. M., Simmons, N. W., and Dounce, A. L., *J. Am. Chem. Soc.*, **74**, 1724 (1952).
16. Lerman, L. S., *Biochim. et Biophys. Acta*, **18**, 132 (1955).
17. Lucy, J. A., and Butler, J. A. V., *Nature*, **174**, 32 (1954).
18. Lucy, J. A., and Butler, J. A. V., *Bull. Soc. Chim. Belg.*, **65**, 133 (1956).
19. Markham, R., and Smith, J. D., *Biochem. J.*, **52**, 565 (1952).
20. Schwander, H., and Signer, R., *Helv. Chim. Acta*, **33**, 1521 (1950).
21. Sevag, M. G., Lackman, D. B., and Smolens, J., *J. Biol. Chem.*, **124**, 425 (1938).
22. Shooter, K. V., and Butler, J. A. V., *Nature*, **175**, 500 (1955).
23. Wacker, A., Trebst, A., Jackerts, D., and Weygand, F., *Z. Naturforsch.*, **9b**, 616 (1954).
24. Weygand, F., Wacker, A., and Dellweg, H., *Z. Naturforsch.*, **7b**, 19 (1952).
25. Zamenhof, S., and Griboff, G., *Nature*, **174**, 306 (1954).
26. Zamenhof, S., Reiner, B., De Giovanni, R., and Rich, K., *J. Biol. Chem.*, **219**, 165 (1956).
27. Zamenhof, S., Rich, K., and De Giovanni, R., *Federation Proc.*, **15**, 390 (1956).

DISCUSSION

DR. FRAENKEL-CONRAT: What levels of RNAase have been tested and not been found to inactivate the preparation? It's the degree of purity of RNAase that I'm interested in.

DR. ZAMENHOF: That was tried in the original paper by Avery, MacLeod, and McCarty. I don't remember the details; but we have used RNAase to remove the RNA from the preparation, and we have found that there is some inactivation because of DNAase present as impurity. Something like one mg. of RNAase per cc. would slowly denature the transforming principle.

DR. LEDERBERG: We just had two papers by Dr. Ephrussi-Taylor and Dr. Hotchkiss on the methodological difficulties of measuring inactivation in such a system, and I wonder if you would comment briefly on the techniques which are used in the determination of activity of treated materials.

DR. ZAMENHOF: The method used was a titration rather than a method of counting the number of transformed cells, though in many cases we have compared the two and found them consistent; so in general we stick to the titration. The titration means that serial dilutions of the transforming principles are made, the sensitive cells in excess are exposed to it, and the lowest concentration of DNA determined at which two out of two samples are still transformed. We have been using these methods since 1951, and we have accumulated a lot of data. We have recently subjected these data to statistical analysis, and we find that if there is a two-fold decrease in activity it doesn't mean anything statistically. A five-fold decrease is significant. You will notice that in our work we encounter 100,000- to 1,000,000-fold decreases.

Dr. LEDERBERG: Do you find the competition effect that was described by the previous speakers?

Dr. ZAMENHOF: Not in this system. Miss Leidy found this effect several years ago, but not in the system where you titrate.

Dr. EPHRUSSI-TAYLOR: You say that you have tested this inactivated material on a number of receptor strains. To what extent are these receptor strains related? Can you test the capsular factor on the same range as you test the streptomycin-resistant factor?

Dr. ZAMENHOF: We find that the degree of inactivation is not dependent upon the choice of receptor.

Dr. EPHRUSSI-TAYLOR: That's not quite the question. I want to know whether you can test the capsular factor and the streptomycin factor on the same strain.

Dr. ZAMENHOF: That is routinely done. The streptomycin factor and the capsular factor are tested on the same receptor stain.

Dr. LURIA: May I point out just one thing in this connection. If you are using a dilution end-point method, unless you have an independent test of the linearity of response with the amount—for example, in double transformed cells—sometimes the shape of the inactivation curve may be less meaningful than in the case where it is tested with a direct count method. Because of different concentrations you may have different numbers of responding cells for the same response.

Dr. ZAMENHOF: That's a very good remark. There are certain ranges which give us results which we cannot interpret. These experiments we repeat. Miss Leidy has done a thorough study of the shape of the curve, and this has been published.

Dr. BENDICH: I wonder whether Dr. Zamenhof or anyone else here would care to comment on the very interesting and curious report of McCarty on the reversible inactivation of the transforming principle by very dilute solutions of ascorbic acid [M. McCarty, *J. Expertl. Med.*, **81**, 501 (1945)]. If I recall the paper, one might conclude there is an oxidation-reduction sensitive system in transforming principle. That reminds me of the thing Dr. Ephrussi-Taylor was mentioning before: the inactivation with succinic peroxide. Is that reversible? I wonder whether McCarty's observation has been repeated and confirmed. There may be something in DNA that nobody suspects—perhaps an oxidation-reduction system reversible by sulfhydryl groups.

Dr. ZAMENHOF: That has been repeated and not confirmed.

Dr. BENDICH: In *Pneumococcus*?

Dr. ZAMENHOF: In *Hemophilus*.

Dr. HOTCHKISS: It is an interesting point. I have tried to repeat it with peroxide which McCarty and Avery inferred was the actual inactivating principle in an ascorbic acid treatment. Neither after treatment with peroxide nor with ascorbic acid was I able to reconstitute with sulfhydryl compounds an active principle in terms of the scoring methods we use now. I recall that in the original work it was necessary, in taking up treated material and testing for reactivation, to reprecipitate; so you might have in this original work a selective concentration of high molecular weight material. Their test was again the dilution end-point—in other words, how many of five cultures at the end-point gave transformation to see where the reaction stops. They used five; I think your two samples are too few.

DR. CHARGAFF: Does ascorbic acid inactivate?

DR. HOTCHKISS: Yes. It does inactivate. It is an ascorbic acid oxidation in the presence of copper and oxygen, and it can be imitated with peroxide.

DR. BENDICH: It is catalyzed by copper. I thought it was also done in the absence of copper.

DR. ZAMENHOF: It can be done in the absence of copper very easily.

DR. WATSON: I would like to ask Dr. Zamenhof what the evidence is for bromouracil going out of the DNA without the DNA reduplicating.

DR. ZAMENHOF: When you grow bacteria in bromouracil medium the growth stops in 7 hours. There is no change in the number of cells, and we determined that the amount of DNA per cell is constant, so there is no *de novo* DNA synthesis. On the other hand, when you plot the curve of incorporation of bromouracil—that is, thymine replacement with time—you find a steep incorporation curve after 7 hours. You can make a very amusing experiment if you suspend the cells in saline containing an excess of thymine but no 5-bromouracil. There is no cell division. After a certain time, the cells are still incorporating 5-bromouracil from inside the cells and not thymine.

DR. PAPIRMEISTER: I would like to ask the group how the DNA gets into the cell. The only reason I bring that up is to find out what the effect is of these various treatments, that you have presented here, on the penetrability of the DNA into the cells, since they have a negative charge. In other words, to rephrase the question, would these agents have the same effect on intracellular DNA as they do here?

DR. ZAMENHOF: Yes, that's a very good question. When I say that the transforming principle is becoming inactive, this may cover a multitude of sins—it may be the inability to penetrate, it may be the inability to displace the existing DNA in the cell, or it may be the inability to act even though present in the genome. Now, Dr. Herriott and Dr. Goodgal have done a very good experiment on penetration of DNA from our strains into the cell, and maybe they'll be willing to say something about it.

DR. LEVINTHAL: I want to ask the people who have been doing UV inactivation whether there is or is not photoreactivation of transforming factor.

DR. ZAMENHOF: We have done this experiment, and there is no photoreactivation.

DR. LURIA: I think we may have to put off the answer to that until Dr. Goodgal takes the floor, because he promised to talk about that.

DR. STENT: Dr. Zamenhof, in the experiments concerned with the specific activities of P^{32} what would be the total activities of P^{32} in the different bases? I would expect, in any case, the specific activity of those DNA constituents which were there in the first place to be rather small.

DR. ZAMENHOF: Yes. The total is small. We calculated it per molecule of bromouracil.

DR. STENT: Yes. Well, what actually is the total P^{32}, let's say in bromouracil compared to adenine?

DR. ZAMENHOF: I couldn't answer that question, because Dr. T. D. Price has done this work; it's in press in *Nature*.

DR. RAVIN: I noticed the two markers that have the least difference with respect to susceptibility to inactivation—the streptomycin character and one of the capsule characters—can come from the same cells.

DR. ZAMENHOF: That is correct.

DR. RAVIN: I wonder whether this difference in susceptibility is a function of whether the markers come from the same cells or from different cells. You have a case of a number of markers coming from the same cell, and they show little or no difference in susceptibility.

DR. ZAMENHOF: The capsular character and the streptomycin character from the same cells of strain b show the biggest difference.

DR. RAVIN: I see.

DR. R. WILLIAMS: I may have missed this in your talk, but when you were testing the effect of the mutagenic agents did you separate the transforming material from the mutagenic agent before applying it to the cells?

DR. ZAMENHOF: Of course, because otherwise it would be just an after-effect of the mutagenic agent.

DR. KAPLAN: Does this mean that the urea would denature the DNA? As I understand it, doesn't urea knock out the x-ray pattern of DNA?

DR. WATSON: No. Urea doesn't do much at room temperature. But if you put DNA in the presence of 6 M urea it will be denatured at a lower temperature.

DR. ZAMENHOF: Well, that makes me wonder, because in our case we can heat DNA to 76° C. in the presence of urea and it doesn't do anything. There is another point which I didn't discuss yet. You may have all kinds of responses to various agents if you start with slightly injured material. If you try to inactivate by x-ray the material which is biologically active, you find that it is about 10 or 100 times more resistant than the material prepared by conventional methods in the literature for getting DNA. This is a very important point. To compare whether something does something or not, we have to use the same standard for the starting material. I don't insist that this standard be transforming activity; but we have to have some standard, because we won't understand each other.

DR. LURIA: Do you mean, Dr. Zamenhof, that you suspect that when you prepare DNA in a way that is not optimal, you obtain DNA which is still transforming but which has already some potential damages, which are more readily amplified by radiation, for example? One might suppose that DNA with breaks in one of the two polynucleotide chains would be more easily breakable by another treatment.

DR. ZAMENHOF: That is correct.

DR. LEDERBERG: I have had the impression that the accessory system for the *Hemophilus* transformation is much simpler than *Pneumococcus*, but I wonder if that's really true. Can you do transformations in a defined medium without serum?

MISS LEIDY: Yes. The medium we use to carry out transformations usually consists of a nutrient broth (lacking X and V growth factor requirements), to which is added DNA, and competent cells were added.

DR. LEDERBERG: The competent cells were not grown on that, of course?

MISS LEIDY: No. They are grown on a broth that in our system contains the X and V factors of heated horse blood.

DR. GOODGAL: We can get transformation in just saline. All you have to do is spin down the cells, resuspend them in saline, and add DNA.

DR. LEDERBERG: Are the cells grown on a non-protein medium?

DR. GOODGAL: No.

DR. ZAMENHOF: Now I would like to mention another study. This one is a study of calf thymus DNA, to avoid objections that what we do is valid only for transforming principles. It is a study of inactivation by heat. The preparation is heated for one hour, then returned to normal or room temperature and the specific viscosity measured. The preparation was prepared like the transforming principle. As a matter of fact, in one case we even added transforming principle to serve as a marker. We found that after all these purifications the DNA of calf thymus was still active in the *Hemophilus* system, because we had these traces of transforming principle which were not destroyed by the methods of preparation. We find that DNA is indeed very stable to heat. Its viscosity starts to decrease only at about 81° C. In one experiment a preparation was subject, previous to heating, to the action of DNAase to the extent of a 2% of viscosity decrease. Now, that's something which is very easy to miss if you make calf thymus DNA and don't inhibit your DNAase properly. This pre-treatment with DNAase produced a marked change in the stability to heat. This is still more pronounced when the initial drop of viscosity was of the order of 4% to 8%. That's also very easy to miss, but such study of the loss of stability to heat reveals that this DNA was indeed injured.

DR. EPHRUSSI-TAYLOR: I would like to clear up the question of the action of urea. I have the impression that Dr. Zamenhof may have misunderstood my remarks about the action of urea. I employed 5 M urea—sometimes for 2 hours, sometimes for 8 hours—at room temperature. Urea has no action whatsoever on biological activity unless the preparation is one which you have reason to believe is aggregated, in which case urea increases activity. The action of urea seems to be uniquely one of dispersing secondary aggregation.

DR. ZAMENHOF: That's how I understood it.

DR. DOTY: I would like to make a passing comment on the effect of urea on DNA. It is now well known from the work of R. Thomas and others that DNA is partially denatured when the salt concentration is too severely reduced in aqueous solution. Mr. Litt in my laboratory has shown that when the counterion concentration (including the sodium ions from DNA itself) is reduced to approximately 10^{-4} $Molar$ the viscosity falls substantially at room temperature and one hour at 40° C. lowers it several fold. At 0.15 $Molar$ salt, however, the viscosity remains constant up to nearly 90° C. (for one-hour exposures). As Dr. Zamenhof first showed, the viscosity falls rapidly at slightly higher temperatures. These observations are consistent with the standard practice of always keeping aqueous solutions of transforming principle "protected" with moderate concentrations of salt. Dr. Rice and I (paper in press) found that at the usual salt concentration (0.1-0.5 $Molar$) the effect of 8 M urea is to lower by 19° the narrow temperature range in which the thermal denaturation takes place. Thus in the presence of salt, DNA that is itself in an undamaged or undenatured state remains stable in the presence of 8 M urea indefinitely at room temperature and can remain unchanged for about one hour at 65-70° C. Now, of course, if concentrated urea is added to a salt-free DNA solution, whose denaturation temperature is already near room temperature, it will depress that critical temperature so that denaturation (similar to that which occurs when saline solutions of DNA are heated above 95° C.) will promptly occur. Thus urea does lower the denaturation temperature of DNA but in the presence of salt the effect is unnoticeable at room temperature.

DR. SPIEGELMAN: I was wondering, Dr. Zamenhof, if you can get UV-resistant strains of your organism.

DR. ZAMENHOF: This is under study.

DR. SPIEGELMAN: You haven't studied the DNA of UV-resistant organisms?

DR. ZAMENHOF: We are doing it now.

DR. BENZER: A question to Dr. Goodgal. On the very last point, is this photoreactivation the same with different characters?

DR. GOODGAL: It has only been measured on one so far.

DR. HOTCHKISS: On that same point, when you say that *Hemophilus* isn't photoreactivable, you mean for growth—that is, photoreactivation of UV killing?

DR. GOODGAL: Yes.

DR. LURIA: What about photoreactivation of the transforming principle in the whole cell? What happens if you radiate this transforming principle, let it get into the cells, and then expose to visible light? Do you get a higher ratio of transformation?

DR. GOODGAL: In the experiment that we tried it didn't work with *Hemophilus*.

DR. LURIA: But in this system you are dealing with the transforming principle from *Hemophilus* and with the extract from *E. coli?*

DR. GOODGAL: That's right.

DR. LURIA: One thing which seems to stand out from the discussion this afternoon is that the molecular size of the DNA involved in transformation seems to be assuming more or less stable, unitarian features. On the other hand, the work of radiation seems to point to the existence of some sort of subunit, which is specifically responsible for certain transformations. Here we meet a problem that is also present in transduction: Are the subunits of sensitivity the units of specificity of the character, or the units of action in whatever phenomena are necessary as prerequisites for transformation, or are they the units of "crossing over" or more generally, of the genetic integration process? There may be all these elements involved when one genetic material is trying to substitute for another.

DR. BENDICH: I think I must take issue with your interpretation or your conclusion that the molecular weight of transforming DNA seems to have taken on a stable character. The total DNA (the total transforming principle isolated from pneumococcus) is a mixture of materials as revealed by experiments that have been described today and in the literature. We have been concerned with this mixture of materials that have come to be called and characterized as DNA. I didn't have time today to go in detail into our fractionation experiments on the various component polynucleotides of the DNA. Together with Dr. H. Pahl, we fractionated a very fine preparation of pneumococcal transforming principle DNA prepared by Dr. Sam Beiser, the results of which I showed earlier today. Various fractions of this material were subjected to preliminary ultracentrifugal analysis in the laboratory of Dr. Alex Rich by Dr. Dan Bradley. He found some of the fractions of the DNA to have a molecular weight in the range of around 6,000,000. The early fractions coming off the column, however, appeared to have much smaller molecular weights. Although it is difficult to assign an exact molecular weight to the early polydisperse fractions, some of these were lower than 400,000. Some of the estimates were even lower than that. There is, however, indirect evidence from our fractionation results that the early fractions from the column come off in regions of salt concentration that coincide with the place where octanucleotides are eluted. These are kind of small. It is indirect evidence, as I indicated, but this fractionation procedure discriminates among molecules of different sizes in the early portions of the chromatogram. Whereas the bulk of the DNA may consist of large molecules, there is still room for smaller pieces.

MISS LEIDY: We have explored the reactivity of the streptomycin-resistance transforming agent in a study of inter- and intra-species transformations in *Hemophilus*. The term species is used with its bacteriological connotations. The degree of reactivity of the transforming agent (DNA) is measured in terms of the ratio of the number of cells transformed to streptomycin-resistant by a heterologous DNA to the number transformed by a homologous DNA.

We have found, as has Dr. Pierre Schaeffer of the Pasteur Institute, that this "hetero-homo" ratio between species of *Hemophilus* is of a low order of magnitude. For example, the frequency of induced streptomycin-resistant cells in *H. influenzae* populations (strain Rd) exposed to the streptomycin-resistance transforming agent derived from populations of *H. influenzae*, *H. parainfluenzae* and *H. suis* is of the order of 1 per 10^3, 1 per 10^6, and 1 per 10^7 respectively.

It is of interest that at least for *H. influenzae* and *H. parainfluenzae*, the "hetero-homo" transformation ratio appears to be relatively constant for a given recipient population. It also appears to be independent of the strain or type source of the heterologous species transforming agent. In other words, for these two species there appears to be a relatively fixed probability of heterospecies transformation, at least for SM resistance, for a given recipient population.

We have also explored the reactivity of the transforming agent derived from cells in which resistance was induced by a heterologous species DNA. Such cells yield an agent which, in its reactivity, is similar to that of the species which has incorporated the transforming agent and not to the species which has donated the agent. However, its degree of reactivity is changed. After passage through the host heterologous species it becomes 4- to 15-fold more efficient in heterospecies transformations.

DR. LURIA: You haven't done any studies as to the ability of different cells to take up the various homologous or heterologous DNA, of the kind that Dr. Goodgal reported?

MISS LEIDY: No.

DR. ZAMENHOF: Am I right that in one case you were able to show that a strain was wrongly classified because it was actually not transformed by heterologous DNA?

MISS LEIDY: We made use of the heterotype/homotype transformation ratio. Margaret Pittman has included another species in the

Hemophilus genus—*H. aegyptius*—that includes the Koch-Weeks bacillus (or conjunctival strains). There has been a controversy as to whether these organisms should be included in the *H. influenzae* forms or not. We received some strains from Dr. Pittman and have just begun working on them; and we have obtained streptomycin-resistant cells from one of them, have prepared the transforming factor, and have given it to *H. influenzae* forms as recipient cells and have found that the proportion of cells transformed is that characteristic of *H. influenzae*. In other words, the ratio is practically one, so this strain may belong to *H. influenzae* rather than a different species.

DR. LURIA: Medical diagnostic laboratories will have to use transformation experiments routinely.

DR. HOTCHKISS: I wonder if Miss Leidy would like to comment about Dr. Schaeffer's work. Also, I would like to speak about the work by MacLeod and coworkers on *Streptococcus* and *Pneumococcus* cross transfers which are giving the same story: poor yield across "species" lines, therefore giving the same picture of compatibility relationships among the different strains.

MISS LEIDY: Dr. Schaeffer had been working with the same strain of *Hemophilus* that we use, the Rd strain, and he has reported that the DNA from a strain of *H. parainfluenzae* can induce resistance in this population of *Hemophilus influenzae*. He came out with the ratio characteristic of what we found for *H. suis* DNA rather than that we found for *H. parainfluenzae*. He did not demonstrate the reciprocal transformation.

DR. LURIA: I may point out something which may be relevant to the matter of efficiency of genetic exchanges among distantly related organisms. The same situation is found in genetic recombination between *Escherichia coli* and all of the Shigellae, in which the same mating system applies as among *E. coli* strains but routinely one finds that all recombination frequencies are between 500 and 5,000 times lower. We do not yet know whether it is a matter of low frequency of mating or of low efficiency of successful mating.

DR. AUSTRIAN: There are some differences in the frequency of transformation that are also intraspecific. One finds non-encapsulated strains of pneumococcus which may be transformed very readily to certain capsular types but with almost negligible efficiency to other capsular types. The significance of such a phenomenon as a guide to speciation must be interpreted somewhat guardedly at the present time.

DR. WOLLMAN: I would like to mention, with reference to Miss Leidy's account of Pierre Schaeffer's work, that he also has recently studied reciprocal transformations and confirms Miss Leidy's results entirely. Whether the recipient strain is *H. influenzae* or *H. parainfluenzae*, the heterospecifically transformed cell retains some of the specificity of the donor. When *H. influenzae*, for instance, is transformed with DNA from a resistant *H. parainfluenzae*, the DNA from the resulting transformants will behave as an *H. influenzae* DNA when tested on *H. influenzae*, but will exhibit a greater efficiency than a normal *H. influenzae* DNA when tested on *H. parainfluenzae*. Schaeffer's interpretation is that the transformation frequency reflects the extent of pairing between the transforming and the bacterial DNA's.

Dr. ZAMENHOF: One of the possible interpretations of these findings is that during the reproduction of DNA of *H. influenzae* in the cells of *H. parainfluenzae* the composition or structure of DNA may change, in that it becomes more sympathetic to the host.

Dr. HARTMAN: I don't think that you need to invoke a requirement for a change in the structure of DNA carrying the specific genetic information you are studying. Although perhaps grossly the same, the genomes of two bacterial species certainly are not identical. The many points at which these small differences in genetic constitution occur may interfere with synapsis, a process which you would almost have to regard as a step in the transformation process. The low efficiency of transformation of a particular locus, found in inter-species tests, may be increased after integration of a marker into a host homologous to the ultimate recipient bacterium. This increased efficiency may result from the replacement of synaptically less efficient genes, linked on the same DNA segment with the gene being analyzed, with genetic material of the recipient species. The portion of the DNA under observation (i.e., one locus) thus may not be "changed" in structure or composition at all.

Dr. EPHRUSSI-TAYLOR: I would like to disagree with Dr. Zamenhof on terminology. I don't think you should call it a radical change in specificity—a vast change—I think you can only call it a genetic recombination.

Dr. ZAMENHOF: Yes, all right. But the point is that it is not a rare change in a DNA molecule due to a typical mutation, but it is rather a change of the bulk of the DNA molecules. It depends on what you want to call it. You put molecules into the cell, and out come different molecules.

MISS LEIDY: If it may be a matter of heterogeneity of DNA so that you have small pieces and large pieces, then for different recipient strains of the same species you should get a constant heterospecies/homospecies ratio. If you find that for one strain the heterospecies/homospecies ratio is .02% and for another strain is something like 2% —wouldn't that imply that with a single heterospecies DNA it is not a matter of selecting extremely small particles that have transforming activity?

Dr. LURIA: If I understood correctly, the point at argument was not so much a matter of selecting small fragments of DNA, but of selecting DNA in which a specific recombination ability has been restricted to regions of different length.

DR. GOODGAL: I have one comment on that point. In the original transformed cell one essentially conserves the old marker as well as introducing a new one; that is, both markers are maintained, as Hotchkiss' experiments show. With *Hemophilus* we showed that those cells which transform actually give off streptomycin-sensitive cells, so that both the transforming DNA and the original streptomycin-sensitive DNA continue to replicate.

DR. AUSTRIAN: I think one must consider the importance of the genome of the donor of the transforming principle as well as the genetic constitution of the recipient. The former factor may play a role both in interspecific and in intraspecific transformations. Miss Leidy and her associates reported (in a paper, as I recall, on new types of *Hemophilus influenzae*) that they had a strain of *H. influenzae* which transformed with great difficulty to capsular type *a* when the type *a* factor came from a wild-type cell. But when the type *a* factor was transferred to an intermediate host, the DNA from that strain transformed the originally refractory strain to type *a* with very high efficiency. I think, as Dr. Hartman pointed out, that minor changes in genetic structure may also influence appreciably the genetic behavior of doubly encapsulated pneumococci in transformation reactions. The genetic structures proximate to those involved in a given reaction may have a considerable effect upon the efficiency of that reaction.

DR. MAZIA: This raises in the mind of one who has not worked with the transforming principle the question whether you know what happens to those cells that are not transformed. If you are firing genetic material at the cells in the form of the DNA solution, you are firing it with a shotgun. The host cells should pick up all sorts of genetic material which might raise havoc with the normal balance of events and appear as the killing of many cells. I realize that you must design your experiments to screen for those that have undergone a given transformation, but what do we know about what happens to the rest?

DR. HOTCHKISS: Since we saw a delay in the division of new transformants, we asked what about all the other cells? If there is some kind of metabolic setback—perhaps a genetic setback—any kind of indigestion at all—there should be a lot of the population besides the known transformants that are set back, although we weren't able to find any signs of them. In fact, these kinetic curves that I have presented show a smooth progress of total cell growth right at the same time one is challenging with the transforming principle.

DR. LURIA: In line with the toughness of cells that receive an intruder, we must remember that you can take bacteria and shoot into them bacteriophage and under the proper conditions—for example, in *Salmonella*—nearly 100% of the cells that have received 40 bacteriophage particles, together with all sorts of other junk that has to be accommodated in their chromosomes, all survive, and even their progeny survive.

Part IV

*VIRUSES AS BEARERS OF HERITABLE
CHARACTERISTICS*

THE VIRULENT Teven PHAGES OF
ESCHERICHIA COLI B

Roger M. Herriott*

*Department of Biochemistry, The Johns Hopkins University,
School of Hygiene and Public Health,
Baltimore, Maryland*

BACTERIAL VIRUSES have proven to be excellent material on which to study the basic biological problems of genetics and replication. This is due primarily to their high efficiency of infection, simplicity and precision of assay, and ease of detecting mutant strains. In addition, essentially pure strains of either host or virus can be obtained in quantity in a relatively short time, and this permits chemical analysis of the various steps.

Although it has been generally supposed that the bacterial transforming factors represent a simpler level of replicating unit than viruses, the papers in this section will show that some of these differences are somewhat illusory. Thus, the nucleic acid of tobacco mosaic virus appears to be able to infect its host in the absence of the viral protein coat (10), and prophage replication in lysogenized cells is limited by the rate of cell division as are transforming factors and other genetic units.

In discussing the virulent phages I limit consideration to the T-even phages of *Escherichia coli* because of personal experience with them and because investigators from so many branches of science have examined this system that it is probably better understood than any other. This review is not intended to be complete and will serve as a preface to the discussion of recent developments which Drs. Delbrück and Stent will cover.

Perhaps a description of the gross features of the T-even coli phages is a useful way to introduce a discussion of this system. The T-even phages are tadpole-shaped viruses made up of approximately equal quantities (14, 37) of protein and deoxyribose nucleic acid (DNA).

* Aided by a grant from the National Foundation for Infantile Paralysis, and from the U. S. Atomic Energy Commission.

That the nucleic acid resides in the head of the phage is suggested by electron microscope pictures (see Figs. 1A and 1B) taken before and after exposure of the phage to osmotic shock (1). This treatment liberates the nucleic acid into the surrounding medium in a highly polymerized and viscous form. Although the residual proteinous "ghost" lacks the faculty for replication, it retains many specific biological functions which are usually associated with the intact phage (13). Thus, the host range specificity, the interference, the "killing" property, the inhibition of pentose nucleic acid synthesis and adaptive enzyme formation (32), and, finally, lysis of the host cell are all properties of both the phage and ghost preparations. By inference this leaves replication and certain other functions to the material released by osmotic shock.

T2 phage infects by first attaching its tail to the host cell (2), after which most of the phage nucleic acid (20) and a small amount of soluble protein (16) pass into the cell. The phage coat, or ghost, remains attached to or embedded in the cell wall. Exposure of infected cells to large shearing forces strips 80 per cent of the ghost protein from the cells without altering the course of the infection (20). This suggests that any influence the ghost exerts on the cell's metabolism is either initiated at the time of infection and that thereafter the ghost

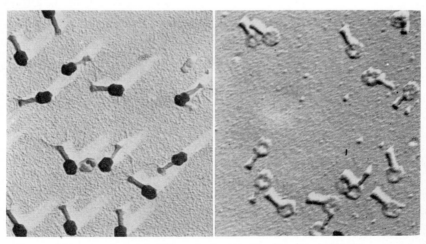

FIG. 1. Electron microscope pictures of: (A) T2 phage, and (B) Ghosts or the protein coats of phage T2 after osmotic shock. Photos taken by Dr. James S. Murphy.

is not important or else that the inhibitory function is associated with the 20 per cent left in the cell wall after shearing.

Passage of the nucleic acid and the soluble protein from the phage coat at the time of infection means, of course, that the unit carrying the phage heredity into the metabolic milieu of the host is not the intact phage but only a fraction of it, as Northrop (30) had suggested. This explains Doermann's observations (5, 6) that no infectious particles could be found in the host soon after infection. We shall be primarily concerned with this "eclipse" period, i.e., the period between infection and the appearance of the first mature particle, for as Hershey and Rotman (23), Doermann and Dissosway (8), and Levinthal and Visconti (26) have found, this is the period during which the hereditary units destined to become phage progeny are determined and formed.

The Metabolic Picture.

We might examine for a moment some of the metabolic changes which occur during the "eclipse" period. Isotopic tracers have been used extensively in this work. In addition, phage nucleic acid and protein can be readily distinguished from the host counterparts. Phage DNA is distinguished by its recently discovered pyrimidine 5-hydroxy-methyl-cytosine (5-HMC) (43), and the phage and bacterial proteins are easily distinguished by serological procedures.

Upon infection of *E. coli* with T-even phages the pentose nucleic acid (PNA) synthesis is reduced to 2-3 per cent (4, 20, 29, 40) of its normal rate and DNA synthesis is held up for several minutes, but protein formation proceeds uninterrupted (4). A number of laboratories (3, 18, 38) working independently have recently brought considerable clarity to this problem. Phage DNA synthesis apparently requires a prior synthesis of protein, for if protein synthesis is blocked at the time of infection by one or another procedure, no phage DNA is formed. If, however, the block is delayed for a few minutes, during which time a small amount of protein is formed, phage DNA is then produced in the usual quantities even if further protein synthesis is again blocked. Using sulfur-35-labelled medium and intermittent introduction and withdrawal ("pulse" experiments) of chloramphenicol, Melechen and Hershey (18) found that much of the protein that is formed in those first few minutes does not appear thereafter in the progeny. Interpretation of this finding will be made later.

In uninhibited infected cells about 50 phage equivalents of viral DNA are formed by the time the first mature intracellular infectious particle is formed (15). This pool of DNA is maintained as the phage continues to be formed. The precursor protein is formed only shortly before maturation of the phage, and the pool size is only half that of the DNA (21).

Synthesis of phage DNA does not carry a prerequisite that the host be able to synthesize *bacterial* DNA, for cells which have lost the latter faculty through treatment with sulfur mustard are nevertheless capable of forming normal quantities of phage, and, of course, this involves DNA synthesis (12). This fact means that for the synthesis of phage DNA the germinal substance of the infecting phage (16) does not need the factor destroyed by mustard.

The Chemical Nature of the Hereditary Unit.

In considering the nature of the material carrying the hereditary information of the phage from cell to cell we find very few unequivocal answers. Analysis of purified preparations of T_2 phage (14, 16) have not revealed the presence of materials in the phage other than protein, DNA, and a small quantity of nucleic acid intermediates; so our interest will be confined to the protein and DNA. There is no way at present of testing directly the effect of the DNA in the absence of protein; but the protein has been tested in the absence of DNA, from which result the effect of the DNA may be inferred. Cells "infected" with the protein ghosts produce DNA and protein (25), but these products do not exhibit the characteristics of phage components (Herriott, unpub.); hence, the phage determinants or factors essential to them were probably eliminated in the preparation of ghosts, and they are very likely in the material that passes into the host on infection. Hershey (16) has shown by isotopic studies that this material, which he calls the "germinal substance," consists of 97 per cent DNA and about 3 per cent soluble protein, but there is no property which permits a decisive assignment of the phage genetic functions to one component in preference to the other. It should be added, however, that the self-complementary nature proposed for DNA by Watson and Crick (41), the linear properties required for genetic material (42), and, of course, the nature of the bacterial transforming factors (24), make DNA the more attractive choice. No appreciable quantity of the isotopically labelled protein is transferred to the progeny (16), whereas upwards of 50 per cent of the nucleic acid phosphorus is transferred (17, 28, 31). However, the relevancy of this information depends on an understanding of the mechanism of replication, and this remains as yet ill-defined.

Before turning to the mechanism of replication, it will be profitable to continue the examination of evidence bearing on the nature of hereditary units in phage. Hershey (18) has pointed out that considerable phage precursor DNA and only small quantities of precursor protein are formed during the eclipse period in which Doermann and Dissosway (8) observed that genetic units and recombinants are formed. In the phenomenon of exclusion or interference another close correlation exists. In this case the genetic units of the superinfecting particle do not appear in the progeny (9), and in a parallel manner the P^{32} of the superinfecting particle is not transferred (11).

While the above results provide suggestive correlations, Stent has supplied some good direct evidence (34, 35). In his work phage labelled with P^{32} of high specific activity was used to infect cells. At various intervals after infection the systems were frozen at low temperatures, and then the effect of P^{32} decay (suicide) on the phage formation of the cell was determined. Phage inactivation developed as a result of the nuclear reaction and not from the effects of the resultant radiant energy. In general, Stent found that one in twelve disintegrations of the P^{32} caused a loss of infectivity for a phage particle, thus confirming earlier studies of Hershey et al. (22). Since at least 97 per cent of the phosphorus of phage is in the DNA (14), this result virtually establishes the essentiality of 8 per cent or more of the DNA. Rescue of some of the genetic markers from the inactive phage was demonstrated (35, 33a) by simultaneously infecting cells with both the inactivated phage and an active one of a different but closely related strain.

Additional strong evidence of the direct relationship between genetic determinants and phage DNA has been furnished by Doermann and his associates (7), who studied the rescue of genetic markers from ultraviolet-inactivated phage. It seems very reasonable, though not proven, that ultraviolet light inactivates the phage by virtue of its action on the nucleic acid. Doermann found that individual markers are only 4 per cent as sensitive as is the phage infectivity, a relation which suggests the size of the marker relative to the sensitive part of the infectious unit. Doermann and his group also made the very important observation that unlinked genetic markers were inactivated independently by ultraviolet light, whereas in the case of linked markers the inactivation of one marker was in general accompanied by a corresponding loss of the other. These studies by Stent and by Doermann constitute the best existing evidence that the genetic structures are associated with the phage DNA.

The Mechanism of Phage Replication.

Several years ago Luria (27) designed an important and ingenious experiment bearing on the mechanism of vegetative phage replication when he studied the distribution of spontaneous mutants in an infected cell population. Analyzing individual cell bursts for the number of mutant phage particles, he found that a few cells contained many copies of the mutant; a fair number had two, three, or four, but most of them had only one. Scoring a large number of experiments showed that the individual clones fell into an exponential distribution. This is strong evidence that daughter units replicate, and it excludes the notion that only the parent serves as a template. The above geometric increase refers only to the genetic units and not to the infectious phage.

Hershey (18) showed that precursor DNA forms sooner than does the precursor protein, whence he concluded that the nucleic acid is probably not formed inside a protein membrane. For some puzzling reason the rate of formation of DNA in these experiments was linear, not exponential. Perhaps a study of the rate of appearance of P^{32}-labeled 5-hydroxymethylcytidilic acid in the DNA of infected synchronized cells would yield a different result.

Some years ago several laboratories (17, 28) found from the use of phosphorus-labeled phage that each cycle of progeny phage received only 30 to 50 per cent of the label from the preceding parent. This was interpreted as meaning that the P^{32} from the parent is distributed randomly in the progeny DNA and not in a specific fraction, for if it were the latter, each succeeding generation would get the same quantity of specific material, not the same percentage. However, Hershey (19) has recently suggested that the failure to transfer 100 per cent is a reflection of the inefficiencies of the many separate steps, and he now proposes that all the DNA is genetically potent. Hershey (21) also studied the transfer of C^{14}-labeled parental DNA to progeny in the presence of excess unlabeled bases. Since the transfer from the parent was equal for all four bases and was not affected by the competing cold bases, Hershey has concluded that the pieces transferred must be large.

Stent and Jerne (36), examining the effect of P³² decay on the infectivity of the progeny, have determined the number of progeny receiving the parental label. They conclude that it is no less than 8 and no more than 25. Interest in this work is based on the assumption that a transfer of label is equivalent to a transfer of nucleic acid. Since single cells produce many more than 25 phage particles, the results of these workers mean that a parental contribution is not required for all phage units. Stent will undoubtedly have much to add to this.

In the P³² suicide studies Stent (34, 34a) made another observation of considerable interest in regard to the mechanism of replication. Using labeled bacteria infected with labeled phage in labeled medium, he found that the bacteria reach a point in their development where the infectivity becomes resistant to nuclear decay. This suggests, of course, that the size of the unit carrying the information has been sharply reduced or that the information has been passed on to some non-phosphorus-containing unit—although other interpretations are also possible.

Finally, Hershey (18) has recently pointed out in a very clear discussion that certain results from his own laboratory as well as those of others (3, 38) suggest that in T_2 phage formation, protein synthesis appears to be a necessary early step to nucleic acid synthesis. Two explanations have been offered. One is that the information in the germinal substance is passed on to another system, e.g., protein, PNA, or both, before there is replication of DNA. Perhaps the enzyme systems needed to form the phage-specific pyrimidine, 5-hydroxymethyl-cytosine, and its glucosidic derivatives (24a, 33, 39) must be produced first, after which the pyrimidine, etc., can be formed and incorporated into phage DNA. Hershey (18) finds it difficult to reconcile this interpretation with the Watson-Crick (41) model of DNA and offers the alternative explanation that phage infection produces a metabolic block which is relieved by the synthesis of protein. Critical to these two explanations is the relationship of the protein synthesized to the genetic units of the phage. If the relationship is close, the DNA may be responsible for formation of the new protein. If there is no direct relationship, Hershey's alternative explanation would gain support. In this connection it may be recalled that all genetic units are bifunctional in that they initiate one or more series of biochemical reactions *in addition to* replicating themselves. The unusual feature of the early protein synthesis, then, is that it represents a case in which one of the other functions is a prerequisite to replication.

SUMMARY

Rescue of genetic determinants following P^{32} decay or ultraviolet inactivation and the relationship of inactivation in linked and unlinked determinants provide the best evidence that genetic information is carried by the DNA fraction of the T-even coli phages.

The mechanism of replication continues to be somewhat elusive, although Luria's analysis of the distribution of spontaneous mutants favors a geometric process.

REFERENCES

1. Anderson, T. F., *Bot. Revs.,* **15**, 464 (1949).
2. Anderson, T. F., *Am. Naturalist,* **86**, 91 (1952).
3. Burton, K., *Biochem. J.,* **62**, 41P (1956).
4. Cohen, S. S., *J. Biol. Chem.,* **174**, 295 (1948).
5. Doermann, A. H., *Carnegie Inst. Wash. Year Book,* **47**, 176 (1948).
6. Doermann, A. H., *J. Gen. Physiol.,* **35**, 645 (1952).
7. Doermann, A. H., Chase, M., and Stahl, F. W., *J. Cell. Comp. Physiol.,* **45** (Suppl. 2), 51 (1955).
8. Doermann, A. H., and Dissosway, C. F. R., *Carnegie Inst. Wash. Year Book,* **48**, 170 (1949).
9. Dulbecco, R., *J. Bacteriol.,* **63**, 209 (1952).
10. Fraenkel-Conrat, H., and Williams, R. C., this volume.
11. French, R. C., Graham, A. F., Lesley, S. M., and vanRooyen, C. E., *J. Bacteriol.,* **64**, 597 (1952).
12. Herriott, R. M., *J. Gen. Physiol.,* **34**, 761 (1951).
13. Herriott, R. M., *J. Bacteriol.* **61**, 752 (1951).
14. Herriott, R. M., and Barlow, J. L., *J. Gen. Physiol.,* **36**, 17 (1952).
15. Hershey, A. D., *J. Gen. Physiol.,* **37**, 1 (1953).
16. Hershey, A. D., *Virology,* **1**, 108 (1955).
17. Hershey, A. D., in *Currents in Biochemical Research* (D. E. Green, ed.), Vol. II, p. 600. Interscience Press, New York (1955).
18. Hershey, A. D., *Brookhaven Symposia in Biol.,* **8** (Mutation), 6 (1956).
19. Hershey, A. D., *Cold Spring Harbor Symposia Quant. Biol.,* **20**, in press.
20. Hershey, A. D., and Chase, M., *J. Gen. Physiol.,* **36**, 39 (1952).
21. Hershey, A. D., Garen, A., Frazer, D. K., Hudis, J. D., *Carnegie Inst. Wash. Year Book,* **53**, 210 (1954).
22. Hershey, A. D., Kamen, M. D., Kennedy, J. W., and Gest, H., *J. Gen. Physiol.,* **34**, 305 (1951).
23. Hershey, A. D., and Rotman, R., *Genetics,* **39**, 169 (1954).
24. Hotchkiss, R. D., in *The Nucleic Acids* (E. Chargaff and J. P. Davidson, eds.), Vol. II, p. 435, Academic Press, New York .(1955).
24a. Jesaitis, M., and Goebel, W. F., *Cold Spring Harbor Symposia Quant. Biol.,* **18**, 205 (1953).
25. Lehman, I. R., and Herriott, R. M., *Federation Proc.,* **13**, 827 (1954).

26. Levinthal, C., and Visconti, N., *Genetics,* **38**, 500 (1953).
27. Luria, S. E., *Cold Spring Harbor Symposia Quant. Biol.,* **16**, 463 (1951).
28. Maaløe, O., and Watson, J. D., *Proc. Natl. Acad. Sci. U. S.,* **37**, 507 (1951).
29. Manson, L. A., *J. Bacteriol.,* **66**, 703 (1953).
30. Northrop, J. H., *J. Gen. Physiol.,* **34**, 715 (1951).
31. Putnam, F. W., and Kozloff, L., *J. Biol. Chem.,* **182**, 243 (1950).
32. Sher, I. H., and Mallette, M. F., *Arch. Biochem. and Biophys.,* **52**, 331 (1954).
33. Sinsheimer, R. L., *Science,* **120**, 551 (1954).
33a. Stahl, F. W., *Virology,* **2**, 206 (1956).
34. Stent, G. S., *Proc. Natl. Acad. Sci. U. S.,* **39**, 1234 (1953).
34a. Stent, G. S., *J. Gen. Physiol.,* **38**, 853 (1955).
35. Stent, G. S., and Fuerst, C. R., *J. Gen. Physiol.,* **38**, 441 (1955).
36. Stent, G. S., and Jerne, N. K., *Proc. Natl. Acad. Sci. U. S.,* **41**, 704 (1955).
37. Taylor, A. R., *J. Biol. Chem.,* **165**, 271 (1946).
38. Tomizawa, J., and Sunakawa, S., *J. Gen. Physiol.,* **39**, 553 (1956).
39. Volkin, E., *J. Am. Chem. Soc.,* **76**, 5892 (1954).
40. Volkin, E., and Astrachan, L., *Virology,* **2**, 149 (1956).
41. Watson, J. D., and Crick, F. H. C., *Cold Spring Harbor Symposia Quant. Biol.,* **18**, 123 (1953).
42. Wright, S., *Physiol. Revs.,* **21**, 487 (1941).
43. Wyatt, G. R., and Cohen, S. S., *Biochem. J.,* **55**, 774 (1953).
44. Zamenhof, S., this volume.

TRANSDUCTION: A COMPARATIVE REVIEW

PHILIP E. HARTMAN*

Leonard Wood Memorial, Department of Bacteriology and Immunology, Harvard Medical School, Boston 15, Massachusetts

THE TERM *transduction* was introduced concurrently with a description of a new type of genetic transfer in bacteria (218, 335). From the beginning, Lederberg has placed a broad interpretation upon the term, viz., to include any process "which differs from sex by the fragmentary nature of the unit of exchange" (227). A number of different systems of hereditary transfer in bacteria thus may be described as transduction under this generic definition. However, it is useful to have a term which will apply to the particular type of genetic transfer first noted by Zinder and Lederberg (335). Therefore, in this review, *transduction will refer only to those processes in which a fragment of the host nuclear genome, other than the genetic material specific for the transmitting phage itself, is carried by bacteriophage particles from one bacterial cell to another.*

In the following sections we will examine, individually, some characteristics of processes underlying genetic transfer in bacteria, at the same time defining and classifying these mechanisms in so far as the data available will allow. Following this descriptive phase, the mechanics and nature of each step in the process of transduction will be reviewed and compared with information obtained from other bacterial systems. Finally, we will outline our current understanding of the genetic structure of bacteria as derived from these multiple approaches.

I. PROCESSES LEADING TO GENETIC RECOMBINATION IN BACTERIA

A. *Mediated by free DNA[1]: Transformation*

We will confine our use of the term *transformation* to those systems in which cell-free and phage-free deoxyribonuclease-sensitive material

---

* Present address: Université Libre de Bruxelles, Auderghem-Brussels, Belgium. During the preparation of this review the author was a Public Health Service Research Fellow of the National Cancer Institute.

[1] All abbreviations and symbols used in this paper are listed in the legend to Fig. 4.

(i.e., DNA), genetically representative of the cell from which it was extracted, is used to transfer genetic characters to recipient bacteria. Data and concepts relating to bacterial transformations have been thoroughly reviewed elsewhere (180, 181, 331), and at this symposium by some of the most active participants in this area of research. Therefore, in the ensuing discussion, only certain specific aspects of the problem pertaining to matters connected or contrasting with transduction will be mentioned.

B. *Phage-mediated genetic transfer*

1. Transduction

a. *Transductions involving many loci which, collectively, encompass a large portion of the bacterial genome.*

The classic paper of Zinder and Lederberg (335) introduced the concept of phage-mediated genetic transfer in *Salmonella typhimurium*. These workers found that bacteriophage lysates contained a filterable agent, inseparable from phage particles, which upon infection of recipient bacteria could confer on them specific genetic characters of the donor bacteria (i.e., of the host cells upon which the phage was last grown). Zinder (335, 333, 334) has reviewed the extensive evidence relating to the identity of phage particles as agents of transduction.

A variety of mutant markers was utilized in the study (e.g., amino acid requirements, fermentative abilities, streptomycin resistance, and serological specificity of flagellar antigens). Although a single lysate was able to transduce a number of different genetic markers in a culture of recipient bacteria, no more than one marker was donated to a single bacterium (335). For a particular marker, one transduction was obtained for approximately 10^6 phage particles. The multipotency of the phage lysate and general independence of transductions for unrelated markers has been demonstrated repeatedly in *Salmonella* (230, 11, 13, 14, 188, 89, 208, 334, 288, 161). Several cases of presumed multiple transduction (21) upon reanalysis have been shown to involve a single genetic determinant at a time, in harmony with the studies cited above (Plough, in discussion to 334).

Several exceptional cases of multiple (joint or linked) transduction have been described for *Salmonella*. Stocker et al. (298) and Kauffmann (208) found that a locus controlling the production of flagella could be simultaneously transduced with that controlling the specificity of a flagellar antigen. Demerec and coworkers (75, 76, 78, 79, 81-84,

161, 329, and unpub.) found that phage prepared from certain mutants produced dual or linked transduction with markers of other mutants exhibiting the same general phenotype (e.g., tryptophan requirement). Otherwise, with one exception (78, 82), transductions were independent.

All known and presumed one-step mutants in *Salmonella* have proven transducible except in *S. typhimurium,* strain LT-2. In this strain markers for resistance to streptomycin, polymyxin, and azide (cited in 42) and a particular adenine marker (329) appear to be non-transducible, even under conditions allowing for phenomic lag. Streptomycin resistance has proved transducible in other strains of *Salmonella* (335, 288, 11, 13).

Lysogenizing phage is generally used for transduction, but clear plaque-forming mutants of these temperate phages may also be used to transduce genetic factors into lysogenic bacteria (334, 324). Not all temperate phages derived from *Salmonella* cultures are capable of demonstrable transduction activity (e.g., 308), but a considerable proportion of them are (e.g., 89, 290). This is in contrast to temperate phages of *Escherichia coli,* where most phage strains appear incapable of this type of transducing (cf. 193). However, two transducing phages have been obtained for *E. coli* (236, 193). These two independently isolated phages are related serologically and produce cross-immunity (193). Lennox found that Pl phage could transduce a number of markers in several *E. coli* strains as well as between *Shigella* and *E. coli* cultures. Several instances were found of joint transduction when markers known by other tests to be closely linked were tested; markers previously indicated as further apart on the chromosome were singly transduced. In addition, Lennox (236) and Jacob (193) found that the gene locus controlling the potentiality for production of lambda phage could be transduced by joint transduction with markers involved in galactose utilization.

Phage with a generalized transducing activity is most commonly prepared by lytic passage through sensitive cells. It is not entirely clear whether phage released from spontaneous or induced lysis of lysogenic cells can carry out this function. Although positive results are suggested (cf. 335, 188, 288), the presence of phage derived from the lysis of sensitive cells in the donor population was not ruled out. The prophage PLT-22-*S. typhimurium* system is weakly inducible, but the ultraviolet dose is critical (cf. 142). It thus is difficult to prepare high titer lysates from these lysogenic bacteria for use in transduction.

Presumed and known recessive traits may be transduced to recipient bacteria, singly or by linkage with other nearby markers (335, 236, 82, 161, 329). Furthermore, the progeny of transduced bacteria exhibit a stable heredity for other mutually exclusive alleles (e.g., 230).

Figs. 1A and 1B schematically illustrate the process of transduction as outlined above and as interpreted further in sections II through IV of this review.

b. *Abortive transduction.*

In the transduction of non-motile cells to motility, the progeny following some transductions form stably motile clones which spread through soft agar ("swarms"). However, Stocker et al. (298) also noted a second type of effect, namely, the production of a variable number of colonies, composed of non-motile cells but separated from the parent streak and appearing as a line of colonies in the agar ("trail phenomenon"). "Trails" appeared about ten times more frequently than "swarms." Only one "trail" could be determined as arising from a single transduction. "Trails" were never branched. "Swarms" never arose from "trails."

Single motile cells have been recovered by micromanipulation from the most distant colony of a "trail" and by transducing non-motile cells in a hanging drop culture and, in a second, originally bacteria-free drop joined to the first, picking up motile cells (296, 227, 232). The motile cells isolated by these procedures present the mode of inheritance depicted in Fig. 2.

The *inherited capacity for the production of motility-conferring organelles* passes along a single cell line. The other daughter cell, formed at each division, may be *phenotypically* motile; it possesses motility-conferring particles which we will here presume to be flagella. The flagellum remains active in the absence of the genetic determiner necessary for its production. Once there is but one flagellum per bacterium, at subsequent fissions this flagellum will be passed on unilinearly to but one of the two progeny ("unilinear transmission," 297).

The line of genetically altered cells thus segregates "semiclones" of weakly motile phenocopies. The stronger motility of the abortively transduced bacterium enables it to move and segregate weakly motile phenocopies and non-motile progeny which are immobilized at new sites in the agar; these are the colonies comprising the "trails."

An analogous phenomenon has been described by Ozeki (271) for transduction of purine loci in *Salmonella*. For technical reasons his

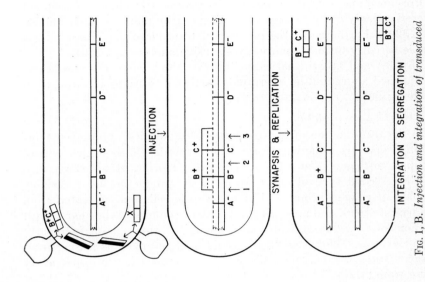

Fig. 1, B. *Injection and integration of transduced genetic material into the recipient cell*

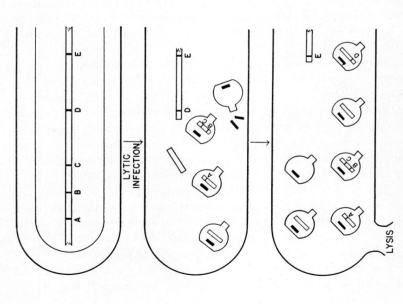

Fig. 1, A. *Incorporation of genetic fragments of the donor bacterial cell into transducing phage*

1, A. The upper part of the figure shows one end of a bacterial cell containing one haploid nucleus within which there is a portion of a single chromosome marked at several gene loci (A–E). Following infection by temperate phage, appropriate sensitive cells may be lysogenized or they may lyse. During the lytic response, the phage genome is replicated (black rods) and incorporated into maturing phage particles. Also during this period, there is a progressive breakdown of the host chromosome. Small fragments of this host genetic material also may be incorporated into phage particles. In the figure this incorporation is depicted as occurring more or less at random and supplementary to incorporation of the phage genome.

It is assumed that the ends of the bacterial chromosomal fragments, in a culture of infected bacteria, will be distributed at random within the short region of the chromosome depicted. A single, small piece is incorporated into any given phage particle. Gene loci will be separated and incorporated into independent phage particles (a) if they are not closely linked (e.g., A & C, A & D, A & E, B & D, B & E, etc.), or (b) if they are closely linked but are separated by a break. In the example shown, B and C are incorporated in a single particle and A and B are separated by a break. But in other cells of the same culture the break may occur between B and C, thus allowing A and B to be incorporated together in one particle while C is separately incorporated into a different particle.

Not all of the phage particles may contain chromosomal fragments nor may all fragments be incorporated before lysis of the cell occurs (e.g., gene locus E). However, loci homologous to E may be incorporated into phage arising from other cells in the population.

1, B. The phage adsorbs to the surface of, and releases its contents into, the recipient bacterium. The phage-specific genetic material (black-and-white rods) and the transduced fragment become separated. If the infection is lytic, the transduced fragment is lost to genetic analysis. If the response is non-lytic (lysogenization or abortive infection), the recipient cell will form a clone which can be analyzed.

Since transduction of single markers occurs with very low frequency and the piece carried by the phage is small when compared with the total host genome, multiple infection does not influence linkage determinations. In the example shown, the recipient bacterium is mutant at five loci (A through E). Most transducing phage particles will carry markers for loci not being examined (e.g., locus X). Also, the chances are negligible of one bacterium adsorbing two independent phage particles, one containing B^+ and the other containing C^+.

The incoming piece synapses with the homologous portion of the host chromosome and undergoes replication when the chromosome is replicated. Crossing over may take place at regions 1, 2, or 3. Two crossovers are required to insert the fragment in the chromosome, except in terminal segments, without causing a deletion of the outer chromosomal segment. If crossing over takes place randomly along the duplicated piece, the opportunity for crossovers between B and C will depend upon the closeness of their positions on the piece (i.e., on the bacterial chromosome). This relative proximity will also presumably play a role in their chances of being incorporated together originally and places a definite limit to the length of the chromosome which can be detected as linked to a single marker (See Fig. 1, A).

In the example shown, crossovers in regions 1 and 2 have occurred, resulting in the integration of B^+ only. In other recipients the events could occur at regions 1 and 3 or at 2 and 3.

A segregation lag for recessives will ensue until the new genotype is separated by cell division from the other nuclei of the cell and from the original chromosome depicted here. The fate of the remaining fragments (bottom cell in figure) is unknown.

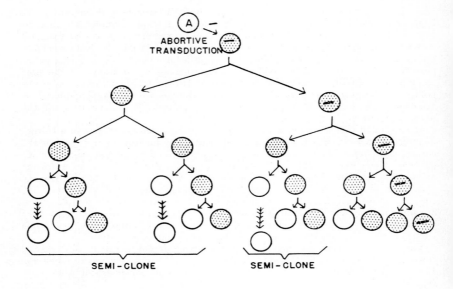

FIG. 2. *Abortive transduction and motility*

The non-motile cell, A, upon infection with transducing phage gains a genetic fragment (black rod) which endows the cell with motility. This property is hereditarily carried only along a single cell line (shaded cells containing black rods); only one of the daughter cells at each division (and, thus, at any one time in the life of the culture) retains the inherited capacity to synthesize motility-conferring particles. This is termed unilinear inheritance. The other daughter cell, formed at each division of the genetically altered cell, is also phenotypically motile. This cell, or sometimes several of its initial progeny (shaded cells), unilinearly transmits the motile phenotype to some of its progeny. "Semi-clones" of phenotypically motile cells (shaded cells) are present in clones derived after each division of the genetically altered bacterium. The non-motile segregants (clear cells) and all of their progeny remain non-motile.

analysis is indirect. Ozeki noted that treatment of certain purine mutants with phage prepared on cells which were wild-type at the given locus produced on certain media large, stably transduced wild-type colonies. After more prolonged incubation, additional small colonies appeared. When a small colony was restreaked on the same or on fresh medium, it again produced no more than one small colony. By this and similar indirect procedures, a unilinear mode of inheritance was demonstrable (271).

c. *Prophage-linked transductions.*

E. coli strain K12 carries the hereditary potential to produce a temperate bacteriophage, lambda (216). This system is inducible by a number of agents (316, 191, 20, 246, 328, 209, 95, 31a, 148, 254). Since sensitive derivatives of K12 are also available (e.g., 216), high-titer phage lysates may readily be prepared either from lysogenic cells or by lytic passage.

The locus, *lyλ*, is the chromosomal site which determines not only maintenance of the lysogenic state for λ phage but also the precise genetic constitution of the phage produced (6, 7, 236, 193). Sexual recombination studies and transductions with unrelated phage have shown that the *lyλ* locus is closely linked to a cluster of galactose markers (see section VI-A; Fig. 4). Although other prophages may presumably occupy a primary and several secondary chromosomal sites (28), the prophage of lambda appears to be specific for the *lyλ* locus (216, 214, 118, others).

Lambda-lysogenic strains can be made to carry a second complementary prophage: (a) after superinfection of lysogenic bacteria with an appropriate lambda mutant (7); (b) after mixed infection of sensitive bacteria with genetically marked phage (193); or (c) after transduction of *lyλ* into lysogenic bacteria, achieved with unrelated phage (193). When a second lambda prophage is introduced by joint transduction with galactose loci, in all cases the galactose marker remains stable and never demonstrably diploid. In about two-thirds of these joint transductions, the transduced lambda prophage also stably replaces its homologue; however, in the remaining third of the cases, *lyλ* is recovered in the diploid condition (193). In doubly lysogenic strains, both lambda prophages are linked to galactose (7).

The doubly lysogenic state is perpetuated in an unstable fashion. Progeny include the original double lysogenic types recombinant for various λ markers or homozygous for some markers originally heterozygous, as well as clones in which only the original prophage remains (8, 193).

Lysogenization with lambda thus usually results in a stable change only at the *lyλ* locus; this locus sometimes exists in a state resembling diploidy, whereas the remainder of the genome remains haploid and unaltered genetically. This propensity for diploidization of the *lyλ* locus is carried through even to linked transduction with nearby markers, which often are dissociable and stably incorporated.

Morse and coworkers (257-259a) found that lambda phage prepared by *lytic* infection did not transduce any genetic traits to receptive bacteria (also see 216). However, one transduction per 10^6-10^7 phage particles could be achieved with lambda prepared from *induced lysogenic* bacteria. The only markers transduced were the galactose markers closely linked with *ly*λ. The specific genetic character of the *gal*² marker transduced was that of the bacteria from which the lambda was obtained.

About one-third of the transduction clones were stable. The other two-thirds of the clones were unstable, segregating about once per thousand divisions. This instability indicated that the transduced marker was not replaced in the genome but, rather, that the bacterial chromosome was heterozygous for a small region. Most often this region was propagated as such. However, it was sometimes reduced with the segregation of haploid clones: (a) most frequently carrying the *gal* markers of the original recipient bacterium; (b) carrying the markers of the transduced fragment; or (c) least frequently (about 1%) carrying a type recombinant for *gal* markers. Other bacteria (about 6% of the total "segregants") were persistent diploids which had become homozygous for the originally heterozygous *gal* marker (259a).

The heterozygosity most often included only the *gal* loci, that is, segregant clones from single sensitive recipients were either all lysogenic (259) or immune (259a). Immune recipients most frequently remained immune, but about 12 per cent of the immune recipients segregated pure for lysogenicity following transduction (259). One example was found where heterozygosity apparently extended over both the *gal* and *ly*λ loci; this heterozygote, derived from an immune recipient, segregated both for *ly*λ and for *gal* (259).

Although the phage yield was low, lysates obtained by induction of these partial heterozygotes ("heterogenotes") produced a high proportion (approaching 100%) of galactose-transducing particles (259, 259a). These phage particles preferentially incorporate the markers of the fragment rather than those of the parental chromosome (259a).

Some aspects of the lambda-galactose transductions are schematically illustrated in Fig. 3.

2. Lysogenization and characters associated with the lysogenic state

As indicated by the preceding discussion, the prophage may be considered as a portion of the *bacterial* genome. It is obvious that lysogenization thus may be taken as a form of genetic transfer akin to trans-

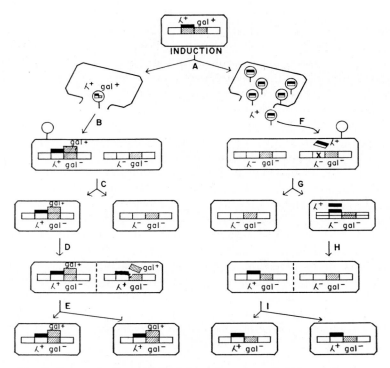

Fig. 3. *Lysogenization with lambda and prophage-linked transductions*

The prophage of lambda phage (λ^+) resides at a chromosomal site closely linked to several galactose loci. When a culture of lambda lysogenic *E. coli* K12 bacteria is induced (A), a considerable number of particles of lambda phage are released upon lysis of the cell. When these phage particles infect sensitive (λ^-) bacteria (F), the phage is reduced to prophage; in this process its genetic material synapses with a region of the bacterial chromosome (G) and the genetic information is incorporated into the replicating bacterial genome (H) at the site specific for the lambda prophage. The prophage is then duplicated and transmitted to bacterial progeny along with the rest of the bacterial chromosome (I). No other genetic characters of the bacterial genome are altered. Some sensitive bacteria may segregate from the infected cell (G and after H) due to the multinucleate nature of the recipient bacterium and, perhaps, to the mode of genetic integration.

An occasional lambda particle (B) may bring into a sensitive cell not only material genetically specific for the phage but, also, some bacterial markers closely linked to the prophage locus. This material *(gal⁺)* synapses with the homologous portion of the recipient genome and may be stably integrated in a manner analogous to that shown in Fig. 1, B. However, in many cases it is perpetuated in the diploid state (D and E). Occasionally, the fragment may be lost from the cell (D), so returning the bacterium to its original haploid condition, except that it is now lysogenic.

duction (also see 259a). However, the special properties of the bacteriophage genome and its level of independent existence are such that lysogenization should be considered separately. F. Jacob is to discuss some aspects of this problem in the present symposium. Therefore I shall here confine the discussion to portions of this subject which influence our concepts of transduction or which at first analysis may be confused with transduction.

It appears that the presence in the genome of prophage not only endows the bacterium with a hereditary capacity for the production of a specific bacteriophage (or abortive development of material related to the bacteriophage), but it also exerts a continuous influence on the metabolism of the host cell, an influence detectable in various cases by diverse means. These alterations in the physiology of the host depend upon the precise genetic constitution of the prophage, as well as the residual genotype of the host in which it resides. Possibly because of its protective advantage for the specific prophage in nature and the sensitivity of its detection, coupled with an early appreciation of its existence, the most commonly found expression of this altered metabolism lies in the phenomenon of immunity to homologous phage. The effects of the prophage are lost by the cells when the prophage, or that portion of its genetic constitution involved in the effect, is lost from the cell.

In engendering immunity and other properties in the lysogenic cell, the action of prophage may be thought of as that of a modifying gene(s) as well as an independent functional group of genetic units. In turn, it is reasonable to assume that the bacterial genome might modify or limit some potential functions of the prophage genome. The bacterial genome might also exert its influence indirectly on the biochemical processes leading to phage maturation and, consequently, on the phenotype of progeny phage.

At first sight, these interactions may be mistaken for transductions, especially for prophage-linked transductions. They are separable only in so far as one is able experimentally to manipulate the separation of the genetic material specific to the phage from other constituents of the genome of the cell in which it resides.

a. *Immunity.* The presence of prophage confers upon the cell an immunity to homologous phage (reviewed in **246**). In many cases, the homologous phage penetrates the cell but is not reduced to prophage and does not undergo replication; the genetic material of the superinfecting phage persists in the cells and is passed to daughter cells, being gradually "diluted out" during growth of the culture (197, 25, 27). In still other cases, homologous phage is not readsorbed to lysogenic cells (43, 37, 36). The receptor for phage adsorption may be absent or, since the change so rapidly follows lysogenization (43), may be present in masked (e.g., 268) form. The means whereby immunity is obtained and ultimately manifested by the lysogenic cell are thus multiple.

Most studies on immunity have been concerned with related phages which differ in but a few specifically selected genetic characters. For these very closely related phages, the prophages may be considered as homologous with respect to the ability to confer immunity and, indeed, exert a gene dosage effect with respect to the level of immunity attained (26). More distantly related phages may also show cross-immunity (cf. 193). However, the data of Groman and Eaton (156) indicate that several more distantly related phages which may undergo genetic recombination do not develop cross-immunity in certain instances. This indicates that the immunity-conferring mechanism may not be due to the presence of a certain prophage but, rather, is an effect exerted by a particular locus, or larger portion, of the phage genome (also see data in 35, 93).

b. *Conversion.* In addition to conferring immunity to homologous phages, the presence of a specific prophage genome in many instances exerts a continuous detectable influence on other phenotypic properties of the host bacterium. The acquisition, by *lysogenization,* of these inherited properties is termed conversion.

The response of the lysogenic culture to certain heterologous phages may be different from that of the parallel non-lysogenic culture. Thus, the lysogenic bacteria may be resistant to the lytic action of a second phage (320, 18, 24, 247, S. Lederberg cited in 247) but not to its host-range mutants (e.g., 4 and previous work cited therein). Lysogenization by a second unrelated phage may be prevented (25, 117). The plaque morphology obtained after heterologous infection with a lytic phage may be altered (18). Lysogenic strains carrying several dissimilar prophages may yield bursts composed of homologous phage only (22, 25). The resistance to a second phage is not a characteristic of the presence of a specific prophage alone, since the prophage may be effective in this respect in one bacterial strain and not in certain derivatives of it or in another strain. Resistance patterns differ in different bacterial strains; and the precise genotype and phenotype of the superinfecting heterologous phage also play a role (S. Lederberg, cited in 247; 317; also see data in 4, 93). The resistance may be due to failure of adsorption (cf. 36) or to some later step in the infectious process (e.g., 317) in which the cell may either be killed or survive, as in immunity. Other effects have been noted by Boyd (337).

Iseki and Sakai (186, 187, 285, 284, 185a) discovered that certain *Salmonella* strains producing the somatic antigens 3,10 could be converted to produce the antigens 3,15 by lysogenization with phage from 3,15-producing bacteria (also see 270, 141). The conversion can also be effected by lysogenization with the particular phages grown on bacteria producing antigens 3,10 (308, 285). By lysogenization with these same phages, bacteria producing somatic antigens 1,3,19 can be converted to produce 1,3,15,19 (188a, 185a).

In addition to the converted cells, non-lysogenic phage-resistant mutants can be obtained from the 3,10-producing bacteria; these resistant mutants appear to possess neither antigen 10 nor 15 (270, 141). The conversion of somatic antigens could explain (a) instances of immunity and instances of resistance to certain heterologous phages where adsorption appears impaired (43, 37, 36), (b) unique antigenic homologies of diverse strains resistant to, but nevertheless still active in the adsorption of, particular phages (e.g., 238, 239), and (c) simultaneous acquisition of resistance to one phage and of sensitivity to another (286).

The opposite antigenic change, i.e., from somatic antigen 15 to 10, can be procured by treatment of 15-producing cells with anti-15 antibody. Since the antibody is prepared against lysogenic cells, it has been suggested that the "conversion" attributed to antibody actually may be due to inactivation of free phage and selection of non-15-producing, non-lysogenic bacteria (308). Indeed, this has been experimentally indicated (188, 188a). Other antigenic alterations, previously reported to be induced by treatment with antisera, may be due to contamination with phage or to effects such as those noted above. Recently, it has been reported that lysogenization with a different phage influences the production of somatic antigen 1 by *Salmonella* (185a-b).

Certain non-toxigenic strains of *Corynebacterium diphtheriae* acquire the ability to produce toxin when infected with particular phages from certain toxigenic strains (137, 138, 276, 277, 175, 177). The conversion to toxigenicity has been shown to be a result of lysogenization with particular phages rather than to selection of preexistent bacterial mutants, lytic action of the phage, etc. (153, 154, 155, 10, 165). Loss of lysogenicity results in loss of toxin production (155). The ability to convert to toxigenicity appears as a discrete genetic character, or characters, separable by recombination from other hereditary markers of the phage (156). The toxigenicity-conferring trait, analogous to other types of conversion noted above, is effective when in combination only with some bacterial strains (275, 178).

Lysogenic strains of *Bacillus megaterium* differ from the parental, nonlysogenic, sensitive bacteria in their colony morphology (91, 185) and growth requirements (90, 63). A similar relationship of colony morphology to the presence of prophage may also exist in *C. diphtheriae* (data in 176, 177). It is possible that Vi-type 1 *Salmonella* with ability to ferment *d*-tartrate may undergo a change with regard to this ability when lysogenized with certain phages (cf. observations in 267).

Further, the functioning of the phage genome in the lysogenized cell, analogous to conversion of other bacterial properties, may possibly effect a change in the bacterial physiology dealing with some aspect of bacterial metabolism utilized in vegetative reproduction of the phage. The phage in this case could be interpreted as affecting indirectly, through conversion, its own modification (see data in 92, 183).

C. *Mediated by Cell Conjugation*

1. Sexual recombination

The first definitive evidence for a coordinated recombination of genetic traits in bacteria stems from the observations of Lederberg and Tatum (233, 217, 303, reviewed in 234) on *E. coli*, strain K12. These, and an increasing number of other workers (see section VI), demonstrated that: (a) a wide variety of genetic traits could undergo recombination; (b) several markers could recombine as the result of a single event, i.e., a large portion of the genome can simultaneously participate in the recombinational event; (c) unselected markers exhibited particular degrees of association and segregation during the recombination process; thus (d) a certain linearity of loci could be derived from the recombination data; (e) recombinant clones usually were pure with regard to unselected markers; (f) recombination involved intimate cell contact; and (g) recombination was a rare event (one recombinant formed per 10^6 bacteria plated).

There were, however, difficulties in the construction of linkage maps based upon the recombination data in that, while some loci could be placed in unambiguous order, this order did not agree with results obtained in other crosses (including reciprocal crosses) or in the same cross when other selective markers were used. In spite of these mapping difficulties, some loci did show a high order of interaction, the anomalies arising mainly from interactions between these and other loci.

The aberrant recombination data are now known or proposed to be the result of several factors; often these complications may be superimposed, one upon the other.

Sexual recombination first involves a union of two cells (see section II). In terms of the subsequent mating process, the two parents are not identical (see section I-C-2). Suffice it to say here: (a) the genetic transfer is from the F^+ or Hfr parent to the F^- parent (i.e., transfer is unidirectional, see section III); (b) markers of the recipient parent predominate among those of the recombinants issuing from the cross; and (c) this "sexual polarity" of the cross is extremely important in analyses of linkage (229, 52, 169, 312, 50, 203, etc.).

An additional factor, and one early considered (see 234, 282) as underlying some of the linkage difficulties, is the possible presence in some of the genetically marked strains of complex chromosomal aberrations. Many of the widely used multiple mutants were obtained in several steps by repeated exposure to x-ray and ultraviolet-irradiation or to nitrogen mustard (cf. 302, 217). This explanation has been abandoned for some aberrant results now known to be due to other factors (229). It may still apply to some K12 derivatives, however (cf. 202, 203, 50).

The conditions of the experiment may bias the recombination values (66, also see 169) or influence the number of recombinants detected (cf. 250, 60). The temperature of incubation is important when a lysogenic donor parent is crossed with a sensitive recipient strain (see section V-A). The number of recombinant colonies on the assay plate and the responses to syntrophy of the parent strains also must be considered (205, 50). Treatment of F^- cells with ethylenediamine tetracetic acid greatly enhances the number of prototrophs obtained (339).

A further complication arises out of what appears to be a "breakage" point (point of rupture $= R$) on the chromosome of the donor parent; R tends to separate otherwise presumably closely linked markers (49, 50). Rupture points with similar properties may occur at a number of sites along the chromosome; different sites are involved in different derivatives from an F+ stock, the appearance of R occurring as a random mutation (202, 203). The rupture point of the donor bacterium leads to a high frequency of transfer of markers "proximal" to it (Hfr strain), thus lowering the *relative frequency of transfer* of distally located markers (203). In crosses involving Hfr donors, only a portion of the haploid complement is interpreted as transferred by most cells during conjugation (203). These interpretations provide that sexual recombination in *E. coli* K12 often may involve a process akin to transduction, except that the former process includes cell conjugation and thus obviates the necessity for an extracellular vector with a more limited genetic transfer capacity (202, 203).

Further complications may arise from postzygotic disturbances in chromosome pairing (e.g., 282, 50, 219) or outright elimination of specific chromosomal regions (e.g., 264, 219, see section V-B). The effects of these disturbances on the recombination process have just begun to be assessed (cf. 50).

Sexual recombination studies have been extended to additional strains of *E. coli* (48, 224, 234, 44, 300, 64-66, 241). Furthermore, Luria (cited in 236) has found that *Shigella dysenteriae* can undergo recombination with Hfr and F+ strains of *E. coli* K12.

Two preliminary notes on recombination between multiply marked mutants of *Pseudomonas* (243, 179) indicate involvement of a system of an order higher than that of transformation and transduction. In addition, S. Yaverbaum (1951, pers. commun.) in extensive tests noted the sporadic appearance of presumed recombinants between mutants of a *Bacillus megaterium* strain (also see 300). The results are of interest in relation to the cytological description of fusion tubules between cells of this strain (67, 70, 71) as well as the amenability of this comparatively large organism to light microscopic analysis (e.g., 72, 67, 68, 69, 31). However, plaques spontaneously form in aged cultures of this strain on complex media (P. Hartman, unpub.), suggestive of lysogenicity (cf. 91, 90). The types of recombinants obtained in successful experiments (see 300) are suggestive of a transduction-like process, perhaps analogous to the genetic transfer noted in *Bacillus* by Brown et al. (40). Forms resembling conjugating bacteria have been noted in other studies (e.g., 88, 319a) but have not been analyzed by genetic methods.

2. F— to F+

F— strains of *E. coli* K12 cannot undergo sexual recombination with one another and appear unable to mutate to a form which is capable of entering into recombination except with F+ strains, or derivatives thereof. F+ cultures are fertile in crosses either with F— strains or, at a lower frequency, with other F+ strains (229, 52, 168, 169).

Cavalli (45) and Hayes (168, 169) isolated from F+ cultures derivatives which showed a high frequency of recombination (Hfr) for some markers. Jacob and Wollman (202, 203) have shown that much of the fertility of F+ cultures is due to the presence in them of spontaneously arising Hfr mutants.

Hfr and some strains of F+ bacteria may be made *phenotypically* F— by strong aeration of the culture (229, 52, 168, 169). In contrast, *hereditarily* F— cells may be selected from the edges of swarms of motile F+ cultures plated on soft agar (Skaar, cited in 264) or by treatment of F+ cells with certain divalent cations (338).

Genetic transfer occurs from the F+ or Hfr donor parent to the F— recipient bacterium (see section III). Ingenious experiments by Jacob et al. (203) have shown that cell conjugation occurs with high frequency between strains of opposite mating type but that, ordinarily, only the F agent (presumably a short chromosomal fragment) passes from the F+ to the F— bacterium. This is the F+ "infection" noted in earlier studies (229, 52, 168, 169, 264). In Hfr strains, the F status of the cell, which now resides at the chromosomal site, *Hfr*, is transmitted with the same low background frequency as other genetic markers distal to it. The mutant locus, *Hfr*, can be recovered in the recombinant progeny derived from the F— cell through the use of appropriate selective markers. *Hfr* acts as a point of rupture ($R = Hfr$) in the chromosome of the donor parent (49, 50). While *Hfr* and markers distal to it are transferred with low frequency, proximally located loci are transferred with extremely high frequency (203).

The high frequency of transfer of the F factor is thus interpreted as comparable to transfer of other genetic elements during sexual recombination, though its precise role in the mechanism of the transfer remains obscure. Other genetic markers may follow the transfer of F+ to the F— recipient cell, but this supplementary transfer peculiarly occurs with very low frequency except in strains carrying an *Hfr* mutation. These interpretations can account for many observations on the K12 mating and recombination system, but further work is required to reconcile them with one observation in particular. Genetic crosses can be performed under conditions excluding infection with the F agent (264) or where transmission of F+ is very low (169). Nevertheless, a high proportion of recombinants are F+ regardless of the selective markers used in their isolation (229, 52, 168, 169) ; these recombinants are presumably derived from the originally F— parent.

F+ transmission and the F+ state of the bacteria are not associated with lysogenicity for lambda (229, 216). The F status of the cell does not affect its activity either as a donor or as a recipient in the transduction of a number of markers in the genome (236).

3. Bacteriocin production

Some bacteria possess the inherited capacity to synthesize specific substances which exert lethal effects on certain other, usually phylogenetically related, bacterial strains (151, 152). These substances (bacteriocins or colicins) differ from one another in their spectra of activity, their rapidity of diffusion on agar and ability to penetrate cellophane, morphology of zones of inhibition on sensitive cells, thermostability, sensitivity to proteolytic enzymes, and specificity in the selection of resistant bacterial variants (see 96, 102, 119, 53).

Many *E. coli* and *Shigella* strains produce bacteriocins (e.g., 158, 157a, 96, 216), but fewer strains have been detected as being lysogenic (216) ; the reverse is true for *Salmonella* strains (110). Bacteriocins are produced by bacteria other than the enterics (e.g., 96, 103, 160, 192, 190).

Some of the bacteriocins have been crudely identified as proteins or polypeptides (170, 159, 160a, 96, others). Recently, Goebel et al. (143) have characterized colicin K as a macromolecule composed of carbohydrate, protein, and lipid, bearing many of the properties of the somatic or 0 antigen of the bacillus.

The bacteriocins become adsorbed to specific receptors of sensitive cells and kill them but do not multiply in series as do bacteriophages on appropriate sensitive host cells (100, 112, 114, 119, 195; also see 246). In most cases the bacteriocin does not cause cell lysis (but see 330). Some of the bacteriocins become adsorbed to receptor complexes common to those utilized by phages (34, 34a, 97, 102, 108, 119, 135, 136), although the receptors may not be structurally identical to those concerned with phage adsorption (cf. 107). Fredericq (111, 114, 119) has compared the killing action of bacteriocins to that exerted by irradiation-inactivated phage and to abortive phage infection.

Colicin K adsorbs to the same receptor as phage T6 of bacteriophage group III (98, 119, 130). It is retained by cellophane and is as thermolabile as bacteriophage III (100). Its adsorption is inactivated by x-rays at the same rate as the adsorption of T6 (212). However, antiserum produced against T6 phage does not inactivate colicin K (113, 143), nor does anti-K serum cross-react with T6 (143). The activity of the colicin, but not that of the phage, is sensitive to treatment with proteases (101, 143).

A number of different bacteriocins may be produced by a single bacterial strain (cf. 96, 53). Similarly, some bacteriocin-producing strains are also lysogenic (29a, 99, 109, 124, 197). With bacteriocins and bacteriophages which utilize common receptors, no correlation was found between bacteria producing colicin K and phage III nor between colicin E and phage II, but there was a positive correlation in the production of colicin B and phage II (109). It should be noted that a negative correlation might be expected if the agents were similar in their basic nature and closely related enough to evidence cross-immunity (e.g., if there exists an intracellular "procolicin" equivalent to, let us say, a certain small segment of a prophage genome).

Like some strains carrying prophages, some bacteriocin-producing strains are inducible (194, 195, 196, 124, 192). Intracellular production of the bacteriocin starts almost immediately after induction, but the bacteriocin is not released into the medium until, after a latent period, mass lysis of the culture ensues. Fredericq (124, 128a) believes that such lysis does not occur unless induction of a prophage occurs concomitantly with the induction of the bacteriocin. In inducible strains which are both lysogenic and bacteriocinogenic, phage production and bacteriocin production show differing ultraviolet sensitivities for their induction (128a; Kaplan et al., cited in 197). Dilution of broth-grown *E. coli* K12 (λ) into synthetic medium following induction does not permit production of lambda (149, 278), but still allows production of a bacteriocin (128a).

The effects of lethal bacteriocin particles on the metabolism of sensitive cells (195, 196, 192) are in some respects similar to those exerted by nucleic-acid-free protein phage ghosts (171, 235, 139). Ghost preparations may contain two types of particles, killing and inhibiting (139, 32). Although some bacteriocin preparations appear to contain killing particles only, some aberrant titration effects have been noted, perhaps indicating a similar heterogeneity in some bacteriocin preparations (e.g., 134). The action of phage ghosts elicits a specific sequence of cytological changes in the sensitive organism (32). These changes differ from those engendered by intact phage (refer in 261). The action of bacteriocins has not been studied cytologically in a comparable system.

After adsorption of bacteriocins, bacteria do not produce bacteriophages to which they are otherwise sensitive (195, 107, 115). This failure in part may be a reflection of the deranged metabolism brought about upon adsorption of the bacteriocin, but it also appears to involve some specificity of action analogous to exclusion by one phage of an unrelated phage (116).

Ordinarily, the potential for bacteriocin production is a stable, inherited trait. The amount of bacteriocin actually elaborated depends upon environmental conditions (170, 159, 59, 144). In a standard environment, one may select variants producing different levels of bacteriocin (cf. 144).

On the other hand, a bacteriocin produced by a derivative of an *E. coli* strain was shown to have changed in its heat stability and antigenic properties but to have retained its host range, i.e., its specificity for adsorption sites or receptors (33). Also, a bacterial strain producing a specific bacteriocin may acquire the ability to release a second, distinct bacteriocin; these strains may be specifically selected for, since they are resistant to certain bacteriophages and to some bacteriocins unrelated to those which they produce (106, 108). Phage-resistant derivatives of colicinogenic strains generally conserve their ability to produce the original bacteriocin (104).

Some bacteriocin-producing strains retain the receptor for specific adsorption of the bacteriocin which they produce, but are now immune to its action (132, 121). Other strains are sensitive to the bacteriocin they produce (190, 283) but may mutate to a resistant form (283).

It has been known for some time that spontaneously occurring resistant mutants may be selected from predominantly sensitive bacterial cultures through the action of virulent, lytic phages (80, 244) or with temperate phages and clear plaque-forming mutants thereof (216). In many cases (for exceptions see discussion above on lysogenization), this resistance is due to the loss or masking of the specific receptor necessary for phage adsorption (e.g., 5, 30, 313, 314, 279, and others). Similarly, bacteria spontaneously (cf. 283) mutate to bacteriocin resistance. Since, as discussed above, some receptors for bacteriocins are common to those utilized by certain phages, either agent may be used for the selection. Just as resistance to phages by loss of adsorptive capacity has been utilized as a standard chromosomal marker in recombination studies (see section VI), so bacteriocin resistance is an inherited trait presumably caused by loss of a specific receptor due to a mutant allele which segregates like other chromosomal markers in recombination tests (129, 130, 119, 120, 204).

In contrast, the inherited *capacity for bacteriocin production* is transmitted to *all* recombinant progeny if the F⁻ parent is the active one and to a majority of the recombinants, independent of the selective markers used, if the F⁺ parent is the bacteriocin producer (131, 132, 120). Further, a high proportion of non-bacteriocinogenic bacteria may acquire the hereditary capacity to produce a specific bacteriocin. This inherited trait is acquired during mixed culture of the strain with certain strains (but not others) that produce the bacteriocin. No other genetic characters were observed to be exchanged in these mixed populations of *E. coli* strains or of *E. coli* and *Shigella sonnei* cultures (121, 126). The genetic transfer was found to occur independently of observable lysogenicity, making improbable a phage-mediated mechanism for the transfer (122, 126). The transfer is "not sensitive to proteases" (Fredericq, pers. commun.).

Transfer of the hereditary capacity for bacteriocin production is achieved only when F⁺ bacteria are mixed with another F⁺ or with an F⁻ strain, and not when two F⁻ strains are mixed (123). Although the F-status of the bacteria plays a role in the transfer, transfer of the bacteriocin-producing capacity of the bacteria is not necessarily accompanied by transfer in the F characteristic of F⁺ cells (as determined by ability to participate in transfer of other bacteriocinogenic properties) (123).

Fredericq (123) has reported that the genetic transfer can be achieved either from F⁺ to F⁻ bacteria, or in the reverse direction. Since the cultures were grown together for relatively long periods, the validity of the F⁻ to F⁺ transfer might be questioned. That the transfer most frequently goes from F⁺ to F⁻ bacteria is indicated by the discovery that bacteriocin production by one parent in some cases decreases fertility and that this effect is most pronounced if the F⁺ parent is the bacteriocinogenic strain (128b). This would be expected if the sensitive F⁻ strain, from which recombinants for chromosomal markers ordinarily arise, are killed by the bacteriocin before genetic transfer and immunity can ensue.

These various findings were originally interpreted by Fredericq as indicating a non-chromosomal inheritance of the potentiality for the production of a specific bacteriocin. The genetic transfer of these extra-chromosomal elements occurred by some unknown process involving intimate cell contact ("transduction"). However, in view of the recent results of Jacob et al. (203), it is equally possible that bacteriocino-genesis is controlled by chromosomal sites which are, like F+, trans-ferred with high frequency during the mating process. If such sites should be demonstrated, a unified picture of fundamentally similar elements could be evolved for genetic transfer during sexual recombina-tion. The existence of simultaneous mutation to phage resistance and bacteriocinogenesis may offer markers for an appropriate genetic analysis.

In addition to the need to elucidate the means of genetic transfer, more effort is required to determine the nature of bacteriocins and their relationship, if any, to bacteriophages and abortive bacteriophage development. The literature contains a large number of articles relat-ing to more or less specific microbial antagonisms (review in 94), as well as reports of "colicins" with strikingly wide spectra (e.g., 59). Also, the elaboration of additional, lytic substances has been reported as accompanying the production of bacteriocins and bacteriophages (287, 184, 272, 273; compare lysins reported in 5, 35, 330). Genetic analysis should provide a powerful tool in extending our knowledge of these substances and the means of their production, whether spon-taneous or induced.

II. Means of Transmission

The infective phage particle, of course, serves to transport its own genetic material from one cell to a new site of synthesis in a susceptible cell. Factors in which immunity and conversion reside are inseparable from lysogenization, that is, they appear as if elicited by factors of the phage genome in cooperation with the residual genome of the host (see section I-B-2).

The phage particle may also transport genetic material other than its own genome. As pointed out by Zinder and Lederberg (335), the phage may act as a more or less passive vector of bacterial hereditary determiners. Like phage infectivity, this genetic transduction is resist-ant to DNAase and is dependent upon phage adsorption (335, others). Extensive data confirm the identity of phage particles as agents in the genetic transfer, both for *Salmonella* transductions (333-335) and for transduction of galactose markers by lambda (259, 259a). We may note again here that, in contrast to conversion, the genetic specificity in transduction is that of the host upon which the phage was last grown.

Brown et al. (40) were able to inactivate with DNAase presumably phage-mediated genetic transfer in *Bacillus* cultures. A similar induced genetic change (transfer of motility), as well as alteration in capsule production, was earlier observed in *Bacillus* spp. and interpreted as a DNA-mediated transformation (252, but see 305). The active agent in the case investigated by Brown et al. (40) could possibly be host DNA, adsorbed to the outer surface of the phage particles (see 57). This externally located DNA might then penetrate the cell at the site of the lesion formed by phage adsorption and injection. It is unlikely that in these experiments (40) DNAase inactivated the genetic material once inside the recipient cells. Although DNAase has been reported as affecting morphology of bacterial growth (87), apparently this enzyme penetrates protoplasts of *Bacillus* spp. poorly, if at all (see 39).

While the phage acts as a vector in transduction, the complete process of transduction may be separated from that of lysogenization by a number of means: (a) the reproductive and lysogenizing capacity of phage is much more rapidly inactivated by radiation and P^{32} disintegration than is the ability of the phage suspension to carry out transduction (142, 304); (b) phage grown at temperatures lower than 37°C. are still infective but have decreased transducing abilities (Table 4 in 334); (c) some progeny comprising the transduction clone are non-lysogenic and sensitive (298, 334); (d) N. Zinder has obtained mutant strains of PLT-22 phage which produce a large proportion of non-lysogenic, sensitive cells in transduction clones (used in 329, 161); (e) lysogenic cells, although immune to the phage they carry, still may adsorb the phage and are transduced by it, though with a lower frequency than are parallel sensitive bacteria (334, 329); (f) a clear plaque type mutant of PLT-22 may transduce cells lysogenic for temperate phage (333, 324), and the transductional progeny remain lysogenic only for the phage originally present (333); (g) transduction occurs in bacterial recipients in which phage infection and lysogenization are abortive (333, 285); (h) PLT-22 phage can be host modified (reviewed in 245) by single passage on cells of *S. gallenarium*, so that only one cell per 10^5 in a culture of *S. typhimurium* yields phage (see 142); and nevertheless, transduction occurs "with about normal frequency" (Zinder, cited in **245**); (i) the phage may lose by mutation its ability to transduce without losing its lysogenizing ability (**334**); and (j) the incubation of recipient bacteria at low temperatures following phage adsorption decreases the number of transductions detected (Plough, pers. commun.; Hartman, unpub.).

In sexual recombination it has been assumed for some time that the transfer of genetic material involved pairing or mating of the bacterial cells proper (e.g., **217, 220, 234, 263**). Bacteria suspended in a common medium but separated by a sintered glass filter could not undergo recombination (**61**). Recently, Lederberg (**226, 227, 228**) has isolated pairs of bacteria actually found in the mating process, confirming his own earlier suspicions. Electron micrographs, made by Dr. T. F. Anderson, of similarly mating pairs were presented by Jacob et al. at the 1956 Cold Spring Harbor Symposium on Quantitative Biology (see **203**).

As mentioned earlier (sections I-C-2 and I-C-3), the F agent and the potentiality for bacteriocin production may also be transferred during cell conjugation. Efforts aimed at the detection of an alteration in the cell surface conducive to cell conjugation (**249**) have so far given negative results in this respect.

III. Unidirectional Nature of the Genetic Transfer

When free DNA is released from a disrupted bacterial cell and serves as transforming principle, it is obvious that the donor cell is destroyed and the genetic event (transformation) is achieved in a unidirectional fashion. Similarly, the donor cell is sacrificed when bacteriophage is prepared, sterilized, and becomes the infective carrier of its own heredity (for lysogenization and conversion or for lytic infection) and a more or less passive tender of foreign genetic elements (transducing fragments).

The incorporation of genetic fragments into multipotent transducing phage may vary during the intracellular growth of the phage. With phage obtained from prematurely lysed cells, the number of transductions obtained per phage (ratio T/P) depends upon the time when lysis is induced and on the environmental conditions (**334**). The T/P either rises or remains constant during the maturation period. The T/P presents "a family of curves bounded at one end by the appearance of mature phage and at the other by the termination of cell lysis. Within this range, some of the markers appear at a maximum by the end, and still others are just ascending when the experiment terminates" (334). The T/P's may reflect a progressive sequence in the breakdown of the host chromosome during phage growth prior to cell lysis (cf. Fig. 1a). Fragments are thence incorporated in a random fashion. An alternative hypothesis, advanced by Bertani (28), suggests that generalized transducing activity resides in "an ability of these phages to move (in a small fraction of the bacterial population) to many different sites scattered all over the genetic complement of the bacterium." Bertani's concept essentially makes all transductions prophage-linked.

In the prophage-linked transduction of galactose markers, transduction is obtained only with phage prepared from induced lysogenic cells, not with phage prepared by lytic infection (259). In the preparation of transducing phage with high activity from induced bacteria diploid for the galactose region, the markers of the small fragment, rather than those of the parental chromosome, usually appear in the phage; the phage yield is low (259, 259a). These and other findings suggest that the prophage-linked and the generalized types of transduction differ in basic mechanisms of incorporation into phage particles. In the former case, it is possible that the entire chromosomal fragment "matures" into an infective phage particle without prior replication of the phage genome *per se* (Fig. 3).

With respect to sexual recombination, the unidirectional nature of the genetic transfer has not always been so obvious as in the above cases. Hayes (166) noted that when one parent (the donor or F+ parent) was killed with streptomycin it could still participate in genetic recombination. These and related data (166-169) led to Hayes' proposal of a new mechanism for genetic recombination involving a unidirectional, partial transfer of genetic material from a donor strain to a recipient strain. Many similar findings relating to this fertility system (section I-C-2) were determined independently by the Lederbergs and Cavalli (229, 52). Lederberg (226-228) has isolated pairs of bacteria in the mating process. The laterally joined cells disjoin after an "hour or so" and, since both usually remain viable, form clones. Recombinants are found with very high frequency among the progeny of the F− cell, but no recombinants are recovered from the clone arising from Hfr parent. In addition, Skaar and Garen (289) showed that DNA-P^{32} is transferred only from Hfr to F− cells; no transfer was detected in the reverse direction.

IV. Composition of the Transferred Genetic Material

A. *Chemical composition*

Research over the past decade has consolidated the identification of transforming principle as DNA (180, 331). On the other hand, only indirect means are available for the chemical characterization of the genetic material transferred in lysogenization, transduction, and sexual recombination. The very indirect evidence indicates that the transmitted genetic specificity resides in DNA. There are no data which would incriminate or exclude other vital accessory substances as participating in these genetic structures.

The hereditary material of the temperate phage particle, like that of lytic phage, appears to be DNA. This conclusion derives from the observations (a) that like analyses of purified lytic phage (e.g., 172), temperate phages show high DNA and protein contents, and negligible amounts of other constituents (e.g., 251); (b) that like lytic phages (174, 173), most or all of the DNA of the phage particle is injected into the recipient cell, whereas the bulk of the protein does not penetrate into it (Garen, cited in 142; also see 146); about 30-40 per cent of the total phage phosphorus is detectably transferred to phage progeny in lytic infection with the temperate phage (Garen and Zinder, cited in 334); and (c) that damage by various treatments (irradiation, P^{32} disintegration, etc.) of temperate phage (e.g., 142) is consistent with the identification of DNA as the hereditary material, comparable to the more extensive evidence (e.g., 291) accumulated for lytic phages.

All published data conform with the view that the genetic elements involved in transduction are also the DNA: (a) the similarities shared by transductions and transformations (cf. 333); (b) the close relationship between the prophage and the bacterial genome and prophage-linked transductions of galactose markers (259, 259a); (c) the transduction of prophages by heterologous phage (236, 193); and (d) the chromosomal nature of the bacterial factors transducible, coupled with an indirect demonstration of the localization of some of these factors in the bacterial nucleus (321, 322), in which DNA is also localized (281, 307, 72, 68, 69, 162, others). Some of these same points may also be brought forward in advancing the thesis that sexual recombination involves a transfer of material containing DNA. In addition, Skaar and Garen (289) have found a transfer of DNA-P^{32} which follows the direction of genetic transfer during recombination. Wollman and

Jacob, in discussion at the 1956 Cold Spring Harbor Symposium on Quantitative Biology, announced that recombinant progeny, arising from F^- bacteria, could be inactivated by P^{32} decay after genetic transfer from labeled Hfr bacteria.

B. *Molecular and genetic size*

The molecular weights of DNA molecules active in transformation have been estimated to be of the order of $5\text{-}10 \times 10^5$ for transformation of single characters (255). For those molecules capable of giving rise to double transformations (182), a molecular weight of $2\text{-}8 \times 10^6$ has been estimated (255).

Studies involving radiation inactivation and inactivation by P^{32} decay indicate that phage infectivity is much more sensitive than the ability of the phage to carry out single transductions (142, 304). The latter potential falls slowly with P^{32} decay (142), but this may be a reflection of the inactivation of phage adsorption or injection. These studies are made all the more striking in view of the ability of phage to transduce the potential for production of one or several unrelated phages (236, 193). If the chemical composition and state of the phage genome and the transducing fragment are similar (with regard to ultraviolet light, see 299), these data indicate that the transduced genetic material has a much smaller total molecular size than that of the material in the phage required to produce lytic or lysogenic infection. The transducible prophage, then, would involve an equally small element. It must differ from mature phage not only in the probable absence of a protective protein coat, but also very likely in the absence of accessory DNA necessary for its infectiousness. It would be of interest to repeat the above general type of P^{32} inactivation experiment using more highly labelled bacterial genetic fragments and linked markers, prophage loci, and recipients such as *hi-22* (section V-B, Fig. 5).

In *Salmonella* transductions, the transducing fragment contained in most phage particles probably involves a section of the host genome at least several gene loci long and very likely much longer (79, 82, 161). A similar complex structure is indicated in work on *E. coli* (236). This orientation of a gene locus on a comparatively large fragment in transduction may allow its incorporation in but one of several possibly homologous sites from which it, once incorporated, could function (cf. situation with regard to flagellar phase antigens in 230, 89). In terms of the total bacterial genome, however, the size of the effective genetic material of the transducing fragment must be small.

It has been noted repeatedly (334, 13, 193, 161) that the observed potency of a bacteriophage lysate varies for transduction of different single markers. Furthermore, in the transduction of two independent markers in *Salmonella*, Plough (pers. commun.) has found that each of two serologically distinct transducing phages are more effective in engendering transduction at one locus than at the second locus of the double auxotroph. Several factors must be postulated in various cases to explain this unequal recovery. These considerations, for the most part, are not mutually exclusive: (a) linkage with a prophage induced in the recipient cell might eliminate a considerable proportion of associated markers (193); (b) a differential incorporation of genetic markers into maturing phage (334); (c) a differential affinity of the prophage of the transducing virus for certain sites of the bacterial genome (based on hypothesis forwarded in 28); (d) a higher frequency of crossing over, leading to a higher proportion of integration of markers in certain portions of the recipient genome (161); (e) the metabolic state of recipient cells (e.g., 161); (f) dominance of the functions of the incoming genetic fragment over the physiological condition imposed upon the cell by the mutant state (see results in 323, 324); or (g) effects of the residual growth and metabolism of recipient bacteria (examples in 161).

In the transduction of galactose markers by the phage lambda, the results of Morse et al. (259a) indicate that the size of the transduced piece extends over the length of at least two galactose loci (section VI-B). Apparently it does not extend as far as the *recT6, lac,* and *gal$_5$* loci (see Fig. 4).

With regard to sexual recombination, in earlier studies it was assumed that a single pair of cells took part in one mating event and that a complete haploid complement was transferred from the donor to the recipient cell. Fredericq and Betz-Bareau (133) have indicated the participation of two F+ and one F− cell in a purportedly single recombinational event, but this conclusion has yet to receive additional confirmation and may represent two successive independent events, possibly one progressing on the assay plate (compare results in 217 and bimodal distribution of colonies in 263). When two Hfr strains, containing genetically different lambda prophages, are mixed with an F− strain, transfer of only one of the types of prophage is detected in any single F— bacterium (203). The existence of bisectored (G. Allen, cited in 231) and mixed-prototroph (50) recombinant colonies indicates that more than one nucleus of a donor bacterium may occasionally participate in a single mating event *or else* that further complications sometimes arise following the initial transfer (e.g., persistence of the diploid state for several generations, 50).

Beginning with the work of Hayes (166-169), it has been suggested that the full genome of the F+ or Hfr parent never reaches the zygote, i.e., that only certain chromosomal fragments of the donor cell are transferred. The hypothesis of partial transfer has received striking support from more recent studies (200, 289, 203). Two groups of workers have detected a progressive, linear transfer of genetic specificity from the Hfr to the F— bacteria until, after 40 to 60 minutes, the transfer has progressed to its limit (327, 289, 203). Markers beyond this limit (the *Hfr* locus or rupture point) are transferred with a low frequency characteristic of the F+ to F— background level of transfer (see sections I-C-1 and I-C-2). The transfer proceeds in the order in which the markers had been previously arranged on the basis of recombination data (see section VI-A). The size of the piece transferred with high frequency in the Hayes Hfr strain (168, 169) has been determined by P^{32} decay as comprising about one-third of the total haploid genome (Wollman and Jacob, discussion at Cold Spring Harbor Symposium on Quantitative Biology, 1956). Since, as noted previously (see section I-C-1), different Hfr strains transfer with high frequency different portions of the genome, other *E. coli* K12 derivatives may transfer greater or lesser portions of the genome than that noted for the Hayes strain.

V. Mode of Incorporation of Transferred Material into Recipient Cells

We have seen that the transfer of nuclear genetic material between bacterial cells is a unidirectional process that usually involves only a portion of one haploid complement of a donor cell. Further examination indicates that only a portion of the transferred material may be retained by the recipient bacteria. Furthermore, this retention is achieved in various ways and in many cases may undergo assortment in subsequent interactions with the chromosome complement already present in the recipient cell.

It should be kept in mind, particularly when growing cultures are used, that the majority of the cells will be multinucleate (**281, 321, 211, 248**, references in **163**, others). This multiplicity of nuclei is evidenced in recipient bacteria by early-division segregation effects in lysogenization (**240, 216, 274**), transduction (**323, 324, 259**), transformation (**181**), and in sexual recombination (Skaar, pers. commun.). The action of temperate phages (see **318**) and other agents (**319**) on nuclear morphology may contribute to complex genetic behavior during early divisions.

There appear to be three general means by which the transferred material enters the heredity of the recipient cell.

A. Functional and genetic persistence without replication— unilinear inheritance

Cells receiving abortive transductions appear to retain the genetic element received from the donor cell. It is passed along through a single cellular line of the progeny (see Fig. 2 and section I-B-1-b). The transduced fragment is sometimes lost from the cell, but it never becomes incorporated into the replicating genetic apparatus of the cell (**298, 227, 271**). Only one abortively transduced cell arises from a single transductional event (**298, 271**). Reversion to the parental type in all but one cell of the clone, and occasionally in the total clone, shows that the genetic homologue of the transduced material is present in the cell, i.e., that it is not replaced by the transduced fragment, which is, therefore, merely added to the preexisting genome. With respect to genetic persistence and pattern of heredity, abortive transductions resemble the type of immunity (see section I-B-2-a) in which the genome of superinfecting homologous phage is passed through a single line of daughter cells but does not replicate (cf. **197, 25, 27**). During sexual recombination this genetically active material of superinfecting (and of vegetative) phage behaves differently from prophage incorporated in the host genome; the genetic material of the superinfecting phage does not appear to be transported from an Hfr to an F⁻ cell (**198**). The cellular site of the genetic material in abortive transduction is unknown (discussed in **227**).

The genetic fragment in an abortively transduced non-motile cell endows it with the ability to manufacture motility-conferring particles which we shall refer to here as flagella. A second type of transmission

is superimposed upon the unilinear inheritance of this synthetic potentiality. Since the flagella, once formed, continue to endow the cell with
motility and are assorted during cell division, a further unilinear transmission of these functional organelles is indicated. These are phenotypically motile cells, semi-clones of which originate at each division
of the genetically potent bacterium (see Fig. 2).

The existence of "satellite" colonies (298, 280) and a small proportion
of certain motile cells in broth cultures of some non-motile strains (297)
indicate that phenotypically motile cells can arise spontaneously. Single
cell pedigrees show that these phenotypically motile cells transmit
motility along one or several single cell lines, in unilinear fashion
(Quadling, in 297). If the non-motile mutants are regarded as having
differing degrees of "leakiness" in the production of a motility-conferring
substance (flagella or flagellar basal granules, see 62, 189), the chance
accumulation of a sufficient level of the intermediate could lead to a
transient ability to produce flagella (cf. 280a). Once produced, the cells
possessing flagella would be expected to transmit these particulate elements in the same way as the phenocopies arising from progeny of cells
which have received an abortive transduction.

Abortive transductions have so far been noted as being carried out
only by phages of the type giving transductions for a variety of
markers in the genome (section I-B-1-a; figures 1a-b). It would not
be surprising were similar phenomena discovered in other systems upon
careful examination and with the realization of critical conditions of
growth, such as those developed for one particular system by Ozeki
(271). For example, not all markers transferred in sexual recombination find their way into the replicating genome. The rate of genetic
transfer can be measured in some cases by the transfer of prophage
lambda from a lysogenic bacterium to a sensitive one. Under certain
conditions the prophage is frequently induced following transfer and
kills the recipient bacterium from which the recombinants must arise.
While this "zygotic induction" has the effect of decreasing below
expectation those markers from the donor parent which are most closely
linked to $ly\lambda$ (198, 326, 125, 127, 203), it can also give a measure of
actual genetic transfer (198, 203). Other workers (216, 259) have not
noted zygotic induction, perhaps because of different conditions under
which the cross was made (cf. 193) or because of differences in the
portion of the genome participating in the high frequency of transfer.

B. *Functional and genetic persistence with replication—diploidization*

Excellent evidence exists for the persistence and replication of varying portions of the bacterial genome in a diploid state following genetic transfer. For the operation of this mechanism, as well as that discussed in the following section (C), a most logical assumption relies upon the synapsis of the transported genetic material with its homologue in the recipient cell. This step rapidly follows genetic transfer in most cases. There are indications, however, that there may be some delay in this step under certain conditions (see 324). The data also indicate that diploidization is rarely, if ever, complete. The diploid genome is relatively unstable; there is a marked tendency for segregation and elimination of the duplicate portions of the chromosome.

Further, the duplicate fragment may interact with the homologous region of the parental chromosome. These interactions are discussed in the following section, C.

In bacteria doubly lysogenic for lambda the prophage locus may persist and be duplicated in the diploid state while the remainder of the chromosome remains haploid (see section I-B-1-c). In lambda-mediated transductions of galactose markers, a like situation occurs except that here the diploid state usually includes a small section of the chromosome nearby the $ly\lambda$ locus (see Fig. 3) and more rarely may include this adjacent region as well as $ly\lambda$ (section I-B-1-c). In transductions encompassing sites over a large portion of the genome, the data (335, others) indicate the absence of, or extremely transient, diploidization. This conclusion should be checked further, in view of the instability of unselected markers (i.e., mixed clones), as noted in transductions with Pl phage (236). With regard to transformations, the system of Hotchkiss and Marmur (182, 181) is amenable to similar examination.

In sexual recombination, certain *E. coli* K12 stocks carrying a presumably nuclear factor, *Het*, form among recombinant prototrophs 5-10 per cent of persistent heterozygotes (220, 222), verified as such by single-cell pedigrees (332). *Het* is effective in inciting diploidy when present either in one or in both parents (220). Heterozygous diploids can be recovered from other crosses, not carrying *Het*, when special techniques are utilized to detect their infrequent occurrence (231, 222). Although segregants of these diploids do not appear to carry a new *Het* mutation (231), the presence of such a change might not have been detected if it had occurred only in F$^+$ cells and appeared in recombinants with a comparatively low frequency.

The diploids segregate spontaneously with a frequency of the order of once per 20 bacterial divisions (Zelle and Lederberg, cited in 222). Ultraviolet irradiation stimulates the production of stable haploid segregants (16), but these are mainly progeny of cells which themselves still remain diploid (231). The K12 diploids can be distinguished cytologically from haploids (231). A possible mechanism for the effect on segregation of ultraviolet light is suggested from further cytological studies of this organism (cf. 209, 163, 278). Similar segregation of the diploid galactose region in progeny from lambda transductions is not achieved with ultraviolet light (259a).

When the K12 diploids segregate, all markers segregate simultaneously (220, 227), and stable progeny are produced which, in some cases (332, 231), are both viable and sometimes contain complementary alleles for certain markers (P. Fried, cited in 282). The minority of the total segregants, however, represent types recombinant between the two haploid strains from which the diploids were constituted. Most segregations from the diploids deviate from a 1:1 expectancy up to as much as 15:1 for some single factors (220-222, 231). Further, when a diploid cell divides, one of the daughter cells is frequently inviable (332).

A partial explanation for these effects may be the regular hemizygous condition of certain loci (*str, mal, gal, ly*λ, and *Hfr*) in otherwise heterozygous cells (220-222, 231, 264). With regard to these loci, the alleles of the F$^-$ parent predominate among the diploids (231, 264). Thus, it would seem that the F polarity of the cross (see I-C-2), and some type of regular post-zygotic "elimination" (234, 226, 227, 231), combine to influence the peculiar composition of these diploids. This composition biases segregation ratios of certain single unselected markers unless appropriate crossover classes are selected for. Lederberg (264, 219) has warned that similar post-zygotic effects may be responsible for aberrant linkage relations calculated from data derived in normal haploid crosses.

We may inquire here as to the existence of evidence for the formation of any true, complete diploids in bacteria. Indeed, Lederberg (222, 223, 231) has found several "exceptions among the exceptions." These bacteria contain the *str* and *mal* loci in homozygous or heterozygous condition. They may be complete diploids, although the published data do not allow one to draw a conclusion in regard to this point yet. This is especially true since it has been indicated that the position and extent of hemizygosity may vary in different diploids (216, Nelson, cited in 50). The more complete diploids presumably arise primarily in diploid × diploid and in diploid ×haploid crosses.

C. Genetic recombination at the chromosomal level—integration

In the preceding discussions we have spoken mainly of recombination as involving *cells*. The emphasis has been placed on genetic transfer and retention of the transferred material in addition to the genome already existing in the recipient bacterium. The situations considered below will focus attention on interactions occurring at the chromosomal level in recipient cells. These interactions will be considered under the title "integration" (200, 203), a term which currently is endowed with but few genetic prejudices as to mechanism. In some cases the evidence indicates that integration may take place by means of crossing over; in other instances integration may be achieved by processes analogous to "gene conversion" (cf. 293 and references cited therein). In all cases, the limited data available do not allow a precise formulation of events at the molecular level.

Demerec (78, 79, 84) and Lederberg (227) have considered several mechanisms for the genetic incorporation occurring during transduction. Demerec (op. cit.) favors the mechanism of crossing over outlined by Belling (17; type B in Fig. 1, ref. 227). My own Fig. 1, B is based on this model. In the model a replica of the transduced fragment is considered to undergo crossing over with the host chromosome at the time of, or following, its own replication. Similar mechanisms may be advanced for the integration of transferred genetic material in *ly*λ-linked transductions of *gal* markers (259a), in sexual recombination (49, 50, 203), and in transformation (181).

Besides these instances of integration, which presumably involve reciprocal exchanges between the gene loci comprising the introduced fragment and its chromosomal homologue, examples exist that indicate a further type of exchange. These involve demonstrations of homozygosity for some, but not all, of the markers persisting in the diploid state and derived from an originally heterozygous individual. This situation has been found for lambda and for *gal* markers as well as for diploids arising after sexual recombination (e.g., 231).

Irradiation of transducing phage particles with appropriate doses of ultraviolet light enhances the number of transductions recovered (333, 142). A like effect is obtained by irradiation of the F+ *donor* parent in sexual recombination (157, 167, 168). This irradiation has the effect of enhancing processes leading to the incorporation of *small* regions of the donor genome into the recipient genome (203). It may also induce mutations to Hfr in the F+ bacteria. Ultraviolet irradiation of lambda phage enhances recombination during subsequent vegetative growth (199); irradiation of only one of the infecting phage stocks introduces a polarity in the cross by increasing its role as a donor of small sections of the chromosome (201). The relations of these grossly similar effects to the mode of integration, in each case, remain to be determined.

VI. Genetic Organization of Hereditary Elements in Bacteria

In the preceding discussion the processes which lead to recombination of bacterial traits have been examined. Much concerning the structure of the host genome has been assumed and stated during the discussion, since these processes of genetic transfer and incorporation are the very tools with which our knowledge of bacterial genetic organization has been deduced. In this section we will examine how instructive these methods have been in elucidating the structure of the bacterial chromosome.

Fig. 4 represents a general scheme for the chromosome of an enteric bacterium. The scheme is based upon genetic studies with *E. coli* K12. The symbols for gene loci are described in the legend of Fig. 4. Data compiled from diverse studies (serological and biochemical, 207; transduction, 236; sexual recombination, Luria cited in 236; bacteriocin production, 121, 126; phage and bacteriocin sensitivity; morphology; etc.) indicate a high degree of phenotypic and genotypic homology among genera of the family *Enterobacteriaceae* (also see 295). Consequently, genetic studies on *E. coli* and *Salmonella* will be discussed together. It might also be noted here that two strains of *S. typhimurium*, LT-2 and LT-7 (335), of diverse origin (see 242), have revealed a strikingly complete genetic homology for one region of the chromosome (161).

A. Gross structure

The following general scheme (Fig. 4) is modified after Cavalli-Sforza and Jinks (50). Although still subject to modification as

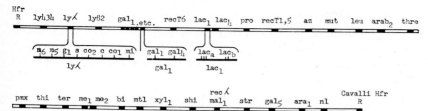

Fig. 4. Order of gene loci on *E. coli* chromosome. Adapted after Cavalli-Sforza and Jinks (50), with additions as cited in the text. Symbols for loci (further description in the text): *arab*—arabinose utilization; *az*—azide resistance; *bi*—biotin synthesis; *gal*—galactose utilization; *Hfr*—high frequency of recombination (point of rupture = *R*), site in Cavalli strain which also acts as a lethal; *lac*—lactose utilization; *leu*—leucine synthesis; *ly*—lysogenicity, prophage loci of phages 434, λ, and 82, respectively; *mal*—maltose utilization; *me*—methionine synthesis; *mtl*—mannitol utilization; *mut*—mutability locus; *nl*—norleucine resistance; *pmx*—polymyxin resistance; *pro*—proline synthesis; *rec*—synthesis of receptors for adsorption of phages T1 and T5, of λ, and of T6, respectively; *shi*—shikimic acid or polyaromatic synthesis; *str*—streptomycin resistance or dependence; *thi*—vitamin B₁ synthesis; *thre*—threonine synthesis; *xyl*—xylose utilization. The nomenclature is a hybrid compromise between that in use for several years for the *E. coli* K12 system and a superior system recently outlined by Demerec (77). Subscript numerals designate the numbers assigned to various loci, except for the *gal* mutants, in which case they refer to individual mutants rather than to loci.

The insert of the *ly*λ locus depicts the arrangement of prophage markers suggested by the studies of Jacob (193). For a full explanation of these markers the reader is referred to the original studies (199, 201, 206, 193). The other inserts are described in the text.

Other abbreviations: DNA—deoxyribonucleic acid; DNAase—deoxyribonuclease.

further data appear, all markers have been placed on a single linkage group. While the recent results of Jacob et al. (203) indicate that linkage relationships may possibly vary in different K12 derivatives, it would seem to me that the arrangement depicted in Fig. 4 is consistent with a large body of evidence. Thus, exceptions may be relatively rare or have as their explanation factors other than the linearity of the genetic organization.

Early studies on *E. coli* K12 (217, 303) demonstrated linkage between the *recT6*, *lac*, *recT1,5*, *leu*, and *thre* loci. Later studies confirmed the linear order given above (231, 282, 50, 203, others). The locus, *recT6*, whose allele confers resistance to phage T6 by the absence of a specific receptor complex (313, 314), appears identical with that locus responsible for the specific receptor for colicin K (130). *Az* is transferred in a manner suggesting its position as between *lac* and *leu*, *thre* (312) and between *recT1,5* and *leu*, *thre* (52a, 46). Only one *az* locus has been detected and no important variability in the degree of one-step resistance to azide has been encountered (51). The transduction experiments of Lennox (236) confirm that *az* is more closely linked than *lac* to *leu, thre*, thus making the order *lac, az, leu, thre*. In addition (236), the *arab₂* marker was placed close to *leu* (as found in sexual crosses, 49, 50) and between *leu* and *thre*. Skaar (288a and in 41) has shown the *mut* locus of Treffers et al. (306) to be near and to the left of *leu*. A *pro* locus lies between *lac* and *leu* (55) and a *pro* marker between *recT1,5* and *recT6* (47), both cases thus indicating the position of a locus (or loci) for proline synthesis between *lac* and *recT1,5*.

Cavalli and Maccacaro (52a) have found at least one locus, or multiple loci, conferring cumulative resistance to chloramphenicol, located between *lac* and *recT1,5*. Markers endowing the cell with resistance to valine are extremely closely linked to *leu* (253, also see 47). A pyridoxine locus lies in the *recT6* to *recT1,5* region (41). A locus giving rise to commonly encountered first-step resistance to chloramphenicol is closely linked to *recT6* (52a).

A *gal* locus was placed in the sequence *gal, lac, recT1,5, thre, leu* by Cavalli (45). *Gal₂* is linked with *Hfr*, a point of rupture in the Cavalli strain (50). Sexual recombination studies have shown that the lambda prophage locus, *lyλ*, is closely linked to a cluster of galactose markers, including *gal₂* (216, 325, 6, 7, 326, 125, 227, others). This linkage has been confirmed by transduction with lambda of *gal* markers, *gal₁, ₂, ₃, ₄, ₅, ₆, ₇, ₈* (257-259a), and also by the utilization of transducing phage with more generalized activity (236, 193). The sequential order of transfer of genetic markers during sexual recombination confirms the order for some loci listed above as derived from recombination data (see 327, 289, 203).

Jacob's transduction and preliminary sexual recombination studies (193) indicate that: (a) the loci for two different prophages (*ly434* and *ly82*) are also close to *lyλ* and a galactose marker; (b) the order of the loci is *ly434, lyλ, ly82, gal*; and (c) some genetic markers of the prophage lambda itself (199, 201, 206, 193) are transduced in conjunction with *gal* more frequently than are others, corresponding to the placement of the phage genome in a linear sequence continuous with that of the bacterial genome (insert, Fig. 4). It is of interest in this respect that the phage lambda (199, 201, 206) and a temperate phage of *B. megaterium* (261a) each carry but a single linkage group, possibly a requisite for lysogenization.

The phenotype of lambda may be host-modified (reviewed in **245**) by a single passage on certain hosts, whether by lytic passage or by release from lysogenic cells (**29, 315**). The ability of the host to modify lambda resides in a locus separate from *lyλ* and behaves as other genetic markers in bacterial crosses (**215, 241**).

Sensitive persistent diploids of K12 (see section V-B) are difficult to lysogenize with lambda but, once lysogenized, segregate lysogenic cells only (**216**). This effect is correlated with the observation that, following certain crosses, the region of the chromosome containing *lyλ* is uniformly present hemizygously in persistent diploids; out of more than **30** markers tested, *mal₁*, *str*, *lyλ*, *Hfr*, and a *gal* locus were hemizygous (**220, 221, 216, 264**). *Gal₅* (weak positive phenotype, e.g. **259a**) and *arab₁* are closely linked; they are both linked to *str* more than to *mal₁* and *xyl* (**265, 266**). These loci have been placed between *str* and the point of rupture (*Hfr = R*) since no linkage with *lac₁* is demonstrable (**50**). The *mal₁* and *recλ* loci have been shown to be equivalent (**215**); *mal₁⁺* is dominant to *mal₁* (**231**). The *mal₁* locus has been shown by sexual recombination (**266, 231**) and transduction (**236**) to be linked closely to a locus which confers streptomycin resistance (*str*). *Str* is linked to, and on the left of, *R* (**50**).

Locus *nl* is closely linked with *gal₅* and *arab₁* (**54**) and more weakly linked with *str* and *mal₁* (**54, 55**). A locus conferring resistance to bacteriocin V is closely linked to this *arab* marker (**131**). Cavalli-Sforza and Jinks (**50**) have placed the probable order of some of these loci as *mal₁*, *str*, *(gal₅, arab₁)*, *R*, *gal₂*.

Sexual crosses indicate linkage of *xyl* to *(str, mal₁)* in the order *xyl*, *mal*, *str* (**52**). *Str* is also linked to a *me* locus (**265, 266, 140**). *Str* shows linkage of decreasing strength with *xyl*, *me*, and *thi* (**50**). Two fermentation loci, *xyl* and *mtl*, are closely linked to each other (**231, 55, 236**) and are linked to *thi* (**50**). Closely linked to *xyl* and *mtl* is a locus whose allele endows the K12 cell with resistance to ultraviolet light (**41**). Skaar (**288a**) has found that polyaromatic *(shi)* locus, when used as a selective marker, is closely linked both with *xyl* and *str*. Similarly, *xyl* and *mtl* have been shown to be linked with *me* (**56**). A marker endowing resistance to phage T3 (Skaar, pers. comm.) and one for radiation resistance (Bryson, unpublished) are probably located between *shi* and *xyl*.

The loci *me₁* and *thi* are closely linked (**169, 312, 52, 231, 55**) and the two *me* loci give few recombinants in crosses (**54, 55**). A *ter* locus (or loci) conferring resistance to terramycin (and also to chloramphenicol) is located between *thi* and *me* (46). A *bi* marker (302) has been little used, since reversions have appeared in the most commonly utilized derivatives originally carrying this mutation. However, *bi* was found to be closely linked to the *thi* and *me* loci (217). *Pmx* is linked, but distal, to *thi* (50).

A mutant *mtl* with alternative requirements (α-aminobutyric acid or isoleucine plus methionine) is tentatively designated between *me* and *xyl* (55). Also, one of possibly multiple sites (27, 28) of P2 prophage is closely linked with *me* in K12 (alpha phage of Fredericq, 118) and also to *xyl* (128). In *E. coli* B, the markers representing a locus, or loci, *recT3,4* and *recT3,4,7*, are linked to a *me* locus (65). An arginine locus lies in the *me-thi* region (288a).

The above considerations demonstrate that there are associations of loci along a linear structure which may be termed the bacterial chromosome. A large variety of specialized functions depends upon specific regions of this linkage group. Within this framework there is a noticeable association of some markers dealing with related functions. For example, this is indicated in Fig. 4 by the proximity of the *ly* loci, the two *lac* loci, and the two *me* loci. However, this correspondence is not complete—witness the position of *gal₅* in relation to the other *gal* markers and the finding that *lyP2* may not be closely linked with *lyλ*. Certain loci (inserts, Fig. 4) appear to be divisible by mutation and recombination. These general observations lead us into a discussion of the fine structure of the bacterial chromosome as determined genetically.

B. Fine structure

In transduction tests between auxotrophic and fermentative mutants of *Salmonella*, Demerec and coworkers (84, 81, 75, 76, 82, 161, 329) have shown that bacteria with presumed *common biochemical deficiencies* are in each case mutant within certain small regions of the chromosome. In general, the mutants of each group produce few or no wild-type recombinants in reciprocal transduction experiments as compared with large numbers recovered after transductions with other mutants or wild-type bacteria. The very closely linked markers, constituting transduction groups (78), are interpreted as sites of mutation within specific gene loci. The mutant loci are thus alleles, or non-identical alleles. Each locus has its own primary discrete function, such as a role in the production of a specific enzyme. The gene locus, therefore, is defined as a *functional unit,* a small length of the bacterial chromosome. It is a *complex unit* which is divisible by mutation and recombination.

Further, mutant alleles producing the same *general* phenotype (e.g., histidine requirement for growth) are in many cases linked with one another. In these cases the apparent sequence of the gene loci on a linkage map parallels precisely the presumed sequence of biochemical reactions leading to the synthesis of the required compound. With such loci in close juxtaposition, it is obvious that both genetic *and* biochemical tests are required for an analysis of allelism. Thus, some phenotypes which we currently indicate as being produced by mutation at a single locus may in the future be shown to involve changes at any one of several functionally differentiated regions within a small chromosomal section. It should be noted that, in spite of this close spatial relationship of the loci on the chromosome, the functioning of individual loci is not *grossly* affected by mutation at sites in nearby loci (161).

Fig. 5 shows a "magnification" of a chromosomal section based on transduction tests in *Salmonella* (161). Following the convenient nomenclature outlined by Demerec (77), each independently obtained histidine auxotroph is designated by a number and, after analysis is sufficient, a capital letter is added to designate the locus *(A–G).* The order of the loci and the chemical reactions they have been associated with are designated with some assurance. The presumed sites of mutation of alleles at each locus, as denoted by mutant numbers, are placed within each locus in a tentative order only (161). All mutants tested which are primarily histidineless fall into one of the seven groups depicted in Fig. 5 (161, 336).

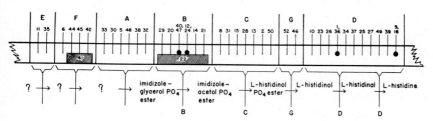

Fig. 5. *Linkage map of the histidine region of the*
Salmonella typhimurium *chromosome*

Probable relation of gene loci (A–G) with enzymatic reactions (A–G) in the proposed primary pathway of L-histidine synthesis. Consult text for further description.

The hatched region shown in Fig. 5 indicates that no wild-type recombinants are recovered in transduction tests with other locus *B* alleles when *hi-22* is used either as donor or as recipient. Several additional mutants of this type, involving other loci, have been described (75, 329). Thus they occur with low frequency among spontaneous mutants selected for any of several nutritional deficiencies (and corresponding loci). In *hi-22* the effect appears to be restricted to a single locus. However, mutants of this type are found with much higher frequency among derivatives mutant at the *cysD* locus; the effect here often appears to extend into a portion of a second locus *(cysC)*, adjacent to the *cysD* locus (Clowes, cited in 76, 336).

Some mutant alleles which do not show evidence of recombination with each other (black circles, Fig. 5) nevertheless can be distinguished by their rates of mutation to prototrophy and the types of mutants obtained (e.g., *hi-9* from *-18*) or by their behavior in transductions with other mutant markers (e.g., *hi-9* from *-18; hi-12* from *-24*). This leaves in the series of mutants examined only *hi-1* and *-36* as probable repetitions of an identical mutation. Still further criteria (e.g., the use of suppressor mutations) might well reveal differences even between these two markers.

The above results may indicate that a mutation sometimes involves a greater than minimal portion of the gene locus, as found to be true in a similar situation for some phage mutants by Benzer (18, 19, this symposium).

As mentioned above, the various mutants comprising a transduction group (alleles of a single, functional locus) show differing, but individually characteristic rates of spontaneous and induced mutation to prototrophy as well as distinctive types of revertants. More extensive analyses of this phenomenon with regard to other *Salmonella* mutants have been made by Z. Hartman (164) and Yura (329). Differences in the non-identical alleles are also demonstrable at the genetic level by differential specificity of suppressor mutations (329, 292). With regard to secondary properties, the alleles are biochemically a heterogeneous group as evidenced, for example (Fig. 5), by the unique temperature sensitivity of *hi-15* or the ability of *hi-32* to grow slowly on purines as an alternative growth requirement (161).

A similar demonstration of non-identical alleles and sequentially linked loci has been made for tryptophan mutants in *Salmonella* (79, 82). This system is technically superior for genetic analysis because the growth responses to biosynthetic intermediates (or compounds closely associated thereto, see **38, 150**) and the presence of linkage to a cystine locus *(cysB)* allow three- and four-point recombination analyses. "The genetic markers controlling tryptophan synthesis in *E. coli* K12 are closely linked to each other and to a marker controlling cysteine synthesis. The ordering of these markers is not yet definite, though there is some evidence not inconsistent with ordering according to the tryptophan biosynthetic sequence" (**237**).

Other instances in *Salmonella* of linked loci controlling steps in biosynthetic sequences are cited by Demerec (**76**). As noted in the previous section, still further situations may be uncovered in further genetic analysis of *E. coli* K12. However, not all complete biosynthetic pathways have as their reflection the same type of sequential genetic arrangement (some exceptions noted in **76**). Certainly, further elucidation of the genetic arrangement will provide a powerful tool for understanding metabolic interactions at the cellular level. The peculiar distribution of related loci in the gram-negative bacteria differs from that observed for analogous loci in *Neurospora* (**15**) and for loci determining sequential biochemical activities in other organisms (examples in **309**).

Ozeki (**271**) finds that abortive transductions in *Salmonella* purine mutants are detected with phage prepared only on *non-allelic* mutants (**329**) or on wild-type bacteria. The abortive transductions are interpreted as functionally analogous to *trans*-heterozygotes for the small region of the chromosome encompassing the mutant allele. It is reasonable to assume that the phenotype of *trans*-heterozygotes, whether heterozygosity is complete or involves only the segment of the chromosome under study, alone may be a valuable tool for tentative decisions concerning allelism. This is a presumptive test only since, while the agreement with transduction and biochemical grouping is excellent in Ozeki's experiments, further complications may arise in other situations.

By transduction tests, Lederberg and Edwards (**230**) found two loci which are implicated in determining the serological specificity of flagella in *Salmonella*. One locus (H_1) controlls the specificity of phase 1 ("specific" phase) and the other locus (H_2) phase 2 ("group" or "nonspecific" phase). Some phase 1 antigens are serologically indistinguishable from phase 2 antigens of other strains; phage prepared on these strains nevertheless transduced the locus of the phase appropriate for the donor (see section IV-B). In single organisms, only one phase (one antigen complex) is expressed at a time. The change in expression from one phase to the other resembles a mutational event; "the rates are such that any (diphasic) culture will tend, as it grows, towards an equilibrium composition in which the specific phase predominates" (294). There appears to be some correlation of the rates of change, back and forth, to the two phases, though that leading to the specific phase is usually the higher (294). Lederberg (225) has reported a correlation "between antigenic state of the donor cells and the transductive competence of phage lysates," a correlation indicating that "the differentiation is based on the H_1 and H_2 loci themselves." Although controlled by presumably single loci, phase antigens are serologically subdivisible. Each flagellum, however, contains the complete antigenic complex (262). Mutation may occur at one of the H loci, and lead to the production of a serologically distinguishable antigen (225; also see "induced phases" in 207). In addition, some cultures are monophasic; these strains may become diphasic following transduction (230). Further properties of flagella and flagellar antigens are reviewed elsewhere (207, 297, 9, 260, 189).

Several loci have been implicated by transduction tests in the production and the functioning of flagella. Without adequate production of the organelles, the antigen-determining loci either are not expressed (298) or possibly are very poorly expressed (see 294). This weak expression may be due to the presence of "leaky" mutant alleles, which allow the formation of a few flagella in the population (see discussion in section V-A). A locus governing the production of flagella is linked to one controlling serological specificity (298, 208). This linkage has enabled Stocker (cited in 334) to map three markers controlling the production of flagella. Motility may also be transferred from *E. coli* K12 to *E. coli* B-K12 hybrids during sexual recombination (141a, 44).

Seven lactose loci have been described for *E. coli* K12 (222, 231, 213). The allele conferring ability to ferment is usually dominant to that responsible for failure of lactose utilization (220). The loci, lac_1 and lac_4, are very closely linked (see Fig. 4) but are genetically dissimilar, as shown in diploids by their wild-type activity when present in the *trans*-configuration (222, 231). Bacteria mutant at the lac_1 locus differ phenotypically from those mutant at lac_4 (222, 231), for lac_1 mutants possess a low residual activity absent in lac_4 mutants (213). Recently it has been found that mutation at lac_1 prevents lactose utilization by eliminating the adaptive synthesis of a galactose permease (y factor, see 256a) which may be concerned with the penetration of lactose into the cell (57a). On the other hand, lac_4 is involved in the adaptive production of β-galactosidase. A third, closely linked locus, *ind*, governs the inducibility of *both* these enzymes (57a), i.e., provided the bacteria are genetically able to form the galactosidase and the permease, both systems will be adaptive (*ind+*) or constitutive (*ind−*). For example, if the bacterial genome contains *ind−* and a mutation at the lac_1 locus, the β-galactosidase is constitutively produced but the cell cannot utilize lactose at an appreciable rate because of its inability to form the permease (see results in 58). A fourth locus, lac_2, also appears to be intimately involved in β-galactosidase activity (57a). Sexual recombination has been demonstrated between non-identical alleles of the lac_1 locus (insert, Fig. 4). These non-identical alleles of lac_1 produce lactose-positive diploids when in the presumed *cis* state, but lactose-negative diploids when in the *trans*-configuration (231, 213). E. M. Lederberg (213) has found that various mutant alleles of lac_1 revert to lactose fermentation at different rates. She has obtained evidence in some cases for the presence of suppressor mutations in the revertants, while in other cases the reversion appears to occur at the locus involved in the original mutation. Additional lactose loci (lac_3, lac_5, lac_6, and lac_7) are apparently neither closely linked with each other nor with lac_1-lac_4. Limited physiological data relating to them have been published (222, 231). It has been reported that *E. coli* K12 may produce a multiplicity of β-galactosidases (2).

Through the use of prophage-linked transductions, Morse et al. (258, 259a) have initiated a study of galactose mutants in *E. coli* K12. All of the mutants used in the study were indistinguishable on eosin, methylene blue, galactose medium and produced *gal+* recombinants in reciprocal transduction experiments. However, gal_1, gal_4, and gal_7 were found to have a weaker lactose positive phenotype than gal_2 and gal_8 (259a). Gal_1 and gal_4 give a negative phenotype in the *trans*-configuration and a positive phenotype in the *cis*-configuration (259a); gal_1 may be assumed to be allelic to gal_4 (insert, Fig. 4). Furthermore, one may infer from the data (259a) that gal_2 and gal_8 give a positive *trans*-heterozygote with gal_1; gal_8 acts similarly when in the *trans*-configuration with gal_4. This indicates that gal_2 and gal_8 are probably non-allelic to gal_1 and gal_4. Thus there appear to be several closely linked *gal* loci. At least one of these loci is divisible by mutation and by recombination. It may be noted here that transduction of loci controlling the potentiality for the formation of adaptive enzymes appears to occur readily even though the donor bacteria are in the unadapted state (data in 335, 11, 12, 164, etc.).

In *E. coli* K12 the markers conferring resistance (*r*) and those conferring partial resistance (*pr*) to phages T1 and T5 (*recT1,5*, Fig. 4) are recessive to the wild-type allele allowing sensitivity. Diploids containing the *r* and *pr* markers in the *trans*-configuration are sensitive, but no crossovers between these markers have been detected in segregant progeny (222, 231). This may indicate the presence of two very closely linked loci, one of them (*pr*) possibly involved in host modification (e.g. 269). On the other hand, the two markers may be allelic; the *pr* mutants might be considered "leaky" mutants, serving to produce particulate receptor sites (313, 314) at a rate low enough to allow adsorption of phage by some cells only (differential receptivity, cf. 310, 311). In a slower dividing or otherwise altered diploid, the dilution of the receptors may not keep up with their synthesis, and thus allow a return of sensitivity. The locus, *recT1,5*, appears to be closely associated with, if not the same as, a locus conferring resistance to bacteriocin B (131). Independent isolates of T1,5-resistant mutants in *E. coli* B, where no partial resistance has been described, are considered as allelic (66). A second locus in K12, concerned with resistance to T1 phage only, is not closely linked with *recT1,5* (217, 220, 222, 231). In *E. coli* B an analogous mutant (80) also usually shows a tryptophan requirement (3, 150). A third locus, giving rise to unstable, mucoid T1-resistant bacteria, is genetically differentiable from the other two resistance loci (217).

All markers endowing high levels of resistance to streptomycin appear to be very closely linked on the *E. coli* K12 chromosome; mutations to streptomycin dependence appear to be allelic to those for resistance (85, 86, 73, 74, 266). The resistance allele is recessive to wild-type sensitive (223). Attempts to obtain bacteria heterozygous for resistance and dependence have failed (51). Strains containing diverse resistance alleles exhibit a number of secondary differences (85, 86, 74, 73). A series of dependent mutants, tested for reversion to streptomycin independence (23), were uniform in showing mutagen susceptibility and in the pattern of a delayed appearance of induced mutants. However, wide differences were found in the rates of mutation (210). Direct "induction of mutation" to streptomycin resistance has been reported (1, 301), and the nuclear nature of the change confirmed by sexual recombination studies (301). A closer examination of this system has indicated that it is highly likely that spontaneous mutation and selection, rather than direct induction, operate in producing the resistant mutants (Szybalski, in 42).

The *mut* locus of Treffers et al. (306) increases the spontaneous rates of mutation of a number of other loci, including *str*. The same *str* locus is involved in mutation whether in a *mut*-containing stock or not (288a). Mutation rates at a *p*-aminobenzoic acid locus (41) and a locus conferring resistance to T2 phage (306) do not appear to be affected by the presence of *mut* in the genome. The close linkage of *mut* to *leu* (Fig. 4) suggests the possibility for its use in obtaining new mutants and a subsequent elimination of *mut* by linked transduction with *leu*. A second highly mutable strain of *E. coli* has been described (145). McClintock (256) has pointed out possible similarities in the action of elements of mutable strains of bacteria and elements governing mutability in maize. Contrariwise, one may speculate that the two systems are basically different and that the *mut* locus is concerned with the production of a substance, such as catalase, which may secondarily affect mutability. This suggestion is in part prompted by the preliminary experiments of Englesberg and Skaar (in 41), which show that the effects of *mut* are greatly decreased in anaerobically grown cultures.

VII. CONCLUSION

Some elementary features of diverse processes involved in the cell-to-cell transfer of hereditary traits in a few bacterial genera have been reviewed. In all cases the evidence indicates that the transfer of the genetic characters is unidirectional. In most, if not all, cases only a portion of the genetic complement is transferred from donor to recipient bacteria. Many transfers very likely involve hereditary material of the bacterial nucleus (chromosome). DNA is implicated as underlying the genetic specificity of the transferred material.

Once transferred to recipient bacteria, the genetic fragments may be carried by the cell in functional form but without being incorporated into the replicating genome. In other instances, the transferred genetic material may synapse with its homologue in the recipient cell. Sometimes these incoming fragments, or replicas of them, are further replicated along with the chromosome of the recipient bacterium. These partial diploids may later segregate, or the genetic material of the diploid portion of the chromosome may undergo recombination by crossing over or by other means (designated as "integration"). In many cases integration rapidly follows genetic transfer, without any detectable persistence of the diploid state.

The convenient methods applicable to bacterial genetics, coupled with the unique features of the types of transfer, have allowed a rapid growth of this new branch of genetics. As yet, the data are mainly of a sketchy and fragmentary nature. In this review, interpretations which are still limited by the available facts have been superimposed on these data. Since most of these interpretations are amenable to further experimental testing, we can be sure that rapid progress will be made in their development and maturation. In spite of these uncertainties, a number of model systems have been developed to a degree which allows the formulation of both theoretical and mechanistic concepts with strong implications for biology in general.

ACKNOWLEDGMENTS

The author wishes to thank various workers, cited in the text and the bibliography, for personal communications and the use of data still in press. The author's own genetic studies were performed while a Research Associate at the Department of Genetics, Carnegie Institution of Washington, Cold Spring Harbor, L. I., N. Y.

REFERENCES

1. Akiba, T., in *Origins of Resistance to Toxic Agents* (M. G. Sevag et al., eds.), 82-85, Academic Press, New York (1955).
2. Aladjem, F., Dubnoff, J., Campbell, D. H., and Bartron, E., *Federation Proc.,* **15**, 209 (1956).
3. Anderson, E. H., *Proc. Natl. Acad. Sci. U. S.,* **32**, 120 (1946).
4. Anderson, E. S., and Fraser, A., *J. Gen. Microbiol.,* **13**, 519 (1955).
5. Anderson, T. F., in *The Nature of the Bacterial Surface* (A. A. Miles and N. W. Pirie, eds.), 76-95, Blackwell Scientific Publications, Oxford (1949).
6. Appleyard, R. K., *Cold Spring Harbor Symposia Quant. Biol.,* **18**, 95 (1953).
7. Appleyard, R. K., *Genetics,* **39**, 429 (1954).
8. Appleyard, R. K., *Genetics,* **39**, 440 (1954).
9. Astbury, W. T., Beighton, E., and Weibull, C., *Symposia Soc. Exptl. Biol.,* **9** *(Fibrous Proteins and Their Biological Significance),* 282 (1955).
10. Barksdale, W. L., and Pappenheimer, A. M., Jr., *J. Bacteriol.,* **67**, 220 (1954).
11. Baron, L. S., *Cold Spring Harbor Symposia Quant. Biol.,* **18**, 271 (1953).
12. Baron, L. S., *Abstr. 3rd Intern. Congr. Biochem.* (Brussels), No. 10-14, p. 89 (1955).
13. Baron, L. S., Formal, S. B., and Spilman, W., *Proc. Soc. Exptl. Biol. Med.,* **83**, 292 (1953).
14. Baron, L. S., Formal, S. B., and Spilman, W., *J. Bacteriol.,* **69**, 177 (1955).

15. Barratt, R. W., Newmeyer, D., Perkins, D. D., and Garnjobst, L., *Advances in Genet.,* **6**, 1 (1954).
16. Beckhorn, E. J., *Carnegie Inst. Wash. Yearbook,* **50**, 190 (1951).
17. Belling, J., *Genetics,* **18**, 388 (1933).
18. Benzer, S., *Proc. Natl. Acad. Sci. U. S.,* **41**, 344 (1955).
19. Benzer, S., *Brookhaven Symposia Biol.,* **8** *(Mutation),* 3-5 (1956).
20. Benzer, S., and Jacob, F., *Ann. inst. Pasteur,* **84**, 186 (1953).
21. Berry, M. E., McCarthy, A. M., and Plough, H. H., *Proc. Natl. Acad. Sci. U. S.,* **38**, 797 (1952).
22. Bertani, G., *J. Bacteriol.,* **62**, 293 (1951).
23. Bertani, G., *Genetics,* **36**, 598 (1951).
24. Bertani, G., *Cold Spring Harbor Symposia Quant. Biol.,* **18**, 65 (1953).
25. Bertani, G., *Ann. inst. Pasteur,* **84**, 273 (1953).
26. Bertani, G., *Genetics,* **38**, 656 (1953).
27. Bertani, G., *J. Bacteriol.,* **67**, 696 (1954).
28. Bertani, G., in *Brookhaven Symp. Biol.,* **8** *(Mutation),* 50-57 (1956).
29. Bertani, G., and Weigle, J. J., *J. Bacteriol.,* **65**, 113 (1953).
29a. Beumer, J., *Compt. rend. soc. biol.,* **142**, 847 (1948).
30. Beumer, J., *Ann. inst. Pasteur,* **84**, 15 (1953).
31. Beutner, E. H., *J. Bacteriol.,* **65**, 619 (1953).
31a. Bird, T. J., and Gots, J. S., *Bacteriol. Proc.,* p. 120 (Abstract) (1956).
32. Bonifas, V., and Kellenberger, E., *Biochim. et Biophys. Acta,* **16**, 330 (1955).
33. Bordet, P., *Rev. immunol.,* **11**, 323 (1947).
34. Bordet, P., *Compt. rend. soc. biol.,* **142**, 257 (1948).
34a. Bordet, P., and Beumer, J., *Bull. acad. roy. med. Belg.,* **14**, 116 (1949).
35. Boyd, J. S. K., *J. Pathol. Bacteriol.,* **62**, 501 (1950).
36. Boyd, J. S. K., *Nature,* **173**, 1050 (1954).
36a. Boyd, J. S. K., *Nature,* **178**, 92 (1956).
37. Bradley, P. L., and Boyd, J. S. K., *J. Pathol. Bacteriol.,* **64**, 891 (1952).
38. Brenner, S., *Proc. Natl. Acad. Sci. U. S.,* **41**, 862 (1955).
39. Brenner, S., *Biochim. et Biophys. Acta,* **18**, 531 (1955).
40. Brown, E. R., Cherry, W. B., Moody, M. D., and Gordon, M. A., *J. Bacteriol.,* **69**, 590 (1955).
41. Bryson, V., Skaar, P. D., Davidson, H., Hadden, J., and Bompiani, G., *Ann. Rept. Biol. Lab., L. I. Biol. Assoc., Cold Spring Harbor,* 16-22 (1955).
42. Bryson, V., and Szybalski, W., *Advances in Genet.,* **7**, 1 (1955).
43. Burnet, F. M., and Lush, D., *Australian J. Exptl. Biol. Med. Sci.,* **14**, 27 (1936).
44. Calef, E., and Cavalli Sforza, L. L., *Ricerca sci.,* **25** (Suppl.), 123-127 (1955).
45. Cavalli-Sforza, L. L., *Boll. ist. sieroterap. milan.,* **29**, 281 (1950).
46. Cavalli, L. L., *Bull. World Health Organization,* **6**, 185 (1952).
47. Cavalli Sforza, L. L., and Calef, E., *Ricerca sci.,* **25** (Suppl.), 129-135 (1955).
48. Cavalli, L. L., and Heslot, H., *Nature,* **164**, 1057 (1949).
49. Cavalli-Sforza, L. L., and Jinks, J. L., *Proc. 9. Intern. Congr. Genet. (Caryologia* **6**, suppl.), Pt. II (1954).
50. Cavalli-Sforza, L. L., and Jinks, J. L., *J. Genet.,* **54**, 87 (1956).
51. Cavalli-Sforza, L. L., and Lederberg, J., *Proc. 6. Intern. Congr. Microbiol.* (Rome), *Rend. ist. super. sanità* (suppl.), 108-142 (1953).
52. Cavalli, L. L., Lederberg, J., and Lederberg, E. M., *J. Gen. Microbiol.,* **8**, 89 (1953).
52a. Cavalli, L. L., and Maccacaro, G. A., *Nature,* **166**, 991 (1950).
53. Chabbert, Y., *Ann. inst. Pasteur,* **79**, 51 (1950).

54. Clowes, R. C., and Rowley, D., *J. Gen. Microbiol.,* **11**, 27 (1954).
55. Clowes, R. C., and Rowley, D., *J. Gen. Microbiol.,* **11**, 250 (1954).
56. Clowes, R. C., and Rowley, D., *J. Gen. Microbiol.,* **12**, iv (Abstract) (1955).
57. Cohen, S. S., *J. Biol. Chem.,* **168**, 511 (1947).
57a. Cohen, G. N., *Ann. inst. Pasteur,* in press.
58. Cohen-Bazire, G., and Jolit, M., *Ann. inst. Pasteur,* **84**, 937 (1953).
59. Cook, M. K., Blackford, V. L., Robbins, M. L., and Paar, L. W., *Antibiotics & Chemotherapy,* **3**, 195 (1953).
60. Corey, A., and Stuart, J. W., *Bacteriol. Proc.,* p. 50 (1956).
61. Davis, B. D., *J. Bacteriol.,* **60**, 507 (1950).
62. Davis, J. S., Winterscheid, L. C., Hartman, P. E., and Mudd, S., *J. Histochem. Cytochem.,* **1**, 123 (1953).
63. de Carlo, M. R., Sarles, W. B., and Knight, S. G., *J. Bacteriol.,* **65**, 53 (1953).
64. de Haan, P. G., *Genetica,* **27**, 293 (1954).
65. de Haan, P. G., *Genetica,* **27**, 300 (1954).
66. de Haan, P. G., *Genetica,* **27**, 364 (1955).
67. DeLamater, E. D., *Cold Spring Harbor Symposia Quant. Biol.,* **16**, 381 (1951).
68. DeLamater, E. D., *Proc. 6. Intern. Congr. Microbiol.* (Rome), *Rend. ist. super. sanità* (suppl.), 108-135 (1953).
69. DeLamater, E. D., *Intern. Rev. Cytol.,* **2**, 158 (1953).
70. DeLamater, E. D., *Bull. Torrey Botan. Club,* **80**, 289 (1953).
71. DeLamater, E. D., and Hunter, M. E., *J. Bacteriol.,* **65**, 739 (1953).
72. DeLamater, E. D., Hunter, M. E., and Mudd, S., *Exptl. Cell Research,* **3** (Suppl. 2), 319-343 (1952).
73. Demerec, M., *Am. Naturalist,* **84**, 5 (1950).
74. Demerec, M., *Genetics,* **36**, 585 (1951).
75. Demerec, M., *Am. Naturalist,* **89**, 5 (1955).
76. Demerec, M., *Cold Spring Harbor Symposia Quant. Biol.* **21**, in press.
77. Demerec, M., *Carnegie Inst. Wash. Publ.,* No. 612, pp. 1-4.
77a. Demerec, M., et al., *Carnegie Inst. Wash. Yearbook,* **55**: in press.
78. Demerec, M., Blomstrand, I., and Demerec, Z. E., *Proc. Natl. Acad. Sci. U. S.,* **41**, 359 (1955).
79. Demerec, M., and Demerec, Z. E., *Brookhaven Symposia Biol.,* **8** *(Mutation),* 75-87 (1956).
80. Demerec, M., and Fano, U., *Genetics,* **30**, 119 (1945).
81. Demerec, M., Hartman, P. E., Moser, H., Kanazir, D., Demerec, Z. E., Fitz-Gerald, P. L., Glover, S. W., Lahr, E. L., Westover, W. E., and Yura, T., *Carnegie Inst. Wash. Yearbook,* **54**, 219 (1955).
82. Demerec, M., and Hartman, Z., *Carnegie Inst. Wash. Publ.,* No. 612, pp. 5-33.
83. Demerec, M., Labrum, E. L., Galinsky, I., Hemmerly, J., Berrie, A. M. M., Hanson, J., Blomstrand, I., and Demerec, Z., *Carnegie Inst. Wash. Yearbook,* **52**, 210 (1953).
84. Demerec, M., Hoser, H., Hemmerly, J., Blomstrand, I., Demerec, Z. E., Fitz-Gerald, P. L., Glover, S. W., Hanson, J. F., Nielsen, F. J., and Yura, T., *Carnegie Inst. Wash. Yearbook,* **53**, 225 (1954).
85. Demerec, M., Wallace, B., Witkin, E. M., and Bertani, G., *Carnegie Inst. Wash. Yearbook,* **48**, 154 (1949).
86. Demerec, M., Witkin, E. M., Catlin, B. W., Flint, J., Belser, W. L., Dissosway, C., Kennedy, F. L., Meyer, N. C., and Schwartz, A., *Carnegie Inst. Wash. Yearbook,* **49**, 144 (1950).
87. Dianzani, M. U., and Vegni, L., *Boll. ist. sieroterap. milan.,* **30**, 123 (1951).

88. Duijn, C. van Jr., *Microscope,* **9**, 29 (1952).
89. Edwards, P. R., Davis, B. R., and Cherry, W. B., *J. Bacteriol.,* **70**, 279 (1955).
90. Ehrlich, H. L., and Knight, S. G., *Nature,* **168**, 658 (1951).
91. Ehrlich, H. L., and Watson, D. W., *J. Bacteriol.,* **58**, 627 (1949).
92. Eisenstark, A., Goldberg, S. S., and Bernstein, L. B., *J. Gen. Microbiol.,* **12**, 402 (1955).
92a. Eisenstark, A., and Kirchner, C., *Rec. Genetics Soc. Amer.,* **25**, 640 (1956).
93. Ferguson, W. W., Juenker, A., and Ferguson, R. A., *Am. J. Hyg.,* **62**, 306 (1955).
94. Florey, H. W., Chain, E., Heatley, N. G., Jennings, M. A., Sanders, A. G., Abraham, E. P., and Florey, M. E., *Antibiotics,* Vol. **I**, pp. 518-536, Oxford Univ. Press, London (1949).
95. Franklin, R., *Biochim. et Biophys. Acta,* **13**, 137 (1954).
96. Fredericq, P., *Rev. belge pathol. et méd. exptl.,* **19** (Suppl. 4), 1-107 (1948).
97. Fredericq, P., *Comp. rend. soc. biol.,* **143**, 1011 (1949).
98. Fredericq, P., *Compt. rend. soc. biol.,* **143**, 1014 (1949).
99. Fredericq, P., *Antonie van Leeuwenhoek J. Microbiol. Serol.,* **16**, 41 (1950).
100. Fredericq, P., *Compt. rend. soc. biol.,* **144**, 437 (1950).
101. Fredericq, P., *Compt. rend. soc. biol.,* **144**, 439 (1950).
102. Fredericq, P., *Bull. acad. roy. méd. Belg.,* **15**, 491 (1950).
103. Fredericq, P., *Compt. rend. soc. biol.,* **144**, 1137 (1950).
104. Fredericq, P., *Compt. rend. soc. biol.,* **144**, 1707 (1950).
106. Fredericq, P., *Compt. rend. soc. biol.,* **145**, 930 (1951).
107. Fredericq, P., *Compt. rend. soc. biol.,* **145**, 1433 (1951).
108. Fredericq, P., *Antonie van Leeuwenhoek J. Microbiol. Serol.,* **17**, 227 (1951).
109. Fredericq, P., *Compt. rend. soc. biol.,* **146**, 154 (1952).
110. Fredericq, P., *Compt. rend. soc. biol.,* **146**, 298 (1952).
111. Fredericq, P., *Bull. soc. chim. biol.,* **34**, 415 (1952).
112. Fredericq, P., *Compt. rend. soc. biol.,* **146**, 1295 (1952).
113. Fredericq, P., *Compt. rend. soc. biol.,* **146**, 1624 (1952).
114. Fredericq, P., *Rev. belge pathol. méd. exptl.,* **22**, 167 (1952).
115. Fredericq, P., *Compt. rend. soc. biol.,* **147**, 357 (1953).
116. Fredericq, P., *Compt. rend. soc. biol.,* **147**, 533 (1953).
117. Fredericq, P., *Compt. rend. soc. biol.,* **147**, 1113 (1953).
118. Fredericq, P., *Compt. rend. soc. biol.,* **147**, 2046 (1953).
119. Fredericq, P., *Ann. inst. Pasteur,* **84**, 294 (1953).
120. Fredericq, P., *Rev. méd. (Liège),* **8**, 456 (1953).
121. Fredericq, P., *Compt. rend. soc. biol.,* **148**, 399 (1954).
122. Fredericq, P., *Compt. rend. soc. biol.,* **148**, 624 (1954).
123. Fredericq, P., *Compt. rend. soc. biol.,* **148**, 746, (1954).
124. Fredericq, P., *Compt. rend. soc. biol.,* **148**, 1276 (1954).
125. Fredericq, P., *Compt. rend. soc. biol.,* **148**, 1501 (1954).
126. Fredericq, P., *Rev. méd. (Liège),* **9**, 150 (1954).
127. Fredericq, P., *Compt. rend. soc. biol.,* **149**, 840 (1955).
128. Fredericq, P., *Ann. soc. roy. sci. méd. et nat. Bruxelles,* **8**, 15 (1955).
128a. Fredericq, P., *Compt. rend. soc. biol.,* **149**, 2028 (1955).
128b. Fredericq, P., *Compt. rend. soc. biol.,* in press.
129. Fredericq, P., and Betz-Bareau, M., *Compt. rend. soc. biol.,* **145**, 1436 (1951).
130. Fredericq, P., and Betz-Bareau, M., *Ann. inst. Pasteur,* **83**, 283 (1952).
131. Fredericq, P., and Betz-Bareau, M., *Compt. rend. soc. biol.,* **147**, 1653 (1953).
132. Fredericq, P., and Betz-Bareau, M., *Compt. rend. soc. biol.,* **147**, 2043 (1953).
133. Fredericq, P., and Betz-Bareau, M., *Compt. rend. soc. biol.,* **148**, 1274 (1954).

134. Fredericq, P., and Delcour, G., *Compt. rend. soc. biol,* **147**, 1310 (1953).
135. Fredericq, P., and Gratia, A., *Compt. rend. soc. biol.,* **143**, 560 (1949).
136. Fredericq, P., and Gratia, A., *Antonie van Leeuwenhoek J. Microbiol. Serol.,* **16**, 119 (1950).
137. Freeman, V. J., *J. Bacteriol.,* **61**, 675 (1951).
138. Freeman, V. J., and Morse, I. U., *J. Bacteriol.,* **63**, 407 (1952).
139. French, R. C., and Siminovitch, L., *Can. J. Microbiol.,* **1**, 757 (1955).
140. Fried, P. J., and Lederberg, J., *Genetics,* **37**, 582 (Abstract) (1952).
141. Fukumi, H., Nojima, T., and Sayama, E., *Japan. J. Med. Sci. Biol.,* **8**, 135 (1955).
141a. Furness, G., and Rowley, D., *J. Gen. Microbiol.,* **12**, v (Abstract) (1955).
142. Garen, A., and Zinder, N. D., *Virology,* **1**, 347 (1955).
143. Goebel, W. F., Barry, G. T., Jesaitis, M. H., and Miller, E. M., *Nature,* **176**, 700 (1955).
144. Goebel, W. F., Barry, G. T., and Shedlovsky, T., *J. Exptl. Med.,* **103**, 577 (1956).
145. Goldstein, A., and Smoot, J. S., *J. Bacteriol.,* **70**, 588 (1955).
146. Goodgal, S. H., *Biochim. et Biophys. Acta,* **19**, 333 (1956).
148. Gots, J. S., Bird, T. J., and Mudd, S., *Biochim. et Biophys. Acta,* **17**, 449 (1955).
149. Gots, J. S., and Hunt, G. R., Jr., *J. Bacteriol.,* **66**, 353 (1953).
150. Gots, J. S., Koh, W. Y., and Hunt, G. R., Jr., *J. Gen. Microbiol.,* **11**, 7 (1954).
151. Gratia, A., *Compt. rend. soc. biol.,* **93**, 1040 (1925).
152. Gratia, A., *Ann. inst. Pasteur,* **48**, 413 (1932).
153. Groman, N. B., *Science,* **117**, 297 (1953).
154. Groman, N. B., *J. Bacteriol.,* **66**, 184 (1953).
155. Groman, N. B., *J. Bacteriol.,* **69**, 9 (1955).
156. Groman, N. B., and Eaton, M., *J. Bacteriol.,* **70**, 637 (1955).
157. Haas, F., Wyss, O., and Stone, W. S., *Proc. Natl. Acad. Sci. U. S.,* **34**, 229 (1948).
157a. Halbert, S. P., *J. Immunol.,* **58**, 153 (1948).
158. Halbert, S. P., and Gravatt, M., *Public Health Repts. (U. S.),* **64**, 313 (1949).
159. Halbert, S. P., and Magnuson, H. J., *J. Immunol.,* **58**, 397 (1948).
160. Halbert, S. P., and Swick, L. S., *Am. J. Ophthalmol.,* **35**, 73 (1952).
160a. Hamon, Y., *Ann. inst. Pasteur,* **88**, 193 (1955); *Compt. rend. acad. sci.,* **242**, 1240 (1956).
161. Hartman, P. E., *Carnegie Inst. Wash. Publ.,* No. 612, pp. 36-61.
162. Hartman, P. E., and Payne, J. I., *J. Bacteriol.,* **68**, 237 (1954).
163. Hartman, P. E., Payne, J. I., and Mudd, S., *J. Bacteriol.,* **70**, 531 (1955).
164. Hartman, Z., *Carnegie Inst. Wash. Publ.,* No. 612, in press.
165. Hatano, M., *J. Bacteriol.,* **71**, 121 (1956).
166. Hayes, W., *Nature,* **169**, 118 (1952).
167. Hayes, W., *Nature,* **169**, 1017 (1952).
168. Hayes, W., *Cold Spring Harbor Symposia Quant. Biol.,* **18**, 75 (1953).
169. Hayes, W., *J. Gen. Microbiol.,* **8**, 72 (1953).
170. Heatley, N. G., and Florey, H. W., *Brit. J. Exptl. Pathol.,* **27**, 378 (1946).
171. Herriott, R. M., *J. Bacteriol.,* **61**, 752 (1951).
172. Herriott, R. M., and Barlow, J. L., *J. Gen. Physiol.,* **36**, 17 (1952).
173. Hershey, A. D., *Virology,* **1**, 108 (1955).
174. Hershey, A. D., and Chase, M., *J. Gen. Physiol.,* **36**, 39 (1952).
175. Hewitt, L. F., *J. Gen. Microbiol.,* **7**, 362 (1952).
176. Hewitt, L. F., *J. Gen. Microbiol.,* **11**, 261 (1954).

177. Hewitt, L. F., *J. Gen. Microbiol.*, **11**, 272 (1954).
178. Hewitt, L. F., *J. Gen. Microbiol.*, **11**, 288 (1954).
178a. Hirota, Y., *Nature*, **178**, 141 (1956).
179. Holloway, B. W., *J. Gen. Microbiol.*, **13**, 572 (1955).
180. Hotchkiss, R. D., *J. Cell. Comp. Physiol.*, **45** (Suppl. 2), pp. 1-22 (1955).
181. Hotchkiss, R. D., in *Enzymes: Units of Biological Structure and Function* (O. H. Gaebler, ed.), pp. 119-130, Academic Press, New York (1956).
182. Hotchkiss, R. D., and Marmur, J., *Proc. Natl. Acad. Sci. U. S.*, **40**, 55 (1954).
183. Hughes, I. M., and Gots, J. S., *Bacteriol. Proc.*, p. 48 (Abstract) (1954).
184. Huppert, J., and Panijel, J., *Compt. rend. acad. sci.*, **238**, 1168 (1954).
185. Ionesco, H., *Compt. rend. acad. sci.*, **237**, 1794 (1953).
185a. Iseki, S., *Japan. J. Genet.*, **30**, 262 (1955).
185b. Iseki, S., and Kashiwagi, K., *Proc. Japan. Acad.*, **31**, 558 (1955).
186. Iseki, S., and Sakai, T., *Proc. Japan. Acad.*, **29**, 121 (1953).
187. Iseki, S., and Sakai, T., *Proc. Japan. Acad.*, **29**, 127 (1953).
188. Iseki, S., and Sakai, T., *Proc. Japan. Acad.*, **30**, 143 (1954).
188a. Iseki, S., and Sakai, T., *Proc. Japan. Acad.*, **30**, 1001 (1954).
189. van Iterson, W., *Proc. 6th Intern. Congr. Microbiol.*, (Rome) *Rend. ist. super sanità* (Suppl.), 24-38 (1953).
190. Ivánovics, G., and Alföldi, L., *Nature*, **174**, 465 (1954).
191. Jacob, F., *Compt. rend. acad. sci.*, **234**, 2238 (1952).
192. Jacob, F., *Ann. inst. Pasteur*, **86**, 149 (1954).
193. Jacob, F., *Virology*, **1**, 207 (1955).
194. Jacob, F., Siminovitch, L., and Wollman, E., *Compt. rend. acad. sci.*, **233**, 1500 (1951).
195. Jacob, F., Siminovitch, L., and Wollman, E., *Ann. inst. Pasteur*, **83**, 295 (1952).
196. Jacob, F., Siminovitch, L., and Wollman, E. L., *Ann. inst. Pasteur*, **84**, 313 (1953).
197. Jacob, F., and Wollman, E. L., *Cold Spring Harbor Symposia Quant. Biol.*, **18**, 101 (1953).
198. Jacob, F., and Wollman, E., *Compt. rend. acad. sci.*, **239**, 317 (1954).
199. Jacob, F., and Wollman, E. L., *Ann. inst. Pasteur*, **87**, 653 (1954).
200. Jacob, F., and Wollman, E. L., *Compt. rend. acad. sci.*, **240**, 2566 (1955).
201. Jacob, F., and Wollman, E.-L., *Ann. inst. Pasteur*, **88**, 724 (1955).
202. Jacob F., and Wollman, E. L., *Compt. rend. acad. sci.*, **242**, 303 (1956).
203. Jacob, F., Wollman, E. L., and Hayes, W., *Cold Spring Harbor Symposia Quant. Biol.*, **21**, in press.
204. Jenkin, C. R., and Rowley, D., *Nature*, **175**, 779 (1955).
205. Jinks, J. L., *Nature*, **170**, 106 (1952).
206. Kaiser, A. D., *Virology*, **1**, 424 (1955).
207. Kauffmann, F., *Enterobacteriaceae*, Ejnar Munksgaard, Copenhagen (1951).
208. Kauffmann, F., *Acta Pathol. Microbiol. Scand.*, **33**, 409 (1953).
209. Kellenberger, E., *Proc. 6th Intern. Congr. Microbiol.* (Rome) *Rend. ist. super sanità*, (suppl.), 45-66 (1953).
210. Labrum, E. L., *Proc. Natl. Acad. Sci. U. S.*, **39**, 280 (1953).
211. Lark, K. G., and Maaløe, O., *Biochim. et Biophys. Acta*, **15**, 345 (1954).
212. Latarjet, R., and Fredericq, P., *Virology*, **1**, 100 (1955).
213. Lederberg, E. M., *Genetics*, **37**, 469 (1952).
214. Lederberg, E. M., *Genetics*, **39**, 978 (Abstract) (1954).
215. Lederberg, E. M., *Genetics*, **40**, 580 (Abstract) (1955).
216. Lederberg, E. M., and Lederberg, J., *Genetics*, **38**, 51 (1953).

217. Lederberg, J., *Genetics,* **32**, 505 (1947).
218. Lederberg, J., *Physiol. Revs.,* **32**, 403 (1952).
219. Lederberg, J., *Science,* **122**, 920 (1955).
220. Lederberg, J., *Proc. Natl. Acad. Sci. U. S.,* **35**, 178 (1949).
221. Lederberg, J., *Genetics,* **35**, 119 (Abstract) (1950).
222. Lederberg, J., in *Genetics in the Twentieth Century* (L. C. Dunn, ed.), pp. 263-289, MacMillan Co., New York (1951).
223. Lederberg, J., *J. Bacteriol.,* **61**, 549 (1951).
224. Lederberg, J., *Science,* **114**, 68 (1951).
225. Lederberg, J., *Genetics,* **39**, 978 (Abstract) (1954).
226. Lederberg, J., in *Perspectives and Horizons in Microbiology* (S. Waksman, ed.), pp. 24-39, Rutgers University Press, New Brunswick (1955).
227. Lederberg, J., *J. Cell. Comp. Physiol.,* **45** (Suppl. 2), 75-107 (1955).
228. Lederberg, J., *J. Bacteriol.,* **71**, 497 (1956).
229. Lederberg, J., Cavalli, L. L., and Lederberg, E. M., *Genetics,* **37**, 720 (1952).
230. Lederberg, J., and Edwards, P. R., *J. Immunol.,* **71**, 232 (1953).
231. Lederberg, J., Lederberg, E. M., Zinder, N. D., and Lively, E. R., *Cold Spring Harbor Symposia Quant. Biol.,* **16**, 413 (1951).
232. Lederberg, J., and Stocker, B. A. D., *Genetics,* **40**, 581 (Abstract) (1955).
233. Lederberg, J., and Tatum, E. L., *Cold Spring Harbor Symposia Quant. Biol.,* **11**, 113 (1946).
234. Lederberg, J., and Tatum, E. L., *Science,* **118**, 169 (1953).
235. Lehman, I. R., and Herriott, R. M., *Federation Proc.,* **13**, 249 (Abstract) (1954).
236. Lennox, E. S., *Virology,* **1**, 190 (1955).
237. Lennox, E. S., Pers. commun. of results by Charles Yanofsky, E. Lennox, and Christina M. Richards (1956).
238. Levine, P., and Frisch, A. W., *J. Infectious Diseases,* **57**, 104 (1935).
239. Levine, P., and Frisch, A. W., *J. Immunol.,* **30**, 63 (1936).
240. Lieb, M., *J. Bacteriol.,* **65**, 642 (1953).
241. Lieb, M., Weigle, J. J., and Kellenberger, E., *J. Bacteriol.,* **69**, 468 (1955).
242. Lilleengen, K., *Acta Pathol. Microbiol. Scand.,* **77** (Suppl.), pp. 68, 75-76 (1948).
243. Loutit, J. S., *Nature,* **176**, 74 (1955).
244. Luria, S. E., *Cold Spring Harbor Symposia Quant. Biol.,* **11**, 130 (1946).
245. Luria, S. E., *Cold Spring Harbor Symposia Quant. Biol.,* **18**, 237 (1953).
246. Lwoff, A., *Bacteriol. Revs.,* **17**, 269 (1953).
247. Lwoff, A., in *Perspectives and Horizons in Microbiology* (S. Waksman, ed.), pp. 12-23, Rutgers University Press, New Brunswick (1955).
248. Maaløe, O., and Lark, K. G., *Colston Papers,* **7**, 159 (1954).
249. Maccacaro, G. A., *Nature,* **176**, 125 (1955).
250. Maccacaro, G. A., and Booth, C. P., *Nature,* **169**, 196 (1952).
251. Mackal, R., Koppelman, R., and Evans, E. A., Jr., *Federation Proc.,* **13**, 257 (Abstract) (1954).
252. Manninger, R., and Nogradi, A., *Experientia,* **4**, 276 (1948).
253. Manten, A., and Rowley, D., *J. Gen. Microbiol.,* **9**, 226 (1953).
254. Marcovich, H., *Ann. inst. Pasteur,* **90**, 303, 458 (1956).
255. Marmur, J., and Fluke, D. J., *Arch. Biochem. and Biophys.,* **57**, 506 (1955).
256. McClintock, B., *Brookhaven Symposia Biol.,* **8** *(Mutation)* 58-74 (1956).
256a. Monod, J., in *Enzymes: Units of Biological Structure and Function* (O. H. Gaebler, ed.), pp. 7-28, 135, Academic Press, New York (1956).
257. Morse, M. L., *Genetics,* **39**, 984 (Abstract) (1954).

258. Morse, M. L., *Genetics*, **40**, 586 (Abstract) (1955).
259. Morse, M. L., Lederberg, E. M., and Lederberg, J., *Genetics*, **41**, 142 (1956).
259a. Morse, M. L., Lederberg, E. M., and Lederberg, J., *Genetics*, in press.
260. Mudd, S., *Ann. Rev. Microbiol.*, **8**, 1 (1954).
261. Mudd, S., Hillier, J., Beutner, E. H., and Hartman, P. E., *Biochim. et Biophys. Acta*, **10**, 153 (1953).
261a. Murphy, J. S., and Gosney, R. L., Jr., *J. Exptl. Med.*, **98**, 657 (1953).
262. Nakaya, R., Uchida, H., and Fukumi, H., *Japan. J. Med. Sci. Biol.* **5**, 467 (1952).
263. Nelson, T. C., *Genetics*, **36**, 162 (1951).
264. Nelson, T. C., and Lederberg, J., *Proc. Natl. Acad. Sci. U. S.*, **40**, 415 (1954).
265. Newcombe, H. B., and Nyholm, M. H., *Am. Naturalist*, **84**, 457 (1950).
266. Newcombe, H. B., and Nyholm, M. H., *Genetics*, **35**, 603 (1950).
267. Nicolle, P., and Hamon, Y., *Ann. inst. Pasteur*, **81**, 614 (1951).
268. Nicolle, P., Jude, A., and Diverneau, G., *Ann. inst. Pasteur*, **84**, 27 (1953).
269. Nojima, T., and Fukumi, H., *Japan. J. Med. Sci. Biol.*, **7**, 385 (1954).
270. Nojima, T., and Fukumi, H., *Japan. J. Med. Sci. Biol.*, **8**, 15 (1955).
271. Ozeki, H., *Carnegie Inst. Wash. Publ.*, No. 612, in press.
272. Panijel, J., and Huppert, J., *Compt. rend. acad. sci.*, **238**, 745, 1452, 2465 (1954).
273. Panijel, J., and Huppert, J., *Compt. rend. acad. sci.*, **242**, 199; *Ann. inst. Pasteur*, **90**, 619 (1956).
274. Parry, W. R., and Edwards, J., *J. Gen. Microbiol.*, **9**, 342 (1953).
275. Parsons, E. I., *Proc. Soc. Exptl. Biol. Med.*, **90**, 91 (1955).
276. Parsons, E. I., and Frobisher, M., Jr., *Proc. Soc. Exptl. Biol. Med.*, **78**, 746 (1951).
277. Parsons, E. I., and Frobisher, M., *Am. J. Public Health*, **43**, 269 (1953).
278. Payne, J. I., Hartman, P. E., Mudd, S., and Liu, C., *J. Bacteriol.*, **70**, 540 (1955).
279. Puck, T. T., in *Dynamics of Virus and Rickettsial Infections* (F. W. Hartman, F. L. Horsfall, Jr., and J. G. Kidd, eds.), pp. 16-29, Blakiston, New York (1954).
280. Quadling, C., and Stocker, B. A. D., *J. Gen. Microbiol.*, **14**, i (Abstract) (1956).
280a. Quadling, C., and Stocker, B. A. D., *Heredity*, **10**, 123 (Abstract) (1956).
281. Robinow, C. F., in *The Bacterial Cell* by R. J. Dubos, Addendum pp. 353-377, Harvard University Press, Cambridge (1945).
282. Rothfels, K. H., *Genetics*, **37**, 297 (1952).
283. Ryan, F. J., Fried, P., and Mukai, F., *Biochim. et Biophys. Acta*, **18**, 131 (1955).
284. Sakai, T., and Iseki, S., *Gunma J. Med. Sci.*, **2**, 235 (1953).
285. Sakai, T., and Iseki, S., *Gunma J. Med. Sci.*, **3**, 195 (1954).
286. Seiffert, W., *Med. Klin. (Munich)*, **19**, 833 (1923).
287. Sertic, V., *Centr. Bakteriol. Parasitenk.*, **I 110**, 125 (1929).
288. Shimizu, E., *Gunma J. Med. Sci.*, **4**, 19 (1955).
288a. Skaar, P. D., *Proc. Natl. Acad. Sci. U. S*, **42**, 245 (1956)
289. Skaar, P. D., and Garen, A., *Genetics*, **40**, 596 (Abstract) (1955).
290. Spilman, W., Baron, L. S., and Formal, S. B., *Bacteriol. Proc.*, p. 51 (Abstract) (1955)
291. Stahl, F. W., *Virology*, **2**, 206 (1956).
292. Starlinger, P., and Kaudewitz, F., *Naturforsch.*, **11b**, 317 (1956).
293. St. Lawrence, P., *Proc. Natl. Acad. Sci. U. S.*, **42**, 189 (1956).

294. Stocker, B. A. D., *J. Hyg.*, **47**, 398 (1949).
295. Stocker, B. A. D., *J. Gen. Microbiol.*, **12**, 375 (1955).
296. Stocker, B. A. D., *Heredity*, **9**, 290 (Abstract) (1955).
297. Stocker, B. A. D., in *Symposia Soc. Gen. Microbiol.*, **6** *(Bacterial Anatomy)*, 19-40 (1956).
298. Stocker, B. A. D., Zinder, N. D., and Lederberg, J., *J. Gen. Microbiol.*, **9**, 410 (1953).
299. Streisinger, G., *Virology*, **2**, 1 (1956).
300. Szybalski, W., *Ann. Rept. Biol. Lab., Long Island Biol. Assoc.*, 27-31 (1954).
301. Szybalski, W., *Antibiotics Annual, 1954-1955*, 174-177 (1955).
302. Tatum, E. L., *Cold Spring Harbor Symposia Quant. Biol.*, **11**, 278 (1946).
303. Tatum, E. L., and Lederberg, J., *J. Bacteriol.*, **53**, 673 (1947).
304. Ting, R. C. Y., and Plough, H. H., *Radiation Research*, **3**, 354 (Abstract) (1955).
305. Tomcsik, J., *Schweiz. Z. allgem. Pathol. u. Bakteriol.*, **13**, 616 (1950).
306. Treffers, H. P., Spinelli, V., and Belser, N. O, *Proc. Natl. Acad. Sci. U. S.*, **40**, 1064 (1954).
307. Tulasne, R., and Vendrely, R., *Nature*, **160**, 225 (1947).
308. Uetake, H., Nakagawa, T., and Akiba, T., *J. Bacteriol.*, **69**, 571 (1955).
309. Wagner, R. P., and Mitchell, H. K., *Genetics and Metabolism*, John Wiley & Sons, New York (1955).
310. Wahl, R., *Ann. inst. Pasteur*, **84**, 51 (1953).
311. Wahl, R., *Ann. inst. Pasteur*, **86**, 729, 589 (1954).
312. Watson, J. D., and Hayes, W., *Proc. Natl. Acad. Sci. U. S.*, **39**, 416 (1953).
313. Weidel, W., *Ann. inst. Pasteur*, **84**, 60 (1953).
314. Weidel, W., *Cold Spring Harbor Symposia Quant. Biol.*, **18**, 155 (1953).
315. Weigle, J. J., and Bertani, G., *Ann. inst. Pasteur*, **84**, 175 (1953).
316. Weigle, J. J., and Delbruck, M., *J. Bacteriol.*, **62**, 301 (1951).
317. Whitfield, J. F., *J. Bacteriol.*, **70**, 125 (1955).
318. Whitfield, J. F., and Murray, R. G. E., *Can. J. Microbiol.*, **1**, 216 (1955).
319. Whitfield, J. F., and Murray, R. G. E., *Can. J. Microbiol.*, **2**, 245 (1956).
319a. Williams, M. A., and Rittenberg, S. C., *Bacteriol. Proc.*, p. 36 (Abstract) (1955).
320. Williams Smith, H., *J. Hyg.*, **46**, 74, 82 (1948).
321. Witkin, E. M., *Cold Spring Harbor Symposia Quant. Biol.*, **16**, 357 (1951).
322. Witkin, E. M., and Fetherston, T. H., *Carnegie Inst. Wash. Yearbook*, **51**, 198 (1952).
323. Witkin, E. M., and Lacy, A. M., *Carnegie Inst. Wash. Yearbook*, **53**, 241 (1954).
324. Witkin, E. M., and Thomas, C. T., *Carnegie Inst. Wash. Yearbook*, **54**, 234 (1955).
325. Wollman, E. L., *Ann. inst. Pasteur*, **84**, 281 (1953).
326. Wollman, E. L., and Jacob, F., *Compt. rend. acad. sci.*, **239**, 455 (1954).
327. Wollman, E. L., and Jacob, F., *Compt. rend. acad. sci.*, **240**, 2449 (1955).
328. Yanofsky, C., *J. Bacteriol.*, **65**, 383 (1953).
329. Yura, T., *Carnegie Inst. Wash. Publ.*, No. 612, pp. 63-75.
330. Zamenhof, S., *J. Bacteriol.*, **49**, 413 (Abstract) (1945).
331. Zamenhof, S., *Progr. Biophys. and Biophys. Chem.*, **6**, 85 (1956).
332. Zelle, M. R., and Lederberg, J., *J. Bacteriol.*, **61**, 351 (1951).
333. Zinder, N. D., *Cold Spring Harbor Symposia Quant. Biol.*, **18**, 261 (1953).
334. Zinder, N. D., *J. Cell. Comp. Physiol.*, **45** (Suppl. 2), 23-49 (1955).
335. Zinder, N. D., and Lederberg, J., *J. Bacteriol.*, **64**, 679 (1952).

Dr. Kalckar: I have a non-aggression pact with Dr. Lederberg not to make schemes, circles or models from what I am going to present. It will just be hard irreducible facts. Perhaps I will be tempted once in a while to talk about the keyboard of a piano, but I will try to do it pianissimo.

Through a fortunate collaboration with Lederberg's group, Dr. Kiyoshi Kurahashi, who at present is working in our laboratory, has put to use some methods which we have designed for studying cellular galactose metabolism, including a class of human galactose-negative mutants comprising a human hereditary metabolic disease called congenital galactosemia. (Kalckar, H. M., Anderson, E. P., and Isselbacher, Kurt J., *Biochimica et Biophysica Acta,* **20**, 262 (1956)). Morse and the Lederbergs have found that a particular lysogenic phage of K12, λ, is able to transduce hereditary units concerned with galactose-metabolism. Morse and Lederberg have described the various galactose negative strains (cf. Morse, Lederberg, E., Lederberg, J.—*Genetics,* in press) in a large paper which is almost a monograph. A few words about the biochemical steps involved. Leloir discovered that the inversion of galactose to glucose takes place on a uridine nucleotide. The equation is simply: UDPG-galactose $\rightleftharpoons$ UDP-glucose. We have isolated the enzyme which catalyzes the incorporation of phosphorylated galactose (a-galactose-1-phosphate or simply PGal) into uridine nucleotide. This incorporation enzyme we call PGal-uridyl transferase, or simply PGal transferase. The inversion enzyme, Galwaldenase, was also purified. (Maxwell E., unpubl. studies (1956)). The steps can be summarized as follows in which URP-PG signifies uridine diphosphoglucose and URP-PP uridine triphosphate.

I	$ATP + Gal \rightarrow ADP + PGal$	Gal kinase (Gal phosphorylation)
II	$PGal + URP\text{-}PG \rightleftharpoons PG + URP\text{-}PGal$	PGal-uridyl transferase (PGal incorporation)
III	$URP\text{-}PGal \rightleftharpoons URP\text{-}PG$	Gal-Waldenase (Gal inversion)
IV	$PP + URP\text{-}PG \rightleftharpoons PG + URP\text{-}PP$	P-G release (PG release)

In human hereditary galactosemia steps I, III and IV are present but step II is either totally absent or in one case present in amounts about 5 per cent of normal; this was studied in erythrocyte lysates as well as in extracts of liver microbiopsies (Anderson, E. P., Kalckar, H. M., and Isselbacher, Kurt, J., unpubl. studies (1956)). We have also studied other tissues and cells but this topic actually touches the problem of differentiation and we will drop that here.

I hope that Dr. Lederberg will elaborate on the genetic intricacies of the story of transduction in *E. coli* K12, which is definitely not my field in spite of my graduation from the Delbrück phage course in 1945.

I shall only mention the features most necessary for what I have in mind bringing up here. According to Morse, Lederberg and Lederberg, strains listed in the table are characterized as follows: The Gal-negatives of the numbers 1, 4, 6 and 7 give, when combined (and this is recombination with λ) mainly Gal-negative strains plus a very low percentage of gal-positive recombinants. They must, therefore, constitute a tune of small intervals when 'played' on the genetic 'keyboard'. Gal-negative number 2 yields by transduction recombination with either 1, 4 or 6 mainly galactose-negative strains, but also at a low percentage gal-positive recombinants. Dr. Kurahashi (K. Kurahashi, *Science*, in press) has shown that the methods outlined for mammalian cell lysates also work well in extracts (prepared by grinding or mechanical vibration) of *E. coli*. The methods seem to constitute a sensitive and specific tool for mapping of the genes concerned with the above-mentioned metabolic steps of galactose metabolism. As will appear from the table 1, Gal-negatives 1, 4, 6, and 7, which are blocks

TABLE 1

THE DISTRIBUTION OF THE GALACTOSE-METABOLIZING
ENZYMES IN *E. coli* MUTANTS

Strains	Kinase	Gal-1-P Trans.	PP Trans.	Waldenase
Gal + (W3100)	+	+	+	+
Gal$_1$ − (W3091)	+	−	+	+
Gal$_2$ − (W3092)	−	+	+	+
Gal$_4$ − (W3094)	+	−	+	+
Gal$_6$ − (W3096)	+	−		+
Gal$_7$ − (W3097)	+	−		+
(W3142)	−	+	+	+

in closely linked alleles, have a block of the same step enzyme. This turns out to be PGal transferase. Conversely the Gal-negative number 2 strain has plenty of this enzyme but lacks the galactokinase which is present in 1, 4 and 6. I encouraged Dr. Kurahashi to make hybrid extracts, i.e., to mix an extract from, let us say, mutant number 1 with an extract from mutant number 2. Such a recombined enzyme mix should be able to bring about incorporation of free galactose into nucleotide. By making hybrid extracts between 1 and 2, and tracking down the incorporation of C^{14} galactose into nucleotides by a method recently developed by us (Anderson and Kalckar, unpubl.), he could show that free galactose can in fact again be metabolized. Strain 1 provides the Gal kinase and strain 2 the PGal transferase.

Table 2 summarizes some of these experiments and some of the controls. It should be emphasized that a mixture of extracts of mutants blocked on genes involved in the synthesis of the same enzyme did not give a significant amount of counts in the nucleotide fractions.

Another strain, W3142, which Morse and the Lederbergs describe as being blocked in a gene further away from the above-mentioned cluster, was found to be galactokinase-negative.

I am especially intrigued with an idea of trying to study incomplete enzymes in hereditary blocks. We have tried to see whether in hereditary galactosemia PGal transferase may have preserved the ability

TABLE 2

GALACTOSE-1-C^{14} INCORPORATED INTO UDPG BY MIXED EXTRACTS OF *E. coli* MUTANTS

Gal + (W3100)	+	−	−	−	−	—	−	−	—	−	—
Gal$_1$ − (W3091)	−	+	−	−	−	+	−	+	+	−	−
Gal$_2$ − (W3092)	−	−	+	−	−	+	+	−	−	+	−
Gal$_4$ − (W3094)	−	−	−	+	−	−	+	+	−	−	+
(W3142)	−	−	−	−	+	−	−	−	+	+	+
Cpm × 10^{-3} of UDPGal formed	33.9	0	0	0	0	37.6	29.6	0	36.2	0	39.8

to exchange PGal with URP-PGal but lost its ability to exchange with the other group, i.e., PGal versus URP-PG. Apparently both activities are lost in the human Gal-mutant. It would be interesting to study the same properties in the Lederberg strains as well as to make attempts to characterize the inactive proteins immunologically, especially the extracts from recombined Gal negative strains.

The lack of incorporation in mixtures of extracts from mutants defective in the same enzyme have served, as just mentioned, as useful controls. The outcome here might be very different if the biological activities of the broken cell preparations were preserved by special measures. What I mean to say is that one should encourage attempts to mix protoplast preparations or other types of lysates which are still capable of synthesizing proteins including PGal transferase. Lysates from strains blocked in an identical enzyme might contain incomplete fragments of the same enzyme which when put together might make the enzyme operate naturally again. Such events might be dismissed as a too unlikely possibility. However, sensitive biochemical assays are now at hand. Moreover, Lederberg has just developed an elegant new technique for obtaining active protoplasts (Lederberg, PNAS, in press). We must first of all remain unprejudiced and not be over duly impressed by predictions about expected stabilities or instabilities, or we shall miss great opportunities.

DR. HARTMAN: It is of interest that, in so far as the limited data overlap, the biochemical data presented by Dr. Kalckar agree perfectly with the genetic results of Morse and the Lederbergs. One way we can test for these "cistrons" is through diploidization of a small chromosomal segment linked with *lambda* prophage or, in sexual recombination, by diploidization of larger regions of the chromosome. As mentioned briefly in my talk, a second method, by which only the critical *trans* configuration may be detected, utilizes abortive transduction (see reference **271**).

Transducing phage, prepared on *non*-allelic mutants or on wild-type bacteria, produces minute colonies in addition to the large colonies composed of true genetic recombinants and characteristic of most intra-locus and inter-locus tests. On the other hand, phage prepared on *allelic* mutants, presumably blocked in the production of the same enzyme, gives no abortive transductions (minute colonies) in *intra*-locus tests. While exceptions to this latter situation have been found, it may be that in these exceptions we are dealing with two or more adjacent loci which more refined analyses will show to differ bio-chemically. The abortive transduction test is applicable to all series of biochemical mutants so far thoroughly examined, including the histidine mutants depicted in my figure 5 (Demerec, et al. 1956 *Carnegie Inst. Wash. Yearbook 55:* In press). There is striking agreement between results with the abortive transduction test and grouping by other transduction methods.

DR. LURIA: I would like to present some data of Lennox that bear on the matter of the amount of genetic material of a bacterial cell that may be transduced by one bacteriophage particle. Using phage P1 and *E. coli* K-12, and examining the well-mapped region of threonine-arabinose-lysine-valine resistance and azide resistance, Lennox finds that all these characters can be transduced by a single particle but the frequency of joint transduction decreases in the same direction as the map distance increases. The frequency of transduction decreases rather slowly as the size of the transduced region increases from *Ara* to *Val*, but much faster when it increases to include *T* or *Az*. The maximum coincidence of transduction has been found to be not more than 1 in 1,000 for the whole region *T* to *Az*. From the work of Drs. Wollman, Jacob, and Hays, there is now a way of measuring quite accurately the proportion of the total bacterial genome that the trans-ductal region encompasses, and it turns out to be somewhere between 1% and 2%. Assuming that the bacterium has on the average two nuclei, that the nuclei are the source of the transduced DNA, and that a single bacteriophage particle has an amount of DNA of the order of 1% that of the bacterial cell, it turns out that the maximum fraction of genetic material that can be transferred by a single phage particle—and this very rarely—is of the same order of magnitude as the fraction of lost DNA that could fit a normal phage particle.

DR. KING: I was just observing the activity of an enzyme lambda waldenase. As you know, the wild type which is found in Greece is always the levo lambda. However, when it is subjected to the action of an enzyme it is converted into the dextro lambda. I have noticed two things: first, there is a very high activity of lambda waldenase here; second, I think that the levo form, the one that occurs in the wild state in Greece, is essentially unstable with respect to the dextro lambda, because all the lambdas that I have seen this morning have been dextro lambda.

DR. LEDERBERG: Would Dr. King define his terms?

DR. KING: λ (levo lambda), ⅄ (dextro lambda).

GENETIC ASPECTS OF LYSOGENY

François Jacob and Elie L. Wollman

Service de Physiologie Microbienne, Institut Pasteur, Paris

Introduction

About six years ago, after a decade of eclipse, the attention of
biologists was drawn back to lysogeny by the work of A. Lwoff. Since
that time, lysogenic bacteria have received considerable attention.
As a matter of fact, they constitute a rather unique example of
healthy cells carrying indefinitely the potentiality of producing viruses.
In lysogenic bacteria, the genetic material of the virus behaves as a
cell constituent endowed with genetic continuity and appears to be
incorporated into the genetic make-up of the host. Lysogeny offers,
therefore, the first experimental evidence in favor of a direct relationship between a cellular gene-like structure and a virus.

Various aspects of lysogeny have been recently reviewed (21, 24, 43).
The present paper aims to recall briefly the general properties of
lysogenic bacteria and to discuss in more detail recent information
which throws some light upon the state of the viral material in
lysogenic bacteria and its relationship with the host bacterium.

The Prophage

It is now well established that bacteria of certain strains are able
to release bacteriophage in the absence of any infection by external
particles. These bacteriophages can be detected through their ability
to multiply on certain other strains of bacteria which are sensitive to
their action. The phages released by lysogenic bacteria are called
temperate phages and they possess a very important property, absent
in virulent phages: temperate phages are able to establish new lysogenic systems, that is, to lysogenize sensitive, previously non-lysogenic
bacteria. When such sensitive bacteria are infected with temperate
phage particles, a certain fraction of the infected bacteria lyses and
liberates phage, but another fraction survives, becomes lysogenic, and
gives rise to lysogenic progeny. Each of their descendants remains
indefinitely able to produce phage, and the phage particles released

by such clones are, in all respects, identical to the one used for the initial infection. Lysogenic clones arising by infection cannot be distinguished from lysogenic strains isolated from natural sources.

Every bacterium of a lysogenic population gives rise to a lysogenic clone, that is, produces cultures in which phage particles can be detected. However, in a lysogenic population, most of the bacteria do not release phages. Phages are produced only by a small fraction of the bacteria and are liberated by bacterial lysis (44).

One is faced, therefore, with the problem of how phage material is propagated in lysogenic bacteria. What happens to a phage which, by infection of a sensitive bacterium, gives rise to a lysogenic system, and which, after many bacterial generations, can reappear as infective particles liberated by the progeny of the original bacterium? No infectious particles can be found by disrupting lysogenic bacteria (9). One is led therefore to conclude that lysogenic bacteria do not contain mature phage particles, but instead must possess a non-infectious unit which carries the information necessary for the production of phage particles. Every individual of a lysogenic population has to contain at least one of these units, for which the term *prophage* has been coined (44). The prophage can be visualized as a non-pathogenic state of the phage whose replication is coordinated with the division of the host and which provides the host with the information necessary for the synthesis of phage particles.

Obviously, any attempt to elucidate the problem of lysogeny requires better knowledge of these specific units endowed with genetic continuity. It is necessary to know how the presence of the prophages can be recognized, what is their composition, and how many of them are present in a bacterium. We intend to describe here the experimental evidence which affords a partial answer to these questions. More specifically, evidence pertaining to the location of prophages within bacteria, as well as their relationships with other cell constituents, will be discussed.

To begin with, we shall summarize the properties of lysogenic bacteria which express phenotypically the presence of a prophage.

Expressions of Lysogeny

Lysogenic bacteria differ from the corresponding non-lysogenic bacteria by two properties. The first one is the *capacity to produce phage.* Since phage production is a lethal process, which results from the development of the prophage, it remains in lysogenic bacteria as a potential character at the bacterial level. The second property of lysogenic bacteria is their *immunity* against the phage they are able to release (homologous phage): upon infection with homologous phage, lysogenic bacteria survive and the infecting particles do not multiply. Immunity may be expressed in every bacterium of a lysogenic population. Indeed, it represents the phenotypic expression of the prophage in the lysogenic system.

These two characters, which allow one to detect the presence of a prophage, will now be considered in turn.

Phage Production.

Spontaneous production. During the exponential multiplication of lysogenic bacteria, the number of free phage particles increases proportionally to the number of bacteria. It can be demonstrated that phage particles are not secreted by living and multiplying bacteria, but are released by the lysis of a small number of bacteria (44). The probability of phage production per bacterium per generation time is rather low, from 10^{-2} to 10^{-5}, and, under given cultural conditions, is constant for a given lysogenic strain. When lysing, a lysogenic bacterium releases the same number of phage particles as a sensitive bacterium infected with the same phage.

Induced production. Phage production occurs spontaneously in an apparently random manner within a few individuals of a lysogenic population. The factors which elicit the spontaneous production of virus particles are unknown. In some strains, the probability of phage production cannot be modified. In other strains it can be increased up to nearly unity by exposing cultures of such lysogenic strains to various agents, as observed by Lwoff, Siminovitch, and Kjeldgaard (46).

This process, called *induction,* is under the control of at least three factors (21, 43). First of all, induction requires the exposure of lysogenic bacteria to the action of an *inducing agent.* Most of the agents which elicit prophage development are known to exhibit mutagenic or carcinogenic activity in other systems. Ultraviolet light (UV) has been the most commonly used. Analysis of UV-induced phage production by lysogenic bacteria carrying two different, but related, prophages has led to the conclusion that prophage development does not result from a direct change in the prophage itself, but from an indirect effect mediated through the bacterium (21). It is not surprising, therefore, that the *physiological conditions* of the bacterial population control the efficiency of the inducing shock. Finally, the existence of a *genetic factor* is shown by the fact that only certain lysogenic systems are inducible. As a rule, inducibility behaves as a property of the prophage, not of the bacterium. The presence of an inducible prophage confers upon its host an increased sensitivity to the lethal action of the inducing agents.

Under suitable conditions, phage production can be initiated in every bacterium of a lysogenic population, even though infective particles could not have been detected, had the bacteria been disrupted before exposure to the inducing agent. Induction therefore demonstrates that the prophage can express its potentiality in every bacterium of a lysogenic population. It thus permits the study of lysogeny, and more especially, of phage development in the absence of infection. This approach has shown that, after exposure of lysogenic bacteria to inducing agents, the features of phage multiplication follow the same steps as infection of sensitive bacteria with the homologous phage (24, 43). Phage production by lysogenic bacteria appears as a consequence of a shift from the prophage, whose replication is balanced with the division of the host, to the so-called vegetative phage, which is not balanced but actively multiplying and in the process of being converted into mature particles.

Immunity.

The presence of the prophage also confers upon its host bacterium the remarkable property of resistance to the infection by homologous phage. This immunity is established against all the mutants of the homologous phage, with the exception of a special class of mutants which, for this reason, have been called virulent (24, 27). As a rule, lysogenic bacteria are able to adsorb the homologous phage particles. Such a superinfection does not alter bacterial growth or division. The genetic material of the superinfecting particles penetrates the bacteria, but does not multiply. It behaves as if it were an inert particle and is diluted out in the course of bacterial multiplication (7, 21). However, the superinfecting phage can enter the vegetative phase and multiply in those bacteria in which prophage develops, either spontaneously or after induction. When lysogenic bacteria, for example, are first induced with ultraviolet light and then superinfected with a mutant of the homologous phage, both types of particles are released upon lysis (24).

Capacity to produce phage and immunity constitute the two criteria by which the presence of a prophage can be detected. When the prophage is lost, both properties disappear. Since phage production results from a disturbance in the equilibrium of the prophage-bacterium system, immunity represents the only permanent expression of the prophage. One may imagine a situation in which the presence of a prophage can be detected only through bacterial immunity, phage particles never being produced. Such conditions are almost completely fulfilled in the case of the so-called defective lysogenic strains which result from mutations of the prophage.

PROPHAGE MUTATIONS

Mutations are known which affect various properties of temperate phages. They occur during vegetative multiplication. Many of these mutations have also been found to occur in homologous prophages.

Among the mutations which can affect the prophage, some are of particular interest because they result in the production of the so-called *defective lysogenic strains*. Such strains can be isolated among the survivors of normal lysogenic bacteria which have been exposed to heavy doses of ultraviolet light. In cultures of these defective lysogenic bacteria, few, if any, infective particles can be detected. After UV induction, the whole of the population lyses in the same manner as a normal lysogenic population, but a very small fraction of the lysed bacteria—10^{-7} or less—produces phage (3, 29). Nevertheless, the lysogenic character of these defective bacteria is clearly demonstrated by the fact that they exhibit the same immunity pattern as their normally lysogenic ancestor. In this case, the expression of the lysogenic character remains lethal for the host, but is not accompanied by the release of infectious particles. Further, if it should happen that defective bacteria are not able to adsorb the homologous phage, their immunity pattern cannot be tested. Obviously, if one were not aware of the origin of such bacteria, their lysogenic character would hardly be recognized.

Genetic analysis of such strains has shown that the defective character can be ascribed to prophage mutations which disturb functions necessary for phage production (29). After UV induction, prophage development is initiated, but the prophage lesion prevents the completion of infectious particles. The rare cases of phage production are due to back mutation of the defective prophage gene to the wild-type allele. The defective mutation can be mapped on the prophage linkage group and it appears that mutations at different loci of the prophage result in alterations of different steps of phage synthesis and morphogenesis (29). With defective lysogenic bacteria, we have therefore a remarkable situation in which the phage genetic material can be indefinitely perpetuated only in the prophage state because lethal alleles prevent phage production. Here, expression of lysogeny results in the disappearance of both the host and the virus. The study of such defective strains might be expected to provide valuable information concerning the genetic determinism and physiology of phage synthesis and morphogenesis.

The Nature of the Prophage

The prophage exhibits the same fundamental genetic properties as the homologous phage. It is endowed with genetic continuity. It can mutate. Furthermore, genetic recombination has been shown to occur among prophages, as will be discussed later. The prophage must therefore contain, in part or in totality, the genetic material of the homologous phage. From experiments of Hershey and Chase (18), it is apparent that the DNA of an infectious phage, but very little or none of its protein, enters the bacterium upon infection. Phage DNA seems, therefore, to possess all the information necessary for the bacterium to make complete phage particles. By definition, the prophage of a lysogenic bacterium is endowed with the same property. Immunological studies have shown that lysogenic bacteria do not contain any known antigen of the homologous phage (48). It seems reasonable, for the time being, to consider that the prophage is made essentially of DNA. No difference has yet been observed between the chemical composition of the DNA of a temperate phage and that of the host bacterium (43).

One may wonder how much of the phage DNA corresponds to the prophage. This seems to be a rather difficult question, because as more information about phage becomes available, the more difficult it is to determine what fraction of the DNA of the phage actually corresponds to its genetic material. On the one hand, it seems that in the T-even phages, only a fraction of the total DNA could constitute the genetic core (40). On the other hand, it is clear from transduction experiments (55) that pieces of DNA which, as far as we can say, seem to have nothing to do with the phage material, can be included within the coat of a temperate phage. For the time being, it is not possible to estimate the relative size of the prophage.

A rather puzzling problem is to know what constitutes the difference between the "physiological" unit, the prophage, whose replication is balanced with that of the host, and the vegetative phage, which brings about the destruction of the host. Such a difference in the behavior of the two types of particles can hardly be ascribed to a difference in the *nature* of the genetic material, but rather in its *activity*. In a lysogenic bacterium, the prophage, presumably composed of DNA, replicates in harmony with the host cell. As far as we know, phage proteins are not synthesized. During the vegetative phase, not only does the phage genetic material replicate at high speed, but phage proteins are also produced. These are the only differences so far known between the lysogenic and the vegetative phases in the life cycle of a phage. It has been shown that the biosynthesis of a protein, such as a colicin, can be lethal (23). For the time being, there is no reason to ascribe the lethal action of the vegetative phage to the unbalanced multiplication of its DNA rather than to the synthesis of a protein.

THE NUMBER OF PROPHAGES

One cannot count directly the number of prophages present in a lysogenic bacterium. However, by a rather indirect method it is possible to estimate this number. The basis for this method rests on two facts. On the one hand, as previously shown, immunity of lysogenic bacteria disappears when the prophage enters the vegetative phase, either spontaneously or after induction. On the other hand, it is known that when bacteria are infected with different ratios of two mutant phages the same ratios are found in the progeny. If now, in lysogenic bacteria, the assumption is made that one prophage plays the same role in phage multiplication as an infecting particle, the number of prophages can be estimated in the following way: bacteria are induced with ultraviolet light, then superinfected with various known multiplicities of a mutant phage, and the composition of the bursts is analysed. If the basic assumption is correct, the number of prophages should be equal to that multiplicity of infection which allows a 1 : 1 ratio in the progeny. In this way, the average number of prophages has been found equivalent to the average number of nuclei per cell (24). An analogous result has also been observed with a non-inducible strain (7). Lysogenic bacteria seem, therefore, to contain one prophage per nucleus.

That a lysogenic bacterium contains a small number of prophages is also supported by the *incompatibility* between mutant prophages. It is known that when sensitive bacteria are successively exposed to the action of two or more *unrelated* temperate phages, lysogenic strains carrying multiple prophages, one of each type, can be isolated. In other words, the presence of one prophage does not alter the ability of a bacterium to be lysogenized with an unrelated temperate phage. The result is quite different, however, when sensitive bacteria are exposed successively to the action of two *mutants* of the same strain of temperate phage. As a rule, such bacteria carry only one type of prophage (6). Bacteria carrying two mutant prophages can occasionally be isolated (3, 7, 22). This incompatibility between mutant prophages indicates that a given type of prophage saturates a limited number of bacterial sites.

CHROMOSOMAL LOCATION OF THE PROPHAGE

If a bacterium is made lysogenic by infection with a temperate phage, it is clear, from the work previously described, that, on the one hand, the lysogenic character is hereditarily perpetuated in the progeny of this bacterium and that, on the other hand, phage is maintained in a non-infectious state, the prophage. Two questions therefore arise. The first one is whether or not the prophage represents the only genetic determinant of lysogeny. The second is the location of the prophage or, in other words, what are the specific bacterial structures which are present at a ratio of one per nucleus and which are saturated by a given type of prophage.

Answers to these questions have been gained through genetic recombination of bacteria. *Escherichia coli* K12 is lysogenic and carries a prophage called λ. However, non-lysogenic clones can be isolated (36). The genetic behavior of the lysogenic character can therefore be studied through crosses between lysogenic (ly^+) and non-lysogenic (ly^-) bacteria.

For a long time, bacterial recombination was restricted to crosses between different strains of *E. coli* K12, in which one recombinant is formed per million of each parental type. Such a low frequency of recombination makes difficult any quantitative work, but, in spite of this difficulty, the genetic analysis of λ lysogeny began with this system and has brought valuable information. In certain crosses, it was observed by Lederberg and Lederberg (38) and by Wollman (51) that the λ-lysogenic character segregates among recombinants and exhibits a strong linkage with another genetic character, galactose fermentation *(Gal)*. Such a result suggests that the lysogenic character is under the control of a nuclear determinant. That this nuclear determinant is the prophage itself is shown by the results of crosses involving two lysogenic strains, each one carrying a different mutant λ prophage. In such a cross, it was first observed by Appleyard (2) that the individual phage characters are linked to the galactose locus. These conclusions have been confirmed by transduction experiments in which pieces of genetic material derived from a λ-lysogenic (or non-lysogenic) donor were transferred, through a transducing phage, into a non-lysogenic (or lysogenic) recipient strain (22).

When opposite mating types F^+ and F^- were discovered in *E. coli* K12 (16, 37), it appeared that λ-lysogeny exhibited an asymmetrical behavior in reciprocal crosses between lysogenic and non-lysogenic bacteria (2, 51). Whereas the ly^- character of the F^+ parent is transmitted to recombinants when the F^- parent is lysogenic, the ly^+ character of the F^+ parent is almost never found among recombinants when the F^- parent is non-lysogenic. Moreover, abnormalities were also observed in the segregation pattern of the galactose character for which linkage with any other character was still unknown. Such a situation was therefore hardly compatible with the expected behavior of a nuclear determinant of lysogeny.

Although we are not primarily interested here in bacterial recombination, it seems necessary to summarize recent advances in this field because they are necessary for understanding the genetic determinism of lysogeny. Many of the difficulties preventing simple genetic mapping, which have been observed in $F^+ \times F^-$ crosses, can now be ascribed to two main causes. On the one hand, bacterial recombination is the result of a partial transfer of genetic material from the donor to the recipient parent (17). On the other hand, recombinants for nutritional characters cannot be formed by F^+ parents, but only by rare mutants arising spontaneously during the growth of F^+ populations (28). These mutants, called Hfr (for high frequency) are able to transfer with high frequency into F^- cells the characters located on a given segment O-R (Fig. 1) of the chromosome, but not characters located on other segments (17).

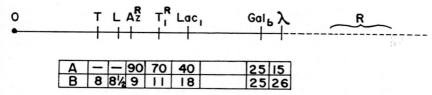

FIG. 1. *Diagrammatic representation of the chromosomal segment which can be transferred from the Hayes Hfr strain to F⁻ bacteria*

This segment carries the following markers: synthesis of threonine (T), leucine (L), resistance to Az (Az^r), to phage T1 ($T1^r$), utilization of lactose (Lac_1), of galactose (Gal_b), λ-lysogeny (λ). O represents the origin or leading locus, R the region of preferential rupture, beyond which no marker of the Hfr, such as resistance to streptomycin (S^r) is transferred to the F⁻ cells. In a cross Hfr $T^+ L^+ Az^s T_1^s Lac_1^+ Gal_b^+ (\lambda)^- S^s \times$ F⁻ $T^- L^- Az^r T_1^r Lac_1^- Gal_b^- (\lambda)^+ S^r$, each marker can be mapped in two ways: A represents the percentage of $T^+ L^+ S^r$ recombinants which carry each of the unselected Hfr markers; B represents the time at which each marker enters the F⁻ cell when the parents are mixed at time O. The distance of R to the genetic markers is unknown.

Experiments, in which the conjugation process between Hfr and F⁻ bacteria was interrupted and the mating pairs separated by agitation in a Waring blendor, have enabled a better understanding of the mating process (53, 54). The O-R segment of the Hfr chromosome is an organized structure containing a linear array of genes. These genes penetrate the F⁻ bacterium in a predetermined order, always the O extremity first, and at a rate slow enough so that the procedure can be interrupted at various times by mechanical treatment. The interruption of the mating process does not prevent the genetic fragment that has already entered the recipient cell from being integrated into a recombinant. In the normal process, spontaneous chromosome breakage can occur in such a way that the amount of the Hfr material transferred into the F⁻ cell varies from one mating pair to another. Bacterial conjugation can therefore be visualized as the injection of a segment carrying a limited number of linked genes, from an Hfr donor into a recipient F⁻ bacterium. In the Hayes Hfr strain (17), used for most of the genetic analysis of lysogeny which will be now summarized, the O-R segment which can be injected involves, among other known markers, the *Gal* and λ loci (Fig. 1).

Let us now examine the information about the determinism of λ-lysogeny which has been obtained from Hfr × F⁻ crosses. First of all, crosses between non-lysogenic strains allow an accurate determination of the linkage between the known markers of the O-R segment, as schematized in Fig. 1. Now, in crosses between non-lysogenic Hfr ly⁻ and lysogenic F⁻ ly⁺, the non-lysogenic ly⁻ character is transferred and segregates among recombinants in the same way as any other marker. It can be located at about 15 recombination units from Gal_b, at one extremity of the transferred segment (52, 54).

In crosses where both parental strains are lysogenic, each one carrying a different mutant λ prophage, the Hfr prophage segregates among recombinants in exactly the same manner as the non-lysogenic character of the previous cross, and the same linkage is found with the other markers (52, 54). From these results we can therefore conclude that the λ prophage occupies a definite position on the K12 linkage group and that, up to now, its behavior in bacterial crosses differs in no way from that of any other genetic marker.

The situation is quite different in reverse crosses between λ-lysogenic Hfr and non-lysogenic F⁻. Here, not only the λ prophage of the Hfr parent is almost never inherited by recombinants, but alterations in the frequency as well as in the genetic composition of recombinants are observed. These abnormalities are the consequences of a phenomenon designated as *zygotic induction* (25, 30).

ZYGOTIC INDUCTION

When lysogenic Hfr are mixed with non-lysogenic F⁻, a number of F⁻ bacteria, corresponding to about half of the input Hfr, lyse and release λ phage particles. Careful analysis of the phenomenon has shown that during the mating process half of the input Hfr cells inject into F⁻ cells a piece of chromosome carrying the prophage λ. The remaining half of the cells inject a shorter segment as a result of spontaneous breakage occurring before the penetration of the λ prophage. Each time the prophage λ enters a non-lysogenic cell, it develops and matures, thus bringing about lysis and destruction of the corresponding zygote. In crosses between Hfr cells infected with λ particles and F⁻ cells, the infecting phages are not transferred into F⁻ cells. In order to be transferred the phage material must be in the prophage state. Each time the prophage λ is transferred into F⁻ cells, it behaves as a lethal character which is immediately expressed (25, 30).

It is obvious that such a phenomenon must lead to distortions of the segregation pattern, since all the zygotes (50%) which have received a big piece of Hfr genetic material carrying *Gal* and λ are destroyed. The only ones (50%) which can survive and give rise to recombinants are those which have received a smaller piece without λ. A certain class of recombinants is therefore eliminated from the crosses. As a result, the more closely a character is linked to the λ-locus, the greater the probability that it will not appear in the recombinants (25, 54).

No similar phenomenon can be demonstrated in crosses involving a lysogenic F⁻ parent, whether or not the Hfr parent is lysogenic. Since no prophage development occurs when the F⁻ parent is lysogenic, in such crosses lysogeny does not lead to genetic distortions. Thus the presence of the prophage in the F⁻ cell confers upon the zygote an immunity against the development of an homologous prophage carried by the genetic piece injected by the Hfr parent. The chromosomal location of the prophage can therefore be demonstrated only when the F⁻ parent is lysogenic, but not in the reciprocal crosses (25, 30).

That lysogeny is under the control of a nuclear determinant and that the only nuclear determinant is the prophage itself, which is located at a specific site of the bacterial chromosome, is therefore unambiguously demonstrated by recombination and transduction experiments. However, when considering the phenomenon of zygotic induction, it is obvious that the prophage does not behave as a normal bacterial gene, since it develops when entering a non-lysogenic F⁻ cell.

Specific Locations of Various Prophages

Let us consider now the location of different prophages within the same host bacterium. It is known that after exposure to several unrelated temperate phages a bacterium is able to carry a wide variety of prophages. Although the compatibility between unrelated prophages suggests that each prophage occupies a different location inside the bacterium, only a genetic analysis makes it possible to check the hypothesis "one prophage, one locus." For this purpose, about 30 different temperate phages, acting on *E. coli* K12, have been isolated from various lysogenic strains. Among these phages, 7 UV-inducible and 7 non-inducible were selected for a genetic study, since cross-immunity was not observed between them (30).

For each prophage two kinds of information can be gained through crosses between lysogenic and non-lysogenic bacteria. On the one hand, when the F⁻ parent is lysogenic and the Hfr is not, the linkage between a prophage and other markers can be measured and, therefore, the location of the prophage on the bacterial linkage group can be accurately determined. On the other hand, when the Hfr parent is lysogenic and the F⁻ is not, one can determine whether or not the development of the prophage is induced by conjugation, and if zygotic induction occurs, one can measure the rate of induction, as well as the time at which the prophage penetrates the F⁻ cell.

Such experiments have been carried out for the 14 selected prophages. Completely different results were found according to whether or not the prophages are UV-inducible (30, 54).

UV-inducible Prophages.

By crosses between non-lysogenic Hfr and lysogenic F⁻, all the 7 UV-inducible prophages can be located on the segment of the bacterial linkage group included between *Gal* and the preferential rupture point *R* of the Hayes Hfr strain. Each of them occupies a definite position and can be mapped to this segment, as shown in Fig. 2, A.

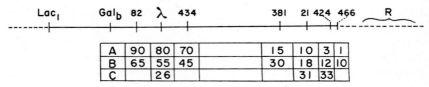

Fɪɢ. 2. *Diagrammatic representation of the Gal region carrying various UV-inducible prophages*

The following UV-inducible prophages: 82, λ, 434, 381, 21, 424, 466 can be located in this respective order on the segment stretching from *Gal*ᵦ to *R* on the Hayes Hfr strain. For each prophage three types of information can be obtained: A represents the percent of *Gal*ᵦ⁺ *ly*⁻ *S*ʳ recombinants in crosses Hfr *Gal*ᵦ⁺ *ly*⁻ *S*ˢ × F⁻ *Gal*ᵦ⁻ *ly*⁺ *S*ʳ. B represents the percent of input Hfr whose mating results in zygotic induction in crosses Hfr *ly*⁺ *S*ˢ × F⁻ *ly*⁻ *S*ʳ. C represents the time at which the prophage enters the F⁻ cell when the parents are mixed at time O. The 7 UV-noninducible prophages which have been studied are located on the segment beyond *R* of the same Hfr strain.

In crosses between lysogenic Hfr and non-lysogenic F⁻, the development of each inducible prophage is induced by conjugation. As a result, the lysogenic character of the Hfr parent is not transmitted to recombinants. However, the rate of zygotic induction—expressed as the percentage of input lysogenic Hfr whose conjugation leads to the lysis of the zygote and phage production—varies widely according to the prophage. The important point is that the rates of zygotic induction found for the various inducible prophages parallel closely their degree of linkage to galactose (Fig. 2, B). Consequently, in such crosses, the distortions produced by the presence of the various prophages in the transmission to recombinants of the most closely linked markers—*Gal, T6,* and *Lac*—follow the same gradient. It must be added that with other Hfr mutants (28) which do not inject the *Gal* region into F⁻ cells, but inject other segments of the bacterial chromosome, zygotic induction is not observed in crosses between Hfr *ly*⁺ and F⁻ *ly*⁻ (30). Finally, the inducible prophages may also be arranged in the same respective order, according to the time at which they enter the F⁻ cells during crosses between Hfr *ly*⁺ and F⁻ *ly*⁻ (Fig. 2, C).

All information gained through reciprocal crosses gives rise to the same conclusion. The 7 UV-inducible prophages are linearly disposed on the *Gal*-R segment of the Hfr bacterial chromosome. Each time a segment of the Hfr chromosome carrying one of the prophages is injected into non-lysogenic F⁻ bacteria, the prophage develops and the zygote is destroyed. The greater the distance of a given prophage from Gal_b, the less frequently it is transferred from Hfr to F⁻ bacteria, possibly because of the increased probability of an interruption in the mating process before the entrance of the prophage into the F⁻ cell. A prophage located close to Gal_b destroys more zygotes and hence produces a greater distortion in the segregation of genetic markers than one located far away from Gal_b.

Non-inducible Prophages.

With the 7 non-inducible prophages, the situation is quite different. None of them is located on the O-R segment of the Hayes Hfr strains. By the use of different Hfr mutants—those which are able to inject other segments of the bacterial linkage group—the non-inducible prophages have been located on other regions, most of them on the segment carrying the maltose, mannitol, and xylose characters. Moreover, none of these non-inducible prophages is induced by conjugation between lysogenic Hfr and non-lysogenic F⁻ bacteria. The lysogenic character is regularly transmitted to recombinants and exhibits the same segregation pattern as the non-lysogenic character in the reverse cross (30).

Such a genetic analysis of various lysogenic characters provides some information about the relationship of the prophage to the bacterium. First of all, each of the various prophages which have been studied occupies a definite locus on the bacterial linkage group. Second, and somewhat unexpectedly, it seems that there exist on the bacterial linkage group several "prophage regions"; the region for UV-inducible prophages is different from the region for non-inducible ones. Such a situation seems to indicate that UV-inducibility is not a property of the prophage, but rather is a property of a given segment of the bacterial chromosome where certain types of prophages are located. In other words, the inducible character of a prophage could be a consequence of its location on the bacterial chromosome and not a specific property of the prophage itself. Finally, in certain crosses, the inducible prophages, once transferred into the zygotes, behave as dominant lethal characters, the expression of which results in the destruction of the zygotes. In contrast, the non-inducible prophages behave in all crosses as any other bacterial character.

LYSOGENIZATION: THE TRANSITION FROM PHAGE TO PROPHAGE

When sensitive bacteria are infected with temperate phages, two different series of events may occur. In a certain fraction of the bacterial population, the infecting phage multiplies and the bacteria lyse. In the other fraction, the infecting particles turn to the prophage state and the bacteria survive. That such a difference in the bacterial response to phage infection is not due to a genetic heterogeneity of either the bacterial or the phage population is shown by the fact that various changes in the cultural conditions, before or after infection, can modify drastically the relative ratio of responses.

Thus, once it has entered a bacterium, the genetic material of a temperate phage has a choice between vegetative multiplication or integration as a prophage. From what is known about the specific location of a given prophage it is clear that, in order to become a prophage, the genetic material of a phage has to reach its specific locus on the bacterial chromosome, where, in some way or other, it becomes incorporated.

The Process of Lysogenization.

In standard conditions, a given temperate phage has a certain probability of becoming a prophage. As already pointed out, this probability can be widely modified by the physiological conditions. However, the study of various systems has shown that the factors which alter the rate of lysogenization differ from one phage-bacterium system to another. It can be either a change in the multiplicity of infection (8) or in temperature (7), or in the metabolism of the host (45). During the "period of choice," stretching from infection to either multiplication or lysogenization, the genetic material of the phage remains in an "intermediary" state. The evidence in favor of such a state stems from the study of the phage properties, which, during this period, differ from those found both in the vegetative and the prophage states (42).

As far as the transformation of phage material into prophage is concerned, it is worth inquiring whether the very material of the infecting particle, or a copy of it, is incorporated into the bacterial chromosome. This question is a particular aspect of a more general problem: do the parental genetic materials contribute their own atoms towards the synthesis of a recombinant chromosome in bacterial transformation, transduction, or recombination, as well as in phage recombination. Attempts to answer this question have been carried out by Stent and Fuerst (49), who have infected bacteria grown in non-radioactive medium with temperate phage λ containing P^{32}. Should the genetic material of the infecting particle itself be incorporated as prophage, then the lysogenic character of the new lysogenic bacteria ought to remain susceptible, at least until the first duplication, to the decay of P^{32} atoms introduced by the infecting phage. Such experiments have shown that, within a few minutes after infection, the lysogenic character becomes insensitive to P^{32} decay. Unfortunately, it has not yet been possible to determine the exact reason for such a rapid change in sensitivity to P^{32} decay. A rapid stabilization might occur either because (a) the prophage contains much less DNA than the free phage, (b) the genetic information is transferred to something else than a nucleic acid, or (c) the prophage is a DNA copy of the infecting phage.

GENETIC FACTORS CONTROLLING THE ABILITY OF A PHAGE TO BECOME A PROPHAGE

Only certain strains of phage, the temperate ones, are able to establish lysogenic systems. The ability of a phage to lysogenize is, therefore, genetically controlled. The plaques formed on sensitive bacteria by temperate phages exhibit a turbid center due to the growth of lysogenized bacteria. In a given strain of temperate phage, mutations

occur which modify lysogenization. Mutants in which the capacity
for lysogenization is decreased or lost form clear (*c*) plaques easy to
identify. The analysis of recombination between such mutants ought
therefore to bring information about factors controlling lysogenization.

Among temperate phages, λ has been the most extensively studied
from the genetic viewpoint (26, 32). Various mutations have been
identified, all of which can be mapped on a single linkage group
(Fig. 3). The irradiation of phage particles with small doses of ultraviolet light before infection increases the rate of recombination (27).
It is therefore possible to analyse accurately the recombination between closely linked markers.

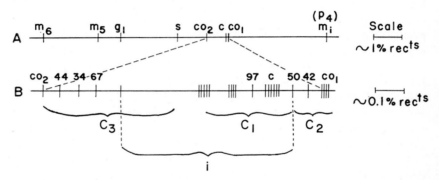

FIG. 3. *Diagrammatic representation of the* λ *linkage-group and its c region*

The upper diagram represents the linear array of the known markers of λ
(ref. 26 and 32). The lower diagram corresponds to a more detailed presentation
of the *c* region (ref. 33). The figures represent various *c* mutations, generally
arising by clusters. The *c* region can be subdivided into three segments c_1, c_2, and
c_3, which apparently correspond to three different functions required in the lysogenization process; *i* represents the segment which controls the immunity pattern.

Various mutations can affect the capacity for lysogenization. The
most important ones, which correspond to the *c* phenotypes, affect
the very process by which the phage is converted into prophage,
whereas other mutations seem to affect the stability of the prophage
in the course of bacterial multiplication. An extensive investigation
of the former has recently been undertaken by Kaiser (33). The *c*
mutants can be subdivided into three classes (*c₁*, *c₂*, *c₃*) according to
their phenotypes, that is, the degree of clearness of the plaques they
form. All of the *c* mutations are located on one segment of the λ
linkage group, this segment comprising about 1/15 of the total genetic

length (Fig. 3). The c_1 mutants, whose ability to lysogenize is not measurable (less than 10^{-5} that of the wild type) are all located in clusters in the median part of the c segment. On this c_1 segment are also located the virulent *(v)* mutations which overcome the immunity conferred by a λ prophage. Mutants of the c_2 and c_3 phenotypes, whose ability for lysogenization is only reduced to about 1/10 to 1/100 that of the wild type, are all located, also in clusters, respectively on c_2 and c_3 segments on each side of c_1 (Fig. 3).

An interesting point about these mutations is that, whereas infection of sensitive bacteria with a given c mutant type leads to little, if any, lysogenization, mixed infection with pairs of mutants belonging to different types *(c_1 + c_2, c_1 + c_3, or c_2 + c_3)* results in a rate of lysogenization equal to that of the wild type, and indicating a cooperation between the two mutants (33). Analogous results have been found independently with another phage-bacterium system (39).

It appears, therefore, that ability to lysogenize is controlled by a given region of the phage linkage group. At least three different functions, each being controlled by a different segment of this region, are involved in the lysogenization process. Alterations in the middle segment probably result in the loss, and alterations in one of the two other segments in the reduction, of the lysogenization ability. The fact that mutants of different types can cooperate for lysogenization would indicate that the series of reactions leading to the establishment of the prophage can occur even when the wild-type alleles are in *trans* position. Such an analysis seems to offer the most promising line of approach to the study of the various steps by which an infecting phage enters the prophage state.

Specificity of the Prophage-Bacterium Linkage

Each of the various temperate phages that a given bacterium can carry as prophages can be defined by two criteria: one, genetic, is the specific location of the prophage on the bacterial chromosome; the other, phenotypic, is the pattern of immunity it confers upon the host. These are indeed the two characteristics of each strain of temperate phages. After lysogenization with various mutants of a phage strain, the resulting prophages appear, on the one hand, to be located exactly at the same place, and on the other hand, to protect the host against infection with any mutant of this phage strain. So far the v mutants seem to offer the only exception to this rule.

The fact that there exists a specific location on the bacterial chromo-some for each type of prophage is indeed quite remarkable. It indicates some kind of relationship between the genetic material of a temperate phage and a given region of the bacterial chromosome. In other words, each strain of temperate phage possesses information allowing its genetic material to settle on its specific locus of the bacterial chromo-some. It appears important therefore to determine how this informa-tion is carried by the phage particle. Although a priori rather difficult, such an analysis has been made possible by the finding that a number of the different UV-inducible phages, which as prophages are differently located on the *Gal*-R segment of the Hayes Hfr (see Fig. 2), are serologically related. After mixed infection of sensitive bacteria with two of these phages, genetic recombination in the vegetative state can be observed (30).

It must be clearly stated that in a cross between two of these phages which are able to exchange certain genetic segments, each type can be individualized only through its immunity pattern. In other words, among the progeny of crosses betwen phages *a* and *b*, the particles of the *a* type, for instance, can be defined exclusively by their ability to form plaques on bacteria lysogenic for *b*, but not on bacteria lysogenic for *a*, and vice versa.

Since many mutations are known and have been mapped in λ (Fig. 3), crosses were carried out between λ and the other phages to which it is serologically related (34). It was found that most of the char-acters of λ, such as plaque size, plaque type, and even host range, located all along the λ linkage group, can be transferred into other phages, except the characters of the *c* region which are known to affect the lysogenizing ability of λ (Fig. 3). The length of the piece in which no recombination is found depends upon the strain of phage which is crossed with λ. With certain phages, this piece is a little longer than the whole *c* region. Hence none of the c_1, c_2, and c_3 markers of λ can be introduced into those phages. With other phage strains, the markers of the c_2 and c_3 region can be transmitted, but not those of the c_1 region (34). The different inducible phages seem, therefore, to be homologous for the major part of their linkage group, except for the *c* region. According to the criterion of immunity, a phage 434 which has received on the left arm of the linkage group all the characters of λ including co_2 (Fig. 3) and on the right arm all the characters of λ including co_1 still remains a 434.

The wild strains of inducible phages used in this study exhibit different immunity patterns, and the corresponding prophages have been located at different sites of the bacterial chromosome. From the previous study, it is clear that the specific immunity, which, for convenience, has been chosen as the test of identity for each phage type, is not under the control of the whole chromosome of this phage but of a short part, the c segment, which is known from other evidence to play a major role in lysogenization. Analogous experiments of phage recombination, in which the various segments of a given phage are gradually replaced by segments of another phage, allow one to determine the segment of the phage chromosome responsible for the specific location of the homologous prophage. Up to now, the results seem to indicate that the c region is also responsible for the location of the prophage. In other words, the prophage 434 having the right and left arms of λ, including co_1 and co_2, but the c_1 region of 434, appears to be located at the 434 site. More detailed analysis will permit us to determine whether or not the locus responsible for immunity can be dissociated from the locus responsible for prophage localization.

The Nature of the Prophage-Chromosome Attachment

The *Gal* region of the bacterial chromosome exhibits a rather peculiar property. It contains a whole series of loci, each of which can select, among a wide variety of phages, the homologous one, can bind it, and thus transform the genetic material of the phage into a prophage. It appears highly desirable to obtain some information about the nature of the bond which links the prophage to its specific bacterial site. Obviously, such a bond is of a special nature, since its formation as well as its breakage can, under suitable conditions, occur with an efficiency of almost 100 per cent. One still knows very little about the nature of this bond, but it constitutes one of the most interesting problems raised by the analysis of lysogeny. It therefore seems worthwhile to discuss the available information as well as the possible ways for obtaining additional evidences.

Addition or Substitution.

The first point is to determine whether a prophage represents a piece of phage material *added* in some way to the bacterial chromosome or one *substituted* for an allelic region of the chromosome present in a non-lysogenic bacterium. For the time being, this last hypothesis appears to be rather unlikely. It is known that in *E. coli,* for example, spontaneous loss of the prophage does not occur at a measurable rate. However, non-lysogenic clones have been obtained from lysogenic strains through various treatments, such as heavy irradiation with ultraviolet light or P^{32} decay. All the clones which are no longer lysogenic are sensitive to the phage released by the lysogenic ancestor. Moreover, infection of these non-lysogenic bacteria by this phage may lead to the establishment of new lysogenic clones, which are undistinguishable from the lysogenic ancestor. On the contrary, it has not been possible, thus far, to obtain lysogenic mutants from non-lysogenic bacteria by any treatment, except of course infection with a temperate phage. No prophage marker can be detected in those bacteria which have lost the lysogenic character. Lysogenization appears therefore to be the acquisition of the genetic material of a phage and the cure of lysogeny to be its loss. It seems likely that the prophage is a structure added in some manner to the bacterial genetic material rather than substituted for an homologous chromosomal segment present in a non-lysogenic cell.

Insertion or Attachment.

If now the prophage is actually an added piece, we have to determine the structural nature of the link tying the prophage to the chromosome. Is the prophage *inserted,* partly or as a whole, into the bacterial chromosome, or is it superimposed in some way on the chromosomal thread, to which it is *attached* at one or more points? Although at first sight rather difficult, it seems likely that an answer could be obtained from certain kinds of experimental evidence.

Bacterial recombination. The first evidence comes from crosses—or transduction—between two lysogenic strains, each of which carries a multiple mutant of the prophage (31). Among selected bacterial recombinants, some are found to carry a recombinant prophage. In order to check whether or not the prophage is in the continuity of the bacterial chromosome, the two bacterial strains have to differ by two other markers, one on each side of the prophage (Fig. 4). If the whole prophage is inserted into the length of the bacterial chromosome, any recombinant carrying a recombinant prophage will be a recombinant for these two bacterial markers (except for rare double cross-overs). If not, recombination of the prophage markers will be more or less independent of the recombination between the two bacterial markers.

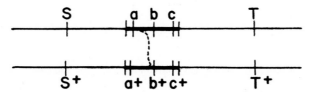

Fɪɢ. 4. *Theoretical representation of prophage recombination in bacterial crosses, according to the hypothesis of the prophages inserted in the bacterial chromosome.*

Each of the parental strains carries a mutant prophage, *abc* or a^+ b^+ c^+. The two bacterial strains also differ by a marker *S* on one side of the prophage and a second marker *T* on the other side. If the prophage is inserted in its totality, as schematized here, prophage recombination should result mostly from single cross-overs inside the prophage. A bacterial recombinant carrying a recombinant prophage should therefore be recombinant for the two markers *S* and *T*. In the experiment reported in Table 1, each of the bacterial strains carries a λ prophage which is genetically labelled by three markers m_1, *co*, and m_5 (*a*, *b* and *c*). The bacterial strains also differ by two characters, Gal_b (*S*) on the left of λ, and *21-lysogeny* (*T*) on the right of λ. The results are not in agreement with the complete insertion hypothesis.

Such an experiment has been performed by crossing Hfr and F⁻ strains, each one carrying a λ prophage labelled with three markers located along the λ linkage group (31). As shown in Table 1, preliminary results indicate that the various recombination patterns of the prophage are more independent of the bacterial recombination than the insertion hypothesis would predict, if prophage recombination is not the result of multiple crossing-over.

In such an experiment, as well as in transduction experiments (22), the λ prophage exhibits a polarity in the sense that the m_1 side of the λ linkage group (see Fig. 3) appears linked to *Gal*. For the time being, any interpretation of this apparent linkage would be premature.

P^{32} *decay.* The lethal action of radiophosphorus decay occurring in bacteria is the basis of another method for an analysis of the relationships of the prophage to the bacterial chromosome. As with phage (19), the decay of P^{32} incorporated into the genetic material of a bacterium destroys its ability to reproduce (14). Now, in the case of lysogenic bacteria, if the prophage were in some way independent of the bacterial chromosome, the killing effect of P^{32} decay should occur independently in each of the genetic materials. Among bacterial survivors of P^{32} decay, one would expect therefore to find non-lysogenic cells. If, on the contrary, the whole prophage were inserted into the bacterial chromosome, any P^{32} distintegration lethal for the prophage

TABLE 1

Recombination of λ Prophages in Crosses Between Two Lysogenic Bacteria

Types of prophage found in recombinants		Number found	
		In the class Gal^+ $(21)^+$	In the class Gal^+ $(21)^-$
Parental types	m_5 co^+ m_i^+ (Hfr type)	276	127
	m_5^+ co m_i (F⁻ type)	57	1
Recombinants	m_5^+ co^+ m_i^+	12	4
	m_5 co m_i	1	0
	m_5 co^+ m_i	3	2
	m_5^+ co m_i^+	1	0
	m_5 co m_i^+	2	0
	m_5^+ co^+ m_i	6	1
Doubly lysogenics	m_5 co^+ m_i^+ and m^+_5 co m_i	3	0
	m_5^+ co^+ m_i and m_5^+ co^+ m_i^+	1	0
	m_5 co^+ m_i and m_5 co^+ m_i^+	1	1

Results of a cross Hfr Gal_b^+ ($λ$ m_5 co^+ m_i^+)⁺ $(21)^-S^s$ × F⁻Gal_b^-($λ$ m_5^+ co m_i) ⁺(21) ⁺S^r. The prophage $λ$ is located at about 20 and the prophage 21 at about 90 recombination units from Gal_b (see Fig. 2). Bacterial recombinants are selected for the characters Gal_b^+ S^r. These recombinants are divided into two classes according to whether or not they are lysogenic for 21. 363 recombinants of the $Gal_b^+(21)^+$ class and 136 recombinants of the $Gal_b^+(21)^-$ class have been re-isolated twice on selective Gal S^r medium and then scored for the phage type they release. For the interpretation of the results, see legend, Fig. 3.

should also be lethal for the bacterium. According to such an hypothesis, one would not expect to find non-lysogenic cells among the bacterial survivors. This type of experiment has been performed with several lysogenic systems, some inducible, the others not (13). Preliminary results are rather different according to the nature of the system. With non-inducible prophages, non-lysogenic cells were not found among several hundred colonies at the survival level of 10^{-5}. On the contrary, with $λ$, or other inducible prophages, non-lysogenic cells were found, and their proportion increased as a function of P^{32} decay. When only one in 10^5 bacteria is still able to form a colony, the fraction of non-lysogenic cells can reach 15 to 20 per cent, a proportion much higher than the 1 or 2 per thousand found after an exposure of the same lysogenic bacteria to a dose of UV or x-rays leaving an identical fraction of survivors.

With non-inducible prophages, it is therefore clear that the fraction of prophage material, if any, which can be inactivated by P^{32} decay independently of the bacterial chromosome is very small. With inducible prophages, the situation is more difficult to interpret. That a selection of non-lysogenic cells, due to a difference to P^{32} decay between lysogenics and non-lysogenics, could account for the results is almost certainly excluded by reconstruction experiments. More difficult to eliminate for the time being is the supposition that the non-lysogenic bacteria arise from a fraction of the population in which prophage development had been induced by radiations and which, at the time of freezing, contain phage genetic material that has already left its chromosomal location and behaves as a unit independent of the chromosome. In order to account for the experimental results, such an hypothesis would require that, once the phage material has left its specific location, the bacterial chromosome is still able to undergo replication. This seems hardly compatible with the notion that a genetic unit as large as the genetic material of a temperate phage is inserted in its totality into the bacterial chromosome.

Relationships Between Closely Located Prophages.

Other interesting information comes from the study of lysogenic bacteria carrying two inducible prophages (34). By successive infections, one can easily obtain lysogenic bacteria carrying two prophages, such as λ and 21, which are not too closely located on the bacterial chromosome (Fig. 2). The situation is quite different with more closely located prophages, such as 82 and λ, or λ and 434 (Fig. 2). When lysogenic bacteria carrying one prophage, λ for example, are infected with 434, most of the surviving bacteria are found to have lost the original λ prophage and to carry only the 434 superinfecting type—or are no longer lysogenic. Only exceptionally can doubly lysogenic strains be isolated.

Now, whereas in crosses or transduction experiments involving singly lysogenic bacteria, the respective location of each single prophage can be determined, in experiments involving a doubly lysogenic strain, both types of prophage segregate together (34). Everything therefore occurs as if, besides their individual link to the bacterial chromosome, both prophages were attached together and behaved as a single unit in bacterial recombination.

In a lysogenic strain carrying two closely located prophages, such as genetically labelled λ and 434, the released phages exhibit a recombination pattern rather different from the one observed after mixed infection of sensitive bacteria with the homologous phages. Among the phages released by doubly lysogenic strains, crossing-over in the c-m_5 region is much more frequent, and in the c-m_1 region less frequent than would be expected from the results of crosses after mixed infection (see Fig. 3). It is not yet possible to ascribe with certainty the recombination pattern observed in doubly lysogenic bacteria to a recombination at the prophage level. But if correct, this hypothesis would indicate some kind of asymmetry between the two prophages such that more opportunities for recombination would be offered to the m_5-c than to the c-m_1 arm of the prophages.

o

o   o

Although some information has thus been obtained concerning the prophage-chromosome relationship, it does not yet allow one to construct a clear picture of how the phage genetic material is tied to its specific locus. There are some indications that, at least in the case of UV-inducible prophages, the phage material is not inserted in its totality into the bacterial chromosome. Further work is necessary before a definite conclusion can be reached, but the various techniques previously described seem to offer possible ways of approach to the solution of this fundamental problem.

Host Modifications Resulting from the Presence of a Prophage

As already described, the lysogenization of sensitive bacteria endows the host with new properties, immunity and capacity to produce phage, which express the presence of the prophage. It is also known from the studies of Zinder and Lederberg (55) that, after infection with certain strains of temperate phages, rare individuals among the survivors acquire new genetic properties. Such changes in hereditary characters result from the transfer of genetic material from a donor to a recipient strain through phage particles which behave as vectors. This process, called transduction, is not specific in the sense that any character of the donor can be transmitted by a small fraction of the phage particles. Transduction will be reviewed in another paper of this symposium.

Other types of host modifications have, however, been reported which appear to be so entangled with the lysogenic character that they must be ascribed to the very presence of a given prophage. Such changes in character seem thus far to be specific and indicate the possibility for a prophage to alter some cellular functions.

The best studied case is the production of toxin by *Corynebacterium diphtheriae* (4, 12). Most of the toxinogenic strains are lysogenic and release phage particles, which are active on certain non-toxinogenic strains. The lysogenic clones which can be isolated after such an infection are all toxinogenic, and the toxinogenic character can be passed from strain to strain by lysogenization. A complete correlation is observed between lysogeny and toxinogeny. However, such a property appears to be restricted to certain strains of temperate phages of *C. diphtheriae*. Recent experiments even suggest that the ability to confer toxinogenicity segregates in crosses between related phages (15). Whether the presence of the suitable prophage induces the synthesis of a new protein or causes to deviate the synthesis of a protein normally present in non-toxinogenic bacteria still remains unsettled.

In other species, the presence of certain prophages can affect various properties of the host such as colonial morphology (20), synthesis of antigens (50), or multiplication of various unrelated phages (1). In *E. coli*, the presence of the λ prophage prevents the multiplication of certain *r* mutants of the T-even phages, and not of other mutants (5). This property is specific for λ and has not been observed with any of the other prophages of *E. coli* K12, even those located very close to λ. It can even be ascribed to the *c* segment of λ (34).

From what is known about the location of the prophage, it is not surprising that the presence of a new piece of genetic material intimately tied to the bacterial chromosome could modify certain characters of the host bacterium. It must be pointed out that we are now able to ascribe such modifications of the bacteria to the presence of a prophage, since we know how to reconstruct artificially such lysogenic systems and to follow the physiological change in the course of lysogenization. It seems therefore quite likely that some other characters of the host bacterium will be found to result from the presence of yet unknown prophage-like structures. It can be safely predicted that more extensive investigations in the field of lysogeny will lead to the discovery that some other changes in bacterial characters are indeed the consequence either of lysogenization or of loss of lysogeny.

PROPHAGE AS A MODEL FOR PROVIRUSES

In the scheme reported previously, lysogeny provides one of the most clear-cut pictures of a determinant added to the genetic make-up of a cell. As a result of such an addition, the host-bacterium and its progeny can be affected in three different ways. First of all, the bacteria can acquire the ability to produce and release phage particles under suitable conditions. Secondly, certain types of addition bring to the host a specific change in cellular functions. Finally, during genetic recombination, the added piece can modify drastically the fate of the zygote and thereby the genetic consequences of conjugation. In conclusion, let us consider in what way lysogeny can provide a model for similar situations observed in other organisms.

Lysogeny and the Problem of the Existence of Proviruses.

In lysogenic bacteria, a specific structure incorporated into the genetic make-up of the host can undergo transition into a pathogenic form, the development of which leads to the death of the host and the liberation of infectious virus particles. Obviously it is tempting to ascribe similar mechanisms to certain cases of "latent viruses" and of cancers, observed in plants or in animals. In other words, one may postulate in plants or in animals the existence of proviruses, analogous to the bacterial prophage. Such proviruses could be visualized as the genetic material of a virus under a non-infectious state, attached to a specific site of a host constituent so that its replication would remain balanced with the cell division. Such a possibility has recently been reviewed (21, 43). It must only be recalled that no evidence in favor of the existence of proviruses in the cells of animals or plants has so far been obtained. A provirus can be demonstrated only with single cells. Recent improvements in cell cultures should provide in the near future the tools for such an investigation.

The presence of a prophage on its chromosomal receptor may modify in a specific and hereditary manner the properties of a bacterium, as exemplified by toxinogenesis in *C. diphtheriae* (12). Thus, two cells, otherwise genetically identical, may exhibit different functional characters, as a consequence of the specific acquisition, by one of them, of an extra piece of genetic material. In maize, factors of unknown origin may apparently settle at various loci and alter gene activity in that region (47). It has already been suggested (11, 47) that such additions to the genome of a cell might be of some value for a possible model of cell differentiation, since recent work in embryology (35) suggests a nuclear basis for certain types of differentiation.

Zygotic Induction and Maternal Inheritance.

Inheritance of a character is said to be matroclinous when such a character is inherited only from the female parent. When a maternally inherited trait is persistent through several generations, this trait is generally considered as being under cytoplasmic control.

In the case of inducible prophages, the inheritance of lysogeny behaves in some ways as a maternally inherited character. In spite of various peculiarities observed in bacterial conjugation, the one-way transfer of genetic material may be compared to a sexual differentiation (17). The Hfr donor bacterium acts as a male gamete which contributes only its genetic material, whereas the F− recipient acts as a female gamete which contributes both its genetic material and cytoplasm to the zygote. In crosses between lysogenic and non-lysogenic bacteria, inducible prophages are inherited by the progeny only when the F− is the lysogenic parent. When carried by the Hfr, the prophage behaves in crosses as a lethal nuclear unit. This is still true when the Hfr parent carries a defective prophage, the induction of which, although lethal for the zygote, does not lead to the production of mature virus particles. If one considers only the zygotes in which the prophage is transferred, these zygotes are destroyed: the cross is sterile. Thus lysogenic bacteria offer a clear example of a nuclear determinant, the transmission of which behaves in a different manner in reciprocal crosses (30).

The question may therefore be raised whether situations of matrocliny in higher organisms could be ascribed to a similar mechanism. If we use phage as a model, we can assume that viral material may be present in a cell in three different states: the provirus, vegetative, and infectious states. The vegetative state may or may not be lethal. The provirus may or may not have a phenotypic expression. According to the various combinations, the development of the proviral material upon fertilization when carried by the male gamete may bring about two kinds of genetic consequence. (1) When the vegetative state has a phenotypic expression, the transition of the provirus into vegetative virus through induction may result either in the destruction of the zygote, that is, lethality, or, as the case may be, in a wide variety of symptoms ranging from viral disease, sterility, to tumors, etc. (2) When the provirus controls a character of the host cell, and provided the vegetative virus has no lethal effect on the zygote, the development of the provirus will lead to the loss of this character in the progeny of such a cross.

It is worth recalling that recognition of a virus is sometimes a difficult task and that, for various reasons, infectious mature particles may well be never detected. It is indeed remarkable that, among classical cases of "cytoplasmic" inheritance, many resemble virus diseases in their expression (10). A well studied case of maternal inheritance in *Drosophila*, that of CO_2 sensitivity, has indeed been proved to be of a viral nature (41). Information gained in the study of CO_2 sensitivity in *Drosophila* parallels to an amazing extent the facts analysed in lysogenic bacteria. It is not as yet possible to say whether or not the model provided by lysogeny could be applied to any of the known cases of maternal inheritance. However, in the light of recent findings about zygotic induction the cytoplasmic nature of the responsible agents might be questioned.

The most striking point revealed by the analysis of lysogenic bacteria is that the genetic material of a virus may be tied to a specific locus of the host and thus behave as a cellular constituent. This cellular constituent may, in turn, develop into a pathogenic form which leads to the destruction of the host cell and the release of infectious particles. Thus, the study of lysogeny throws a new light upon the origin and the nature of viruses, since it indicates an intimate relationship between the genetic material of the virus and that of the host cell.

SUMMARY

(1) Lysogenic bacteria contain the genetic material of a phage in a non-infectious state, the prophage. The prophage confers upon its host the capacity to produce phage and also immunity against infection with that phage.

(2) The prophage can be affected by various mutations which prevent the completion of phage particles.

(3) A lysogenic bacterium contains one prophage per nucleus. The prophage is the only genetic determinant of lysogeny. It is located at a specific site of the bacterial chromosome. Each of 14 different prophages acting on *E. coli* K12 occupies a specific location on the bac-

terial chromosome. This can be demonstrated by crosses between non-lysogenic Hfr and lysogenic F⁻ bacteria.

(4) The 7 UV-inducible prophages which have been studied are located on one segment of the bacterial chromosome, whereas the non-inducible prophages are all located on other segments.

(5) In crosses between lysogenic Hfr and non-lysogenic F⁻ bacteria, the UV-inducible prophages develop each time they are transferred from the Hfr to the F⁻ parent. This "zygotic induction" results in the destruction of those zygotes into which the prophage of the Hfr parent has been transferred. In such crosses, genetic distortions are observed, and the lysogenic character of the Hfr parent is not inherited by the recombinants. The non-UV-inducible prophages are not induced by the conjugation and behave normally in crosses.

(6) The ability of a temperate phage to lysogenize is under the control of a short segment of its linkage-group, called the *c* segment.

(7) Genetic recombination has been shown to occur among various UV-inducible phages acting on *E. coli* K12. Genetic analysis indicates that the *c* segment controls the immunity pattern and, so far as we know, the specific location of each prophage on the bacterial chromosome.

(8) Lysogenization corresponds to the incorporation of phage genetic material into the genetic make-up of the host. This process appears more likely to be the result of an addition of the phage genetic material to the bacterial chromosome than of its substitution for an allelic segment. Preliminary results would indicate that, at least in the case of inducible prophages, the phage material is not inserted in its totality in the bacterial chromosome.

(9) The presence of certain prophages can cause specific modifications in some functions of the host.

ACKNOWLEDGMENT

The authors wish to express their thanks for helpful criticisms to Drs. C. Fuerst, H. Halvorson, D. Kaiser, A. Lwoff, and J. Monod.

REFERENCES

1. Anderson, E. S., and Fraser, A., *J. gen. Microbiol.,* **13**, 519 (1955).
2. Appleyard, R. K., *Genetics,* **39**, 429 (1953).
3. Appleyard, R. K., *Genetics,* **39**, 440 (1953).
4. Barksdale, W. L., and Pappenheimer, A. M., Jr., *J. Bacteriol.,* **67**, 220 (1954).
5. Benzer, S., *Proc. Natl. Acad. Sci. U. S.,* **41**, 344 (1955).
6. Bertani, G., *Ann. inst. Pasteur,* **84**, 273 (1953).
7. Bertani, G., *Cold Spring Harbor Symposia Quant. Biol.,* **18**, 65 (1953).

8. Boyd, J. S. K., *J. Pathol. Bacteriol.*, **63**, 445 (1951).
9. Burnet, F. M., and McKee, M., *Australian J. Exptl. Biol. Med. Sci.*, **6**, 277 (1929).
10. Caspari, E., *Advances in Genet.*, **2**, 1 (1948).
11. Ephrussi, B., in *Enzymes; Units of Biological Structure and Function,* (O. H. Gaebler, ed.), p. 29, Academic Press, New York (1955).
12. Freeman, V. J., *J. Bacteriol.*, **61**, 675 (1951).
13. Fuerst, C. R., Jacob, F., and Wollman, E. L., unpub.
14. Fuerst, C. R., and Stent, G. S., *Biochim. et Biophys. Acta,* in press.
15. Groman, N. B., and Eaton, M., *J. Bacteriol.*, **70**, 637 (1955).
16. Hayes, W., *J. gen. Microbiol.*, **8**, 72 (1952).
17. Hayes, W., *Cold Spring Harbor Symposia Quant. Biol.*, **18**, 75 (1953).
18. Hershey, A. D., and Chase, M., *J. Gen. Physiol.*, **36**, 39 (1952).
19. Hershey, A. D., Kamen, M. D., Kennedy, J. W., and Gest, H., *J. Gen. Physiol.*. **34**, 305 (1951).
20. Ionesco, H., *Compt. Rend. Acad. Sci. Paris*, **237**, 1794 (1953).
21. Jacob, F., *Les Bactéries Lysogènes et la Notion de Provirus,* Masson, Paris (1954).
22. Jacob, F., *Virology,* **1**, 207 (1955).
23. Jacob, F., Siminovitch, L., and Wollman, E. L., *Ann. inst. Pasteur,* **83**, 295 (1952).
24. Jacob, F., and Wollman, E. L., *Cold Spring Harbor Symposia Quant. Biol.,* **18** 101 (1953).
25. Jacob, F., and Wollman, E. L., *Compt. Rend. Acad. Sci. Paris,* **239**, 317 (1954).
26. Jacob, F., and Wollman, E. L., *Ann. inst. Pasteur,* **87**, 653 (1954).
27. Jacob, F., and Wollman, E. L., *Ann. inst. Pasteur,* **88**, 724 (1955).
28. Jacob, F., and Wollman, E. L., *Compt. Rend. Acad. Sci. Paris,* **242**, 303 (1956).
29. Jacob, F., and Wollman, E. L., *Ann. inst. Pasteur,* **90**, 282 (1956).
30. Jacob, F., and Wollman, E. L., *Ann. inst. Pasteur,* in press.
31. Jacob, F., and Wollman, E. L., unpub.
32. Kaiser, A. D., *Virology,* **1**, 424 (1955).
33. Kaiser, A. D., *Compt. Rend. Acad. Sci. Paris,* **242**, 3129 (1955).
34. Kaiser, A. D., and Jacob, F., unpub.
35. King, T. J., and Briggs, R., *Proc. Natl. Acad. Sci. U. S.,* **41**, 321 (1955).
36. Lederberg, E. M., *Genetics,* **36**, 500 (1951).
37. Lederberg, J., Cavalli, L. L., and Lederberg, E. M., *Genetics,* **37**, 720 (1952).
38. Lederberg, E. M., and Lederberg, J., *Genetics,* **38**, 51 (1953).
39. Levine, M., pers. commun.
40. Levinthal, C., *Proc. Natl. Acad. Sci. U. S.,* **42**, 394 (1956).
41. L'Héritier, P., in *Problèmes Actuels de Virologie,* Masson, Paris (1954).
42. Lieb, M., *J. Bacteriol.*, **65**, 642 (1953).
43. Lwoff, A., *Bact. Revs.*, **17**, 269 (1953).
44. Lwoff, A., and Gutmann, A., *Ann. inst. Pasteur,* **78**, 711 (1950).
45. Lwoff, A., Kaplan, A. S., and Ritz, E., *Ann. inst. Pasteur,* **86**, 127 (1954).
46. Lwoff, A., Siminovitch, L., and Kjeldgaard, N., *Ann. inst. Pasteur,* **79**, 815 (1950).
47. McClintock, B., *Cold Spring Harbor Symposia Quant. Biol.*, **16**, 13 (1951).
48. Miller, E. M., and Goebel, W. F., *J. Exptl. Med.*, **100**, 525 (1954).
49. Stent, G., and Fuerst, C. R., unpub.
50. Uetake, H., Nakagawa, T., and Akiba, T., *J. Bacteriol.*, **69**, 571 (1955).
51. Wollman, E. L., *Ann. inst. Pasteur,* **84**, 281 (1953).
52. Wollman, E. L., and Jacob, F., *Compt. Rend. Acad. Sci. Paris,* **239**, 455 (1954).

53. Wollman, E. L., and Jacob, F., *Compt. Rend. Acad. Sci. Paris,* **240**, 2449 (1955).
54. Wollman, E. L., and Jacob, F., *Ann. inst. Pasteur,* in press.
55. Zinder, N. D., and Lederberg, J., *J. Bacteriol.,* **64**, 679 (1952).

DISCUSSION

DR. M. LEVINE: Working with the same system that Dr. Hartman works with, phage PLT 22 and *Salmonella typhimurium,* we have been studying the mutations from wild temperate phage, which produces turbid plaques, to the mutant forms of phage which produce clear plaques. Temperate stocks of this phage contain one clear plaque-forming mutant in about 1,000 phage particles. As Dr. Jacob has already mentioned, we too can classify these mutants into three groups; c_1, c_2 and c_3, the wild type being c^+ (Levine, M., *Genetics,* **40**: 582, 1955).

One group of clear mutants, c_3, allows bacterial cell survival at levels of 50% or more. These are temperature mutants despite the fact that they produce clear plaques. The remaining types, c_1 and c_2, lyse 99% of the infected cells. The c_1 mutants either do not lysogenize by themselves or lysogenize at very low levels, something in the order of 10^{-3}. The c_2 mutants are good virulent phages. The c_1 and c_2 mutant types can be distinguished on the basis of mixed infection. A mixed infection between any mutant of group c_1 and any of group c_2, instead of lysing 99% of the cells (as these two types will do individually), will give as many as 90% of the cells surviving and producing stably lysogenic cells.

Crosses between the three mutant phages have been carried out and both the phage progeny from those cells which lyse and the prophage progeny of those cells which are lysogenized have been studied. Using the cross of phages c_1 and c_2 as an example, we find at lysis in addition to both parental types, wild-type temperate recombinants and recombination between the c characters and plaque morphology traits. Taking all the data together, the results of lysis show the three c characters to be under the genetic control of three closely linked loci. Dr. Kaiser has found a similar situation in the phage lambda. All the lysogenic bacteria arising from this cross carry prophage bearing the c_1 marker; c_2 never appears as prophage. These c_1 prophages may show recombination for the plaque morphology characters of the c_2 parent, suggesting that genetic recombination may precede prophage fixation.

An analysis of the early development of clones which will give rise to lysogenic bacteria as a result of mixed infection with phages c_1 and c_2 show some interesting phenomena. The developing clone can segregate into three cell types; sensitive cells, lysogenic cells, and cells that lyse. The lysogenic cells all carry c_1 prophages. The cells that lyse liberate only c_2 phages.

We interpret these data to mean that on mixed infection with c_1 and c_2 particles a decision may be made to lysogenize. As the clone enlarges segregation of these phage elements into the different fission products takes place. A cell receiving no phage element becomes sensitive, a cell getting c_1 will be lysogenic, and cells receiving c_2 phage elements will lyse. This indicates that mutant phages of the c_2 type have lost the ability to integrate into the bacterial genome while retaining the ability to help c_1 phages integrate.

We have adopted the tentative working hypothesis that a series of reaction steps are necessary for the establishment of lysogeny. The wild type can carry out all these steps and can produce a lysogenic cell. The mutants are blocked at different steps in the sequence of reactions, but when put into the same cell they can complement one another and give rise to a lysogenic bacterium.

We are now carrying out mixed infections with modified phage of one type (modified in some way so that its growth in bacteria is inhibited) and normal phage of another type. We are getting information which may allow us to order the steps in the sequence and begin to define some of these reactions.

Dr. Herriott: I want to say that I am very much impressed by the triple check on the sequence of characters. I wonder how many genetic maps have had the cross-checking of this sort. This gives great strength to the validity of the procedures.

Dr. Luria: I would like to point out that using 14 prophages, 7 UV-inducible and 7-UV-non-inducible in this collection, it has been possible to locate them in 2 specific regions of the map of this bacterium. The question that immediately comes to mind is: would it be possible by using other sensitive indicators to locate more phages and to map as prophages other areas of the genome of the bacterium? How much of the genome of the bacterium will be reducible to potential prophages? It is possible that there are certain regions that on phylogenetic grounds are specific carriers of potential prophages. This is, I think, very important in understanding the organization and evolution of the genetic material of the bacteria.

Dr. Jacob: This is indeed a very important question, but it requires more than 14 phages.

Dr. Maaløe: I would like to ask Dr. Jacob whether or not he has found within a given group of prophages any difference in the resistant pattern to UV or any other inducing agent.

Dr. Jacob: Yes; there are some different degrees of, say, UV-inducibility and UV-resistance, but there doesn't seem to be any order. I mean there are things which are less inducible here and more inducible there, but there is no definite order.

Dr. Maaløe: I wasn't thinking so much of the UV-inducibility, but rather of UV-resistance or heat resistance of the free phage.

Dr. Jacob: There are already differences of heat sensitivity among the various mutants of the same phage, lambda for example.

THE NATURE OF THE PROGENY OF VIRUS
RECONSTITUTED FROM PROTEIN AND
NUCLEIC ACID OF DIFFERENT STRAINS
OF TOBACCO MOSAIC VIRUS *

H. Fraenkel-Conrat, Beatrice A. Singer, and Robley C. Williams
Virus Laboratory, University of California, Berkeley, California

Methods have been described for the separation of tobacco mosaic virus protein and nucleic acid. It has also been demonstrated that the protein and nucleic acid components interact under appropriate conditions of pH concentration, and time, to form particles which in physicochemical respects resemble the original virus and which are likewise able to cause infection (4). Since no or almost no infectivity could be detected in each component, or in instantaneously diluted mixtures of these, the interpretation was at first adopted that reconstitution of rods also evoked regeneration of viral activity, which would thus depend upon the presence and the structure of the two-component particle.

Further studies have revealed that the nucleic acid fraction, while free from significant contamination with virus rods, is actually not free of virus activity. This activity, however, easily escapes detection, owing to its great instability, particularly in 0.1 M phosphate, the solvent commonly used in assaying tobacco mosaic virus for its infectivity. As more was gradually learned about the properties of this activity of the nucleic acid, it became easier to detect it and measure it reliably, and to differentiate it from that of tobacco mosaic virus (TMV). Our conclusion that infectivity is a property of the nucleic acid per se (2) was reached separately in Schramm's laboratory (5).

If the nucleic acid alone was active, what significance was there to the activity of virus particles reconstituted from it and the protein? I will enumerate a few points of such significance. In the first place,

* Aided by a grant from the National Foundation for Infantile Paralysis and research grant No. C-2245 from the National Cancer Institute of the National Institutes of Health, Public Health Service.

historically, reconstituted activity was the primary observation, and probably was a necessary stepping-stone toward a recognition of nucleic acid infectivity. Reconstitution from the two pure components, uncontaminated by virus, was also a prerequisite to the acceptance of the validity of later data when virus activity was found to be slightly increased in mixtures of less pure components (6). Secondly, reconstitution yields a stable infectious agent which is much easier to detect and handle than the infectious nucleic acid. Thirdly, reconstitution has, in our hands, given higher activity than could be demonstrated in the nucleic acid alone, though this may only be due to the lability of the latter in the unwrapped form. Yet "yields" of the order of 10 per cent are to a chemist much more satisfying than recovery of only about 0.1 to 1 per cent of the original activity. And we have in some recent reconstitution experiments obtained reaction mixtures with specific activities of 10 to 25 per cent of that of native tobacco mosaic virus, while of the nucleic acid we need of the order of a hundred times as much to evoke the same number of lesions as tobacco mosaic virus, or 2000 times as much in terms of its nucleic acid. Fourthly, the fact that reconstitution permits the encasing of nucleic acid from one strain of tobacco mosaic virus within protein from another has supplied definitive proof that the activity obtained upon reconstitution is actually due to the newly formed particles. For it was found that the infectivity was selectively inhibited by antiserum to the strain that supplies the protein component, but not by antiserum to the strain that supplies the nucleic acid (3). Furthermore, the genetic role of each of the components could be studied only through the use of such reconstituted particles.

The value of reconstitution both in opening up a new field of study and in supplying a powerful spade with which to till it appears thus evident. On the other hand, we can now gracefully retreat from a position which we have never held or expressed. Life was not here created in test tubes, since the nucleic acid alone shows "signs of life" similar to those of the original virus.

PROGENY OF VIRUS COMPOSED OF NUCLEIC ACID AND PROTEIN OF DIFFERENT STRAINS

The approach to the nature of viral inheritance listed under the fourth point above, namely, the study of the progeny of mixed virus prepared from the nucleic acid and protein of different strains, has occupied much of our time during the past year. The first conclusion was easily reached, and is well in line with what one would predict if the nucleic acid *per se* is an infectious agent, a fact which only evolved concomitantly. This conclusion was that the nucleic acid alone seemed to be the genetic determinant. The symptomatology of mixed virus infection was always that of the parent supplying the nucleic acid (Table 1), and the chemical characteristics of the progeny (where they

TABLE 1

NATURE OF DISEASE PRODUCED WITH RECONSTITUTED VIRUS OR NUCLEIC ACID OF DIFFERENT STRAINS OF TOBACCO MOSAIC VIRUS

| Nucleic Acid | Strain supplying | Disease Symptoms† |
	Protein	
TMV	Masked	TMV
TMV	HR	TMV
Masked	TMV	Masked
YA	TMV	YA
YA	Masked	YA
HR	TMV	HR
HR	Masked	HR
TMV	TMV	TMV
HR	HR	HR
HR	—	HR
TMV	—	TMV

† In Turkish tobacco TMV, YA, and HR give systemic infection of different appearance; Masked gives no symptoms, but its presence can be demonstrated by transfer to another host. In *Nicotiana sylvestris*, TMV and Masked give a systemic disease, while HR and YA give local lesions only. In *N. glutinosa* HR gives small local lesions with little necrosis and pigmentation, and is strikingly different from the spreading lesions produced by other strains.

could be studied fruitfully) were those of the same parent virus. However, detailed study has revealed some minor differences, and our tentative conclusion at present is that the protein may after all have a minor influence in the replication process. This possibility is naturally no more excluded by the infectivity of pure nucleic acid than is bisexual fertilization excluded by the occurrence of parthenogenesis.

Now what are these minor differences between mixed virus progeny and its nucleic acid parent? To answer this question, I will have to describe to you the two strains which were used for most of this work. While most strains of tobacco mosaic virus are chemically almost indistinguishable, a strain isolated by Holmes from ribgrass (HR) differs from common tobacco mosaic virus and most other strains markedly in its amino acid composition, and particularly in possessing histidine and methionine, both absent from tobacco mosaic virus. The HR strain is also immunologically more distinct from tobacco mosaic virus than other strains. Strain HR, furthermore, shows pronounced plant pathological differences from tobacco mosaic virus (Table 1), and, when isolated in the customary manner, shows a lower specific infectivity (about 5 per cent of that of common TMV). When it proved possible to produce mixed virus (hybrids) between this HR strain and common tobacco mosaic virus, these mixed viruses obviously represented the object of choice for detailed study. Batches of progeny have been prepared from single lesions of the following infectious agents: (a) HR nucleic acid + TMV protein; (b) TMV nucleic acid + HR protein; (c) HR nucleic acid + HR protein; (d) TMV nucleic acid + TMV protein; (e) HR nucleic acid alone; (f) TMV nucleic acid alone; and finally, the undegraded HR and TMV virus (Table 2). Six separate preparations of the first hybrid (HR nucleic acid + TMV protein) have now been propagated. The symptoms were always those characteristic of HR, whether the hybrid or its progeny

TABLE 2

LIST OF SINGLE LESION PROGENY PREPARATIONS*

Inoculum Reconstituted Virus	Nature and Activity of		
	Progeny I		Progeny II
HR nucleic acid——→ +TMV protein	HR** (6 preps.): (nucleic acid)——→HR** (14)——→U.I.† (30, 30, 20, 5, 6)		
		→Strain a (55)——→U.I.	
TMV nucleic acid——→ +HR protein	(TMV) (3 preps.) (100, 60, 80)		
HR nucleic acid——→ +HR protein	HR (2 preps.) (18, 3)		
TMV nucleic acid——→ +TMV protein	TMV		
HR nucleic acid——→	HR (2 preps.) (12, 12)———————————→U.I.		
	——→Strain b (12)————————————→U.I.		
TMV nucleic acid——→	(TMV) ——————————————————→U.I.		
HR virus———————→	HR (5, 5, 4, 5, 3, 6, 13)		
TMV virus——————→	TMV		

* Figures in parentheses represent specific activities, expressed as percentages of TMV assayed simultaneously.

† U.I., Under investigation.

** Resembles HR closely, yet shows consistent small differences in some amino acids.

was used as an inoculum. However, a difference was noted in the specific activity of most of these progeny preparations. This activity was 20 to 30 per cent of that of TMV, and not 5 to 13 per cent, as observed with pure HR. Amino acid analyses were then performed, and the progeny was found to resemble HR closely in almost all amino acids, and in particular in containing histidine and methionine, the two amino acids which are absent from TMV. However, a few amino acids differ slightly in strain HR and the hybrid progeny, and while some of these happen to belong to the group for which the analytical technique is less than perfect, one, viz., glycine, is not problematic, and this amino acid we have found to be about 10 per cent lower in amount in each of 4 hybrid preparations, each of which was analyzed in duplicate (Fig. 1). These findings certainly suggest a constitutive difference between the hybrid progeny and the original HR virus that supplied the nucleic acid. And the fact that concordant results have been obtained with many preparations appears to rule out random mutation.

When one such preparation of the progeny of the first hybrid was further propagated from a single lesion, as customary, a more striking difference was observed. The resultant virus was appreciably more active than the parent stock, and approached that of tobacco mosaic virus quite closely. Also its symptoms resembled those of HR on some hosts and of TMV on other hosts. Finally, its amino acid composition was markedly different from that of either HR or TMV (Fig. 1, strain a). In this case, we believe that we are dealing with an accidental variant, unless or until we should find this change to occur repeatedly under the same conditions. Only one related experiment has been completed at this time, one in which a lesion produced by the nucleic acid of the same preparation of hybrid progeny was used as source for further propagation. And here no definite differences were found between the inoculated and harvested virus.

The other combination (TMV nucleic acid + HR protein) has produced progeny which was not markedly different from tobacco mosaic virus, but this pair has not yet been studied to a similar extent as the above. Progeny from HR nucleic acid has been repeatedly prepared and found to resemble HR closely. However, upon one instance a mutation was again observed, with markedly unusual symptomatology and greatly different amino acid composition (Fig. 1, strain b). It is noteworthy that the accidental mutants obtained in the course of this work show much more marked changes in chemical and biological

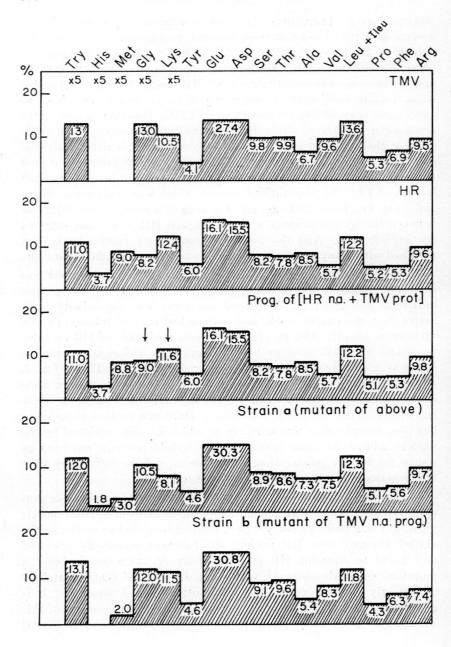

characteristics than does that minor variant that appears to be regularly produced when propagating the chemically prepared hybrid with HR nucleic acid and TMV protein.

In regard to the origin of the new strains, the question arises whether the manipulation of the nucleic acid plays a causative role in their formation. It must be noted that one of the two observed mutants was not the product of a chemically treated inoculum, but of the virus isolated from such an inoculum. But this question will probably only resolve itself after many single-lesion propagations of TMV, HR, and their manhandled nucleic acids have been performed and a definite mutation rate has been established for each.

Progeny of Virus Containing Two Different Nucleic Acids

We have now summarized our findings concerning the progeny of viral nucleic acid, and of mixed virus containing protein from a different strain. The conclusion, now based on 6 strain mixtures, is that the progeny is always very similar to the virus supplying the nucleic acid, although reconstitution may evoke small genetic changes. The appearance of mutants at a seemingly unusually high rate appears of interest, but does not represent an important advance in our search for "tailor-made" strains of desirable qualities. Another approach to this aim has been investigated which appears to have more factual basis and thus more promise for success. This is the use of a mixture of two nucleic acid preparations derived from different strains in reconstitution experiments. If infectious virus particles carrying both types of nucleic acid are formed in such experiments, they might well propagate as a new strain of predictable intermediate properties. Obviously, such experiments can only hope to succeed if the active component in our nucleic acid preparation is not an undegraded multistrand complex of the entire nucleic acid complement of one virus rod. Fortunately we have recently obtained what appears to be good evidence (see below) that this is not the case, and that reconstitution thus involves an aggregation of both protein and nucleic acid subunits. Now to the

Fig. 1. Approximate amino acid composition of TMV, of HR, of the progeny of the virus reconstituted from TMV-protein and HR nucleic acid, and of two mutants obtained in the course of this work. Some of these values will be corrected in a forthcoming publication.

Values are not corrected for moisture, nor for losses during hydrolysis. Most values were obtained by the DNP-method of Levy, and some by a new technique of combined chromatography and colorimetry.

results of these mixed nucleic acid hybridization experiments. We have had no difficulty in obtaining infectious material upon reconstituting tobacco mosaic virus protein with a mixture of equal amounts of nucleic acid from HR and TMV. A considerable number of the resulting single lesions have been propagated on those host plants that should help in identifying the nature of the virus in such lesions. The results were no more bewildering than might have been expected. Thus typical TMV as well as typical HR symptoms were obtained, as well as several mixed or intermediate responses. If one were willing to assume that a single lesion represents progeny of a single virus particle (as we assumed when starting these experiments), then the mixed symptoms observed on many plants were an indication of success. However, since this assumption appears not to be justified the mixed symptoms may well be due to double infection with both types of viruses. Actually, it was possible to isolate "pure cultures" of each of the component strains. This could be interpreted as evidence that the mixture of two types of nucleic acid had been unscrambled in the course of reconstitution, and that the two types of infectious particles were formed which would then be expected, namely, HR nucleic acid + TMV protein (HR-like) and TMV nucleic acid + TMV protein (TMV-like). However, the results could also signify that mixed nucleic acid hybrid particles had actually been produced, and that they in turn had yielded progeny consisting of a mixture of pure TMV and HR rods, as well as the hoped-for cross, according to a sort of Mendelian pattern. This will be a difficult problem to unravel. At present we are inclined to favor the latter concept, since the mixed symptoms have occurred more frequently than one would expect for the occurrence of coincidentally double infected lesions. But control experiments with mixtures of the two virus strains are in progress to ascertain the probability of such double-barreled lesions. Up to the present we have not found any such "impure" lesions. The case for experimentally produced heterogeneity within many particles is thus strengthened. However, it seems that a reversion to the original strains would deprive the as yet somewhat hypothetical "mixed strain" of any medicinal or other usefulness. It would nevertheless be of some importance to establish its fleeting existence, since it would contribute a little to our understanding of the mechanism of replication. For if mixed nucleic acid particles in the cell lead to the replication of the two separate components, then they must disintegrate intracellularly to the same molecular weight level at which they were isolated, studied, and mixed. This would bring an interesting biological phenomenon more definitely into the realm of physicochemical study.

NATURE OF ACTIVITY OF NUCLEIC ACID

This discussion has led us back to its starting point: the chemical nature of the infectivity of nucleic acid preparations. Evidence that this infectivity is not due to contaminating virus is based on the following observations.

1. Tobacco mosaic virus can be almost quantitatively sedimented in the ultracentrifuge under suitable conditions, and with particular efficiency in the presence of nucleic acid (Table 3). Yet the number of

TABLE 3

SEDIMENTABILITY OF TOBACCO MOSAIC VIRUS FROM DILUTE SOLUTIONS*

TMV μg./ml.	Nucleic Acid μg./ml.	Percentage of Infectivity in		
		Solution	Drain	Pellet
50	—	0.2	18	82
5	—	0.04	43	57
5	2500	0	4	96
1	—	2	21	77
1	500	0.05	2	98
1	400	0.02	2	98
1	160	0	50	50
1	—	41	40	19

* Centrifuged for 2 hours with refrigeration at 40,000 r.p.m. in a 40-rotor with nylon adaptors to fit 2 ml. tubes. "Solution" is the bulk of the sample, poured off rapidly after arrest of the centrifuge, "drain" the last 0.1-0.2 ml., and "pellet" the material that adheres to the bottom of the tube, when resuspended in water.

virus particles that can be sedimented from active nucleic acid preparations ranges from zero to about 1 per cent of the number required for the infectivity observed.

2. Tobacco mosaic virus is specifically inhibited by high dilutions of rabbit anti-TMV-serum, or preferably the γ-globulin fraction of such sera, but the nucleic acid activity is resistant to such treatment.

3. The nucleic acid activity is very sensitive to the presence of salt, quite in contrast to TMV. Incubation in the best assay medium, 0.1 M pH 6.8 phosphate (1 hour at 36° C.), has been used as a routine criterion for the differentiation of the two types of activities. But

other 0.1 M ionic media are as effective in inactivating the nucleic acid; at 0.01 M concentration most of the activity is retained, as it is in water, and 0.001 M salts may actually protect the infectivity. In all those tests, the samples are diluted with 0.1 M phosphate at 0° C. just prior to assay (Fig. 2).

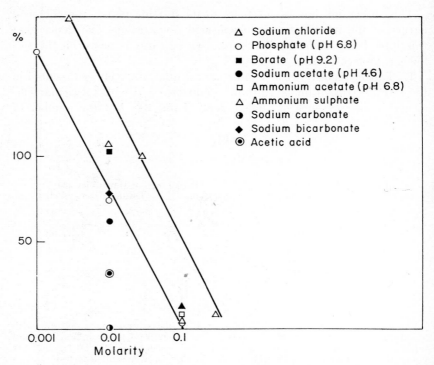

FIG. 2. Percentage of activity of nucleic acid treated for 1 hr. at 36° C. with various buffers and salts, compared to water (also incubated) as 100 per cent.

4. While all previous criteria indicate differences in the nature of the infectivity of tobacco mosaic virus and nucleic acid preparations, the effect of enzymes seems to indicate that the activity of the latter is not only different from that of tobacco mosaic virus, but is due specifically to the ribonucleic acid in these preparations. For it was found that the infectivity of the nucleic acid is extraordinarily sensitive to ribonuclease, and is abolished in 2 hours at 36°C. at an enzyme-substrate ratio of one to a hundred million. Considerably

higher concentrations (a hundred and a thousand fold) are needed of deoxyribonuclease or of trypsin to achieve inactivation.

Thus many-fold evidence is at hand that nucleic acid preparations contain infectious components of non-viral, and most probably of ribonucleic acid, character. A working hypothesis which we originally favored is that the active component represents a small fraction of high molecular weight, possibly corresponding to the entire nucleic acid core of one virus particle (molecular weight about 3×10^6). This concept appears to be held by Schramm (5). However, we can find no experimental evidence favoring this hypothesis. Recent experiments actually appear to indicate that the infectivity is associated with material of comparatively low, or average, molecular weight. In these experiments the nucleic acid was ultracentrifuged in the same narrow tubes which favor quantitative sedimentation of tobacco mosaic virus from dilute solutions. Samples were then taken from the top, middle, and bottom sections of the tube, and analyzed for nucleic acid concentration and infectivity. The efficacy of centrifugation was indicated by the concentration gradient, the bottom sample being about four times as concentrated as the top. Yet the specific infectivity of the nucleic acid was the same in the top and in the bottom sections (Table 4). It would

TABLE 4

EFFECT OF ULTRACENTRIFUGATION ON ACTIVITY OF NUCLEIC ACID

Exp. No.	Fraction	Concentration mg./ml.	Lesions/h.l.*
I	Nucleic acid, once ultracentrifuged	5.6	25
	2 × ultracentrifuged	5.6	25
	3 × ultracentrifuged	2.6	23
II	Nucleic acid, once ultracentrifuged	1.25	52
	Same, 2 × centrifuged, top 25%	1.0	30
	Same, 2 × centrifuged, bottom 20%.	1.7	18
III	Nucleic acid, once ultracentrifuged	5.2	154
	Same, 2 × centrifuged, top 25%	3.2	74
	Same, 2 × centrifuged, middle 60%	4.9	102
	Same, 2 × centrifuged, bottom 15%	8.3	73
IV	Nucleic acid, once centrifuged	4.0	30
	Same, 2 × centrifuged, top 13%	1.0	24
	Same, 2 × centrifuged, bottom 25%	3.2	24
	Same, ammonium acetate, top 10%	0.8	34
	Same, ammonium acetate, bottom 25%	3.0	21

* Lesions per half leaf at 20-25 μg./ml. in Holmes necrotic-type tobacco.

thus appear that the typical TMV nucleic acid to which a molecular weight of about 200,000 to 300,000 has been ascribed (1) is infectious, to the extent that its intramolecular bonding has not been disturbed in the course of release from the virus and subsequent purification. High ionic strength appears to favor this loss of "native" structure, but variations in pH are less harmful (Fig. 2).

These studies concerning the nature and structure of infectious nucleic acid are only in their beginning phases, and I have brought you right up to date in regard to our work. It will be a long time before anyone will attempt to decipher in chemical terms the code transmitting the "information" carried by these relatively simple, and yet so formidable, molecules. All we hope to do at present is to determine the length of the message and the nature of the material that it is written on.

REFERENCES

1. Cohen, S. S., and Stanley, W. M., *J. Biol. Chem.*, **144**, 589 (1942).
2. Fraenkel-Conrat, H., *J. Am. Chem. Soc.*, **78**, 882 (1956).
3. Fraenkel-Conrat, H., and Singer, Beatrice A., unpub.
4. Fraenkel-Conrat, H., and Williams, Robley C., *Proc. Natl. Acad. Sci. U. S.*, **41**, 690 (1955).
5. Gierer, A., and Schramm, G., *Nature,* **177**, 702 (1956).
6. Lippincott, J. A., and Commoner, B., *Biochim. et Biophys. Acta,* **19**, 198 (1956).

DISCUSSION

DR. SCHRAMM: The idea of the reconstitution of virus from its constituents and building blocks is an idea which has had us fascinated for a long time. I think we did the first experiment about 15 years ago. At that time we found that we could separate the protein from the nucleic acid and that from this protein we could again prepare the virus rods. At that very early time, the role of nucleic acids in the biosynthesis of proteins was not known to us. At that time we were disappointed that we had no activity in this reconstructed rod. Naturally this was because there was no nucleic acid inside the rods. This protein—we call it a single protein—has a molecular weight of about 90,000; and by changing pH's you can prepare from the rod those interesting intermediates which look like doughnuts, and these stick together to make these rods. If you change the pH to 5 you have only the rods and very few of the doughnut intermediates. From that time on, as the role of nucleic acids in biosynthesis became more and more obvious we tried to combine this nucleic acid from different preparations with protein, and we have published many unsuccessful experiments in this direction. We believe that this failure was due to the preparation of the RNA. It seems to us that the RNA is the more sensitive part of the particle, and so we developed a new method for the preparation of the RNA which permitted us to prepare it at low temperatures and in a very short time. This method consists of extracting the protein by phenol. The protein is very soluble in the phenol, giving a phenol phase, and of course the pure RNA remains in the aqueous phase. Working with this RNA preparation, we found that the infectivity of this RNA was very high, and so we carried out many experiments to show that the infectivity is not due to any contamination of protein by a property of RNA itself. Before I come to this biological activity, I should like to make some remarks about the physicochemical activity of the RNA. This RNA which we obtained by the phenol method is stable for only a very short time. We have enough data to make a determination of the molecular weight. The sedimentation constant is greater than 25 Svedbergs, and the intrinsic viscosity is about 140 cubic cm. per gram. From this one can see we have a molecular weight higher than 2 million. We believe that shortly after preparation we have the intact core of the virus. One can calculate the particle weight of the virus core from the molecular weight as about 2.5 million. I think there is only a bit of degradation by our method, but after a few days this value drops to a molecular weight of about 60,000. Now, we have investigated the biological activity of this high molecular weight preparation, and have recorded and published activities of about 2% by weight; but now I have received a letter from my laboratory, and we have found that the activity depends upon the kind of buffer you use for the bioassays. At pH 6 you have an activity of about 2%. That means that 2 mg. of TMV is equivalent to 100 mg. of nucleic acid. At pH 8 we have an activity of about 5%, and at pH 10 we have an activity of about 13% by weight. I think this may be a little higher activity than for the preparation made by Dr. Fraenkel-Conrat, who used mostly the detergent method. Also, we got very good fibers in the electron microscope from this preparation. The diameter is not very homogeneous. The molecules tend to aggregate both longitudinally and transversely. These fibers are much longer than the TMV itself. From my experiments it is clear that the activity is not due to any contamination of the protein. I think that we have good evidence, as Dr. Fraenkel-Conrat has shown, that the RNA itself is infective and that it is itself a genetic material. The RNA is a genetic material in TMV, just as the DNA is in the transforming principle, and serves as the genetic material for the bacteriophage in transduction. Another question is: Can the activity of the RNA be increased or enhanced by combining it with protein? We have carried out such experiments, and we have never found any increase in infectivity by combining our RNA preparation with an RNA preparation made by the methods of Dr. Fraenkel-Conrat or Dr. Robley Williams. I will say that it doesn't mean too much. I hear from other laboratories that combination experiments of this kind are not successful every time. Maybe some factors are involved such that sometimes you get reconstitution and sometimes you don't. I think we must be very careful about this reconstitution experiment. It is very easy if you have some nucleic acid to attach some protein on the outside of it, and it is very easy to make rods that have the same appearance as TMV; but that is not reconstitution, I think. Then we know from x-ray investigations of Miss Franklin and others that there is a very peculiar arrangement of the subunits around this core, and it seems to be not so very easy to achieve the right arrangement here. I could believe that, if you coat some RNA with some HR protein and you put antibodies in this mixture, the core is carried down as a precipitate even if there is no reaction of the RNA with the antibodies. Another thing which we have to bring up is that the activity of the TMV depends upon the buffer solution and the external medium. We know, further, that if we combine the virus particle with detergent we get inactivation, and it is possible to remove the detergent by dialysis and obtain active rods again. So I think we should be very careful and have good proof before we speak of reconstitution. You can expect if you combine the protein and the core that you will have a higher infectivity. We know, of course, that the protein stabilizes the activity, and there may be some other protective function of the protein—for instance, against RNAase activity from the cell. I think it would be very fruitful to repeat these reconstitution experiments, and I think (as Dr. Fraenkel-Conrat said) that these experiments are very stimulating and give us an insight into many biological problems.

DR. SINSHEIMER: In a sedimentation pattern, using ultraviolet optics, of the RNA of TMV prepared by brief heating in salt and then rapid cooling—actually freezing—and keeping at 1° in all the preparations, it is seen that the preparation actually does possess primarily a single boundary—actually about 85% of the material is in the leading edge, which has a sedimentation constant of 36 Svedbergs. Electron micrographs show that this material is rod-like in shape. This rod is about 280 Å long and 70 Å in diameter. These rods are about all we see in these preparations, and we believe they are what Dr. Schramm suggests is the nucleic acid core.

DR. STANLEY: I think it ought to be emphasized that Dr. Fraenkel-Conrat and Dr. Schramm have made their nucleic acid preparations by two completely different techniques, one involving detergent and the other involving phenolization, and yet they both end up with biologically active preparations, and they are not too far different so far as sizes are concerned. The important point is that this has been done completely independently in this country and in Germany. The reconstitution story, I think, is quite clear to me, but the most important aspect of this thing is that you can get a biologically active RNA which will induce its own replication and simultaneously with that its own specific protein, which apparently stabilizes the nucleic acid and the biological activity. Dr. Fraenkel-Conrat didn't have time to go into this stabilization, but it is apparently true. We are now attempting to find out the difference between the phenolized preparations and the detergent preparations, because in our hands and in Dr. Schramm's hands one is unstable and will not reconstitute a virus, whereas the other one does. I think the answer to this problem will come out before long.

Dr. Spiegelman: I am a little bit worried about this inactivation with DNAase. Did you do it in the presence of citrate? Did you compare its action in the presence of carrier substrate and in the presence of magnesium?

Dr. Fraenkel-Conrat: We have tried it, but the results have been erratic.

Dr. Spiegelman: That might give you a way of providing convincing proof that there was contamination in this preparation by RNAase.

Dr. Volkin: I wonder if you have any evidence whether the recombination or reconstitution has to be specific between the plant virus RNA and plant virus protein, or whether you might have tried some non-plant-virus RNA's to see whether they were incorporated into the protein shell.

Dr. Fraenkel-Conrat: That has been done in our laboratory with a variety of nucleic acids by J. E. Smith and Roger Hart. Practically any nucleic acid can become incorporated into the protein, but then there is no activity and the length seems to be limited. You get rods of all lengths, as you do with protein alone, only at a somewhat higher pH. Whereas when you have the right nucleic acid you get rods that group up to the size of 300 mμ and then stop; there is not a single one beyond that size, so there is something size-determining and activity-giving in the right nucleic acid.

Dr. Kaplan: I was wondering, Dr. Fraenkel-Conrat, in these experiments where you compared the nucleic acid of the HR and the TMV with the whole virus whether there is any difference in infectivity between the HR and the TMV. Is there a possibility that the TMV is a more infective particle than the HR?

Dr. Fraenkel-Conrat: The activity of the HR nucleic acid is as high as the TMV nucleic acid, and therefore when you use TMV-HR nucleic acid for reconstituting you end up with preparations which are more active after reconstituting than the virus which supplied the nucleic acid originally. It seems to me that the differences in specific activity of the different viruses are due to the protein coat affecting the ease of entering into the cell, or something. The activity of the nucleic acids of all strains seems to be of the same order.

Dr. Rich: You imply from your experiments with mixed strains that there may be several infective or self-duplicating units per TMV rod. If one lesion arises from one infective rod, couldn't you mix active

TMV-RNA with an inactive or synthetic RNA so that there are fewer infective units per rod. This might show up as either a smaller lesion or fewer TMV units per lesion.

DR. FRAENKEL-CONRAT: It hasn't been tried yet.

DR. LURIA: Would it be correct to conclude from the evidence presented today that the essential thing is to have the full length of the nucleic acid and that the function of the protein is to keep the full length intact? Would the people working in this field be willing to subscribe to this working hypothesis?

DR. FRAENKEL-CONRAT: There is no evidence against it, but neither has it been proved. It would explain the 3,000 Å units, which is otherwise difficult to explain.

DR. SCHRAMM: We have done experiments in our Institute that show that the activity goes down at the same sedimentation rate as the high molecular weight particles; yet there are some differences that yet need to be cleared up. It is fascinating to assume that the RNA determines the length of the virus, but I am not sure that is so. I think there is some mystery about this very, very specific length.

DR. ZAMENHOF: Dr. Fraenkel-Conrat, you mentioned that the nucleic acid of the RNA which has been tampered with seems to have a higher mutation rate than normal. That would be very important. What is the nature of the tampering, and how sure are you of this higher mutation rate?

DR. FRAENKEL-CONRAT: We have observed two new strains. One was the progeny of nucleic acid which had been made by our technique, so the tampering involved precipitation by alcohol, and detergent treatment at pH 8.5 and 50°. The other one cropped up as a progeny of such a preparation. Virus was inoculated, propagated from a single lesion, and we got back a different strain. Thus the tampering can be in one generation or a thousand generations removed, but actually we have too little data to say much. In working with nucleic acid and taking it apart in 20 some progeny preparations, two of them gave new strains, which seemed to be high but not high enough to analyze statistically.

DR. N. SIMMONS: I don't want to terminate this discussion, but I think there is a lesson to be drawn from the Mayflower Baking Company's slogan, "When you walk the road of life, brother, whatever be your goal, keep your eye upon the doughnut and not upon the hole."

DR. SEYMOUR COHEN: I just thought it relevant to comment on the apparent size or the molecular weight of the RNA of a small spherical virus. The total RNA content of all the viruses is about the same—that is, a sphere-like turnip yellow mosaic virus has about the same RNA charge as tobacco mosaic virus, and the weight of the RNA charge of 6×10^{23} virus particles is about 2½ million. When one degrades turnip yellow mosaic virus by very gentle methods, one finds a very low molecular weight for the turnip yellow virus ribonucleic acid. Dr. Smith and Dr. Markham have found by end-group analysis a molecular weight of about 17,000, and we have found a size of about 35,000 to 50,000 by kinetic studies, so that one has actually in turnip yellow mosaic virus approximately 50 particles of small molecular weight, in contrast to the long core of large RNA particles which one finds in the tobacco mosaic virus.

Part V

*NUCLEIC ACIDS—CHEMICAL COMPOSITION
AND STRUCTURE*

BASE COMPOSITION OF DEOXYPENTOSE AND PENTOSE NUCLEIC ACIDS IN VARIOUS SPECIES

ERWIN CHARGAFF

Cell Chemistry Laboratory, Department of Biochemistry,
College of Physicians and Surgeons, Columbia University,
New York

INTRODUCTION

WHEN LISTENING to all these wonderful papers at this Symposium, from which it appeared to me that almost all the riddles of life were riddles no longer, I began to dream of what might have gone on at an International Congress of Pure and Applied Alchemy held sometime in the 15th Century. What was said there I could not reproduce; but I am sure of one thing: no one got up and said he could not make gold. Another thought that occurred to me was that in the Tower of Babel one language would not have been heard, namely Babylonian. Our sciences have lost a commonly or mutually intelligible language; and whatever dictionaries there are, they give wrong translations. When we go from the level of structure and cellular organization to that of molecules and their interactions, the same words often have entirely different connotations. In speaking, for instance, of a coil, how far is it from what the morphologist sees to what the crystallographer infers? And if there is no other difference between the splitting of chromosomes and the duplication of double strands of DNA, could it not be that the one does take place and the other probably does not? Furthermore, each science has equipped itself with a specific fire-extinguisher to dampen the enthusiasm of the other; so that if one screams "Speculation!" the other retorts with "Artifact!"

There can be little doubt that the nucleic acids are occupying the center of biochemical attention at this moment—too much so, in my opinion, since this had to be done at the expense of other very worthy cell constituents, such as the proteins, the polysaccharides, the lipids. I should like to end these introductory remarks by quoting a few words from a recent review article (3). "The spectator who has followed the development of our knowledge of nucleic acids in the past

521

few years cannot help feeling that the stage is set for a grand finale. Many an acrobat has announced the 'salto mortale' to a gasping audience; and though often only a graceful pirouette could be seen, 'tamen est laudanda voluntas.' But I believe that the deeper we get, the darker it becomes. It is true, the temptation is almost overwhelming to pour all into one pot: growth, and its change from benign to malignant; bacterial transformations; the transmission of hereditary properties; the multiplication of virus and phage; the synthesis of inducible enzymes; the differentiation of tissues; the formation of antibodies—everywhere an interplay between nucleic acids and proteins, a spinning wheel in which the thread makes the spindle and the spindle the thread. But if it is hard to recognize the similarities between what is ostensibly dissimilar, it is even more difficult to make out the differences between what appears so similar; and moderation still is among the tools of our science."

In the following remarks I shall, wherever possible, refer to the pages of the recently published treatise on the nucleic acids (5). Deoxypentose nucleic acids will be abbreviated as DNA, pentose nucleic acids as PNA.

BASES IN NUCLEIC ACIDS

DNA, according to the species of origin, may contain four or five nitrogenous constituents. Adenine, guanine, and thymine seem to occur in all, and cytosine in most, specimens (4). 5-Methylcytosine occasionally replaces a portion of the cytosine, more so in plant than in animal DNA and not at all in microbial DNA. 5-Hydroxymethylcytosine substitutes entirely for cytosine in coliphage DNA of the even varieties. Under exceptional circumstances 6-N-methyladenine occurs in partial replacement of thymine (7). The existence of trace constituents cannot be excluded.

PNA is even less varied in the list of its constituents (14). No exception to the exclusive occurrence of adenine, guanine, cytosine, and uracil has, thus far, been found. It is remarkable, also in view of the many discussions on the biological interconversion of DNA and PNA, that wheat germ, whose DNA is notoriously rich in 5-methylcytosine, does not appear to incorporate this pyrimidine into its PNA (12).

Uniform as the inventory of nucleic acid constituents appears to be, the proportions of these constituents often vary very considerably in specimens from different sources, and they vary perhaps over a wider range in DNA than in PNA. For analytical details the recent compilations (4, 14) should be consulted. I should like to limit myself here to a few remarks bearing more directly on the theme of this Symposium.

NUCLEIC ACIDS AS HIGH POLYMERS

If we assume that the magic capacity of which there is so much talk in these days, namely, "biological information," is carried by the nucleic acids by virtue of specific nucleotide sequences and by the proteins through a specific arrangement of amino acids, we shall immediately notice a fundamental difference between these two types of polymers. The insertion of a different amino acid molecule into the polypeptide chain requires the cleavage of the peptide linkage. In a nucleic acid the superstructure of glycosidically bound nitrogenous constituents could, at any rate theoretically, be modified without the breakage of the poly-sugar phosphate backbone. It is, however, noteworthy that enzymes capable of attacking, or exchanging, the purines and pyrimidines in a polynucleotide chain have not yet been observed.

One could put it in another way by saying that the ideal monomer of a protein consists of one molecular species, an amino acid; that of a nucleic acid, the nucleotide, of three: base, sugar, phosphoric acid. Even the lack of a proper terminology emphasizes this difference. We have no name to classify high polymers of the type to which the poly-sugar phosphate backbone of a nucleic acid belongs, i.e., substances in which molecules are linked to each other through bridges of a different chemical character, as in this instance the pentoses by phosphoric acid. I have little doubt that this type of mixed polymer is not limited to the nucleic acids.[1]

DEOXYPENTOSE NUCLEIC ACIDS

The evidence, far from all-embracing, of the architectural principles holding DNA together, viz., 5':3' phosphate bridges, has been reviewed recently (1). Faults in this structure cannot be excluded, nor is the position, or even the existence, of a terminal phosphate group rigorously proved. Whether cyclic polynucleotides occur under circumstances has not been determined. The assertion that the sugar is always deoxyribose

[1] There could be several acceptable designations, based on derivations from the Greek, for this type of bridge polymer: *gephyrides,* "bridge compounds"; *peronides,* "clasp compounds"; *desmotides,* "link compounds"; or *plektides,* "plait compounds."

rests on no firmer foundation than the identification of ribose as the only sugar of PNA. The chemistry of this subject is unusually rich in magnificent, though ill-founded, generalizations.

The composition of DNA has been discussed recently in great detail (4). The findings indicate that there exists a very large number of different nucleic acids which can be distinguished by different proportions, and hence by differences in the sequence, of the component nucleotides. In the two most extreme cases the disymmetry ratio $(A + T/G + C)^2$ varies from 0.4 to 1.9. Despite these far-reaching divergences several regularities that appear to be characteristic of all DNA have been known for something like seven years (2). They are: (a) $A = T$; (b) $G = C$; (c) $A + G = C + T$; and, therefore, (d) $A + C = G + T$, i.e., (6-Am = 6-K).

PENTOSE NUCLEIC ACIDS

With the exception of the PNA of plant viruses, which in my opinion occupy a special position among the nucleoproteins, it is highly questionable whether the analysis of isolated PNA preparations offers much hope for an understanding of their specificity. In the experience of our laboratory it is extremely difficult, and in some cases impossible, to prepare several specimens from the same animal or microbial source that are as closely similar in composition as the DNA of a given species. We have pointed out recently how close the conjugation of PNA with proteins is in many instances and how tenaciously pentose nucleoproteins resist complete deproteinization (9).

It was, for this reason, only after we had relinquished the analysis of isolated PNA and had transferred our attention to the nucleotide distribution in total crude pentose nucleoproteins that the comparison of different preparations and the establishment of compositional regularities became possible (8, 9). It appears that PNA, when analyzed in the form of undegraded nucleoprotein, shows one, and only one, of the regularities characteristic of DNA, namely, 6-Am = 6-K, i.e., $A + C = G + U$. This regularity does not, however, seem to apply to certain plant viruses. Table 1 illustrates a few characteristic instances.

---

[2] Abbreviations: A, G, C, T, U stand for adenine, guanine, cytosine, thymine, uracil, respectively, or for the corresponding nucleotides. 6-Am denotes nucleotides carrying an amino group in 6 position (adenylic and cytidylic acids), 6-K those having a 6-oxo group (guanylic and thymidylic or uridylic acids). Pu indicates purine nucleotides; Py, pyrimidine nucleotides.

TABLE 1

Nucleotide Ratios in Pentose Nucleoproteins

Source	Pu/Py	A+U/G+C	6-Am/6-K
Ox liver [a]	0.80	0.63	1.04
Rat kidney [a]	0.96	0.66	1.00
Cytoplasm of rat liver and kidney [a]	0.99	0.62	0.93
Paracentrotus lividus, eggs and embryos [b]	1.08	0.77	0.99
Wheat germ [c]	1.07	0.76	1.00
Yeast [a]	1.00	1.12	0.93
Escherichia coli [a]	1.18	0.87	1.00
Mycobacterium phlei [a]	1.06	0.73	0.93
Azotobacter vinelandii [d]	1.21	0.78	1.00

[a] Taken from Elson and Chargaff (9).
[b] Taken from Elson et al. (10).
[c] Taken from Lipshitz and Chargaff (12).
[d] Taken from Lombard and Chargaff (13).

Remarks on the Meaning of Regularities, on Nucleotide Sequence and on Fractionation

Is there any sense—one might ask—in searching for regularities in nucleic acid composition? Has not the old tetranucleotide hypothesis, defunct but not forgotten, done enough mischief? Is Nature nothing but an interior decorator's dream? Granted all that—and our easygoing cryptographers deserve to be discomfited, as they surely will. But if there is any meaning to a concept of biological information that can be transcribed in chemical terms, the existence of regularities of the sort mentioned before may, as I have pointed out recently (3), furnish us the only clue to systems through which such information is preserved or—and this is more important—transmitted. The precise features of this transfer can hardly be discerned at this time; the unbelievable amount of male handicraft spent on getting inept models out of difficulties appears to me as wasted.

If we consider the one regularity that almost all nucleic acids appear to share, namely, the presence in them of an equal number of nucleotides having a 6-amino group and of those having a 6-keto group, the most satisfactory construction that could impose this uniformity is one in which two polynucleotide chains are bonded to a polypeptide chain, so that each peptide carbonyl is linked by a hydrogen bond to the 6-amino group of adenine or cytosine and each peptide amino group to the 6-keto group of guanine or uracil (or thymine). Such a relationship has been discussed for PNA in detail in a recent paper (9). It is for the moment, of course, purely hypothetical. Whether in DNA the other pairing principles mentioned above are a secondary consequence, not applicable to PNA, of the 6-Am to 6-K relationship or whether they indicate an entirely different structural arrangement in the two types of nucleic acid, cannot yet be said. It will, however, be clear that I should prefer to consider the protein moiety of a nucleoprotein as not merely an ornamental or protective supplement.

Methods for the determination of nucleotide sequence remain one of the most urgent problems in nucleic acid chemistry. It is, however, obvious that sequence cannot be the sole agent of biological information. Even if the arrangement of an entire polynucleotide could be written, a third dimension would be lacking: the operative three-dimensional shape of the molecular aggregate, in which perhaps not only numerous nucleic acid molecules take part, but also proteins and possibly even other polymers (polysaccharides, lipids, etc.). The ease with which preparations of transforming principles can be inactivated makes it improbable that nucleotide sequence in itself can be the only determinant; and a similar conclusion would apply to the amino acid sequence in many proteins. Thus far, sequence analysis has yielded only fragmentary results. The work on PNA will be discussed by others. I should like to limit myself to the mere mention of previous studies in our laboratory on apurinic acid and similar degradation products (4, 11), on the enzymic breakdown of DNA and PNA (4, 6, 14) and on the mechanism of the formation of nucleoside-3:5-diphosphates from DNA (15, and unpub. studies with H. S. Shapiro). In general, it can be said that, in both DNA and PNA, purine nucleotides have a greater chance to be next to, or near, other purine nucleotides than next to pyrimidine nucleotides; in other words, there is some evidence of bunching. In addition, as yet unpublished work of Shapiro has shown that it is sometimes possible to distinguish between DNA specimens of similar composition if they are derived from different species.

There can be little doubt that the sequence analysis of DNA would have been pursued with greater vigor if the last few years had not provided so much evidence that DNA preparations can be fractionated into many fractions of a regularly graded nucleotide composition. I have no time to go into these questions here, but may end by referring to several papers in which this problem is reviewed (4, 12, 16).

REFERENCES

1. Brown, D. M., and Todd, A. R., in ref. 5, **1**, 409 (1955).
2. Chargaff, E., *Experientia,* **6**, 201 (1950).
3. Chargaff, E., *Rend. ist. Lombardo Sci. Pt. I,* **89**, 101 (1955).
4. Chargaff, E., in ref. 5, **1**, 307 (1955).
5. Chargaff, E., and J. D. Davidson, eds., *The Nucleic Acids,* 2 vols., Academic Press, New York (1955).
6. Chargaff, E., and Shapiro, H. S., *Exptl. Cell Research,* **3** (Suppl.), 64 (1955).
7. Dunn, D. B., and Smith, J. D., *Nature,* **175**, 336 (1955).
8. Elson, D., and Chargaff, E., *Nature,* **173**, 1037 (1954).
9. Elson, D., and Chargaff, E., *Biochim. et Biophys. Acta,* **17**, 367 (1955).
10. Elson, D., Gustafson, T., and Chargaff, E., *J. Biol. Chem.,* **209**, 285 (1954).
11. Hodes, M. E., and Chargaff, E., *Biochim. et Biophys. Acta* (in press).
12. Lipshitz, R., and Chargaff, E., *Biochim. et Biophys. Acta,* **19**, 256 (1956).
13. Lombard, A., and Chargaff, E., *Biochim. et Biophys. Acta,* **20**, 585 (1956).
14. Magasanik, B., in ref. 5, **1**, 373 (1955).
15. Shapiro, H. S., and Chargaff, E., *Federation Proc.,* **15**, 352 (1956).
16. Spitnik, P., Lipshitz, R., and Chargaff, E., *J. Biol. Chem.,* **215**, 765 (1955).

DISCUSSION

DR. MATTHEWS: As Dr. Chargaff has pointed out, we have no information at present about the sequence of nucleotides in RNA and DNA chains. Under these conditions speculation can work freely. One idea has been that a triplet of nucleotides in a polynucleotide might define the position of one amino acid in a polypeptide. At present we cannot do anything in the way of nucleotide sequence determination to test this hypothesis, but we can look at the composition of nucleic acids and associated proteins in cases where the composition of one is unusual. We already have one example of this. The plant virus turnip yellow mosaic virus has 37% of cytidylic acid in its RNA. The protein of this virus has recently been analysed by Markham and Rees, and it contains as the highest constituent about 10% of serine. Ten per cent is not an unusually large amount for the most abundant amino acid in a protein. Looking for another example of unusual composition we examined the silk gland in the silk moth *Philosamia ricini.* Silk proteins contain about 45% glycine. The silk gland is very rich in RNA. If this RNA is acting as a template for the silk proteins we might expect unusual base ratios, or at least ratios differing from the RNA's of a tissue of more mixed function. We have determined the base ratios for the RNA of the silk gland and the gut, which is an organ of diverse functions (Table 1). Organs were obtained from larvae in the last instar.

The RNA's from the two sources were very similar in composition and not at all unusual. This is not what we would expect at first sight if the triplet idea was correct. However, with only two RNA—protein comparisons we cannot prove or disprove any hypothesis. It may be worthwhile looking for further examples of unusual composition in nucleic acids and the proteins associated with them.

TABLE 1

Molar Ratios of Bases in the RNA's from the Silk Gland and the
Gut of the Silk Moth *Philosamia ricini*

	Silk Gland	Gut
Guanine	1.26	1.30
Adenine	0.95	0.99
Cytosine	1.03	0.94
Uracil	0.76	0.77
Ratio G + U/A + C	1.02	1.07

DR. McELROY: Have there been other comparisons made with an end-group analysis to the molecular weight determined by other methods?

DR. SEYMOUR COHEN: The only comparison that has been made is in the turnip yellow system, in which Drs. Smith and Markham obtained a value of 15,000 to 17,000 and we have obtained an average value of about twice that. In this connection I would like to bring up the very interesting recent results of Dr. Warner and Dr. Ochoa in which they obtained a pairing of polyadenine nucleotides and polyuridine nucleotides. This also seems to fit in with the apparent pairing of the various bases via the 6-amino—6-hydroxyl groups which Dr. Chargaff's analysis seems to point to. One would like to know whether this is at all possible. In other words, we may have actually seen an aggregation, and what Dr. Smith has observed with the RNA of turnip yellow mosaic virus may be the actual ends of the chains. We have seen the two chains going together. I don't know whether this is true or not, but it seems reasonable.

DR. CHARGAFF: I think that before long, Dr. Crick, you will retreat from this untenable position of dinucleotides entering the template. Once you relinquish the idea that monomers only are lined up on the template, you will notice that you get into all the troubles that those got into who tried to explain protein synthesis by the assembly of oligopeptides. If you have to have a template, mononucleotides are your best bet. You see, you would have had to have a Maxwellian demon in each cell which would really direct the methylcytidylic acid to go next to guanylic acid before they are incorporated into DNA; a sort of a higher cellular intelligence unlikely to find outside of Cambridge. I have recently reviewed the evidence from Smith and Sinsheimer that methyl cytosine has a remarkable tendency to lie next to guanine and that it shows a highly uneven distribution with respect to cytosine in DNA fractions (*Symp. Soc. Exp. Biol.*, **9**, 32 (1955)). This we could explain if we assumed—and it won't fit into your hypothesis—that the neighboring and not the opposite base directed the incorporation. Then you would end up with an infinite number of determinants in the directing template. Now, maybe this could be so. But if it were, at the same time I am afraid you would have to erase your beautiful hypothesis.

Dr. Bendich: I think there is a more serious objection than whether 5-methyl cytosine fits in at random or not, and that is whether or not in all instances the specific pairing unity ratio principle is maintained. I think it's a question again of stressing a point that Professor Chargaff made that we are dealing with impure materials, i.e., mixtures of polynucleotides. A very important point then is whether one is separating the component parts of the mixture, and studying only certain parts thereof. With our anion exchange system we were able to obtain a number of calf thymus DNA fractions from the column and we performed a number of base analyses on some of them. Some fractions were eluted in the neutral salt region, and others were obtained at elevated values of pH, from 8.9 to 11. The original material has an adenine to thymine ratio of 1.03 and guanine to cytosine of one. A selection of some of the data (given in the accompanying table) shows significant deviations from unity ratio with fractions of DNA obtained by this method, which we believe has a much higher resolution than some of the other fractionation methods which have been described in the literature. These analyses are plus or minus less than 0.02, so that these are real deviations from unity ratios. It should be recognized that these nucleic acids are hopeless mixtures, and we should seriously consider methods of higher resolution to separate the many components thereof. If we have a 10% deviation from unity base ratio in a DNA of molecular weight as high as 6 million, it would mean then that there could be several hundred bases (out of a grand total of 20,000) which are naked—that is to say, that on one side of the hypothetical double helical chain there might be several hundred bases without any specifically-paired partners on the other side. These are more serious objections than whether 5-methyl cytosine fits in or not.

Dr. Ochoa: I would like to add a comment to the point that was made before—namely, about the chain length of ribonucleic acids and the molecular weight as determined by physical methods. Dr. John Smith himself, as he mentioned before, has done end-group assays of several polynucleotides synthesized by polynucleotide phosphorylase, and we have calculated molecular weights in this way. Dr. Warner has carried out centrifugal studies on these polynucleotides. We don't yet have enough data for a molecular weight based on sedimentation, but the results are clear-cut enough so that we can say that there is a very marked discrepancy. For example, take what we call the AGUC polymer which contains all of the bases, it has an average chain length, I believe, of about 30 units, and its molecular weight on this basis should be about 9,000; yet by sedimentation we can say that the molecular weight is over 70,000. That is also the case with other synthetic polynucleotides. I would like to ask Dr. Smith the question whether the chain length of TMV has been determined and whether one finds similar discrepancies.

BASE COMPOSITION OF COLUMN FRACTIONS OF CALF THYMUS DNA

Fraction Number	Composition of Eluent		Molar Base Composition (Adenine = 1.00)			AD THY	GU CYT	Recovery per cent
	NaCl Molarity	NH$_3$ Molarity	Thymine	Guanine	Cytosine			
Original			0.97	0.77	0.77	1.03	1.00	95
50-54	0.25		0.91	0.61	0.81	1.10	0.75	91
55-57	0.30		0.88	0.64	0.84	1.14	0.76	89
197	2	0.1	0.88	0.67	0.74	1.14	0.91	89
199-200	2	0.1	0.95	0.64	0.74	1.05	0.87	98
236-237	2	0.25	0.98	0.63	0.74	1.02	0.85	100
242	2	0.45	0.98	0.78	0.78	1.02	1.00	99
244	2	0.53	0.94	0.86	0.90	1.06	0.96	104
I	0.29-0.40		1.01	0.64	0.74	0.99	0.91	
III		pH10-10.8	1.03	0.83	0.77	0.97	1.08	
IV		0.5N NaOH	0.99	0.78	0.79	1.01	0.99	

Dr. Smith: Nucleic acid of the Cambridge strain of TMV has a chain length of almost 50 nucleotide residues, but no physical studies of molecular weight have been made on nucleic acid from this strain.

Dr. Ochoa: If I may say just a few more words, a further point of information comes from the results of the analysis of *Azotobacter* RNA mentioned by Dr. Chargaff. He pointed out to me that the analysis was done on whole cells, and it is interesting to note that these analyses are very close to those obtained by Dr. Smellie in our laboratory on RNA isolated from *Azotobacter*.

Dr. Butler: This discrepancy between the molecular weight and end-group analysis is not very surprising, but one would like to know, of course, under what conditions the sedimentation value was estimated. In our experience RNA aggregates very easily and so could complicate the determination.

Dr. Ochoa: I might say, Dr. Butler, that Dr. Warner had similar results with our synthetic polynucleotides. There is clear-cut evidence for aggregation, and presumably the differences in chain-length and sedimentation are due to that factor.

Dr. Buchanan: Dr. Roland Beers, who has been working at M.I.T. on polynucleotide phosphorylase, finds that he can get almost any molecular weight or polynucleotide he wants to, depending upon how he chooses to isolate the material after the enzymatic reaction. This is more a function of the care he takes in isolating the polynucleotide than it is of any other one factor. He can get values of 2 million when light scattering was used as the method of determining the molecular weight of his sample of polynucleotide.

Dr. Ochoa: Yes, that's true, but there you have already started with purified enzyme and the method of isolation of the polynucleotides is very mild. All we do to isolate the polynucleotides is to add alcohol at $0°C$. at the end of the reaction.

THE STRUCTURE OF DNA

F. H. C. CRICK

*The Medical Research Council Unit for the
Study of the Molecular Structure of Biological Systems,
The Cavendish Laboratory, Cambridge, England*

THE STRUCTURE proposed for DNA (deoxyribonucleic acid) has been described before (for a review, see Jordan, 21) and will only be outlined here. It consists of two polynucleotide chains running in opposite directions and twined round one another. The two chains are held together by hydrogen bonds between the bases, each base being joined to a companion base on the other chain. This pairing of bases is specific, adenine going with thymine, and guanine with cytosine. The structure is not only found in extracted DNA from a wide variety of sources, but is also present in intact biological material such as sperm heads and bacteriophage (36).

The x-ray work up to 1954 has already been briefly summarized, with references (6). Since then, the group at King's College, London, under Dr. M. H. F. Wilkins have published an interim report (17) on their studies of the B form of DNA and on their work on nucleoprotamine. Two reviews (9, 37) have also appeared; the one by Wilkins (37) touching on the very recent work of his group on nucleohistone. Some studies of the B form of DNA have also been carried out by Wykoff (38), who has shown that the B structure obtained by stretching the A form is slightly different from that produced by swelling it. The King's College group have obtained the B form in a crystalline state, and in particular, have shown that the lithium salt gives a good lattice (37).

According to Wilkins (37), the structure is now firmly established. The detailed structure described by Crick and Watson (8) has been shown to have too large a diameter, and a drawing has been given of an improved model which is in fairly good agreement with the x-ray data. No coordinates have so far been published.* (It should be noted

* Dr. Wilkins has offered to make his provisional coordinates available to anyone who would like to have them.

that there is some minor disagreement between Wykoff and the King's College group.) The published work on the A form is even more preliminary. This is unfortunate, as the ultimate test of a model must be its agreement with the very beautiful and detailed pictures which Wilkins and his coworkers have obtained from the A form. It is encouraging to learn that isomorphous replacements of Na, K, and Rb ions have been possible (37). The full publication of the experimental data, together with the coordinates of the proposed models and their calculated Fourier transforms is awaited with interest.

There have been two independent suggestions (19, 24) that the polynucleotide chains of the DNA structure are paranemically coiled; that is to say, that the two chains are not truly intertwined, but merely lie side by side in an intimate but distorted embrace. Gamow (19) does not use the term paranemic coiling to describe his proposal, but his suggestion that "the long helical molecule is wound into a coil possessing the same repetition period as the original helix" is a description of paranemic coiling. This has already been discussed and rejected (35), as being very difficult to reconcile with the data. The two authors putting forth this idea are apparently unaware of the convention that for a structure to be given serious consideration it must be possible to build a scale model of it having acceptable bond distances and angles— inspiration by itself is not enough. Until a satisfactory model has been presented this idea must be regarded as incorrect.

The experimental evidence, other than the x-ray data, which supports the double helical model, falls into two classes: the chemical evidence, and the physico-chemical evidence. The chemical evidence shows that the molar ratio of adenine/thymine and of guanine/cytosine + 5-methyl cytosine are very close to unity for all sources of DNA. This striking experimental fact was originally pointed out by Chargaff. The latest evidence is reviewed by Chargaff elsewhere in this volume (3).

Unusual Bases

One feature of the recent analytical data which appears to be causing a certain amount of confusion is the occurrence in DNA of various bases other than the usual four. The replacement of cytosine by 5-hydroxymethyl cytosine (probably with glucose attached) in the T-even phages presents no problem, since it will fit into the structure without difficulty. The smaller amount of 5-methyl cytosine which occurs in the DNA of various organisms is again not a structural problem, since it appears to replace cytosine, in the sense that the molar sum of cytosine and 5-methyl cytosine is closely equal to the number of moles of guanine. The same applies to the very small amounts of 6-methyl aminopurine (15) found in certain bacteria. However, the larger amounts of this base which apparently replace thymine in the thymineless mutant T15⁻ of *Escherichia coli*, when growing without a supply of thymine (14), do constitute a problem; but the effect is lethal to the cells and the DNA may well be abnormal.

A possible explanation of this peculiar behavior is suggested by the data on 5-methyl cytosine. This base does not replace cytosine at random, since it has been shown that different fractions of DNA have large variations in the cytosine/5-methyl cytosine ratio (3, 4, 25). However, it has been found that 5-methyl cytosine occurs almost entirely next to guanine (30-32).

This relationship suggests that the precursors of DNA are not mononucleotides (or related molecules) but resemble dinucleotides or higher nucleotides. Applying this idea to the case of 6-methyl aminopurine, one might surmise that 6-methyl aminopurine (denoted by X) is incorporated not by itself, but attached to some other nucleotide, probably thymidylic acid (denoted by T) either as XT or as TX, and that, in particular, it goes into places which would normally accommodate TT. The amounts incorporated are crudely compatible with this idea. This hypothesis has the unusual advantage of being testable—for example, by analyzing the various amounts of various dinucleotides, from a partial digest, which contains X. In general, whenever an unusual base is incorporated into DNA it would be well worth-while to see if it occurs with certain preferred neighbors (including the ends of the polynucleotide chains).

PHYSICAL CHEMICAL EVIDENCE

There is now much physical evidence to support a two-chain structure. Briefly, this includes the titration curve (20-23, 27), which suggests that the bases form hydrogen bonds, and that these are bonds within the structure, since the titration hysteresis persists to very low dilutions (22); the shape and size of the molecule in solution, obtained from a combination of light scattering, viscosity, and sedimentation measurements (12, 28), which show that DNA in solution is highly extended, but not completely straight, and that its diameter is compatible with the double helix model (12); and also studies of the rates at which the structure is broken down by gamma rays (5), acid (34), or enzymatic attack (33), which are consistent with there being two strands in the DNA, so that the molecule does not come apart until there are breaks in both backbones almost opposite one another (opposite to within two nucleotides, according to Thomas, 33).

The claim of Alexander and Stacey (1) to have separated the two chains by the use of various treatments, such as exposure to 4 M urea, has not been accepted by other workers (12). Similarly the suggestion of Dekker and Schachman (10) that there were occasional breaks (say 1 in 50) in the phosphate-sugar backbone has not been supported by the recent evidence (27, 33, 34), which seems to show that breaks, if they exist at all, must occur only very infrequently (less than 1 in 500, say).

GENERAL REMARKS

It is important to notice the combination of symmetry and pseudo-symmetry, and of repetition and non-repetition, in the DNA structure. The phosphate-sugar backbone repeats regularly, both chemically and structurally. This repetition necessarily implies that the phosphate-sugar groups are related by symmetry, in this case by a screw axis, and it is this which makes the backbone a simple helix. Again, the two separate phosphate-sugar backbones are related to each other by symmetry, in this case by two-fold rotation axes perpendicular to the fiber axis.

The arrangement of the bases, however, does not repeat, and only shows pseudosymmetry; that is, the region occupied by a pair of bases is fixed, and successive regions are related to each other by symmetry, but there is no restriction on which pair of bases occurs at any point, as long as one of the allowed pairs is used.

There are many different ways of pairing the four common bases, using two hydrogen bonds, and these have recently been systematically described by Donohue (11). As far as we know, these are all equally likely in solution. The base pairing described is the only satisfactory way which allows all four bases to occur on one chain, and which will fit the x-ray data. It remains to be seen whether there are other structural reasons (e.g., that the glycosidic bond must point roughly toward the axis) which favor the particular pairing suggested.

It should be noted that while x-ray diffraction shows that a substantial portion of the DNA must be in the double helix form it is an extremely poor method for deciding how much of the DNA is in this configuration. The titration curve and the analytical data suggest that the great majority of bases are paired. However, as has been stressed before (35), it seems certain that the molecule is folded in its biological condition, and there may conceivably be occasional regions where the configuration is somewhat modified. Before this idea becomes too popular, however, it would be nice to have some positive (rather than indirect) evidence for it.

REPLICATION AND GENE ACTION

The function of DNA is outside the scope of this paper, but there have recently been a number of suggestions for mechanisms which are based on features of the molecular structure. For example, the mechanism of Lockingen and DeBusk (26) depends on the presence of breaks in the backbones, which are now thought to be absent, or at least very rare. The suggestion of Block (2) depends upon being able to turn over the bases—as does the scheme of Dounce, Morrison, and Monty (13) for RNA. This may be possible for adenine, but molecular models suggest that it is difficult if not impossible to do it for guanine, thymine, and cytosine because the resulting van der Waals contact would be too close (between the pyrimidine O, in position 2, and the ribose ring oxygen, or between the NH_2 of guanine and the adjacent sugar). The suggestion of Schwartz (29), that aromatic amino acids are sandwiched between pairs of bases, can be criticized (apart from the rather doubtful idea that 5-membered rings attract only 5-membered rings, and 6-membered rings only 6-membered rings) on the ground that it seems unlikely that such a model could be constructed, since the argument that the bases can be packed 7 Å apart is based on a misconception of the structure.

In both these cases, it would have been better if the authors had attempted to build scale models* to show that their ideas were structurally feasible.

Incidentally, it is possible to produce schemes similar to that of Block by separating the base-pairs by *rotating* one of the DNA chains about the fiber axis, relative to the other. This is structurally possible if the bases are not too close to the axis of the molecule, but this may not normally be the case (17, 36).

* A recent comment that "Real Research is done at the Bench and not playing about with Metal Models," should be ignored here.

Although not directly supported by the experimental evidence, it seems very probable that the two phosphate-sugar backbones run in opposite directions and are related by two-fold axes. This means that if we regard the sequence of base pairs as a code, there is nothing in the structure to tell us in which direction to read it, *except* the sequence of the bases themselves. Thus, a code of the type described by Gamow (18) does not specify the *direction* of the polypeptide chain for which the DNA is supposed to be coding. For example, the sequence gly-ala-leu would correspond in his code to the same piece of DNA as would leu-ala-gly, using the usual convention. There are several ways out of the dilemma—for example, that the base-sequence makes "sense" if read one way and "nonsense" if read the other—but the point is a fundamental one and should not be overlooked.

It has been pointed out elsewhere (7) that the most obvious way in which the sequence of bases could express itself in terms of physical chemistry is in the patterns of sites for hydrogen bonding presented by the structure. The significance of 6-methylaminopurine in this respect should be noted, since the introduction of the methyl group changes this pattern radically, at least on the inner surfaces of the structure.

NUCLEOPROTEIN

Essentially all the x-ray work on nucleoprotein has been done by Wilkins and his coworkers (17, 37). Much of it is still in a very preliminary stage.

Nucleoprotamine.

The evidence suggests that the protamine chain is wound helically round the DNA structure in the *smaller* of the two grooves between the backbones (17). Models show (17) that an extended polyarginine chain can be fitted in there without difficulty, with the positively charged basic groups of the side-chains going alternately up and down to the negatively charged phosphate groups of the DNA backbones. In nucleoprotamine there appears to be one arginine for every phosphate, yet only two-thirds of the protamine side-chains are basic. This suggests that the polypeptide chain is folded whenever the non-polar amino acids occur. Model building shows (17) that it is difficult to construct a fold with one non-polar residue, but relatively easy with two in succession. The data on the amino acid sequence (16) show that the non-polar residues do indeed occur in pairs. It is not yet clear whether the interaction between the non-polar residues and the bases of the DNA structure is specific or non-specific, nor whether the non-polar folds go inwards or outwards (17).

Nucleohistone.

The main features of the preliminary x-ray work (37) are that (1) the DNA—or at least part of it—maintains its characteristic structure; and that (2) some larger repeating structure is also present. These results are obtained with nuclei, swollen in water and drawn into fibers, and also with artificial combinations of DNA with (lysine-rich) histone. One equatorial spacing (of about 60 Å) changes little on drying; another, around 40 Å, alters with humidity. The significance of these results is not yet clear. Their main importance is to show that nucleohistone has a structure of some sort.

ACKNOWLEDGMENT

I should like to thank Dr. M. H. F. Wilkins for allowing me to read the manuscript of his latest paper (37) before publication.

REFERENCES

1. Alexander, P., and Stacey, K. A., *Biochem. J.,* **60**, 194 (1955).
2. Block, D. P., *Proc. Natl. Acad. Sci. U. S.,* **41**, 1058 (1955).
3. Chargaff, E., this volume.
4. Chargaff, E., Crampton, C. F., and Lipshitz, R., *Nature,* **172**, 289 (1953).
5. Cox, R. A., Overend, W. G., Peacocke, A. R., and Wilson, S., *Nature,* **176**, 919 (1955).
6. Crick, F. H. C., *Proc. Natl. Acad. Sci. U. S.,* **40**, 756 (1954).
7. Crick, F. H. C., *Biochem. Soc. Symposia* (in press).
8. Crick, F. H. C., and Watson, J. D., *Proc. Roy. Soc. (Lond.),* A, **223**, 80 (1954).
9. Crick, F. H. C., and Watson, J. D., *Rend. ist. Lombardo Sci., Pt. I.,* **89**, 52 (1955).
10. Dekker, C. A., and Schachman, H. K., *Proc. Natl. Acad. Sci. U. S.,* **40**, 894 (1954).
11. Donohue, J., *Proc. Natl. Acad. Sci. U. S.,* **42**, 60 (1956).
12. Doty, P., *Intern. Congr. Biochem.,* **3** (Brussels, 1955), 135 (1956).
13. Dounce, A. L., Morrison, M., and Monty, K. J., *Nature,* **176**, 597 (1955).
14. Dunn, D. B., and Smith, J. D., *Nature,* **175**, 336 (1955).
15. Dunn, D. B., and Smith, J. D., *Biochem. J.,* **60**, XVII (1955).
16. Felix, K., Fischer, H., and Krekels, A., *Progr. Biophys. and Biophys. Chem,* **6**, 1 (1956).
17. Feughelman, M., Langridge, R., Seeds, W. E., Stokes, A. R., Wilson, H. R., Hooper, C. W., Wilkins, M. H. F., Barclay, R. K., and Hamilton, L. D., *Nature,* **175**, 834 (1955).
18. Gamow, G., *Kgl. Danske Videnskab. Selskab, Biol. Medd.,* **22**, 1 (1954).

19. Gamow, G., *Proc. Natl. Acad. Sci. U. S.*, **41**, 7 (1955).
20. Gulland, J. M., Jordan, D. O., and Taylor, H. F. W., *J. Chem. Soc.*, 1131 (1947).
21. Jordan, D. O., in *The Nucleic Acids*, Vol. I (E. Chargaff and J. N. Davidson, eds.), Academic Press, New York (1955).
22. Jordan, D. O., Mathieson, A. R., and Matty, Sheila, *J. Chem. Soc.*, 154 and 158 (1956).
23. Lea, W. A., and Peacocke, A. R., *J. Chem. Soc.*, 3361 (1951).
24. Linser, H., *Biochim. et Biophys. Acta*, **16**, 295 (1955).
25. Lipshitz, R., and Chargaff, E., *Biochim. et Biophys. Acta*, **19**, 256 (1956).
26. Lockinger, L. S., and DeBusk, A. G., *Proc. Natl. Acad. Sci. U. S.*, **41**, 925 (1955).
27. Peacocke, A. R., *J. Chem. Soc.* (in press).
28. Sadron, C., *Intern. Congr. Biochem.*, **3** (Brussels, 1955), 125 (1956).
29. Schwartz, D., *Proc. Natl. Acad. Sci. U. S.*, **41**, 300 (1955).
30. Sinsheimer, R. L., *J. Biol. Chem.*, **208**, 445 (1954).
31. Sinsheimer, R. L., *J. Biol. Chem.*, **215**, 579 (1955).
32. Smith, J. D., and Markham, R., *Nature*, **170**, 120 (1952).
33. Thomas, C. A., *J. Am. Chem. Soc.*, **78**, 1861 (1956).
34. Thomas, C. A., and Doty, P., *J. Am. Chem. Soc.*, **78**, 1854 (1956).
35. Watson, J. D., and Crick, F. H. C., *Cold Spring Harbor Symposia Quant. Biol.*, **18**, 123 (1953).
36. Wilkins, M. H. F., Seeds, W. E., Stokes, A. R., and Wilson, H. R., *Nature*, **172**, 759 (1953).
37. Wilkins, M. H. F., *Biochem. Soc. Symposia* (in press).
38. Wykoff, H. W., Thesis, Mass. Inst. Technology (1955).

THE PHYSICAL HETEROGENEITY OF DNA

J. A. V. BUTLER AND K. V. SHOOTER

Chester Beatty Research Institute,
Fulham Road,
London S. W. 3, England

IF DNA IS the genetic material it obviously must carry an enormous variety of characteristics. The fractionation of DNA by various means examined by Chargaff (2), Brown and Watson (1) and Lucy and Butler (4, 5), has yielded fractions of different composition indicating that chemical heterogeneity does occur. Physical heterogeneity has been observed in our observations with the ultracentrifuge at very low concentration, in which a wide range of sedimentation constants, often extending from S = 10 to 40 or more, is observed in a single specimen (6, 7). This range of sedimentation constants seems to be quite real and it is possible to separate DNA's with higher and lower sedimentation constants by centrifuging in the preparative centrifuge (Fig. 1) (8).

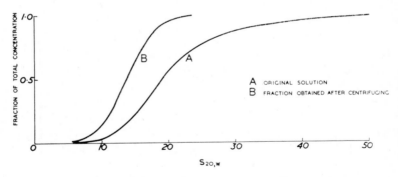

FIG. 1.   Fractionation of calf thymus DNA by centrifuging.

The distribution of sedimentation coefficients observed, however, is found to depend on the preparative procedures used. When DNA is isolated by the detergent process of Dounce and Simmons (3), it is found that its characteristics are very similar to that of a solution of the nucleoprotein in 2.5 M salt solutions (Fig. 2). However, the Sevag

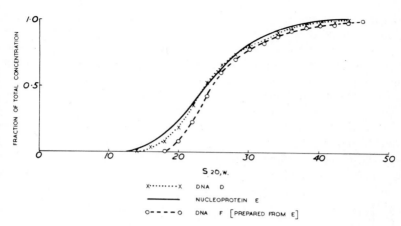

FIG. 2. Sedimentation characteristics of DNA obtained by adding 2.5 *M* NaCl to nucleoprotein and after precipitation.

process was found to yield DNA specimens with lower average sedimentation constants.

It is obvious, then, that there must be a considerable variation of particle configuration in the specimens of DNA as prepared. This does not seem to be correlated with composition in any way, as the fractionation by composition does not yield specimens with very different sedimentation constants (4, 5). It has not yet been possible to prepare DNA specimens by fractional centrifugation in sufficient quantity to determine their composition.

We may ask what is the origin of the different configurations. There must be a considerable variety of shapes, but we have not yet been able to make a comparison of the sedimentation behavior with light-scattering molecular weights. It might be noted that in light-scattering investigations efficient centrifugation procedures are undertaken with the object of removing "dust," and this probably has a marked influence on the molecular weights of the specimens studied.

At present we are unable to draw any conclusions about the nature of the configurations of the DNA particles. The results are not compatible with a system of fairly straight rods of constant diameter and different lengths. It may be that some kind of aggregation occurs, with the result that we have clusters of particles of different sizes. The nature of the distribution is not markedly dependent on the method of dissolving the specimen. Addition of bivalent salts such as calcium chloride has very little effect; and this is also true of complexing agents such as versene. It can be concluded that if aggregates exist they are not formed by association through ion bridges. The question of protein is a more difficult one. All our specimens contain protein, which is not removed by repeated treatment with detergent. It could well be that this protein holds the DNA in particular configurations. It will be of considerable interest to discover the nature and mode of binding of this residual protein. DNA from T_2 bacteriophage prepared by Dr. Loveless of the Chester Beatty Research Institute (Fig. 3) has also been examined. It shows a fairly wide range of sedimentation coefficients, though not so wide as that from beef thymus DNA.

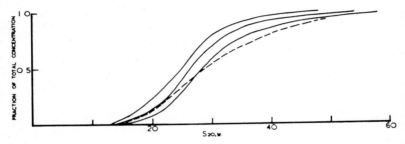

Fig. 3. Sedimentation characteristics of three preparations of T2 phage DNA (unbroken lines) and beef thymus nucleoprotein (TNA 23) (dotted line).

Finally, it may be useful to say something about the action of heat on DNA solutions (9). A short period of heating (15 mins.) at 100° C. in salt solutions causes a limited decrease of the sedimentation constant, together with a great decrease of viscosity. It is impossible to interpret this except as due to a decrease of molecular weight (to 1/4 or 1/6 of the original). However, heating in water, especially when continued, causes much more extensive degradation, and the average sedimentation drops into the region of 4-6.5. The question arises as to whether this degradation is due to breaks in the nucleotide chains originally present, or whether they are produced by hydrolysis during the heating. It is very difficult to detect the minute amounts of chemical change which would be sufficient to be responsible for the decreases of molecular weight which are observed. If it is a slow hydrolytic process which causes the breaks, there is no reason why it should not continue until extensive hydrolysis can be observed.

REFERENCES

1. Brown, G. L., and Watson, M., *Nature,* **172**, 339 (1953).
2. Chargaff, E., *Nature,* **172**, 289 (1953).
3. Kay, E. R. M., Simmons, N. S., and Dounce, A. L., *J. Am. Chem. Soc.,* **74**, 1724 (1952).
4. Lucy, J. A., and Butler, J. A. V., *Nature,* **174**, 32 (1954).
5. Lucy, J. A., and Butler, J. A. V., *Bull. soc. chim. Belges,* **65**, 133 (1956).
6. Shooter, K. V., and Butler, J. A. V., *Nature,* **175**, 500 (1955).
7. Shooter, K. V., and Butler, J. A. V., *Trans. Faraday Soc.,* **52**, 734 (1956).
8. Shooter, K. V., and Butler, J. A. V., *Nature,* **177**, 1033 (1956).
9. Shooter, K. V., Pain, R. H., and Butler, J. A. V., *Biochim. et Biophys. Acta,* **20**, 497 (1956).

DISCUSSION

DR. ALLFREY: I would like to point out that concerning nucleo-histones, at least as they exist in nuclei, there are linkages which should be kept in mind other than those between histone and DNA. To cite an instance of that, if you take thymus nuclei and remove all the DNA using DNAase, the histone remains in the nucleus bound to other proteins.

DR. G. SCHMIDT: I think the only analysis of liver nucleohistone was reported in a paper by Luck in one of the recent issues of the *Journal of Biological Chemistry.* If one calculates the number of basic groups, one finds an almost exact equivalence to the number of phosphate groups in the nucleic acid. This would be perhaps interesting to Dr. Crick, because the distances between basic amino acids in the histone moiety would certainly be very different from those in protamines.

DR. DAVIDSON: I have two comments to make on the nucleohistones. From the analysis of thymus material the proportion of basic amino acid is only enough to satisfy 85% to 90% of the phosphate groups of the nucleic acid, and the sodium content in the isolated material would satisfy the remaining phosphate groups. The presence of these free phosphate groups is also indicated by dye binding of bases, and the suggestion that these groups are free is conceded by other people in the field. Of the histones surrounding the nucleic acid, they are not homogeneous, but they all contain approximately 25% basic amino acids, on molar ratios—in other words, ¾ of them are nonbasic residues. That means that, if you are going to propose any sort of regular structure in order to get such a high proportion of the phosphate groups satisfied by the available basic amino acids, then the fit will not reasonably go into the narrow groove or the deeper groove on the nucleic acid and you would anticipate an increased diameter of the nucleohistone.

DR. SCHACHMAN: We have been following this tremendous poly-dispersity with respect to sedimentation rate which is exhibited by most preparations of thymus DNA: and we too have fractionated this material by centrifugal methods. We reasoned that it should be possible to decide whether the polydispersity observed in the ultracentrifuge is due to heterogeneity of the molecules with respect to shape or molecular weight or whether there is heterogeneity with regard both to shape and weight. The way one goes about this is to determine whether the material that sediments more closely does so because the molecules are more stretched out and therefore experience more frictional resistance to movement in a centrifugal field. Solutions of molecules which are very elongated will have a higher viscosity than a solution containing more compactly coiled macromolecules. The results of preliminary experiments performed with Dr. V. Schumaker show that the fraction containing the more slowly sedimenting particles is not more viscous but, on the contrary, is less viscous than equivalent concentrations of the unfractionated materials or the more rapidly sedimenting fraction. The bulk of our preliminary evidence indicates that we are dealing with polydispersity mainly with regard to molecular weight, although it isn't clear that the difference in viscosity between a leading and trailing material can be accounted for solely by differences in molecular weight. It seems likely that variations in shape from particle to particle have to be considered as well. The next part of my comments, I think, ought to deal with the DNA isolated from phage, about which we shall hear more tomorrow. Dr. S. S. Cohen has obtained a series of DNA preparations from different phages and these samples have been examined in the ultracentrifuge by the same techniques. The results can be summarized by saying that the material by and large is more homogeneous than the DNA from calf thymus and, more importantly, the phage DNA is much larger. It is not only more rapidly sedimenting, but is also more viscous and its dependence of viscosity on shear gradient is also greater than that observed for thymus DNA. The molecular weights calculated from these data turn out to be in the neighborhood of 25×10^6 as contrasted with only 6 or 7×10^6 for thymus DNA. When you get to thinking about molecular weights of such polydisperse material I think it is fair to say that the molecular weight distribution is more important than just some average molecular weight. In fact, with this high degree of polydispersity it seems as if even the average molecular weight deduced from light-scattering studies will require further revision, and it seems fair to summarize by stating that we do not know the molecular weight of DNA at all. The importance of knowledge of the molecular weight of DNA is perhaps the subject of another discussion, but I wanted only to emphasize our ignorance even in this area.

Before I sit down I would like to make a few comments about the remarks of Dr. Crick on the subject of interruptions in DNA. Dekker and I pointed out some time ago that we should be able to obtain information of relevance to the two-strand model proposed by Watson and Crick by a detailed examination of the kinetics of degradation of DNA by the enzyme, deoxyribonuclease. Upon reviewing the literature we found that the one thing that stood out in apparent contradiction to the model was the end-group analysis about which we have already had some discussion with regard to RNA. The end-group analysis for DNA is much worse than it is for RNA, and the only decent end-group analysis at that time appeared to be the results of titration studies which were interpreted as indicating a group dissociating with the apparent constant of a secondary phosphoryl group—i.e., originating from monoesterified and therefore terminal phosphate groups. At that time those people who performed the titration studies concluded that there was one such terminal phosphate group for every 30 to 50 nucleotides. If this were the case, then obviously the two-strand model would require some modification. The modification proposed at the time involved the addition of short branches to the backbone structure. This seemed unappealing to us for the reasons that Dr. Smith already mentioned concerning the instability of triesterified phosphate groups. So we proposed just making some cuts in the two-strand model in order to explain the data. We looked around to see if there was any other pertinent information on this subject and focussed our attention on the reported heat degradation of DNA and the making of apurinic acid. Accordingly we did some heating experiments, and from a combination of ultracentrifugal and viscosimetric data concluded that DNA was broken down by heating for fifteen minutes at 100° C. and pH 7.5. It seems unlikely to us that phosphodiester bonds are being broken during this treatment, but "unlikely" is far from "certain." We therefore did some experiments to detect the hydrogen ions which would have been liberated had there been hydrolysis of phosphodiester bonds, and we were unable to detect such hydrogen ions. This does not mean, however, that there was no hydrolysis. We did all our heating experiments, by design, in the absence of salt or at low ionic strengths even though DNA at such low ionic strengths loses its biological activity. The reason for this, of course, was that we wanted electrostatic repulsion to be manifested so that the individual pieces would come apart if, indeed, DNA is made up of smaller molecules held together by secondary forces. The heating experiments, I think, are satisfactory, but I for one am in no better position than I was a year ago to conclude that these experiments can be interpreted to mean that there are breaks or interruptions in the backbone structure of DNA. The next part of our studies has been directed toward finding out whether the enzyme kinetics give any information regarding interruptions. Let us now forget interruptions and deal with the enzyme kinetics briefly. First, we have to tell DNAase how to act. We have no objection to doing this but we must always bear in mind that we really do not know whether the enzyme follows our instructions. In any case we work on the assumptions that DNAase breaks only a single bond at a time and that the enzyme acts completely at random. Schumaker has shown that appropriate treatment of the data can lead directly to a determination of the number of strands. This follows because a single enzymatic splitting of a phosphodiester bond is 100% effective in creating a fission in a single-strand molecule. In contrast, if we have a two-strand structure, at least two attacks by the enzyme are needed, and they must be combined in a certain fashion, to cause splitting of the macromolecule. From measurements of the change in viscosity of a DNA solution as a function of the number of bonds broken by the enzyme we made the necessary calculation and came out with the unhappy answer that the macromolecules are made of 1.5 strands. In searching for an explanation as to why the answer was neither one nor two strands, we find many ways of getting out of this dilemma. One of them is to imagine the creation of a little flexibility in the macromolecule due to the splitting of a bond in one strand, thereby causing the viscosity to drop not by fission but by increased flexibility. Another way of explaining this, and the one to which we look forward with some enthusiasm, was to consider the question whether an interrupted two-strand model would have a number somewhere between one and two. If you calculate how many interruptions are needed to explain the difference between 2 and 1.5 we find, and Thomas independently has obtained similar results, that there are only a few such breaks necessary to account for the enzyme kinetics in terms of a two-strand model. There are still some difficulties in interpreting the enzyme kinetics, but, nonetheless, at this moment it looks as if this approach indicates that there are not many interruptions. If interruptions exist, the only way of demonstrating them would be through the use of specific end-group methods. This could be done with some phosphomonoesterase which would detect terminal phosphate groups. Until we have such a method with adequate controls to make certain that the enzyme is pure and attacking only known types of bonds, I see no way of answering this problem.

DR. MONTY: Dr. Butler has suggested that protein bridges between DNA molecules may be responsible in part for the more rapidly sedimenting fractions of his DNA preparations. In this connection I would like to describe briefly the results of some experiments carried out by Dr. Dounce and myself during the past few years. Our work has been primarily with rat liver, but there are indications that these considerations are rather generally applicable to animal tissues, at least, and perhaps to living systems in general. It is our conclusion that DNA does not exist normally as a free chemical compound, but rather is combined with protein through some linkage which appears to be more than simple ionic or hydrogen bonding.

The material remaining after the quantitative removal of globulins and histones from isolated cell nuclei is what we refer to as deoxyribonucleoprotein. One might expect this preparation to be contaminated by such materials as the constituents of the nuclear membrane, but thus far our attempts to detect and remove such possible contaminants have been unsuccessful. This nucleoprotein is decidedly different from, and not to be confused with, the nucleohistones and nucleoprotamines.

The deoxyribonucleoprotein apparently cannot be separated into its two components—DNA and protein—without the mediation of mild hydrolysis. Heating at 100° C. for seven minutes in the presence of dilute acid, dilute alkali, or even at neutrality, causes disruption of the molecule to yield free, high-polymer DNA and free protein. The bonds uniting the DNA to protein thus appear to be rather labile. The molecule can be similarly destroyed, interestingly enough to the geneticist perhaps, by low doses of ionizing radiation (*J. Biophys. Biochem. Cytol.*, **1**, 155-160, 1955). Approximately 1000 r of x-rays will cause almost complete cleavage of the DNA from the protein, judging by our criteria.

Our measurements of the integrity of the nucleoprotein are based upon the elastic properties of its solutions. At concentrations far below the levels where the viscosity of the DNA becomes significant, the nucleoprotein solutions are firm, elastic gels. DNA, you may remember, has a practical limit of solubility at about 0.25%, above which concentrations a stiff, non-fluid gel is obtained. The nucleoprotein gels will refuse to flow at concentrations which are only one one-hundredth of this value. In very dilute solutions, the elasticity of the nucleoprotein is displayed by a tendency to recoil from a swirling motion. The solution appears to wind up, and then unwind when the swirling force is removed. By measuring the dilution required to destroy this recoil-ability, we are able to estimate the destruction of the DNA-protein bonds in the radiation-susceptibility experiments. This is not as fine a measure of nucleoprotein destruction as we would like to have, but it was the most sensitive method available at the time.

Another point about the hydrolytic destruction of the deoxyribonucleoprotein, and the most likely reason for the failures to recognize its existence in the past, concerns its susceptibility to enzymatic attack. There exists within the soluble internal phase of mitochondria an enzyme, or a series of enzymes, which will quickly cause the dissociation of the nucleoprotein into its constituent molecular sub-species (*J. Biophys. Biochem. Cytol.*, **1**, 139-153, 1955). This enzyme system is most active around pH 6, a very common pH for cytochemical investigations. If damage to the mitochondria is incurred during the preparation of an homogenate, the enzymes are released, and profound degradation of the nucleoprotein can result. The final products of this attack are free protein and DNA.

The protein constituents of the deoxyribonucleoprotein appear to be the lipoproteins commonly recognized as nuclear constituents, and these have been studied in the past by a number of laboratories. There are two classes of these proteins, rcognizable by their different solubility properties, released by the hydrolytic cleavage of the nucleoprotein. Histones do not seem to be involved.

Since the attachment of DNA to protein is relatively stable at pH values around neutrality and at moderate temperatures, it has been possible to separate degradation products, produced by the action of enzymes on the nucleoprotein, which appear to contain both amino acids (presumably as peptides) and nucleotides (presumably as oligo-nucleotides). This was accomplished as follows. Deoxyribonucleo-protein was treated successively with crystalline pancreatic trypsin, chymotrypsin, and DNAase. The products of this degradation, after removal of the enzymes, were examined by paper electrophoresis. Bands of material were found which did not migrate with the expected mobil-ity of free peptides or nucleotides, and which contained both nucleo-tides and amino acids, as judged by the ultraviolet absorption spectra and tests with the ninhydrin reagent. These zones very probably con-tain the "points of attachment" between the DNA and the protein. It is hoped that further work with these degradation products will ultimately identify the type of bond that is involved.

I should also like to insert a comment about the isolation of DNA. Detergents are commonly used today to aid in obtaining protein-free presentations of DNA. In our experience, the dissociation of DNA from the lipoproteins by anionic detergents is slow without the hydro-lytic assistance of either the mitochondrial enzyme system or heat. It is likely that many of these detergent methods depend upon the action of these enzymes, rather than on some catalytic power of the detergent, to rupture the bonds between protein and DNA. The isolation procedures which involve precipitation of protein at an organic solvent interface do not release DNA from the nucleoprotein. Sevag (*J. Biol. Chem.*, **124**, 425-436, 1938) observed that mild hydrolysis in bicarbonate solutions would shorten the duration of his procedure, and greatly increase the yields of DNA. At any rate, it appears that a method for the isolation of DNA must provide for the hydrolytic cleavage of the DNA-protein bonds as well as for the subsequent precipitation of protein.

A final comment about the size of the nucleoprotein molecule might be of interest. The centrifugation of very dilute solutions of the nucleoprotein in strong salt solutions results in the recovery of the nucleoprotein as a concentrated gel in the bottom of the tube. This may be done, for example, with only 700 g in about ½ hour. This very high sedimentation rate would suggest either that we did not have a true solution to start with, or that the molecular weight of the nucleoprotein is extremely high. Our experiences with these "solu-tions" lead us to favor the latter interpretation. One is tempted to postulate, then, that DNA exists in nature in a huge macromolecular polymer with protein. Such a macromolecule could be of use in explain-ing several attributes of the chromosome, as, for example, its "coiled-thread" morphology and the exact retention of gene order along its length.

DR. DOUNCE: I would like to add to Dr. Monty's comments about the destruction of the nucleoprotein by mitochondrial factors. We originally doubted (*J. Biophys. Biochem. Cytol.*, **1**, 155-160, 1955) that the mitochondrial enzyme system in question could be deoxyribo-nuclease, since a rather highly polymerized DNA could still be isolated from cell nuclei after the action of these enzymes, and since DNAase I acting at pH 7.0 would not liberate all of the DNA from the chromosomal protein, even when used repeatedly in relatively high concentrations. We have, however, been forced to revise this conclusion, as the result of subsequent studies showing that a component, at least, of the mitochondrial enzyme system is activated by magnesium, that the crystalline DNAase I on isolated nuclei at pH 6.0 closely resembles the action of the mitochondrial enzyme system, and that the fibrous DNA isolated from nuclei exposed to the mitochondrial enzyme system may be somewhat depolymerized. Our results are briefly as follows:

1. The mitochondrial enzyme system, or at least one of its components, requires a divalent metal (we have used magnesium) for activity. The enzyme in question cannot, therefore, be DNAase II, but it might be DNAase I if other properties were found to be in agreement with the known properties of the latter enzyme.

2. At least 98 per cent of the DNA can be liberated from the "residual" protein of the nuclei at pH 6.0 by properly diluted DNAase I, yielding on purification a fibrous product essentially free from protein, which is not highly depolymerized. At pH 7.0, DNAase I will not liberate more than 85 per cent of the DNA of nuclei which contain the latter substance in the firmly bound state, even on repeated applications of the enzyme, and the DNA that is removed is very extensively depolymerized.

3. Fibrous DNA isolated from nuclei previously exposed to the action of the mitochondrial enzyme system is also partially but not extensively depolymerized, as was ascertained from a study of its viscosity under various conditions, and is very similar to or identical with the fibrous DNA isolated from nuclei obtained at pH 4.0 after treatment with DNAase I at pH 6.0.

Thus it now seems very probable that the mitochondrial enzyme responsible to an important extent for the detachment of DNA from protein of the cell nucleus is DNAase I, although we have not excluded the possibility that other enzymes may also be involved. At pH 6.0 this enzyme appears to cleave mainly internucleotide bonds which are close to the points of attachment of the DNA to the protein, leaving short oligonucleotide stubs still attached to the protein. The lack of extensive depolymerization of the DNA forces us to conclude that internucleotide bonds more distant from the points of attachment of the DNA to the protein must be to a considerable extent protected against the action of the DNAase, perhaps because of condensation of protein on the DNA fibers at pH 6.0. On the other hand, at pH 7.0 internucleotide bonds close to points of attachment of the DNA to the protein seem less sensitive to attack by the enzyme than those which are more distant. At pH 7.0 we cannot expect to find a condensation of protein other than histone on the DNA fibers, and histone itself for some reason does not appear to complex strongly with the DNA except possibly in physiological saline. This situation may explain the apparent increase in exposure to DNAase I of internucleotide bonds distant from points of attachment of protein to DNA, that seems to occur when the pH is raised from 6.0 to 7.0.

It is more difficult to see why the enzyme should attack internucleotide bonds close to the points of attachment of DNA to protein more readily at pH 6.0 where the chromatin of the nuclei is condensed, than at pH 7.0 where the chromatin is in the form of a gel in the case of nuclei containing firmly bound DNA. Possibly the gel itself offers some steric hindrance to action of the enzyme.

The idea of a stable attachment of DNA to the residual protein of nuclei (or chromosomes) at the present time is slowly gaining ground, although many investigators still seem to doubt the validity of this concept. Kirby believes that the attachment is through metal (*Biochem. J.*, **62**, 31, 1956). We have as yet no direct evidence as to the type of bond involved, except that, as Dr. Monty has stated, it is labile to heat in the presence of dilute acid or alkali, and thus conceivably could be a phosphoamide bond. It seems clear, however, that most of the phosphate groups of the DNA molecule are not involved in bond formation of this sort, and we suspect attachment of the DNA to protein only at one or both ends of the DNA chain.

I want to make just one additional comment on the action of detergents. We have tried to chop the nucleic acid off from the residual protein in isolated nuclei by detergent at pH 7 and at room temperature, but even though we let the reaction run from 90 to 100 hours, we got very poor splitting. However when the pH was lowered a little (to about 6.2), the detergent did slowly liberate the DNA. I am inclined to think this was due to the action of the detergent itself rather than to the DNAase, because DNAase seems to have no activity in the presence of the detergent at pH 6.2, although there is some activity at pH 7.

Dr. Doty: As a result of the distributions of sedimentation constant found by Professors Butler and Schachman, Dr. Simmons and I have undertaken a brief study of fractions separated in the bucket rotor under identical conditions. This offers a test of whether the sedimentation distribution reflects primarily a distribution of molecular weights or rather of configurations amongst DNA molecules of essentially uniform molecular weight. In the former case the intrinsic viscosity of the supernatant would have fallen relative to the original solution; for the latter case—polydispersity with respect to configuration—it would have risen. The former turned out to be the case, but the effect was not as large as might have been expected. For example, when only 15% of the DNA remained in the supernatant its intrinsic viscosity was only about 25% lower than that of the original DNA.

We do not believe this is consistent with the observed sedimentation distributions being entirely due to molecular weight polydispersity. Going back to Dr. Crick's talk, I might mention that Mr. Zubay in our laboratory has isolated a nucleoprotein from thymus which we believe for the first time was made up of one DNA molecule plus the attending protein. It has a molecular weight of about 18 million and is slightly more than half protein. It turns out to have a configuration in solution identical with that of the DNA after the protein is removed, and its diameter is about double that of ordinary DNA. This is inviting material for further work along these lines.

X-RAY STUDIES ON RNA AND THE
SYNTHETIC POLYRIBONUCLEOTIDES

J. D. WATSON *

*The Medical Research Council Unit for the Study of the
Structure of Biological Systems, The Cavendish Laboratory,
Cambridge, England*

IN THIS ARTICLE, I shall summarize some recent experimental work pertaining to the structure of ribonucleic acid (RNA). Much of this work has been done by Alexander Rich, partly at the National Institutes of Health and partly in collaboration with Francis Crick and myself at the Cavendish Laboratory. More recently we have been joined by David Davies, working also at the National Institutes of Health.

Two years ago, Rich and I (5) reported the details of x-ray diagrams from oriented RNA fibers and emphasized that our experimental data were inadequate to allow a serious proposal for the basic configuration of the RNA molecule. The striking feature of the RNA x-ray diagram was its resemblance to the deoxyribonucleic acid (DNA) pattern (3, 6). The poor quality of the diagram, however, precluded any decision as to whether the similarity was accidental or whether we were dealing again with a two-stranded helical molecule. At that time we hoped that preparation of RNA by more gentle techniques would result in improved x-ray photographs, but in this respect we have been disappointed. It is possible that none of these techniques are yet mild enough to prevent denaturation of a "native" RNA molecule, but it is also conceivable that RNA exists in a highly ordered configuration only when it is combined with protein. We thus began to question whether it would be possible to establish the RNA structure by x-ray techniques.

Fortunately, the problem was transformed by the enzymatic synthesis of polyribonucleotides by Ochoa and his coworkers (4). Soon

* On leave from the Biology Department, Harvard University. Supported by a grant from the National Science Foundation.

after their discovery, Rich obtained x-ray diffraction photographs which immediately provided several very useful facts. Firstly, the x-ray diagrams of poly-AU (the co-polymer of adenylic acid and uridylic acids) and poly-AGCU (the co-polymer of all four ribonucleotides) are identical to those obtained from natural RNA. Secondly, the diagrams obtained from the pure polymers poly-A (adenylic acid) and poly-C (cytidylic acid) show similarities to the RNA diagram. Fiber diagrams have not yet been obtained from poly-G (guanylic acid) or poly-U (uridylic acid). Moreover, the fiber diagrams of poly-A and poly-C give indications of highly ordered structures. Some of the reflexions are quite sharp when compared to the diffuse bands of the RNA picture. This is a very encouraging result, for it suggests that the structures of the pure polymers can be solved by x-ray methods. We have therefore concentrated our efforts on these compounds. Most of our work has been with poly-A, largely because of the greater availability of its monomeric precursor.

In Fig. 1 is shown the diffraction pattern of poly-A fiber prepared from material synthesized enzymatically by Drs. R. Markham and D. Lipkin. The main feature to observe is the relative absence of meridional reflexions. This suggests a helical molecule. Only one reflexion appears to be truly meridional (3.75Å); and by helical diffraction theory (2), this tells us that the fiber axis translation between nucleotide residues on a given chain is 3.75Å. The repeat along the fiber axis is at about 15Å. Each chain thus contains approximately four nucleotides per fiber axis repeat. The innermost equatorial reflexion is at 15.6Å, which suggests a crystallographic unit cell with approximately that diameter. Unfortunately, we are not yet able to index the equatorial reflexions, since the second observed reflexion at about 7.8Å is most likely a second order of the 15.6Å reflexion. We thus cannot tell if the crystallographic units are hexagonally (or pseudo-hexagonally) close-packed or whether a tetragonal arrangement is present. In either case, however, the size of the unit cell indicates that more than one polynucleotide chain is present. Only two-chain or three-chain models need be considered, and three-chain models appear most improbable on density grounds. Even if we assume the larger hexagonal cell, three chains could only be present if the fiber possessed a density around 1.80. This is clearly incompatible with the measured density of 1.58. We thus conclude that two chains are found in the crystallographic unit cell.

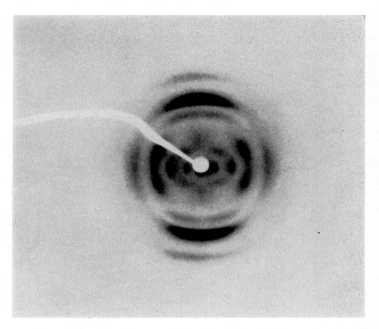

Fig. 1.   X-ray diffraction photograph of poly-A fiber. CuK α radiation. Flat film at 2 cm. fiber to film distance. The fiber axis is vertical, and the very strong meridional reflexion is at 3.75Å.

The symmetry of the helical diffraction absences restricts the possible polynucleotide configurations to two main classes. In the first, each chain has approximately a four-fold screw axis and a pitch of about 15Å. Two such chains are found in each unit cell, and they do not coil around each other but lie side by side. In the alternative class, the two chains coil around a common axis and are related by a parallel diad. Each chain has a pitch of about 30Å and the 15Å fiber axis repeat results from running the chains in the same direction. To attempt to distinguish between these two categories, we have constructed a number of specific molecular models and compared their predicted x-ray patterns with those actually observed.

Up till now, we have failed to find a satisfactory model of the first type. Though we can build a variety of models with a four-fold screw and a pitch of 15Å, their effective diameter tends to be about 10Å, and we have been unable to devise a specific model which directly gives a 15.6Å equatorial reflexion. Moreover, in none of our models have we found a satisfactory way to form hydrogen bonds involving either the amino group of adenine or the free hydroxyl group of ribose. We have been able to form satisfactory hydrogen bonds only with models that are markedly incompatible with the x-ray diagram. Even when we relax the requirement of suitable hydrogen bonding the agreement with the x-ray data (excluding the 15.6Å equatorial) is only fair.

On the contrary, we have been able to construct an intertwined chain model which appears more satisfactory, both from a-priori structural grounds and from considerations of the x-ray diffraction pattern. In this poly-A model, the sugar-phosphate backbone is on the outside of the molecule and the bases point toward the central axis. (Alternative models with the backbones in the center are very unlikely because of charge repulsions between neighboring phosphate groups.) The two chains are related by a parallel diad and two hydrogen bonds join together pairs of adenine residues at the same level. The hydrogen bonds run from the amino nitrogen in position 10 to the free nitrogen in position 7. The hydrogen atoms point almost directly toward the acceptor nitrogen atoms, and it is of interest that a similar arrangement was found by Broomhead (1) in crystals of adenine hydrochloride. Only one of the hydrogen atoms of the amino groups is involved in the base pairing, and it is possible that the second hydrogen atom will form an additional hydrogen bond to one of the non-esterified oxygen atoms in the phosphate group of the opposing chain. Formation of this second bond brings the phosphate group relatively close to the central axis and gives the molecule an effective radius of about 8Å. Because the thickness of a purine base (3.4Å) is less than the longitudinal translation (3.75Å), optimal van der Waals contact between adjacent bases is achieved by slightly tilting the bases in the direction of the pitch of the helix.

Though this model appears quite promising, we must emphasize that our work is still in a preliminary stage. We have not yet made a detailed comparison between the predicted and observed x-ray intensities. These calculations are now in progress. The preliminary results seem encouraging when compared to our more detailed calculations of four-fold screw models. We are also preparing various salts of poly-A in order to see if the cation influences the x-ray pattern. If changes are observed, we may be able to locate the cation and provide additional evidence for testing proposed models.

It is difficult to comment on RNA until the structure of poly-A is established. We will list, however, the reasons why we believe that the structures of the two are closely related: (1) Fibers of both poly-A and RNA are negatively birefringent. This fact suggests an approximately perpendicular arrangement of the bases with respect to the fiber axis. Likewise, both diffraction patterns show strong meridional (near?) reflexions in the 3Å-4Å region. This again indicates a perpendicular orientation of the bases. (2) Both diffraction photographs show systematic absences on the meridian. These absences are in the same regions and suggest a similar helical arrangement. (3) The first obvious layer in both poly-A and RNA is at about 15Å. On both patterns we find a prominent non-meridional reflexion about 45° from the meridian. (4) Both photographs show a strong reflexion on or near the equator in the 5Å region. This is the strongest reflexion from a dry RNA fiber, while in poly-A, its strength is second only to the very strong 3.75Å meridional reflexion. The only striking difference between the two patterns is that RNA has two strong meridional (near?) reflexions (3.3Å and 3.8Å) whereas poly-A gives only one 3.75Å reflexion. Here it is of interest that the strongest reflexions in the poly-C diagram are a 3.3Å meridional reflexion (or near meridional) and a 5Å equatorial (or near equatorial) reflexion (Rich, unpub.).

Thus if the structure of poly-A is a two-stranded hydrogen-bonded helix, it seems most likely that RNA will also be a two-stranded intertwined helix. We do not see, however, how such a structure could form regular hydrogen bonds. Not only do the purines and pyrimidines have different sizes, but in addition we must postulate a correspondence in sequence between opposing chains. It is thus possible that the RNA structure is very irregular and that the observed configuration results largely from the tendency of the backbone to assume a configuration similar to that of DNA. Such questions seem best deferred until the structures of the pure polymers are better understood.

REFERENCES

1. Broomhead, J., *Acta Cryst.*, **2**, 64 (1949).
2. Cochran, W., Crick, F. H. C., and Vand, V., *Acta Cryst.*, **5**, 581 (1952).
3. Franklin, R. E., and Gosling, R. G., *Nature,* **171**, 740 (1953).
4. Grunberg-Manago, M., Ortiz, R. J., and Ochoa, S., *Biochim. et Biophys. Acta,* **20**, 269 (1956).
5. Rich, A., and Watson, J. D., *Proc. Natl. Acad. Sci. U. S.,* **40**, 739 (1954).
6. Wilkins, M. H. F., Stokes, A. E., and Wilson, H. R., *Nature,* **171**, 738 (1953).

THE STRUCTURE OF SYNTHETIC POLYRIBONUCLEOTIDES AND THE SPONTANEOUS FORMATION OF A NEW TWO-STRANDED HELICAL MOLECULE

Alexander Rich

*National Institutes of Health,
Bethesda, Maryland*

Introduction

Most of our detailed knowledge about the configuration of biologically important macromolecules comes from x-ray diffraction studies. Using this method, it has been possible to obtain remarkably precise information about deoxyribose nucleic acid (DNA), which is of fundamental importance in understanding the chemical basis of heredity.

A basic understanding of molecular mechanisms in heredity requires a knowledge of the molecular configuration of ribose nucleic acid (RNA) in addition to that of DNA. Not only is RNA important in protein synthetic reactions, but it also acts as a carrier of genetic information in the plant and smaller animal viruses.

However, in marked contrast to DNA, knowledge about the molecular configuration of RNA is rudimentary. Successful x-ray diffraction studies require oriented molecules, either in crystals or in fibers. It has been impossible to obtain well-oriented RNA specimens which produce sharply defined diffraction photographs. Thus, the prospects for solving its structure directly have not been promising.

However, the recent synthesis of polyribonucleotides by Ochoa and his collaborators (3) has radically altered the pace of structural studies. These molecules have the same nucleotide units and covalent backbone as those found in native RNA. They act as substrates for a variety of enzymes which act on RNA itself. Thus it is apparent that these molecules might have molecular configurations similar to that of RNA, and could act as model substances for studying RNA. With these polymers, it became possible to control the composition as well as the chain length of the constituent molecules. This has led in many cases to well-oriented x-ray diffraction photographs. Some of the results obtained by studying them will be described here.

POLYADENYLIC ACID (A)

Polyadenylic acid can be polymerized to form viscous, high molecular weight material. From concentrated solutions it is possible to pull glassy birefringent fibers ($\Delta n = -0.08$) which are brittle and produce an oriented x-ray diffraction pattern. Some features of this pattern are similar to those found in an oriented RNA diffraction pattern, and this suggests that their structures may not be entirely dissimilar. The structure of polyadenylic acid has not been fully worked out yet. The status of the problem has been described in more detail by J. D. Watson in this symposium.

POLYURIDYLIC ACID (U)

Polyuridylic acid can be pulled into fibers which are not birefringent. These produce an amorphous diffraction pattern indicating that there is virtually no repetitive structural organization in these molecules.

POLY AU

It is possible to make mixed polymers by adding two or more nucleotide diphosphates to the reaction mixture. If both adenosine diphosphate and uridine diphosphate are added, an AU polymer is formed. It has been demonstrated by enzymatic digestion (3) that this is not a block copolymer but is rather an intimate mixture of A and U residues. From a viscous solution it is possible to pull fibers which are negatively birefringent ($\Delta n = -0.06$) and these yield an x-ray diffraction pattern similar in all details to that yielded by a variety of native RNA's (4, 7). Although these patterns are better oriented than those produced by RNA, they are still not of a sufficiently high quality to make possible a direct structural interpretation. Nonetheless, it is significant that both patterns are identical, since it demonstrates that the synthetic polymers can assume a configuration identical to that of the native molecule. This tends to confirm the chemical work carried out on the covalent polymer backbone and underlines the importance of carrying out structural studies on the synthetic polyribonucleotides.

It should be noted here that a polymer composed of all the four nucleotides found in native RNA produces the same diffraction pattern as that produced by AU and by native RNA (4).

Poly A + Poly U

Of great genetic interest is the reaction between polyadenylic acid and polyuridylic acid: when these two substances are mixed in solution, they spontaneously form a two-stranded helical molecule which is similar in many respects to DNA!

Warner (8) first reported a drop in optical density when these two compounds were mixed. In experiments carried out with Dr. D. R. Davies (5), we mixed these materials together and observed a very rapid increase in viscosity. It was then possible to draw very long, tough fibers which were strongly negatively birefringent, (Δn = −0.10). If these fibers are stretched, they neck down and start to lose their birefringence. By vigorous stretching it is possible to change the sign of the birefringence to positive. This phenomenon has been observed with both DNA and RNA (6, 10).

These fibers produce a well-oriented x-ray diffraction pattern (Fig. 1), with a distribution of intensity which is characteristically helical. The equator of this diffraction photograph shows that the molecules

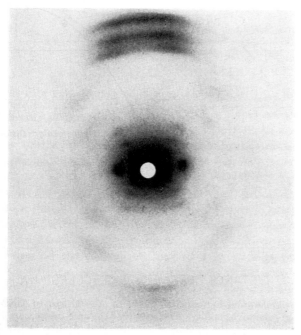

Fig. 1. X-ray diffraction pattern of mixed polyadenylic acid and polyuridylic acid (A + U) at 90% relative humidity. The fiber was tipped slightly from the vertical to show the splitting of the higher layer lines.

It is possible, however, to make an alternative interpretation of the diffraction photograph by assuming that the backbone chains are anti-parallel but that the molecule has a larger diameter than DNA. It is anticipated that further studies of the Fourier transforms of these two possible structures will permit us to distinguish between them.

The over-all similarity between the diffraction pattern produced by this synthetic molecule and that produced by DNA resolves one of the long-standing questions concerning the configuration which a ribonucleic acid backbone may adopt. Despite an earlier suggestion to the contrary (9), the additional hydroxyl group in the ribose residue does not prevent the backbone from assuming a configuration similar to that seen in DNA. It is therefore possible that the underlying mechanism for molecular duplication of RNA is identical to that which occurs with DNA. Further work on the intracellular configurations of RNA will be necessary before this suggestion can be fully evaluated.

Many of the problems which arise in understanding the molecular duplication of DNA are concerned with the energetics and the mechanism for separating the two polynucleotide chains. A very useful model system for studying such interactions is the combination of polyadenylic and polyuridylic acids, since it forms a similar helical molecule utilizing specific interactions.

REFERENCES

1. Feughelman, M., Langridge, R., Seeds, W. E., Stokes, A. R., Wilson, H. R., Hooper, C. W., Wilkins, M. H. F., Barclay, R. K., and Hamilton, L. D., *Nature,* **175**, 834 (1955).
2. Franklin, R. E., and Gosling, R. G., *Nature,* **171**, 740 (1953).
3. Grunberg-Manago, M., Ortiz, P. J., and Ochoa, S., *Science,* **122**, 907 (1955).
4. Rich, A., unpub.
5. Rich, A., and Davies, D. R., *J. Am. Chem. Soc.,* **78**, 3548 (1956).
6. Rich, A., and Watson, J. D., *Nature,* **173**, 995 (1954).
7. Rich, A., and Watson, J. D., *Proc. Natl. Acad. Sci. U. S.,* **40**, 759 (1954).
8. Warner, R. C., *Federation Proc.,* **15**, 379 (1956).
9. Watson, J. D., and Crick, F. H. C., *Nature,* **171**, 737 (1953).
10. Wilkins, M. H. F., Gosling, R. G., and Seeds, W. E., *Nature,* **167**, 759 (1951).
11. Wilkins, M. H. F., Stokes, A. R., and Wilson, H. R., *Nature,* **171**, 738 (1953).

DISCUSSION

DR. WARNER: I would like to make just a few comments on this AU interaction in solution. The experiments which I want to mention were done with the A polymer and the U polymer, each of which had a molecular weight in the order of 80,000. The first experiment was simply to examine a mixture of these two substances electrophoretically under circumstances in which there is a substantial mobility difference between the samples when examined alone. Under these conditions we found that the mixed sample migrated as a single peak with an electrophoretic homogeneity approximately the same as the separated samples but with an intermediate mobility. On finding that, we next did the same kind of experiment with centrifugation. Whereas at concentrations of around ½% each of these had a sedimentation constant of around 2½, when A and U are mixed the sedimentation constant rises to approximately 6 with no trace of the slower sedimenting material. Then we also examined the ultraviolet absorption, and I might just indicate what these curves look like. I think it's well known to all of you that, if one observes the nucleic acid at its maximum absorption and then compares the absorption with that of its component nucleotides obtained by hydrolysis of this sample, the absorption maximum of the mononucleotide curve is considerably higher than that of the nucleic acid. This has been known as the hyperchromic effect. The nucleic acid peak varies anywhere from 60% to 90% of that of the mononucleotide level. This same difference is shown by the A polymer by itself. The A polymer has an absorption of about 70% of that of the adenylic acid. The U polymer doesn't show it at all, which is a matter of some interest but not quite related to this problem. We did a mixture experiment of the same kind as before. This can be represented by 3 curves: a curve for the mixture of the A and U nucleotides, which has the highest absorption maximum; a curve representing the summation of maximum for the A polymer and the U polymer taken separately, lower than the first; and, finally, the observed curve for the mixed A and U polymers, actually found to be lower than the predicted one. The total drop is about half the nucleotide level, or somewhat greater than is observed in any naturally occurring nucleic acid; so there is evidence here for a strong interaction in solution, which is obviously similar to the kind which Dr. Rich is describing in fibers. I would say that this kind of interaction is obviously at the base of the difference between the molecular weight as calculated from end-group analysis and physical analysis as was discussed a little while ago. We might look at the properties of the A polymer, since Dr. Rich has suggested that this may also be in the form of a double-stranded helix in the oriented fiber. If the interaction resulting in such a helix persisted in solution, we might expect to find a weight average molecular weight of about twice the value predicted by end-group analysis. However, since all of the polynucleotides show a distribution of size, the available data are not good enough to decide this point. The number average molecular weight as determined by Dr. Smith for one sample by end-group analysis is around 80,000. Our own sedimentation work doesn't go to low enough concentrations to really answer this question, but Dr. Doty has examined this same sample by light scattering and found a value of around 140,000 for the weight average molecular weight. Although this is in the neighborhood of twice the value that Dr. Smith obtained, I do not think this is evidence for this kind of association in solution because the material is sufficiently heterogeneous, so that a ratio of weight average to number average molecular weight of 2 might be expected without association. While the existence of a hyperchromic effect for the A polymer by itself indicates base interaction, it may be presumed that this is on an intramolecular basis.

DR. FRANKLIN: I want to say a few words about RNA in tobacco mosaic virus, because there have been quite a number of references to a nucleic acid *core* in TMV whereas our x-ray diffraction studies show clearly that the RNA is not, in fact, in the center of the TMV particle. This emerges in about 6 different ways from the analysis of the x-ray diffraction diagrams. I shall describe only one of these ways.

From measurements of the equatorial x-ray scattering of TMV and of a heavy-atom derivative of TMV it is possible to deduce the radial density distribution in the virus particle; that is, one can determine the mean density at any given distance from the particle axis. This was first done by Casper (*Nature*, **177**, 928, 1956) with the aid of a lead derivative of TMV, and was repeated by us (*Ciba Symp.*, in press) using a mercury derivative. The results show that the intact TMV particle is hollow; there is a hole of radius about 20 Å along the particle axis. Proceeding outwards from the axis, the first density peak occurs at a radius of about 25 Å, and a much higher peak occurs at 40 Å. Other peaks occur at larger radii, but none is as strong as the 40 Å radius peak.

We then made a similar series of measurements on repolymerized RNA-free TMV protein provided by Dr. Schramm. The radial density distribution which we obtained for this material differed significantly from that of intact TMV *only* in the region of the 40 Å peak. The 40 Å peak of TMV was, in fact replaced by a sharp *minimum* at exactly this radius. This can only mean that the RNA—or, more precisely, the phosphate-sugar backbone of the RNA molecule—lies at a radial distance of about 40 Å from the axis in the TMV particle. That is, the RNA in TMV is deeply embedded in the virus protein, and lies at a position approximately half-way between the particle axis and the particle surface.

The same conclusion can be reached independently from an analysis of the x-ray scattering on any of six different layer-lines in the x-ray diagrams of normal TMV and RNA-free TMV protein.

IMPORTANCE OF HELICES IN MOLECULES
OF BIOLOGICAL ORIGIN

BARBARA W. LOW

Harvard Medical School, Boston, Massachusetts

IN DISCUSSING this topic the prime problem is obviously to define "importance"; that is, to differentiate between questions concerning the existence or the prevalence of helices in molecules of biological origin, and questions concerning the biological significance of any helices which may occur. This is really the old and fundamental question of the relationship between structure and function. We can say something about the prevalence of helices in biologically important molecules, but questions concerning their significance can in general only be answered by tentative inference and speculation.

Helical structures have been recognized in keratin (26, 28), collagen (8), and DNA (38) as well as in polyglycine (12) and some synthetic polypeptides (4, 9, 39). [The pleated sheet structures of silk fibroin (24) and β-keratin may be regarded as degenerate helices.]

SOME FEATURES OF POLYPEPTIDE AND POLYNUCLEOTIDE HELICAL STRUCTURES

All the helical structures so far described arise from the application of rigid chemical specifications of the kind first described in detail by Pauling, Corey, and Branson (27) for polypeptide chain configurations. The precise dimensions of the monomer unit of the chain must first be defined. The nature of the intra- or inter-chain bonding between units can then be specified, and the requirement imposed that identical chain units should all be structurally equivalent. When identical chain elements are arranged so that one common operation serves to translate the first unit position into the second and the nth into the $(n+1)^{th}$ the resulting structure is a helix.

In polypeptide and polynucleotide helices the structures are maintained by the formation of the maximum possible number of strong intra- or inter-chain hydrogen bonds. In the units of polypeptide and polynucleotide chains we may identify two separate parts: (a) the backbone chain residue; and (b) the side-chain residue R (e.g., CH_3 alanyl) for a protein, and a nucleotide for DNA.

In the Watson and Crick (38) model for the DNA structure, the hydrogen bonds are located between side-chain nucleotide residues, and the structure depends on specific ordered and repeating nucleotide sequences. In the collagen model (29) the hydrogen bonding is between units of the chain residue, but the particular chain configurations are dependent upon the stereochemistry of certain specific side-chain residues arranged in ordered and repeating sequence. Thus DNA and collagen model structures are both completely defined.

The α helix, the pleated sheet structures, and all the helices of the "α" and "γ" series are essentially backbone chain structures. That is, they may be formed with a completely random sequence of naturally occurring amino-acid side-chain residues (except prolyl or half-cystine). Further, there is a certain flexibility in the wrap-up angle of α helices which can markedly affect the spatial relationship between side-chain groups spaced several residues apart. Discussions of detailed stereochemistry of the "α" and "γ" series of helical structures will be found elsewhere (18, 21, 22, 23).

Studies of the relative stability of different helices have shown that the α helix structure is the most stable backbone-chain configuration (13). The effects of specific residue sequences on the stability of the backbone-chain configuration can be calculated for hypothetical sequences (19b, 20). As Schellman (37) has shown, uncharged and hydrocarbon side-chains will both generally tend to stabilize a stable helical configuration. Interactions between charged side-chains may disrupt a region of helical array if they enhance the free energy of unfolding of the whole chain array. Three well-defined situations can be recognized: (1) prolyl residues introduce a stereochemical discontinuity, and cannot be fitted into the smooth sequence of an α-helix (22); (2) inter- and intra-chain cystine cross-linkages may disrupt α-helix structures; and (3) hypothetical sequences can be invoked which could give rise to a more stable local configuration than a simple α-helix structure with unbound side-chain groups (19b).

THE PREVALENCE OF HELICAL STRUCTURES IN THE PROTEINS AND IN DNA

Drawn-out fibers of DNA are extremely well oriented. X-ray diffraction patterns of these fibers indicate that the structure is helical. The

Watson-Crick model (38) appears to fit the experimental data extremely well. Unless the fiber orientation is an artifact arising from the preparative procedure employed, then most of the native structure must have a helical configuration of the type described.

An analogous situation exists in considering the collagen structure. The model structure proposed appears to fit the experimental data extremely well. We must conclude therefore that "helices" of this kind are a fundamental feature of the collagen structure. A fundamental relationship between the correct model structure and the function of collagen must certainly exist.

The evidence in support of the α-helix structure in keratin is in general diverse and formidable. In order to fit the experimental data the primitive α-helices must be distorted into a coiled coil with a pitch angle of about $20°$. In the model these coiled coils pack together to give a rope-like structure with each α-helix a single strand in the complete cable. Side-chain interactions or interaction between side-chains and the carboxyl or amino groups of the amide residue have been suggested as probable causes of the local variation in hydrogen bond length which would lead to "coiled coil distortion" (25). An alternative explanation given by Crick (10) would relate the systematic distortion of the helices to more economical dovetail packing of side-chain residues. Whether the formation of a coiled coil is attributed to such systematic steric effects or to more general polar and nonpolar side-chain residue interactions, the coiled coil proposed has the advantage of explaining the observed diffraction effects.

Although extensive regions of α-helix configuration certainly occur in keratin, we have no knowledge of the amino-acid residue sequences within these regions, nor any information concerning the relative distribution of prolyl or cystine side-chains.

The chains in α-keratin are held together by cystine disulfide linkages. The α-β transformation in the k-m-e-f group of fibrous proteins is usually considered to take place without -S-S- link breakdown. If the interchain cystine linkages are disposed at random, the α-β transformation could not take place without breaking the disulfide linkages (3). Indeed, simple steric hindrance effects of neighboring side-chains would appear to make the transformation extremely difficult, even if the disulfide linkages are located in positions favorable to forming the stretched-out (β) configuration. This difficulty can be avoided by consigning most of the -S-S- linkages to the non-oriented regions of the peptide chain. Polarized infra-red radiation studies of keratin show rather low dichroism (1). They do suggest that keratin must contain regions of unknown structure as well as regions where the α-helix structure predominates.

Globular Proteins.

Detailed structural studies have been made on only a very few globular proteins. These proteins, of lower than average molecular weight, may not be truly representative of their class. The most general study of protein structure is that of Arndt and Riley. The x-ray scattering distribution from a large number of globular proteins, studied as amorphous powders, can be compared with the interference intensity function calculated from the parameters of any well-defined chain configuration. Arndt and Riley's studies using this method show that the left-handed (α_1) helix is the most plausible predominant chain configuration in seventeen globular proteins, and that the helical regions are associated in some sort of relatively compact array (2, 30, 31).

Early studies of the vector structures (Patterson series) of hemoglobin appeared to support this conclusion. A grossly over-simplified picture of a globular protein, as derived at that time, represented it as a close-packed array of rod-like cylindrical regions of high electron density, in which lengths of polypeptide chain were coiled or folded into a regular chain configuration. In considering the agreement between a simple model of this kind and the experimental data for hemoglobin, both Bragg, Howells, and Perutz (5) and Crick (11) have shown that the model is oversimplified.

To fit the experimental data, some deviations are necessary from this simple structure—that is, chains 25 to 30 Å in length with an α-helix configuration cannot all be stacked parallel; irregularities must occur. Several different kinds of irregularities can be postulated: (1) short lengths of chain in an α-helix configuration may be imperfectly aligned so that as a group the coiled chains zigzag about the over-all axial direction; (2) short lengths of α-helix may be followed by regions in which the specific local molecular configuration is not associated with any regular peptide chain configuration.

A striking piece of evidence for the existence of regions of regular chain configuration in hemoglobin is, of course, the 1.5 Å spacing observed by Perutz (28). Polarized infra-red radiation studies of some crystalline proteins confirm the hypothesis of oriented regions of ordered chain configuration (14, 15).

Electron density projections have been published recently for the two globular proteins hemoglobin (6) and ribonuclease (17). Both projections are complex and do not appear to correspond to the incompletely resolved view of parallel regions of coiled chains, whether seen along their length or "end-on." Such a correspondence would, however, arise only (1) if the molecular configuration were very simple, with intramolecular regions of α-helix all packed parallel to each other, and (2) if the intermolecular packing in the crystal structure maintained one common chain direction for all the molecules in the unit cell. The possibility of non-parallel packing either within or between molecules cannot be ruled out.

In insulin (21) preliminary studies of the peak distribution in the vector structure tend to support a simple α-helix model for the molecule with parallel intra- and inter-molecular packing of the α-helices. The complete two-dimensional structure of insulin has been established by Sanger and his associates (7, 32, 33, 34, 35, 36).

The chemical structure imposes recognized limitations on helical models. The $-C_{(\beta)}$-S- (half-cystine) residues on the A_6 and A_{11} α-carbon positions are too far removed in space on a simple α-helix structure to permit the formation of an $A\begin{bmatrix} 11 \\ 6 \end{bmatrix}$ intrachain disulfide bond. A simple continuous α-helix structure is thus ruled out for the A chain of insulin. This limitation does not impose intrinsic restrictions on the configuration of the terminal segments of the A chain. Both these two parts of the A chain and the whole of the B chain may be in the α-helix configuration without affecting the inter-chain cystine linkages. If the specific configuration of the pentapeptide loop is irregular, then intrachain hydrogen bonds between peptide CO-NH residues cannot be formed. If we ask whether there is any configuration for this region of the chain which would permit some intrachain hydrogen bonding, or whether it is possible to maintain the α-helix configuration in at least some part of the $A\begin{bmatrix} 11 \\ 6 \end{bmatrix}$ loop, then these problems can be studied using scale atomic models.

Several model structures have been proposed for insulin (19a, 20, 22), all based on the assumption that the α-helix will predominate except in a region of the intrachain disulfide bond A $\left.\begin{smallmatrix}6\\ \\11\end{smallmatrix}\right]$. Linderstrøm-Lang's recent study (19a) has led him to conclude that the regions of α-helix structure, if they exist, are restricted to the regions of the molecule between interchain disulfide linkages A $\begin{smallmatrix}7\text{———}7\\20\text{———}19\end{smallmatrix}$ B.

There is one technique which has already provided a powerful tool in the identification of helical structures in some fibrous proteins. Use of the optical diffractometer (16) permits the direct and detailed comparisons of the Fraunhofer diffraction pattern of a given model structure with the observed x-ray diffraction patterns. This study of optical transforms may be employed at several different levels of resolution. It can be employed (a) to establish the molecular shape and orientation, (b) to recognize the presence and establish the orientation of regions of regular polypeptide chain configuration in the molecule, and (c) to study the detailed molecular stereochemistry.

This method is now being used by Dr. P. R. Pinnock in our laboratory in the systematic search for regions of helical structure in insulin. It should be possible to establish whether a large part of the insulin molecule is in the α-helix configuration and to do this with some certainty whether or not the helical regions are all parallel to each other. The evidence concerning the existence of α-helices in some globular proteins is conflicting. Here, obviously, the prime need is for more information.

Speculations Concerning the Biological Importance of Helical Structures

Speculations in this field are almost inevitably anthropomorphic. Some of us expect to find in biological mechanisms efficiency, simplicity, and elegance. Others regard the process of evolution more casually, and, while agreeing that a particular molecule does perform a certain function, would not say that the molecule was built to do this job, but rather that it now does the job after multiple evolutionary modifications.

It may well be that biological mechanisms are the most efficient, simple, and elegant possible under the complex conditions in which they occur. Unfortunately, we rarely know much about the detailed conditions under which biological mechanisms operate.

DNA.

The determination of the detailed stereochemistry of the DNA unit of structure is a magnificent achievement. Furthermore, unless the function of DNA is wholly associated with the rather small disoriented fraction, then it must derive in some way from the ordered configuration.

This conclusion does not imply in any way that a single double-strand unit of the Watson-Crick model is the prime operator or the complete unit template in any or all of the functional processes of DNA. Recently, mechanisms have been devised for the transfer of information from nucleic acid to protein. Many of these employ one single, two-strand helical unit of DNA structure and directly depend on its detailed stereochemistry.

We do not, however, know the size of the functional unit of DNA in the chromosomes or viruses. Is it not possible that one double strand of a DNA molecule may be only a very small part of the complex topography of a single functional unit, which may involve several helical units of DNA and perhaps sometimes protein molecules as well?

The helical structure of the DNA unit is obviously of prime biological importance. The precise role of a single structural unit has not yet been established.

Collagen.

Similar considerations arise in discussions of the collagen structure. A fundamental relationship between the correct model structure and the function of collagen must certainly exist. The function of collagen appears to be the provision of architectural support and some mechanical flexibility. Here it seems certain that the function of collagen depends both on the detailed stereochemistry of a single helical unit and on the way in which the units are packed together. Until the packing arrangement is known in detail, the separate role of one individual helix cannot be described.

Keratin.

Although keratin is undoubtedly made up of extensive regions of α-helix, the problems involved in attempting to consider their biological importance, are complex. There are several reasons for this: (1) appreciable regions of non-helical structure may occur in keratin; (2) a notable feature of the α-keratin structure is the presence of inter-chain disulfide bonds, and when these are broken, the α-helix structure cannot be maintained; (3) the α-helix is not a completely defined configuration, and we do not know with which residue sequences the regions of α-helix configuration are associated. α-Helices provide necessary mechanical stability. The detailed properties of the fibers themselves must be equally dependent upon the way in which the helices are joined and packed together. The properties of a woven fabric depend both on the fiber used and on the weave.

Globular Proteins.

There is some evidence that regions of α-helix configuration may exist in a few globular proteins. This has been discussed briefly above and in some detail elsewhere (21, 22). We can profitably ask whether on chemical grounds we might expect to find α-helices in the globular proteins, and if so what role they might be expected to play.

In globular proteins the stable discrete unit is a single molecule. The native state of the globular molecule is related to a specific intramolecular configuration, the loss of which is associated with loss of biological specificity. Ordered and disordered regions of chain configuration are confined within and establish the unique three-dimensional molecular structure. Globular proteins are almost always shorter than the model structure which would be derived if peptide chains of average length (calculated from end-group determinations) were each coiled into a single cylindrical α-helix structure and then stacked together in close-packed array. Reactive sites or groups on a globular protein molecule are reactants in certain specific chemical reactions— usually when the protein is in aqueous solution. These sites must be accessible; they probably have a complex, highly specific, three-dimensional structure.

Most globular proteins are labile structures and become denatured when they are attacked by certain reagents or are subject to conditions under which covalent bonds of the primary chemical structure remain, at least initially, unbroken. Prolonged exposure to hydrogen-bond-breaking reagents usually results in some irreversible denaturation. This would appear to suggest that the molecule is not the most thermodynamically stable one. This reasoning may, however, be invalid. After irreversible denaturation of a protein preparation, molecular aggregation occurs when the original conditions are restored. The molecular aggregates are held together by intermolecular bonds.

A single molecule which has been wholly or partially "opened up" might either (a) refold back into the original native configuration or into another configuration, or (b) interact with one or more molecules to form an aggregate. The number of ways in which reactions of the latter type may occur is probably infinite. The evidence would strongly suggest that these reactions predominate.

The presence of intramolecular disulfide linkage will inhibit the degree of "opening-up." A molecule which contains many disulfide linkages might be expected to follow path (a). In general, protein molecules which are extensively cross-linked by disulfide groups can be renatured more readily than can molecules with few intramolecular covalent cross-linkages.

The significant feature of irreversible denaturation is the finding that the native configuration of the single disperse protein molecule is not usually lost in favor of another configuration for the single molecule alone, but in favor of an aggregate of several molecules.

This does not mean that after extensive unfolding a single protein molecule alone would, necessarily, regain its native configuration. It simply emphasizes that many experimental studies of denaturation are not capable of resolving this question.

We do not know whether the configuration of a protein molecule is adopted de novo after protein synthesis is completed, or whether separate parts of the molecule, synthesized and held on a template in some specific configuration, are joined together in situ. It is very difficult to draw satisfactory conclusions about the thermodynamic stability of proteins. We do know that the stability of the protein molecule is adequate for its physiological functions. Apart from special features related to the specific role of each individual protein, the structures of all globular proteins have two further important properties: (a) they are soluble in physiological media, and (b) they do not aggregate under physiological conditions. In spite of their widely different amino-acid residue composition, the structures of all globular proteins satisfy these three prime requirements.

The α-helix provides the most stable backbone-chain configuration. Therefore if regions of α-helix do exist generally in globular proteins, we may suppose that they make an important contribution to the over-all molecular stability. In many proteins the principal reactive sites appear to be situated at the molecular surface. Under these circumstances we may perhaps suppose that those regions of molecule not normally accessible to physiological reagents provide stability for the molecule as a whole. α-Helices would be excellent for this purpose. I should like to speculate that we will find regions of α-helices particularly in many of the larger protein molecules and that their architectural function will be to stabilize and maintain the special configuration of the reactive sites.

ACKNOWLEDGMENT

I am very grateful to Dr. Margaret J. Hunter for her helpful criticisms during the preparation of this paper.

REFERENCES

1. Ambrose, E. J., and Elliott, A., *Proc. Roy. Soc. (London)*, **A206**, 206 (1951).
2. Arndt, U. W., and Riley, D. P., *Trans. Roy. Soc. (London)*, **A249**, 409 (1955).
3. Astbury, W. T., *Proc. Roy. Soc. (London)*, **B141**, 1 (1953).
4. Bamford, C. H., Brown, L., Elliott, A., Hanby, W. E., and Trotter, I. F., *Nature*, **169**, 357 (1952).
5. Bragg, W. L., Howells, E. R., and Perutz, M. F., *Acta Cryst.*, **5**, 136 (1952).
6. Bragg, W. L., and Perutz, M. F., *Proc. Roy. Soc. (London)*, **A225**, 315 (1954).
7. Brown, H., Sanger, F., and Kitai, R., *Biochem. J. (London)*, **60**, 556 (1955).
8. Cohen, C., and Bear, R. S., *J. Am. Chem. Soc.*, **75**, 2783 (1953).
9. Cochran, W., and Crick, F. H. C., *Nature*, **167**, 2053 (1951).
10. Crick, F. H. C., *Nature*, **170**, 882 (1952).
11. Crick, F. H. C., *Acta Cryst.*, **5**, 381 (1952).
12. Crick, F. H. C., and Rich, A., *Nature*, **176**, 780 (1955).
13. Donohue, J., *Proc. Natl. Acad. Sci. U. S.*, **39**, 470 (1953).
14. Elliott, A., *Proc. Roy. Soc. (London)*, **A211**, 490 (1952).
15. Elliott, A., and Ambrose, E. J., *Discussions Faraday Soc.*, **9**, 246 (1950).
16. Hanson, A. W., Lipson, H., and Taylor, C. A., *Proc. Roy. Soc. (London)*, **A218**, 371 (1953).
17. Harker, D., in *Advances in Biological and Medical Physics.* (J. H. Lawrence and C. A. Tobias, eds.), Chapter 1, Academic Press, New York (1956).
18. Kendrew, J. C., and Perutz, M. F., in *Haemoglobin* (F. J. W. Roughton and J. C. Kendrew, eds.), p. 161, Butterworth, London, and Interscience, New York (1949).
19a. Linderstrøm-Lang, K., in *Peptide Chemistry: Report of a Symposium held by the Chemical Society March 30, 1955,* The Chemical Society, London, 1955; A. Hvidt and K. Linderstrøm-Lang, *Compt. rend. trav. lab. Carlsberg, Sér. chim.*, **29**, 385 (1955).
19b. Lindley, H., *Biochim. et Biophys. Acta*, **18**, 194 (1955).
20. Lindley, H., and Rollett, J. S., *Biochim. et Biophys. Acta*, **18**, 183 (1955).
21. Low, B. W., in *The Proteins* (H. Neurath and K. Bailey, eds.), Vol. 1, Part A, Chap. 4, Academic Press, New York (1953).

22. Low, B. W., and Edsall, J. T., in *Currents in Biochemical Research* (D. E. Green, ed.), p. 378, Interscience, New York (1956).

23. Low, B. W., and Grenville-Wells, H. J., *Proc. Natl. Acad. Sci. U. S.*, **39**, 785 (1953).

24. Marsh, R. E., Corey, R. B., and Pauling, L., *Biochim. et Biophys. Acta*, **16**, 1 (1955).

25. Pauling, L., in *Les Protéines: Rapports et Discussions* (R. Stoops, ed.), p. 63, Inst. Intern. Chimie Solvay, Brussels (1953).

26. Pauling, L., and Corey, R. B., *Proc. Natl. Acad. Sci. U. S.*, **37**, 235-285, 729 (1951).

27. Pauling, L., Corey, R. B., and Branson, H. R., *Proc. Natl. Acad. Sci. U. S.*, **37**, 205 (1951).

28. Perutz, M. F., *Nature*, **167**, 1053 (1951).

29. Rich, A., and Crick, F. H. C., *Nature*, **176**, 915 (1955).

30. Riley, D. P., and Arndt, U. W., *Nature*, **169**, 138 (1952).

31. Riley, D. P., and Arndt, U. W., *Proc. Roy. Soc. (London)*, **B141**, 93 (1952).

32. Sanger, F., *Advances in Protein Chem.*, **7**, 1 (1952).

33. Sanger, F., Smith, L. F., and Kitai, R., *Biochem. J. (London)*, **58**, vi (1954).

34. Sanger, F., and Thompson, E. O. P., *Biochem. J. (London)*, **53**, 353, 366 (1953).

35. Sanger, F., Thompson, E. O. P., and Kitai, R., *Biochem. J. (London)*, **59**, 509 (1954).

36. Sanger, F., and Tuppy, H., *Biochem. J. (London)*, **49**, 463, 481 (1951).

37. Schellman, J. A., *Compt. rend. trav. lab. Carlsberg, Ser. chim.*, **29**, 223, 230 (1955).

38. Watson, J. D., and Crick, F. H. C., *Nature*, **171**, 737 (1953).

39. Yakel, J. L., Jr., *Acta Cryst.*, **6**, 724 (1953).

DISCUSSION

DR. HARKER: I like very much having helices important, but there must be a real reason for some things being globular and others being fibrous. When things are fibrous it is because a unit repeats, and in general when a unit repeats it almost always produces spirals. There are not only the alpha helices in proteins and the DNA spirals; there are also helices, such as Waugh got in polymers of insulin molecules. Now, in globular proteins it's a very different thing. A globular protein develops because of some necessity in a biological system which requires it. It is easy to think in terms of helices, because they are obvious in some biological systems, but I don't think this creates any obligation on the part of the molecules; these molecules may be built up of units in essentially different arrangements. I think there are small molecules, like insulin and ribonuclease, which cannot be made of systematic spirals. They must be very complicated jobs indeed. May it not also be that some of the nucleic acids occurring in the more or less globular viruses are not built on spirals but are built in some more complicated way?

DR. RICH: On your last point, I would like to comment on the evidence concerning the RNA in globular viruses. It's just like the RNA from other sources, and, although we don't know its structure, it's probably helical.

DR. HARKER: You pulled it out into fibers, didn't you?

DR. RICH: Yes, but I do not believe that the structure is so labile that it will change during that operation.

DR. DOTY: Dr. Yang and I have been using polypeptides prepared by Dr. Blout to "calibrate" optical rotation and rotary dispersion in terms of the fraction of helical configuration present. This is possible because these synthetic polypeptides exist as complete helices in some solvents and as randomly coiled chains in others. With this background we would interpret the observed rotary behavior of proteins such as insulin and serum albumin as resulting from roughly 30% helical configuration. This appears to be consistent with what Dr. Low has told us.

Part VI

*SYNTHESIS OF NUCLEOTIDES AND
NUCLEIC ACIDS*

PATHWAYS OF ENZYMATIC SYNTHESIS OF NUCLEOTIDES AND POLYNUCLEOTIDES *

ARTHUR KORNBERG

Department of Microbiology,
Washington University School of Medicine,
St. Louis, Missouri

Nucleotides are the building blocks of coenzymes and, more pertinent in this symposium, of nucleic acids. How nucleotides are formed from simpler molecular units and in turn are assembled into the more complex coenzymes and polynucleotides remains a fascinating jigsaw puzzle. The solution to this puzzle has been approached by nutritional, genetic, and isotopic tracer studies with intact cells. The results of such studies have provided interesting phenomena which eventually must be explained by any proposed biosynthetic pathways. But by themselves these studies have not defined any mechanism and have even on occasion presented pieces of other, accessory, puzzles. The objective of approaches that will be emphasized here is the isolation from cells of separate enzymes, each of which effects a single, chemically rational step. These steps taken in order should lead to the total synthesis of complex nucleotides. To assume real significance, the rates and conditions under which a synthetic pathway operates must ultimately be reconciled with the observations made with intact cells.

The topics to be considered in this report are as follows:

I. Ribonucleotide synthesis
   A. Ribose phosphates
   B. Purine nucleotides

---

* For excellent reviews on this subject which have appeared in recent years, references 9, 10, 22, 27, 40, 64, 95, 98, 105, and 111 should be consulted.

The abbreviations used in this paper are: inorganic pyrophosphate, PP; phosphate, P; inorganic orthophosphate, P_i; 5-phosphoribosylpyrophosphate, PRPP; adenosine triphosphate, ATP or ARPPP; adenosine diphosphate, ADP; thymidine triphosphate, TTP; thymidine diphosphate, TDP; uridine triphosphate, UTP; uridine diphosphate, UDP; guanosine diphosphate, GDP; deoxyribonucleic acid, DNA; deoxyribonuclease, DNAase; ribonucleic acid, RNA; diphosphopyridine nucleotide, DPN.

I. Ribonucleotide Synthesis

Because of their importance as coenzymes in electron transport and in carbohydrate metabolism, the ribonucleotides (of which adenosine-5'-phosphate is an example, Fig. 1) were recognized early and their biosynthesis is much better understood than that of deoxyribonucleotides (of which thymidine-5'-phosphate is an example, Fig. 1).* It is for this reason that these two groups of nucleotides are considered separately.

We now know that there are several pathways of nucleotide synthesis in nature, and it has also become clear that alternative pathways may

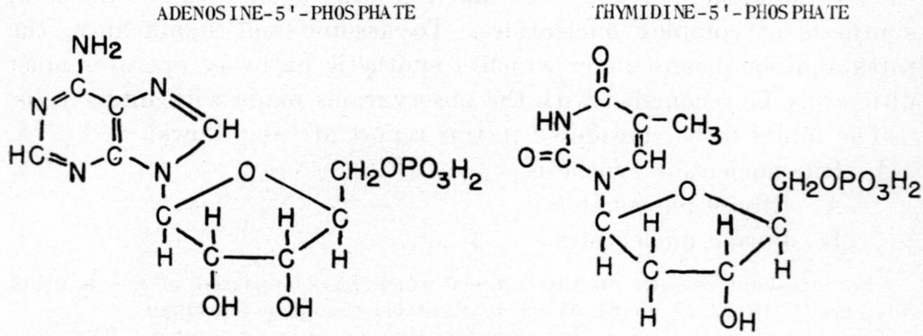

Fig. 1

* The D-furanoside structures, drawn in this review, should be viewed as having the C—O—C bridge facing the reader with the substituents on carbons 1 and 5 facing down.

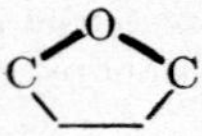

exist in a single cell. For simplicity the pathways of nucleotide synthesis may be grouped in two categories, (a) *de novo* or "do-it-yourself" pathways, in which the cell requires only ammonia, phosphate, and simple carbon sources (Figs. 2, 3), and (b) *salvage* path-

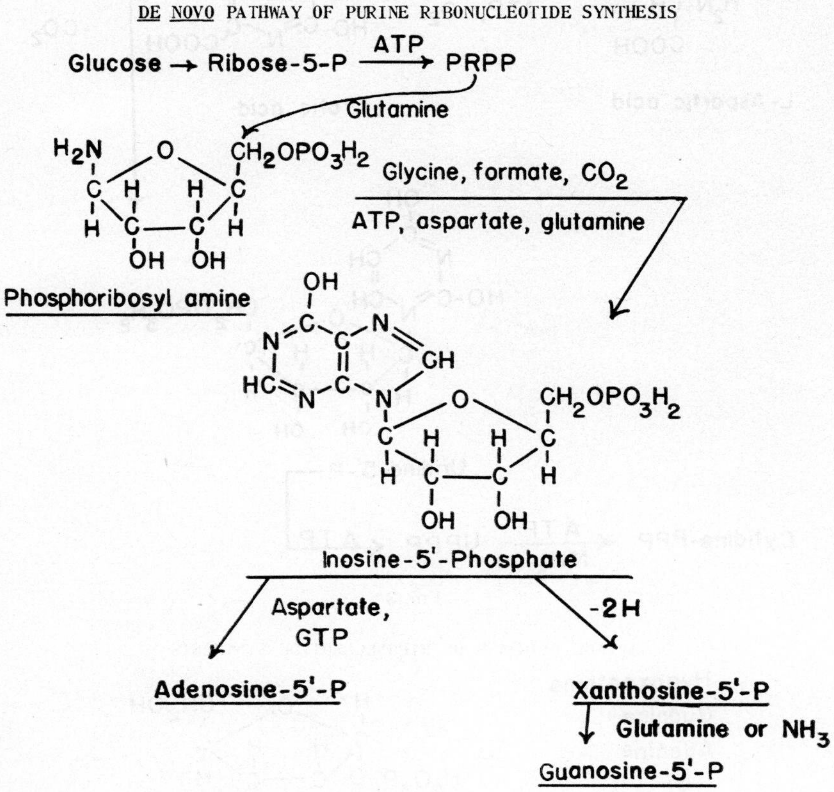

DE NOVO PATHWAY OF PURINE RIBONUCLEOTIDE SYNTHESIS

Fig. 2

ways in which some of the component parts, viz., purines, pyrimidines, nucleosides, are derived from the soil, the liquid medium, the intestinal tract, or from degradative processes within the cell (Fig. 4).

A. *Ribose Phosphates.*

There are three compounds of special interest, ribose-5-phosphate and two of its derivatives, ribose-1-phosphate and 5-phosphoribosyl-pyrophosphate (PRPP).

DE NOVO PATHWAY OF PYRIMIDINE RIBONUCLEOTIDE SYNTHESIS

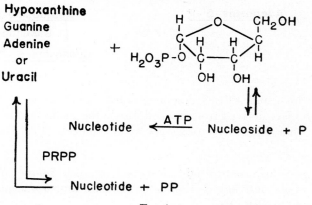

$$\text{L-Aspartic acid} \xrightarrow[\text{ATP, O}_2]{\text{NH}_3\text{, CO}_2} \text{Orotic acid} \xrightarrow[-\text{CO}_2]{\text{PRPP,}}$$

Uridine-5'-P

$$\text{Cytidine-PPP} \xleftarrow[\text{NH}_3]{\text{ATP}} \text{UPPP} \xleftarrow{\text{ATP}} \text{Uridine-5'-P}$$

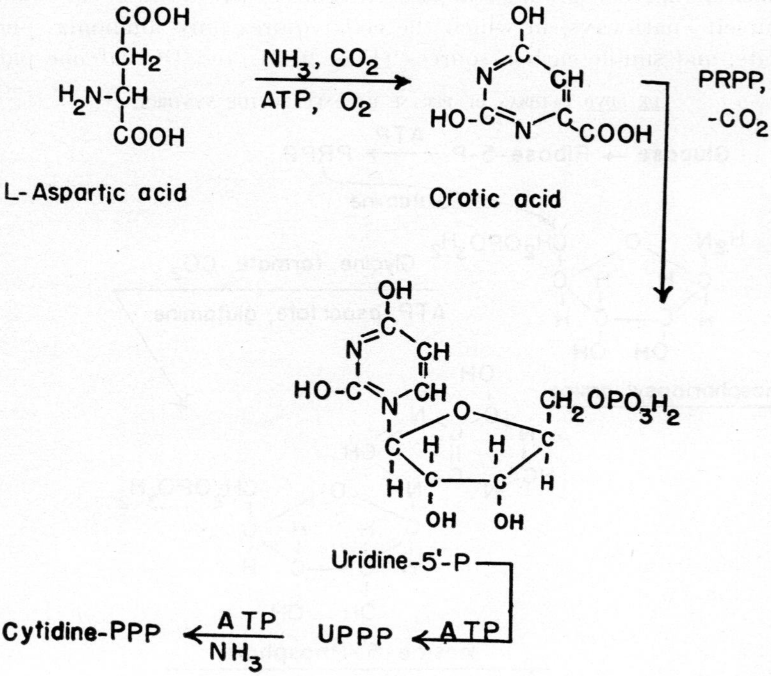

Fig. 3

SALVAGE PATHWAYS OF RIBONUCLEOTIDE SYNTHESIS

Hypoxanthine
Guanine
Adenine
  or
Uracil

$+$

$$\text{Nucleotide} \xleftarrow{\text{ATP}} \text{Nucleoside} + \text{P}$$

PRPP

$$\text{Nucleotide} + \text{PP}$$

Fig. 4

Ribose-5-phosphate may be formed by an oxidative pathway from glucose-6-phosphate via 6-phosphogluconate and ribulose-5-phosphate (41) (Fig. 5), by an anaerobic pathway from fructose-6-phosphate (96) (Fig. 5), from ribose and ATP by the action of kinases (2a, 17, 20, 64, 104), or from ribose-1-phosphate by phosphoribomutase action (2, 35, 46, 48, 109).

Of these four possible routes, the two originating from glucose are the most commonly used; the relative predominance of the oxidative and anaerobic pathways varies among different cells and is directly influenced by a variety of factors (27). Direct phosphorylation of ribose is of quantitative importance when this sugar is available as a substrate or provided by hydrolysis of nucleosides. Nucleosides salvaged by phosphorolysis (see below) can yield ribose-5-phosphate via ribose-1-phosphate.

Ribose-1-phosphate is produced by the phosphorolysis of nucleosides (23, 46, 49, 50, 88, 89), and as already mentioned is reversibly formed from ribose-5-phosphate. No direct origin of ribose-1-phosphate by kinase action or from glucose is known.

Phosphoribosylpyrophosphate is formed by the donation of a pyrophosphate group by ATP to carbon 1 of ribose-5-phosphate through the action of a kinase (57, 58, 101), according to the equation:

$$\text{ATP} + \text{ribose-5-P} \rightarrow \text{PRPP} + \text{adenosine-5'-P}.$$

PRPP is the activated pentose phosphate which reacts with pyrimidines and purines to produce nucleotides directly, and combines with glutamine to form 5-phosphoribosylamine, the ribotide precursor of purine nucleotides. The formation of PRPP from ATP and ribose-5-phosphate has been observed to be of widespread occurrence. While PRPP can be derived by pyrophosphorolysis of nucleotides (reversal of their synthesis, see below), such a reaction could lead only to an exchange of the nitrogenous bases, but no net synthesis of ribotides.

B. *Purine Nucleotides.*

Thus far there is no evidence for synthesis *de novo* of free purines and, except in what appear to be the less common circumstances, purine nucleotides are not made by the salvage pathway. The steps of what is then the more universal pathway (*de novo* pathway, see Fig. 2) have been worked out by Buchanan (10, 66, 67, 78, 110, 112)

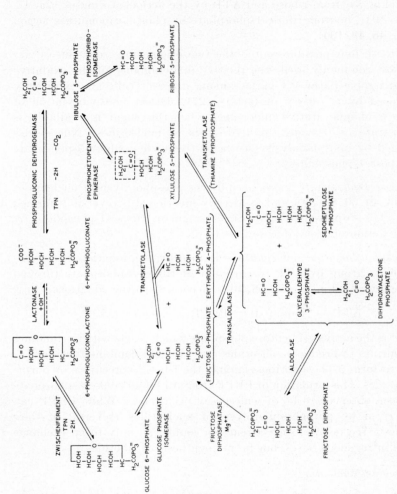

FIG. 5. Glucose-6-phosphate metabolism by the pentose phosphate pathway. (After Horecker and Mehler (40).)

and Greenberg (28, 29, 30) and their colleagues. They have defined a series of some ten discrete enzymatic reactions involving the initial formation of a simple amino ribotide, then the addition of glycine, and then of formate so as to yield formyl glycinamide ribotide. This is followed by ring closure yielding the imidazole ribotide. Reaction with glutamine, demonstrated to be the enzymatic locus of azaserine inhibition (37), leads to an amino imidazole. The addition first of carbon dioxide and then of the amino group of aspartate yields amino-carboxamide ribotide. The only lacking element of the purine ring, carbon 2, is incorporated by a formyl group transfer followed by ring closure, yielding inosinic acid. Of considerable interest from the standpoint of comparative biochemistry are the studies of Rabinowitz and Barker (90, 91, 92, 93) showing that the degradation of free purines by anaerobes isolated from soil follows in remarkably close detail the pattern described for purine nucleotide synthesis in higher animals. Inosine-5'-phosphate is the key intermediate from which adenosine-5'-phosphate (1, 15, 16, 69) and guanosine-5'-phosphate (1, 4, 63, 84) are formed.

The salvage pathway (see Fig. 4) has been observed in artificially produced microbial mutants and naturally occurring species of heterotrophic cells, as well as in cells which are also capable of synthesis *de novo*. A common, but I believe erroneous, impression that this is the major pathway of nucleotide synthesis stems from the popular use of mutants, microbiologic assays, emphasis on fastidious pathogenic species and the "sparing" effect of the salvage pathway in cells carrying out synthesis *de novo*. The utilization of free purines (see Fig. 4) is predominantly by reaction with PRPP to form nucleotides directly (51, 59), but they may also be converted to nucleotides via the nucleosides. The purine nucleosides produced by nucleoside phosphorylase or by nucleotidase action may in some instances be converted to 5'-nucleotides by the action of ATP and specific kinases (12, 31, 61). The specificity of the adenosine kinase is noteworthy; only adenosine and 2'-aminoadenosine (2, 6-diaminopurine riboside), among a group of closely related nucleosides, were substrates for an enzyme studied in yeast (61).

Nucleotide synthesis by phosphatase transfer is of great interest but is of doubtful importance, in view of the nonspecificity and high concentration of nucleosides required (8).

C. *Pyrimidine Nucleotides.*

Unlike the biosynthesis of purine nucleotides, the principal pathway of pyrimidine nucleotide formation involves the intermediate formation of a free base, orotic acid (see Fig. 3). Orotic acid is synthesized from aspartic acid by way of ureidosuccinic and dihydroorotic acids (44, 70, 100). It is then converted to orotidine-5′-phosphate by reaction with PRPP and finally is decarboxylated to yield uridine-5′-phosphate (42, 43, 71, 73). The accumulation of orotic acid and orotidine by certain *Neurospora* mutants (82, 83) may be due to a relative lack of orotidine-5′-phosphate decarboxylase. Thus, piling up of orotidine-5′-phosphate might inhibit utilization of orotic acid, and the action of phosphatases on orotidine-5′-phosphate would also lead to the accumulation of orotidine. Formation of cytosine nucleotides occurs by amination of uridine-5′-triphosphate (68).

The existence of species of lactobacilli, mutants of *Escherichia coli* and other species which specifically require uracil for growth and fail to respond to orotic acid led us to examine the nature of the pyrimidine nucleotide-forming systems in these organisms. Dr. Irving Crawford was able to show (19) (Table 1) that *Lactobacillus bulgaricus*, which

TABLE 1

PYRIMIDINE NUCLEOTIDE SYNTHESIS IN LACTOBACILLI

Species	Growth Factor		Uridine−5′−P synthesis from	
	Orotic Acid	Uracil	Orotic Acid	Uracil
			units/mg.	
L. bulgaricus 09	+	−	0.8	0.0
*L. arabinosus**	−	+	0.0	1.0
*L. arabinosus***	−	−	1.9	1.5
L. bifidus	+	+	0.6	2.4
L. leichmanii	+	+	0.8	2.6

* During early growth phase.
** During later growth phase.

requires orotic acid (113, 114), has a PRPP-orotic acid pyrophosphorylase like that described for yeast and liver, while *L. arabinosus* during a uracil-requiring phase of its growth has a specific uracil-PRPP pyrophosphorylase. *L. bifidus* and *L. leichmanii*, which respond to either pyrimidine, were found to have both enzymes. Similar results have been recently reported by Canellakis (11). The source of uracil for the nutrition of these cells is very likely in the enzymatic hydrolysate of ribonucleic acid furnished by the environment. Whether uracil is ever produced by cells is still uncertain. Attempts to demonstrate its synthesis by a route analogous to that of orotic acid may prove successful.

Another salvage of uracil may be by way of a uridine phosphorylase—found in *E. coli* (88, 89) and in liver (11, 13)—followed by phosphorylation by ATP. A kinase for uridine has been observed in yeast extracts (Kornberg, unpub.) and in liver (11). Phosphorolysis of cytidine has not yet been convincingly demonstrated (64).

D. *Nucleoside Di- and Tri-phosphates.*

Nucleotides, from a biosynthetic sense, are almost always inert. It is the addition of one or two phosphates to bring them to the nucleoside di- or tri-phosphate stage that endows them with activity as coenzyme and nucleic acid precursors. Several enzymatic reactions were known for the phosphorylation of nucleoside diphosphates to the triphosphates, but until two years ago there was with one exception no enzymatic pathway known for the phosphorylation of a nucleoside monophosphate (that is a nucleotide) to the nucleoside diphosphate stage. The only known example was adenylate kinase (myokinase) (18, 45), which is strictly specific for the adenine nucleotides. There were a number of reasons for expecting that some way of forming the other nucleoside di- and tri-phosphates existed. A variety of purine and pyrimidine nucleoside di- and tri-phosphates had been found to occur in natural materials (7, 75, 106); uridine triphosphate was known to function in the synthesis of the uridine coenzymes (87); and studies of coenzyme synthesis created an impression that nucleoside-5'-triphosphates would prove to be the precursors of polynucleotides (54). Recently, the formation of UTP has been shown to be brought about by liver enzyme preparations from uridylate and ATP (57). An enzyme was found in yeast (72, 74) which effected a transphosphorylation between adenosine, uridine, and guanosine nucleosides:

$$\text{Uridine-5'-P} + \text{ATP} \rightleftarrows \text{UDP} + \text{ADP}$$
$$\text{Adenosine-5'-P} + \text{UTP} \rightleftarrows \text{ADP} + \text{UDP}$$
$$\text{Uridine-5'-P} + \text{UTP} \rightleftarrows 2\text{ UDP}$$
$$\text{Guanosine-5'-P} + \text{ATP} \rightleftarrows \text{GDP} + \text{ADP}.$$

The mechanisms may be summarized by the general equations,

$$\text{Nucleoside-P} + \textit{nucleoside}\text{-PPP} \rightleftarrows \text{nucleoside-PP} + \textit{nucleoside}\text{-PP}$$
$$2\ \text{nucleoside-PP} \rightleftarrows \text{nucleoside-P} + \text{nucleoside-PPP}$$
$$2\ \textit{nucleoside}\text{-PP} \rightleftarrows \textit{nucleoside}\text{-P} + \textit{nucleoside}\text{-PPP}.$$

Essentially similar conclusions were reached simultaneously in several laboratories (38, 85, 108).

II. Deoxyribonucleotide Synthesis

Knowledge about the formation of deoxyribonucleotides is meager compared with what is known about ribonucleotide synthesis. There are two principal questions and these derive from the distinguishing structural characteristics of the deoxynucleotides. What is the origin of the deoxypentose units and how are the methylated pyrimidines (thymine and methylcytosine) formed?

A. *Deoxyribose Phosphates.*

Racker discovered an aldolase in *E. coli* and in animal tissues which condenses, reversibly, glyceraldehyde-3-phosphate and acetaldehyde (94). Through the action of a mutase (24, 81) deoxyribose-1-phosphate is formed, and may then react with purines or pyrimidines by a nucleoside phosphorylase step (Fig. 6). A limitation of the aldolase reaction

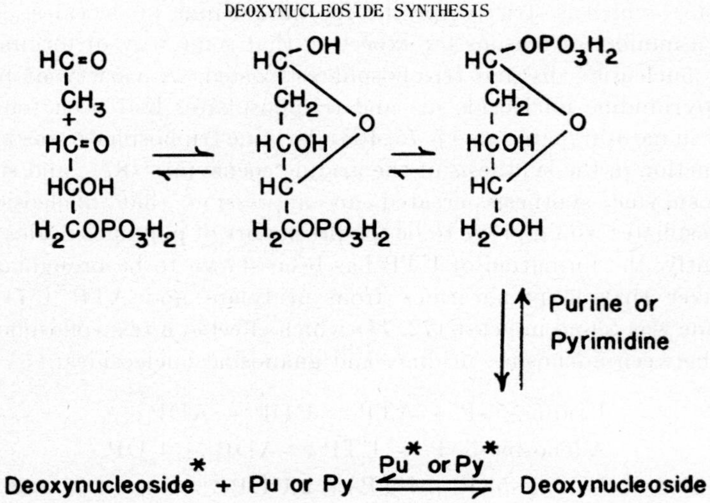

DEOXYNUCLEOSIDE SYNTHESIS

Deoxynucleoside* + Pu or Py $\rightleftharpoons$ Deoxynucleoside

Fig. 6

is the high dissociation constant of acetaldehyde for the enzyme. The concentrations of acetaldehyde in cells do not appear to be sufficient to provide adequate rates for this reaction, and Racker suggested that an aldehyde derivative of purines and pyrimidines may prove to be the true precursor. Another and perhaps more likely function for this enzyme is the utilization for the energy needs of the cell of deoxyribose-5-phosphate derived from deoxynucleosides.

With the finding of PRPP as the activated pentose phosphate in ribonucleotide synthesis, hope was aroused that an analogous pyrophosphoryl derivative of deoxyribose-5-phosphate would be found to occupy a key place in deoxynucleotide synthesis. Such a derivative might be expected to be even more unstable than deoxyribose-1-phosphate, and indirect methods were therefore used to find it. For example, a kinase reaction of deoxyribose-5-phosphate with $ARPP^{32}P^{32}$ should lead after brief acid treatment to a liberation of radioactive inorganic phosphate; the latter can be readily differentiated from $ARPP^{32}P^{32}$ by its failure to be adsorbed to Norit.

$$ARPP^{32}P^{32} + \text{deoxyribose-5-P} \xrightarrow{\text{kinase}} P^{32}P^{32}\text{-deoxyribose-5-P}$$

$$\xrightarrow{\text{acid}} P^{32}P^{32} + \text{deoxyribose-5-P}$$

A deoxyribose-5-P-dependent liberation of P^{32} from $ARPP^{32}P^{32}$ was sought in a number of cell extracts and eventually was found in *E. coli*. However, this reaction proved to be nothing more than the liberation of glyceraldehyde-3-phosphate from deoxyribose-5-phosphate by Racker's aldolase and a subsequent rapid exchange of the terminal P of ATP with the inorganic phosphate buffer through the action of glyceraldehyde-3-phosphate dehydrogenase and 3-phosphoglyceric acid kinase. To date, no evidence has appeared for a deoxyribose analog of PRPP.

B. *Deoxynucleosides.*

A purine deoxynucleoside phosphorylase reaction like that observed for the ribonucleosides, and carried out by what may even be the same enzyme, was found by Friedkin and Kalckar (21, 24) in liver and by Manson and Lampen in thymus and *E. coli* (81). Likewise, a phosphorolysis of pyrimidine deoxynucleosides has been observed with liver preparations. Both uracil and thymine, but not cytosine, react with deoxyribose-1-phosphate to yield the corresponding nucleosides.

Another mechanism for forming a wide variety of deoxynucleosides is the deoxynucleoside transglycosylase of MacNutt (79). This enzyme, found in a number of bacterial species, effects an exchange of free purine or pyrimidine bases with those found in a deoxynucleoside without the intervention of phosphorolysis or hydrolysis. While no net synthesis of nucleoside results, this reaction explains how a number of different, and even unnatural, deoxyribosides can satisfy the deoxynucleoside growth requirements of certain bacteria.

C. *Thymidine Nucleotide.*

For many years the deoxynucleotides were known only as a result of the degradation of DNA by phosphodiesterase action and only relatively recently were shown by Carter (14) to be 5′-phosphate esters. The observation that thymidine-5′-phosphate may be produced from thymidine by the action of ATP and an *E. coli* enzyme came as a result of attempts to determine how thymidine was incorporated into DNA (56). The studies of Friedkin (26) had shown thymidine to be an effective precursor of DNA thymine in suspensions of chick embryonic tissue cells or bone marrow, and Reichard and Estborn (99) had demonstrated with intact animals that N^{15}-labeled thymidine and deoxycytidine are utilized for DNA synthesis.

In our first experiments with C^{14}-thymidine (kindly provided by Dr. Morris Friedkin) we found that extracts of *E. coli*, with added ATP, converted thymidine to an acid-insoluble, DNAase-sensitive material and also to three distinct acid-soluble nucleotides (Table 2). One of these was identified as thymidine-5′-phosphate, and the other two, on the basis of their chromatographic behavior, were presumed to be thymidine di- and tri-phosphate. The thymidine kinase was

TABLE 2

THYMIDINE CONVERSION TO NUCLEOTIDES AND DNA

Fraction	0 minutes	60 minutes
	c.p.m.	
Acid-insoluble ("DNA")	32	196
" —DNAase-treated	35	30
Acid-soluble		
Thymidine-5′-P	1,000	17,100
"TDP"	500	9,500
"TTP"	100	2,300

Thymidine-C^{14}, 1 μmole, 4×10^5 c.p.m.

partially purified, but the requirement for an exceptionally high concentration of ATP has thus far prevented a reliable balance study of this reaction. Thymidine does have a high affinity for the enzyme and so its conversion to thymidine-5'-phosphate can be made essentially complete. Deoxyuridine is also phosphorylated by this enzyme preparation at a rate about one-third that of thymidine. While thymidine, and probably other deoxynucleosides, can be converted to nucleotides by this type of kinase action, the main route of deoxynucleotide synthesis probably lies elsewhere. As proposed for the ribonucleotides, the nucleoside kinase may for the most part represent a salvage operation.

Current studies of Dr. M. Friedkin, presented elsewhere in this volume, describe an avenue of thymidine-5'-phosphate synthesis that should bring us closer to an important *de novo* pathway. Deoxyuridine-5'-phosphate and serine in the presence of an *E. coli* enzyme preparation are converted to thymidine-5'-phosphate. The requirement for serine may be replaced by hydroxymethyl tetrahydrofolic acid. The intimate mechanism of this transfer reaction as well as the biosynthetic pathway of deoxyuridine-5'-phosphate synthesis now loom as major objectives in these studies.

D. *Deoxynucleoside Di- and Tri-Phosphates.*

Enzymatic formation of the di- and tri-phosphates of deoxyadenosine and the pyrimidine deoxyribonucleosides has been reported (37a, 104a), and the occurrence of pyrimidine deoxynucleoside di- and tri-phosphates in thymus extracts has also been observed (89a). We have found and purified a kinase from *E. coli* which in the presence of an excess of ATP converts thymidylate, deoxycytidylate, deoxyadenylate, and deoxyguanylate to the respective nucleoside triphosphates. These have been isolated by anion-exchange chromatography and yield analyses of base:total P:acid-labile P of 1:3:2. We have presumed that the mechanism for their synthesis resembles the one described for the ribonucleotide kinase, but this is still a question for study. Of great interest is the failure of this enzyme to phosphorylate deoxyuridine-5'-phosphate, an observation which may help explain why uracil nucleotides are not found in DNA.

E. *Hypothetical Scheme for Deoxynucleotide Synthesis.*

A rather simple scheme is one involving a direct reduction of purine and pyrimidine ribonucleotides to the deoxynucleotides (Fig. 7). That

HYPOTHETICAL PATHWAY OF DEOXYNUCLEOTIDE SYNTHESIS

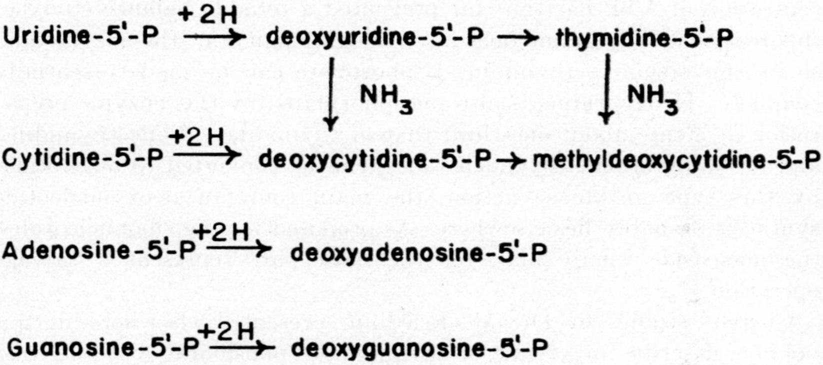

$$\text{Uridine-5'-P} \xrightarrow{+2H} \text{deoxyuridine-5'-P} \longrightarrow \text{thymidine-5'-P}$$

$$\downarrow NH_3 \qquad\qquad\qquad \downarrow NH_3$$

$$\text{Cytidine-5'-P} \xrightarrow{+2H} \text{deoxycytidine-5'-P} \longrightarrow \text{methyldeoxycytidine-5'-P}$$

$$\text{Adenosine-5'-P} \xrightarrow{+2H} \text{deoxyadenosine-5'-P}$$

$$\text{Guanosine-5'-P} \xrightarrow{+2H} \text{deoxyguanosine-5'-P}$$

Fig. 7

simplicity in a hypothetical biochemical scheme is not necessarily a virtue is a lesson we have learned many times over. However, results showing ribonucleotides to be effective DNA precursors led Hammarsten et al. (36) some years ago to make the suggestion of a direct conversion of the ribo to the deoxy derivatives. The demonstration by Rose and Schweigert (103) that C[14]-randomly-labeled cytidine is incorporated as a unit into DNA (with the thymidine and deoxycytidine each maintaining the same relative C[14] distribution between base and sugar as the cytidine) and its recent confirmation by Roll et al. (102) provide additional support for this suggestion.

The above-mentioned studies of Dr. Friedkin, which demonstrate the enzymatic conversion of deoxyuridine-5'-phosphate to thymidine-5'-phosphate, are a further indication that the reduction step can precede the methylation. Possible pathways for the synthesis of other deoxynucleotides considered in Fig. 7 have no experimental basis as yet. The findings of Friedkin and Roberts (25) that deoxyuridine is a good precursor of DNA thymidine and those of Reichard (97) that deoxyuridine is a better DNA precursor than 5-methyluridine in the whole rat also suggest a pathway involving deoxyuridine-5'-phosphate as an intermediate.

III. Coenzyme Synthesis

While a consideration of the enzymatic synthesis of coenzymes in this symposium may seem to have only a remote relationship to the subject of gene biochemistry, it does represent the origin of my interest in nucleic acid biosynthesis and the orientation of much of my thinking and work toward that goal. Aside from this minor personal reason, the key reaction in coenzyme biosynthesis, based on the reactivity of the 5'-phosphoryl nucleoside group of a nucleoside triphosphate (viz., ATP, UTP) or of nucleoside diphosphate derivatives (i.e., coenzymes), may be instructive with respect to polynucleotide synthesis.

The synthesis of DPN (52, 53, 60) may be pictured as a nucleophilic attack (62) on ATP by nicotinamide mononucleotide (Fig. 8). The synthesis of flavin adenine dinucleotide (FAD) (107) and of coenzyme A (CoA) (39) may be regarded as quite similar (Fig. 9). Berg's (5, 6)

NUCLEOPHILIC ATTACK OF NICOTINAMIDE MONONUCLEOTIDE ON ATP

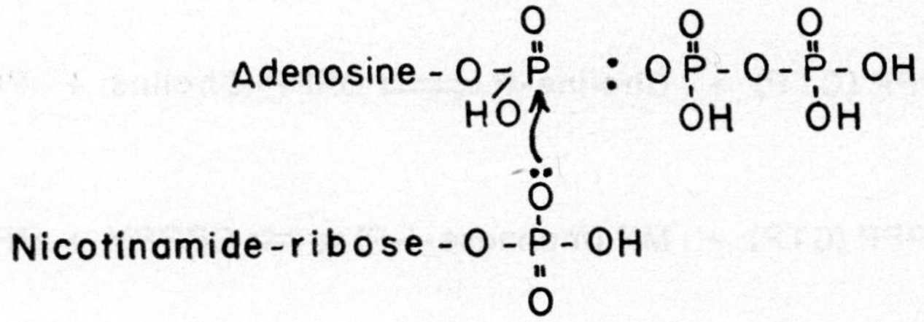

FIG. 8

ADENINE NUCLEOTIDE COENZYME SYNTHESIS

1. ARPPP (ATP) + NRP (nicotinamide mononucleotide) $\rightleftharpoons$ ARPPRN (DPN) + PP

2. ARPPP + FRP (riboflavin-P) $\rightleftharpoons$ ARPPRF (FAD) + PP

3. ARPPP + Pantetheine-P $\rightleftharpoons$ ARPP-Pantetheine + PP

   $\xrightarrow{\text{ATP}}$ ARPP-Pantetheine (CoA)
   P

4. ARPPP + RCH₂COOH $\rightleftharpoons$ ARPOCCH₂R + PP
                                              ‖
                                              O

   or   or

   RCHNH₂COOH   ARPOCCHNH₂R + PP
                                    ‖
                                    O

FIG. 9

demonstration that the activation of fatty acids and amino acids by ATP leads to the formation of adenyl acylates may be formulated as another closely related mechanism. What has been described here for adenosine nucleotides seems to apply with equal force to the triphosphate coenzyme precursors of the uridine (87), cytidine (47), and guanosine (86) nucleotide coenzymes (Fig. 10).

URIDINE, CYTIDINE, AND GUANOSINE NUCLEOTIDE COENZYME SYNTHESIS

1. URPPP(UTP) + G-P (glucose-1-P) ⇌ URPPG (UDPG) + PP

2. URPPP + Gal-P (galactose-1-P) ⇌ URPPGal + PP

3. CRPPP (CTP) + Choline-P ⇌ CRPP-Choline + PP

4. GRPPP (GTP) + MP (mannose-1-P) ⇌ GRPPM + PP

Fig. 10

On the basis of these reactions, the lengthening of a polynucleotide chain by reaction with a nucleoside di- or triphosphate may also be regarded as a nucleophilic attack on the 5'-phosphoryl group by the oxygen of the alcohol group (at carbon 3) of the pentose (Fig. 11). In mechanism A, a polynucleotide chain (or acceptor group) ends as a triphosphate and the addition of an ATP molecule to this end leads to displacement of inorganic pyrophosphate from the acceptor. (It is immaterial at this point whether the reactive component is ADP with phosphorolytic reactions or ATP with pyrophosphorolytic reactions.) In mechanism B, ATP adds to the sugar end of the acceptor, with the displacement of pyrophosphate from ATP.

IV. Ribonucleic Acid Synthesis

Our studies on nucleotide and coenzyme synthesis led to attempts to convert ribonucleoside triphosphate to polyribonucleotides. Dr. U. Z. Littauer and I (76, 77) were able to show that extracts from *E. coli* converted C^{14}-adenine-labeled ATP to an acid-insoluble nucleotide and that the addition of adenylate kinase increased the rate of the

HYPOTHETICAL SCHEMES OF POLYNUCLEOTIDE CHAIN INCREASE

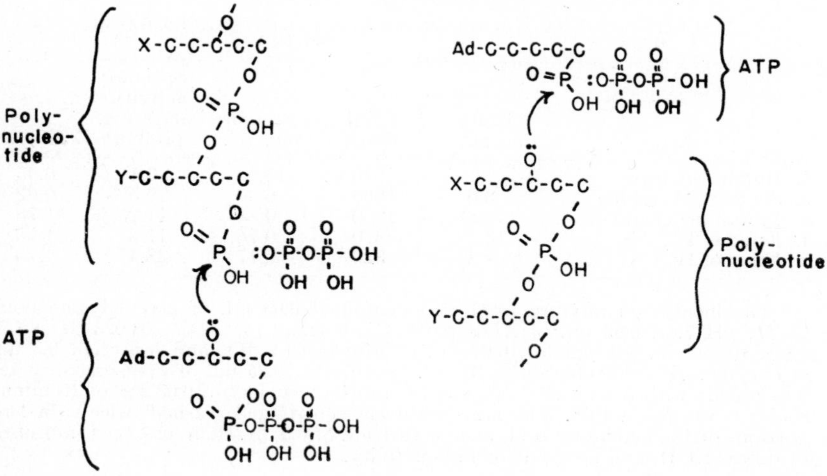

Fig. 11

reaction. The important discovery made at this time by Ochoa and coworkers (32-34) that nucleoside diphosphates are polymerized by an enzyme from *Azotobacter vinelandii* made it clear that in our *E. coli* system ADP rather than ATP was the reactive component.

The enzyme was purified from extracts of *E. coli* prepared by sonic disruption of the cells. As seen in Table 3, a considerable purification was achieved, and as judged by ultraviolet absorption very little, if any, nucleic acid remained.

The product of the ADP reaction is insoluble at pH 3.5, forming a transparent, gel-like precipitate which dissolves at neutral pH to give a highly viscous solution from which fine threads can be drawn. The ultraviolet absorption spectrum shows λ280/λ260 and λ250/λ260 values of 0.32 and 0.93, respectively, as compared with near normal values of 0.14 and 0.84 after alkaline hydrolysis. The product from ADP is resistant to RNAase action.

A balance study of the reaction (Table 4) indicated that ADP, and also UDP and CDP, were polymerized with a concomitant liberation of inorganic orthophosphate. For reasons that are still obscure, GDP

TABLE 3

Purification of Ribopolynucleotide-Synthesizing Enzyme

Step	Units per ml. *	Total units	Protein mg./ml.	Specific activity units/mg. protein	λ280/λ260
1. 10-min. sonicate	1.1	670	10.9	0.1	0.55
2. Sonicate of residue	3.0	1860	6.90	0.5	0.62
3. Protamine eluate	9.8	1960	0.88	11.2	1.75
4. Ethanol I	13.1	870	0.76	17.3	1.75
5. Ethanol II	4.8	320	0.17	28.4	1.75

* The incubation mixture (0.25 ml.) contained 0.05 ml. of glycylglycine buffer (1 M, pH 7.4), 0.02 ml. of ADP (0.04 M), 0.02 ml. of ADP (0.0023 M, 8-C^{14}, 7.8 × 10^5 c.p.m. per μmole), 0.01 ml. of $MgCl_2$ (0.1 M), and less than 0.3 unit of enzyme. After incubation at 37° C. for 10 min., 0.25 ml. of 7% perchloric acid was added; with the purified enzyme fractions a "carrier" of 0.03 ml. of 10-minute sonicate was also added. The precipitate was centrifuged, washed twice with 1-ml. portions of 1% perchloric acid, once with 1 ml. of 0.01 N HCl, dissolved in 0.40 ml. of dilute KOH, and assayed for radioactivity.

is inert in the purified enzyme system. Similar results have been reported by Beers (3) with an enzyme from *Micrococcus lysodeikticus*.

The reaction is readily reversed by inorganic phosphate (Table 5). In view of this evidence, the reaction may be formulated by the equation:

$$\text{n nucleoside-PP} \rightleftarrows \text{(nucleoside-P)}_n + \text{n P}_i$$

and thus is an example of the reaction described by Grunberg-Manago and Ochoa for the enzyme from *A. vinelandii*. As in their studies, we observed an exchange of inorganic P^{32} with ADP in the presence of the enzyme. However, the ratio of ADP incorporation activity to ADP-orthophosphate exchange activity was more than four-fold greater in the purified fraction than in a crude sonicate. By the addition of an early fraction, which by itself was devoid of activity, the P^{32}-ADP exchange could be increased by about four-fold (Table 6); the rate of ADP incorporation was not affected. This "activator" is nondialyzable, heat-stable, and resistant to RNAase and DNAase. The nature of this material and how it modifies the kinetics of the reaction are still unknown. Of interest too, in view of the known susceptibility of polyuridylate to ribonuclease, is the failure of this enzyme to influence the P^{32}-UDP exchange. It is clear that much remains to

TABLE 4

BALANCE STUDY OF ADP, UDP, CDP, AND GDP INCORPORATION INTO POLYNUCLEOTIDES

	ADP		UDP		CDP		GDP	
	Acid soluble	Polymer	Acid soluble	Polymer	Acid soluble	Polymer	Acid soluble	Polymer
Orthophosphate, Δ μmole	+0.42	—	+0.21	—	+0.44	—	0.0	—
Acid-labile phosphate, Δ μmole	-0.38	—	-0.21	—	-0.44	—	0.0	0.0
Total phosphate, Δ μmole	—	+0.41	—	—	—	—	—	0.0
*U.V. density, Δ μmole	-0.36	+0.39	-0.25	+0.28	-0.44	+0.43	0.0	0.0
Pentose, Δ μmole	—	+0.36	—	—	—	—	—	—
Radioactivity, % incorporation	—	57	—	30	—	60	0	—
Acid-labile phosphate, % lost	52	—	32	—	—	—	—	—

* Measurement of the polymer was made after hydrolysis in 1 N KOH for 15 hours.

TABLE 5

POLYADENYLATE BREAKDOWN

Phosphate concentration	Polymer breakdown
$M \times 10^{-4}$	% of original
* 0.64 (0 min.)	0
* 0.64 (60 min.)	14
4.40 "	29
19.0 "	96
38.0 "	99

* Present in the reaction mixture without added phosphate.

TABLE 6

P³²-ADP EXCHANGE COMPARED TO POLYMER FORMATION

Enzyme fraction	Ratio of ADP incorporation to		Activation ratio column 1/column 2
	P_i exchange without activator	P_i exchange with activator	
10-min. sonicate	0.5	0.5	1.0
Sonicate of residue	1.1	1.1	1.0
Protamine eluate	3.3	1.4	2.5
Ethanol I	2.3	0.9	2.5
Ethanol II	2.3	0.6	3.8

be learned about the intimate mechanism of the component events in the polymerization reaction.

Since the polyribonucleotide phosphorylases thus far described assemble long polymers of a single nucleotide and assemble mixed nucleotides in an apparently indiscriminate way, one of the most important questions still confronting us is the problem of how a cell synthesizes a specific RNA. Unfortunately, the separation and characterization of ribonucleic acids is still at an early stage and little more can be said than that several RNA-rich fractions possess biological activity and that there are suggestive analytical differences between RNA's from different cells (80). The plant viruses and certain animal viruses which are considered to be ribonucleoproteins represent immediate objectives for determination of the biologic activity of enzymatically synthesized polymers. What appears to be another functional RNA is the inhibitor of DNAase which is widely distributed and has a remarkable degree of specificity. For example, the DNAase inhibitor of *E. coli,* which almost completely masks DNAase activity in *E. coli* extracts, does not affect the activity of pancreatic DNAase. Assays of the DNAase inhibitor activity of the synthetic polymers indicate only a slight activity and one which is directed nonspecifically against both the *E. coli* and pancreatic DNAases (77).

V. Deoxyribonucleic Acid Synthesis

To understand the chemical events in the development of a bacterial virus, to define the biochemical reactions in bacterial transformation or, in short, to formulate the chemical basis for most genetic phenomena, a knowledge of the pathways of DNA biosynthesis is essential. I should like to turn now to a consideration of our attempts to define the steps leading to DNA synthesis. In view of a report of these studies at the meeting of the Federated Societies in April (55, 56) and some clarifying results since then, I shall present the whole chronologic, and at times illogical, development of this story.

We had observed the conversion by *E. coli* extracts of thymidine into thymidine nucleotides (see Table 2) and to a substance showing the chemical properties commonly attributed to DNA. Fractionation of the *E. coli* extracts led to the separation of a number of enzymes which appeared to convert thymidine by successive kinase steps to thymidine-5′-phosphate, TTP, and an acid-insoluble nucleic acid fraction (Fig. 12). From the results shown in Table 7 it appears that, even with a crude enzyme preparation, thymidine-5′-P is a more favorable substrate than thymidine, and TTP in turn appears to be

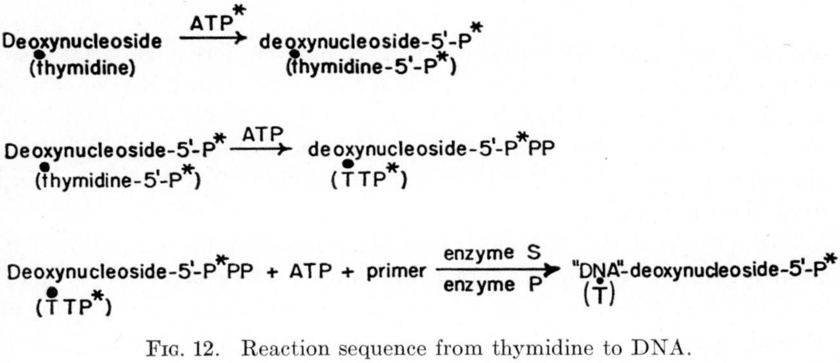

Deoxynucleoside $\xrightarrow{\text{ATP}^*}$ deoxynucleoside-5′-P*
(thymidine) (thymidine-5′-P*)

Deoxynucleoside-5′-P* $\xrightarrow{\text{ATP}}$ deoxynucleoside-5′-P*PP
(thymidine-5′-P*) (TTP*)

Deoxynucleoside-5′-P*PP + ATP + primer $\xrightarrow[\text{enzyme P}]{\text{enzyme S}}$ "DNA"-deoxynucleoside-5′-P*
(TTP*) (T)

Fig. 12. Reaction sequence from thymidine to DNA.

TABLE 7

REACTION RATES WITH CRUDE AND PURIFIED ENZYME PREPARATIONS

Substrate	Crude	Purified
	mμmoles DNA-P$_i$/mg. protein/hr.	
Thymidine	0.2	<4
Thymidine-5'-P	0.5	9
Thymidine-5'-PPP	1.6	97

The crude enzyme consists of two fractions prepared by fractionation of an *E. coli* extract (obtained by sonic disintegration) with streptomycin: a supernatant fraction, S, and a redissolved precipitate, P. In the purified system, the S and P enzymes have each been purified more than 100-fold, using TTP as the substrate.

a more immediate precursor of the product than thymidine-5'-P. In an assay with enzyme fractions purified with TTP as substrate, thymidine conversion to DNA was not detectable and thymidine-5'-P was only about one-tenth as effective a substrate as TTP.

The TTP (labeled with P^{32} in the acid-stable phosphate or with C^{14} in the thymine) which became acid-insoluble was shown to be part of a DNA or closely related molecule (Table 8). Treatment of the

TABLE 8

CHARACTERISTICS OF THE PRODUCT

Product	c.p.m.
Acid-insoluble product	274
DNAase-treated	13
RNAase-treated	240
NaOH (1 N), 18 hours at 37° C.	214
Perchloric acid (0.01 N), 5 min. at 100° C.	232
Perchloric acid (0.04 N), 5 min. at 100° C.	82

product with crystalline pancreatic DNAase rendered essentially all of the radioactivity acid-soluble, while treatment with RNAase, strong alkali, or dilute acid had little or no effect. Exposure to somewhat stronger acid led to a solubilization of the radioactive material, with an approximately parallel release of ultraviolet-absorbing material from the precipitate.

The nature of the polymerization reaction remains the subject of greatest interest to us. As shown in Table 9, the conversion of TTP to "DNA" required ATP, a heat-stable DNA-containing fraction, at present regarded as a "primer," and two enzyme fractions (called

TABLE 9

Requirements of the Purified System

Extracts of *E. coli* B prepared by sonic disintegration were treated with strepto-mycin to yield a precipitate (fraction SP) and a supernatant fluid (fraction SS). Ammonium sulfate, gel, and acid fractionation procedures applied to fractions SP and SS yielded fractions P and S, respectively. *E. coli* DNA was prepared by heating fraction SP (optical density at 260 mμ = 15) at 70° C. for 10 minutes. To produce "primer," 0.1 ml. of *E. coli* DNA was combined with 40 μg. of fraction SP; after 1 hour of 37° C. in the presence of 5×10^{-3} M MgCl$_2$, the mixture was heated for 10 minutes at 80° C. The complete system contained (in 0.3 ml.) 0.014 μmole of TTP (1.5×10^6 c.p.m./μmole), 0.1 μmole of ATP, 0.10 ml. of "primer," 10 μg. of fraction S, 1 μg. of fraction P, 1 μmole of MgCl$_2$, and 20 μmoles of glycine buffer, pH 9.2. After incubation for 30 minutes at 37° C., 0.05 ml. of crude *E. coli* extract ("carrier") and 0.3 ml. of 7 per cent perchloric acid were added. The precipitate was washed and its radioactivity was measured.

	mμmoles DNA-P$_i$/hr.
Complete system	1.48
No ATP	0.20
No "primer"	0.11
No enzyme fraction S	0.07
No enzyme fraction P	0.04

S and P), each of which has been purified more than 100-fold. At this time studies with TDP indicated that it could replace TTP and that it had the same requirements for its incorporation into DNA. A decision as to the more immediate precursor requires further purifica-tion of the system.

To determine whether the other deoxynucleotides found in DNA react in a manner similar to thymidine-5′-phosphate, the deoxynucleo-side-5′-triphosphates of adenine, guanine, and cytosine were prepared. The P^{32}-labeled deoxynucleoside-5′-phosphates were obtained by enzymatic digestion of DNA derived from *E. coli* grown in a P^{32}-containing medium and then phosphorylated to the triphosphate stage by the partially purified kinase. As shown in Table 10, utilization of the triphosphates of adenine, guanine, and cytosine deoxynucleotides for DNA synthesis occurred at rates approximately equal to those for TTP in crude enzyme fractions, but at appreciably slower rates with the purified enzymes, purified, that is, for TTP polymerization. Mixtures of these triphosphates, each tested at concentrations near enzyme saturation, gave additive or superadditive rates of incorpora-tion, a result showing a facilitation of polymerization by such mixtures. The dependence on "primer" even with a mixture of the four nucleo-tides is noteworthy.

TABLE 10

<small>Conversion of Four Deoxynucleoside Triphosphates</small>

The incubation mixtures and assays were as described in Table 9 except that (1) the concentrations of deoxynucleoside triphosphates were 1.5 × 10⁻⁵ *M*, and (2) the crude enzymes were 60 μg of fraction SP and 240 μg of fraction SS.

Triphosphates	Tested with crude enzymes	Tested with purified enzymes (for TTP)
	mμmoles DNA-P³²/hr.	
Thymidine (T)	0.8	5.48
Deoxyguanosine (G)	0.6	0.98
Deoxycytidine (C)	0.8	1.44
Deoxyadenosine (A)	0.6	1.28
T + G	2.2	14.6
T + G + C	4.4	19.6
T + G + C + A	6.4	22.0 *
T + G + C + A (no "primer")	2.0	0.28

* 65 per cent conversion of substrate.

Our studies during the past few weeks have given us a little more insight into the nature of the terminal reaction. We continued to use as an assay the incorporation of TTP³² into DNA. Purification of the "primer" showed us that it consisted of two components: one has proved to be a nondialyzable, DNAase-sensitive substance indistinguishable from DNA, and the other is a dialyzable, acid-soluble fraction which can be replaced by an exhaustive DNAase-diesterase digest of DNA. Chromatography of this digest resolved it into three components, coinciding with deoxycytidylic, deoxyadenylic, and deoxyguanylic acid-containing fractions, each inactive by itself but active when combined.

These results have led to the demonstration of the absolute need for all four deoxynucleoside *triphosphates* and a considerable simplification of the enzyme system (Table 11). ATP and the enzyme fraction S are no longer required and do not influence the reaction. The previous requirement for ATP and enzyme fraction S (see Table 9) was presumably to provide the deoxynucleoside triphosphates not added to the incubation mixture. It is apparent from the data that in the absence of ATP and fraction S, no detectable reaction occurs when any one of the triphosphates is omitted. Mg⁺⁺ and DNA are also essential.

Preliminary results now indicate a net synthesis of DNA (Table 12). In experiment I, the precipitation of DNA was incomplete due to the

TABLE 11

Requirements for TTP Incorporation into "DNA"

	mμmoles
Complete system *	0.50
Omit C,G,A	0.00
" C	0.00
" G	0.00
" A	0.00
" Mg++	0.00
" DNA	0.00
DNA pretreated with DNAase	0.00
Add ATP (100 mμmoles)	0.54
Add ADP (100 mμmoles)	0.50
Add S enzyme	0.49

* 5 mμmoles of each deoxynucleoside triphosphate (TTP $= 1.5 \times 10^6$ c.p.m./μmole), 1 μmole of $MgCl_2$, 3μg. of P enzyme, 5μg. of DNA; 30 minutes at 37° C. C, G, and A stand for the triphosphates of deoxycytidine, deoxyguanosine, and deoxyadenosine, respectively.

TABLE 12

Net Synthesis of DNA

	Control **	Exptl.	Δ
	mμmoles		
Exp. I *			
P32	3	104	101
U.V.	37	109	72
Deoxypentose	42	130	88
Exp. II			
P32	1.9	18.3	16.2
U.V.	21.4	31.6	10.2

* DNA precipitation incomplete.
** Deoxyadenosine triphosphate omitted.
The P32 value is a measure of deoxynucleotide incorporation into DNA; the U.V. value is calculated using the molar absorption coefficient of thymus DNA. The reaction mixtures were similar to those in Table 11, but larger in scale and incubated for 60 minutes.

lack of addition of a "carrier" or coprecipitant. In experiment II, the addition of albumin resulted in a quantitative precipitation of the DNA; extraction with hot perchloric acid eliminated interference by albumin with the optical density value at 260 mμ. However, the ultraviolet absorption values are only approximate because the correct absorption coefficient of the product is not known.

The release of inorganic pyrophosphate during the course of the reaction (Table 13) and the inability of thymidine diphosphate to replace thymidine triphosphate (Table 14) point to the triphosphates as the immediate precursors of DNA. The reaction does not appear readily reversible, as judged by the failure of inorganic pyrophosphate at high concentrations (1×10^{-3} M) to prevent or markedly inhibit the DNA synthesis reaction.

We know relatively little about this enzyme reaction and the nature of the DNA product. We must learn more about methods of sequential and end-group analysis of DNA. The overriding question remains: How is biologically specific DNA formed? Nevertheless, the relative simplicity of the DNA-forming system described now makes a number of experiments feasible. The enzymatic synthesis of a bacterial transforming factor, once regarded beyond experimental reach, has now become an immediate objective.

IN SUMMARY, we have reasonably good evidence that the 5'-nucleoside di- or tri-phosphates are the immediate precursors in the enzymatic formation of a nucleic acid polymer. In the case of the ribonucleotides, pathways of purine and pyrimidine nucleotide formation are fairly

TABLE 13

PYROPHOSPHATE RELEASE FROM TTP

	Control *	Exptl.	Δ
		mμmoles	
DNA-C^{14}	1	21	20
$P_i{}^{32}$	8	12	4
$P^{32}P^{32}$	2	21	19

* Deoxyadenosinetriphosphate omitted.

The TTP was labeled with C^{14} in the thymine and P^{32} in the terminal two phosphate groups. The incubation mixtures were similar to those in Table 11, but larger in scale and incubated for 60 minutes. $P_i{}^{32}$ and $P^{32}P^{32}$ were separated and determined by chromatography on Dowex-1 chloride columns.

TABLE 14

INABILITY OF THYMIDINE DIPHOSPHATE TO
REPLACE THYMIDINE TRIPHOSPHATE

	mμmole DNA-P^{32}
Complete system *	0.65
No TTP	0.06
TTP replaced by TDP	0.06

* The labeled substrate was deoxy-ARP^{32}PP; the reaction mixtures and incubation conditions were similar to those in Table 11.

well understood. While the pathways of deoxynucleotide synthesis have not been described, there is a hope that the demonstration of a mechanism of direct reduction of the ribonucleotides will lead to a simple solution. In our current studies of DNA synthesis we are dealing with a moderately purified protein fraction which appears to increase the size of a DNA chain. It does so only under the remarkable condition that all four of the deoxynucleoside triphosphates be present.

ACKNOWLEDGMENT

The unpublished results on the enzymatic synthesis of DNA come from the joint efforts of Dr. I. R. Lehman, supported by an American Cancer Society Fellowship, Dr. M. J. Bessman, a fellow of the Public Health Service, and Mr. E. S. Simms. Grants to me from the Public Health Service and the National Science Foundation have made the work of this laboratory possible.

REFERENCES

1. Abrams, R., and Bentley, M., *J. Am. Chem. Soc.,* **77**, 4179 (1955).
2. Abrams, A., and Klenow, H., *Arch. Biochem. and Biophys.,* **34**, 285 (1951).
2a. Agranoff, B. W., and Brady, R. O., *J. Biol. Chem.,* **219**, 221 (1956).
3. Beers, R. F., Jr., *Nature,* **177**, 790 (1956).
4. Bentley, M., and Abrams, R., *Federation Proc.,* **15**, 218 (1956).
5. Berg, P., *J. Am. Chem. Soc.,* **77**, 3163 (1955).
6. Berg, P., and Newton, G., *Federation Proc.,* **15**, 219 (1956).
7. Bergkvist, R., and Deutsch, A., *Acta Chem. Scand.,* **7**, 1307 (1953).
8. Brawerman, G., and Chargaff, E., *J. Am. Chem. Soc.,* **75**, 2020, 4113 (1953).
9. Brown, G. B., and Roll, P. M., in *The Nucleic Acids* (Chargaff, E., and Davidson, J. N., eds.), II, 341, Academic Press, New York (1955).
10. Buchanan, J. M., in *Phosphorus Metabolism* (McElroy, W. D., and Glass, B., eds.), II, 406, Johns Hopkins Press, Baltimore (1952).
11. Canellakis, E. S., *Federation Proc.,* **15**, 229 (1956).
12. Caputto, R., *J. Biol. Chem.,* **189**, 801 (1951).
13. Cardini, C. E., Paladini, A. C., Caputto, R., and Leloir, L. F., *Acta physiol. Latinoamer.,* **1**, 57 (1950).
14. Carter, C. E., *J. Am. Chem. Soc.,* **73**, 1537 (1951).
15. Carter, C. E., *Federation Proc.,* **15**, 230 (1956).
16. Carter, C. E., and Cohen, L. H., *J. Am. Chem. Soc.,* **77**, 499 (1955).
17. Cohen, S. S., Scott, D. B. M., and Lanning, M., *Federation Proc.,* **10**, 173 (1951).
18. Colowick, S. P., and Kalckar, H. M., *J. Biol. Chem.,* **148**, 117 (1943).
19. Crawford, I., and Kornberg, A., unpub.
20. DeLey, J., quoted by G. E. Glock, *Bull. assoc. diplômés microbiol. fac. pharm. Nancy,* p. 1 (1952).
21. Friedkin, M., *J. Biol. Chem.,* **184**, 449 (1950).
22. Friedkin, M., *J. Cell. Comp. Physiol.,* **41**, Supp. 1, 261 (1953).
23. Friedkin, M., *J. Biol. Chem.,* **209**, 295 (1954).

24. Friedkin, M., and Kalckar, H. M., *J. Biol. Chem.*, **184**, 437 (1950).
25. Friedkin, M., and Roberts, D., *Federation Proc.*, **14**, 215 (1955).
26. Friedkin, M., Tilson, D., and Roberts, D., *Federation Proc.*, **13**, 214 (1954).
27. Glock, G. E., in *The Nucleic Acids* (Chargaff, E., and Davidson, J. N., eds.), II, 248, Academic Press, New York (1955).
28. Goldthwait, D. A., *Federation Proc.*, **15**, 263 (1956).
29. Goldthwait, D. A., Greenberg, G. R., and Peabody, R. A., *Biochim. et Biophys. Acta,* **18**, 148 (1955).
30. Greenberg, G. R., *Federation Proc.*, **13**, 745 (1954).
31. Greenberg, G. R., *J. Biol. Chem.*, **219**, 423 (1956).
32. Grunberg-Manago, M., and Ochoa, S., *J. Am. Chem. Soc.*, **77**, 3165 (1955).
33. Grunberg-Manago, M., Ortiz, P. J., and Ochoa, S., *Science,* **122**, 907 (1955).
34. Grunberg-Manago, M., Ortiz, P. J., and Ochoa, S., *Biochim. et Biophys. Acta,* **20**, 269 (1956).
35. Guarino, A. J., and Sable, H. Z., *J. Biol. Chem.*, **215**, 515 (1955).
36. Hammarsten, E., Reichard, P., and Saluste, E., *J. Biol. Chem.*, **183**, 105 (1950).
37. Hartman, S. C., Levenberg, B., and Buchanan, J. M., *J. Am. Chem. Soc.*, **77**, 501 (1955).
37a. Hecht, L. I., Potter, V. R., and Herbert, E., *Biochim. et Biophys. Acta,* **15**, 134 (1954).
38. Herbert, E., Potter, V. R., and Takagi, Y., *J. Biol. Chem.*, **213**, 923 (1955).
39. Hoagland, M. B., and Novelli, G. D., *J. Biol. Chem.*, **207**, 767 (1954).
40. Horecker, B. L., and Mehler, A. H., *Ann. Revs. Biochem.*, **24**, 207 (1955).
41. Horecker, B. L., Smyrniotis, P. Z., and Seegmiller, J. E., *J. Biol. Chem.*, **193**, 383 (1951).
42. Hurlbert, R. B., and Potter, V. R., *J. Biol. Chem.*, **209**, 1 (1954).
43. Hurlbert, R. B., and Reichard, P., *Acta Chem. Scand.*, **9**, 251 (1955).
44. Jones, M. E., Spector, L., and Lipmann, F., *J. Am. Chem. Soc.*, **77**, 819 (1955).
45. Kalckar, H. M., *J. Biol. Chem.*, **148**, 127 (1943).
46. Kalckar, H. M., *J. Biol. Chem.*, **167**, 477 (1947).
47. Kennedy, E. P., and Weiss, S. B., *J. Am. Chem. Soc.*, **77**, 250 (1955).
48. Klenow, H., *Arch. Biochem. and Biophys.*, **46**, 186 (1953).
49. Korn, E. D., and Buchanan, J. M., *J. Biol. Chem.*, **217**, 183 (1955).
50. Korn, E. D., Charalampous, F. C., and Buchanan, J. M., *J. Am. Chem. Soc.*, **75**, 3610 (1953).
51. Korn, E. D., Remy, C. N., Wasilejko, H. C., and Buchanan, J. M., *J. Biol. Chem.*, **217**, 875 (1955).
52. Kornberg, A., *J. Biol. Chem.*, **176**, 1475 (1948).
53. Kornberg, A., *J. Biol. Chem.*, **182**, 779 (1950).
54. Kornberg, A., in *Phosphorus Metabolism* (McElroy, W. D., and Glass, B., eds.), I, 392, Johns Hopkins Press, Baltimore (1951).
55. Kornberg, A., Lehman, I. R., Bessman, M. J., and Simms, E. S., *Biochim. et Biophys. Acta,* **21**, 197 (1956).
56. Kornberg, A., Lehman, I. R., and Simms, E. S., *Federation Proc.*, **15**, 291 (1956).
57. Kornberg, A., Lieberman, I., and Simms, E. S., *J. Am. Chem. Soc.*, **76**, 2027 (1954).
58. Kornberg, A., Lieberman, I., and Simms, E. S., *J. Biol. Chem.*, **215**, 389 (1955).
59. Kornberg, A., Lieberman, I., and Simms, E. S., *J. Biol. Chem.*, **215**, 417 (1955).
60. Kornberg, A., and Pricer, W. E., Jr., *J. Biol. Chem.*, **191**, 535 (1951).
61. Kornberg, A., and Pricer, W. E., Jr., *J. Biol. Chem.*, **193**, 481 (1951).

62. Koshland, D. E., Jr., in *The Mechanism of Enzyme Action* (McElroy, W. D., and Glass, B., eds.), 608, Johns Hopkins Press, Baltimore (1954).
63. Lagerkvist, U., *Acta Chem. Scand.,* **9**, 1028 (1955).
64. Lampen, J. O., in *Phosphorus Metabolism* (McElroy, W. D., and Glass, B., eds.), II, 363, Johns Hopkins Press, Baltimore (1952).
65. Lampen, J. O., *J. Cell. Comp. Physiol.,* **41**, Suppl. 1, 183 (1953).
66. Levenberg, B., and Buchanan, J. M., *J. Am. Chem. Soc.,* **78**, 504 (1956).
67. Levenberg, B., and Melnick, I., *Federation Proc.,* **15**, 117 (1956).
68. Lieberman, I., *J. Am. Chem. Soc.,* **77**, 2661 (1955).
69. Lieberman, I., *J. Am. Chem. Soc.,* **78**, 251 (1956).
70. Lieberman, I., and Kornberg, A., *Biochim. et Biophys. Acta,* **12**, 223 (1953); *J. Biol. Chem.,* **207**, 911 (1954); *ibid.,* **212**, 909 (1955).
71. Lieberman, I., Kornberg, A., and Simms, E. S., *J. Am. Chem. Soc.,* **76**, 2844 (1954).
72. Lieberman, I., Kornberg, A., and Simms, E. S., *J. Am. Chem. Soc.,* **76**, 3608 (1954).
73. Lieberman, I., Kornberg, A., and Simms, E. S., *J. Biol. Chem.,* **215**, 403 (1955).
74. Lieberman, I., Kornberg, A., and Simms, E. S., *J. Biol. Chem.,* **215**, 429 (1955).
75. Lipton, S. H., Morell, S. A., Frieden, A., and Bock, R. M., *J. Am. Chem. Soc.,* **75**, 5449 (1953).
76. Littauer, U. Z., *Federation Proc.,* **15**, 302 (1956).
77. Littauer, U. Z., and Kornberg, A., unpub.
78. Lukens, L. N., and Buchanan, J. M., *Federation Proc.,* **15**, 305 (1956).
79. MacNutt, W. S., *Biochem. J. (London),* **50**, 384 (1952).
80. Magasanik, B., in *The Nucleic Acids* (Chargaff, E., and Davidson, J. N., eds.), I, 373, Academic Press, New York (1955).
81. Manson, L. A., and Lampen, J. O., *J. Biol. Chem.,* **191**, 95 (1951); *ibid.,* **193**, 539 (1951).
82. Michelson, A. M., Drell, W., and Mitchell, H. K., *Proc. Natl. Acad. Sci. U. S.,* **37**, 396 (1951).
83. Mitchell, H. K., Houlahan, M. B., and Nyc, J. F., *J. Biol. Chem.,* **172**, 525 (1948).
84. Moyed, H. S., and Magasanik, B., *Federation Proc.,* **15**, 318 (1956).
85. Munch-Petersen, A., *Acta Chem. Scand.,* **8**, 1102 (1954).
86. Munch-Petersen, A., *Arch. Biochem. and Biophys.,* **55**, 592 (1955).
87. Munch-Petersen, A., Kalckar, H. M., Cutolo, E., and Smith, E. E. B., *Nature,* **172**, 1036 (1953).
88. Paege, L. M., and Schlenk, F., *Arch. Biochem.,* **28**, 348 (1950).
89. Paege, L. M., and Schlenk, F., *Arch. Biochem. and Biophys.,* **40**, 42 (1952).
89a. Potter, R. L., and Schlesinger, S., *J. Am. Chem. Soc.,* **77**, 6714 (1955).
90. Rabinowitz, J. C., *J. Biol. Chem.,* **218**, 175 (1956).
91. Rabinowitz, J. C., and Barker, H. A., *J. Biol. Chem.,* **281**, 147, 161 (1956).
92. Rabinowitz, J. C., and Pricer, W. E., Jr., *Federation Proc.,* **15**, 332 (1956).
93. Rabinowitz, J. C., and Pricer, W. E., Jr., *J. Biol. Chem.,* **218**, 189 (1956).
94. Racker, E., *J. Biol. Chem.,* **196**, 347 (1952).
95. Racker, E., *Advances in Enzymol.,* **15**, 141 (1954).
96. Racker, E., de la Haba, G., and Leder, I. G., *Arch. Biochem. and Biophys.,* **48**, 238 (1954).
97. Reichard, P., *Acta Chem. Scand.,* **9**, 1275 (1955).

98. Reichard, P., in *The Nucleic Acids* (Chargaff, E., and Davidson, J. N., eds.), II, 277, Academic Press, New York (1955).
99. Reichard, P., and Estborn, B., *J. Biol. Chem.*, **188**, 839 (1951).
100. Reichard, P., Smith, L. H., and Hanshoff, G., *Acta Chem. Scand.*, **9**, 1010 (1955).
101. Remy, C. N., Remy, W. T., and Buchanan, J. M., *J. Biol. Chem.*, **217**, 885 (1955).
102. Roll, P. M., Weinfeld, H., and Carroll, E., *J. Biol. Chem.*, **220**, 455 (1956).
103. Rose, I. A., and Schweigert, B. S., *J. Biol. Chem.*, **202**, 635 (1953).
104. Sable, H. Z., *Biochim. et Biophys. Acta*, **8**, 687 (1952).
104a. Sable, H. Z., Wilber, P. B., Cohen, A. E., and Kane, M. R., *Biochim. et Biophys. Acta,* **13**, 156 (1954).
105. Schlenk, F., in *The Nucleic Acids* (Chargaff, E., and Davidson, J. N., eds.), II, 309, Academic Press, New York (1955).
106. Schmitz, H., Hurlbert, R. B., and Potter, V. R., *J. Biol. Chem.*, **209**, 41 (1954).
107. Schrecker, A. W., and Kornberg, A., *J. Biol. Chem.*, **182**, 795 (1950).
108. Strominger, J. L., Heppel, L. A., and Maxwell, E. S., *Arch. Biochem. and Biophys.*, **52**, 488 (1954).
109. Wajzer, J., and Baron, F., *Bull. soc. chim. biol.*, **31**, 750 (1949).
110. Warren, L., and Flaks, J. G., *Federation Proc.*, **15**, 379 (1956).
111. Welch, A. D., in *Enzymes: Units of Biological Structure and Function* (Gaebler, O. H., ed.), Academic Press, New York (1956).
112. Williams, W. J., and Buchanan, J. M., *J. Biol. Chem.*, **203**, 583 (1953).
113. Wright, L. D., Driscoll, C. A., Miller, C. S., and Skeggs, H. R., *Proc. Soc. Exptl. Biol. Med.*, **84**, 716 (1953).
114. Wright, L. D., Miller, C. S., and Driscoll, C. A., *Proc. Soc. Exptl. Biol. Med.*, **86**, 215 (1954).

THE ENZYMATIC CONVERSION OF DEOXYURIDYLIC ACID TO THYMIDYLIC ACID AND THE PARTICIPATION OF TETRAHYDROFOLIC ACID

MORRIS FRIEDKIN AND ARTHUR KORNBERG

Departments of Pharmacology and Microbiology,
Washington University School of Medicine,
St. Louis, Missouri

THE SEQUENCE of reactions by which the thymidine of deoxyribonucleic acid (DNA) arises is unique in that it involves constituents, thymine and deoxyribose, not found among the known nucleotide synthetic pathways. Tracer studies have provided a profile of the over-all pattern of reactions which lead to the biosynthesis of the thymine of DNA. The pyrimidine bases of thymidine (14, 4), deoxycytidine (14), or deoxyuridine (3, 13) can serve as precursors of DNA thymine. Furthermore, the hydroxymethyl group of serine (2), formate (17), or formaldehyde (10) is the precursor of the 5-methyl group of thymine by a pathway in which folic acid compounds appear to play an important role. It is the mechanism of this methylation which is the subject of the present report.

It is not surprising that the presence of 5-methylcytosine and 5-hydroxymethylcytosine in certain DNA's has led to suggestions for sequences in which cytosine (as part of an undetermined structure) may be the primary acceptor of a one-carbon unit at position 5 and that upon deamination this would result in the formation of thymine. The observation that uracil-C^{14} deoxyriboside is a precursor of the thymidine of DNA and *not* of the deoxycytidine of several species (3, 13) showed clearly that a uracil-containing compound could be a methyl acceptor, however. It was further found that the utilization of deoxyuridine for thymidine synthesis was effectively blocked by low concentrations of Aminopterin, the powerful folic acid antagonist (3). The antimetabolic effects of Aminopterin on the utilization of one-carbon donors have been known for some time (5, 17).

Studies were initiated with cell-free extracts of *Escherichia coli*, in which it was hoped that the methylation of deoxyuridine could be demonstrated. Our main emphasis was placed on the preparation of

609

the nucleotides of deoxyuridine, on the assumption that the conversion to thymidine occurred with a phosphorylated form of the nucleoside.

The enzymatic kinase reactions by which thymidine is converted to thymidylic acid and subsequently to thymidine triphosphate (TTP) (9) were reinvestigated with deoxyuridine as phosphate acceptor from ATP. Although deoxyuridine was converted to deoxyuridylic acid, the subsequent phosphorylations to deoxyuridine triphosphate were not catalyzed by the *E. coli* enzyme which rapidly converts thymidylic acid to TTP. This specificity, which perhaps explains why thymine and not uracil is a component of DNA, was made the basis of a new assay for the methylation of deoxyuridylic acid:

deoxyuridine-5'-P^{32} (phosphomonoesterase-susceptible)
↓ methylation reactions
thymidine-5'-P^{32} (phosphomonoesterase-susceptible)
↓ ATP + thymidylic acid kinase
thymidine-5'-P^{32}-P-P (TTP) (phosphomonoesterase-resistant).

The working hypothesis was that only after methylation of deoxyuridylic acid to thymidylic acid could the specific thymidylic acid kinase catalyze phosphorylation to TTP. The assay consisted of counting TTP as a charcoal-adsorbable P^{32}-containing nucleotide resistant to the action of prostatic phosphomonoesterase. The phosphomonoesterase dephosphorylates deoxyuridylic acid and thymidylic acid but not TTP. Charcoal adsorbs nucleotides but not inorganic orthophosphate.

Employing this assay we found that P^{32}-labeled deoxyuridylic acid was converted to TTP by crude *E. coli* preparations. When the bacterial extracts were treated for the removal of cofactors by passage over a Dowex-1 formate column, the enzymatic activity was markedly diminished, but could be restored by the addition of a boiled extract of *E. coli*.

It was reasoned at this point that tetrahydrofolic acid (THFA), which is known to be involved in several transfer reactions (6, 1, 15, 12), might be the factor in the boiled extract which was activating the methylation of deoxyuridylic acid. Jaenicke (7) has shown that the β-carbon of serine is transferred to THFA with the probable formation of N^{10}-hydroxymethyl THFA. From this work one might expect that N^{10}-hydroxymethyl THFA by reductive reactions could result in the formation of methyl groups.

The effect of boiled bacterial extract could be replaced by synthetic THFA (8) in incubation mixtures containing deoxyuridylic acid, serine, ATP, Mg^{++}, thymidylic acid kinase, and Dowex-1-formate-treated extracts of *E. coli*. Furthermore, in the absence of serine (which acts as a methyl donor in the bacterial system), synthetic N^{10}-hydroxymethyl THFA (7) could act as a methyl donor. These effects are shown in Table 1.

TABLE 1

CONVERSION OF DEOXYURIDYLIC ACID TO THYMIDINE TRIPHOSPHATE

	c.p.m on Norit
Exp. 1	
Complete system	1650
zero time	24
minus THFA	47
" serine	480
" ATP	51
" extract	212
" Mg^{++}	30
" pyridoxal phosphate	1500
Exp. 2	
a) Complete system	
+ serine + THFA	1870
− serine + THFA	470
b) Complete system	
+ serine + hydroxymethyl THFA	1650
− serine + hydroxymethyl THFA	1210

The complete system (325 μliters; pH 7.4) contained 0.011 μmole of deoxyuridine-5'-phosphate labeled with P^{32} (2900 c.p.m.), 2.3 μmoles of ATP, 5.7 μmoles of $MgCl_2$, 11.4 μmoles of L-serine, 0.1 μmole of THFA or N^{10}-hydroxymethyl THFA, 0.5 μmole of cysteine, 2.5 μmoles of inorganic orthophosphate, 0.1 μmole of pyridoxal phosphate, 21 μmoles of TRIS, thymidylate kinase, and an extract of *E. coli* treated with Dowex-1 formate. The mixtures were incubated at 37° C. for 60 minutes and then heated at 100° C. for 3 minutes. Each mixture was then adjusted to pH 4.6 with acetate buffer, treated with semen phosphatase for 30 minutes, adsorbed on Norit A, and counted in a gas-flow chamber.

Two procedures were used to substantiate the conclusion that a methylation of deoxyuridylic acid had indeed occurred. First, an incubated reaction mixture containing deoxyuridylic acid-2-C^{14} (similar to that in Table 1, Exp. 1) was subjected to acid-hydrolysis, phosphomonoesterase action, and then to paper chromatography (butanol: ammonia:water). The thymidine zone ($R_F = 0.50$) contained about 90 per cent of the radioactivity; about 10 per cent of the radioactivity was detectable in the deoxyuridine area ($R_F = 0.36$); and no counts

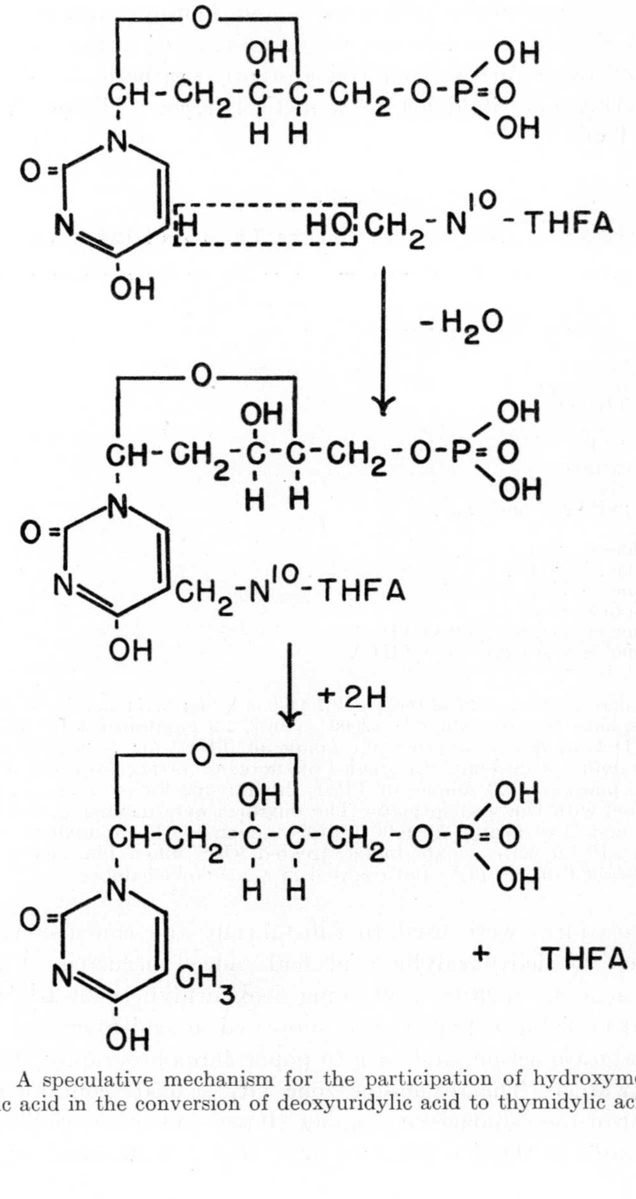

FIG. 1. A speculative mechanism for the participation of hydroxymethyltetrahydrofolic acid in the conversion of deoxyuridylic acid to thymidylic acid.

were found in the hydroxymethyl deoxyuridine area ($R_F = 0.24$). Second, a similar reaction mixture containing P^{32}-labeled deoxyuridylic acid was incubated and then adsorbed on a Dowex-1-chloride column. Inorganic phosphate, deoxyuridylate, and ATP were eluted in succession with 0.01 N HCl—0.1 M NaCl. The TTP zone, eluted with 0.01 N HCl—0.3 M NaCl, contained 35 per cent of the counts, a value consistent with that obtained by the assay for phosphomonoesterase-resistant, Norit-adsorbable radioactivity. The requirement for THFA and the partial dependence on the presence of serine are consistent with the conclusion that a conversion of deoxyuridylic acid to thymidylic acid had taken place.

A chemical reaction described for N-hydroxymethyl compounds with β-diketones in which water is split out (11) may be instructive with respect to the enzymatic methylation of deoxyuridylic acid. This would involve the condensation of deoxyuridylic acid with hydroxymethyl THFA as shown in Fig. 1. The hypothetical intermediate thus formed would yield thymidylic acid and THFA by a process of reductive cleavage similar to that described for the formation of acetic acid from glycine (16). This speculative sequence of reactions is consistent with the isotopic data of Elwyn and Sprinson (2) which indicate that the hydroxymethyl group of serine, doubly labeled with C^{14} and deuterium, is transferred to the 5 position of thymine with a minimum of 1.5 atoms of deuterium per atom of carbon.

ACKNOWLEDGMENT

This investigation was supported in part by research grants from the National Institutes of Health and the National Science Foundation. We are also grateful to Dr. Lothar Jaenicke for giving us information regarding the preparation of tetrahydrofolic acid and of hydroxymethyl tetrahydrofolic acid prior to publication.

REFERENCES

1. Blakley, R. L., *Biochem. J.*, **58**, 448 (1954).
2. Elwyn, D., and Sprinson, D. B., *J. Biol. Chem.*, **207**, 467 (1954).
3. Friedkin, M., and Roberts, D., *Federation Proc.*, **14**, 215 (1955) ; *J. Biol. Chem.*, **220**, 653 (1956).
4. Friedkin, M., Tilson, D., and Roberts, D., *Federation Proc.*, **13**, 214 (1954) ; *J. Biol. Chem.*, **220**, 627 (1956).
5. Goldthwait, D. A., and Bendich, A., *J. Biol. Chem.*, **196**, 841 (1952).
6. Greenberg, G. R., *Federation Proc.*, **13**, 745 (1954).
7. Jaenicke, L., *Federation Proc.*, **15**, 281 (1956).

8. Jaenicke, L., and Greenberg, G. R., *Biochemical Preparations,* in press.
9. Kornberg, A., Lehman, I. R., and Simms, E. S., *Federation Proc.,* **15**, 291 (1956); Kornberg, A., Lehman, I. R., Bessman, M. J., and Simms, E. S., *Biochim. et Biophys. Acta,* **21**, 197 (1956).
10. Lowy, B. A., Brown, G. B., and Rachele, J. R., *J. Biol. Chem.,* **220**, 325 (1956).
11. Monti, L., *Gazz. chim. ital.,* **60**, 39 (1930); [*Chem. Abstr.,* **24**, 4013 (1930)].
12. Rabinowitz, J. C., and Pricer, W. E., Jr., *J. Am. Chem. Soc.,* **78**, 1513 (1956).
13. Reichard, P., *Acta Chem. Scand.,* **9**, 1275 (1955).
14. Reichard, P., and Estborn, B., *J. Biol. Chem.,* **188**, 839 (1951).
15. Sagers, R. D., Beck, J. V., Gruber, W., and Gunsalus, I. C., *J. Am. Chem. Soc.,* **78**, 694 (1956).
16. Stadtman, T. C., and Elliott, P., *J. Am. Chem. Soc.,* **78**, 2020 (1956).
17. Totter, J. R., and Best, A. N., *Arch. Biochem. and Biophys.,* **54**, 318 (1955).

POLYNUCLEOTIDE SYNTHESIS *

SEVERO OCHOA

Department of Biochemistry, New York University College of Medicine, New York, N. Y.

and

LEON A. HEPPEL

National Institutes of Arthritis and Metabolic Diseases, National Institutes of Health, United States Public Health Service, Bethesda, Maryland

UNTIL RECENTLY the mechanisms of synthesis of the polynucleotide chains of nucleic acids had remained obscure despite notable advances in our understanding of the enzymatic mechanisms involved in the synthesis of the mononucleotides, the purine and pyrimidine bases, and the sugar moieties.

As previously reported (16-18, 32), an enzyme isolated, and partially purified, from the microorganism *Azotobacter vinelandii* catalyzes the synthesis of highly polymerized ribonucleotides from 5′-nucleoside diphosphates, with release of orthophosphate. The reaction requires Mg^{++} and is reversible. Chemical and enzymatic degradation of the synthetic polynucleotides has shown that they are made up of 5′-mononucleotide residues linked to one another through 3′-phosphoribose ester bonds as in RNA.[1] It has been shown that the enzyme is able to catalyze the phosphorolytic cleavage of polynucleotide chains to form 5′-nucleoside diphosphates. Thus, in analogy with polysaccha-

* The experimental work reported in this paper was aided by grants from the U. S. Public Health Service, the American Cancer Society, the Rockefeller Foundation, and the Office of Naval Research, as well as by generous gifts of 5′-ribonucleoside diphosphates from the Sigma Chemical Company and the Pabst Laboratories and of 5′-deoxyribonucleoside monophosphates from the California Foundation for Biochemical Research.

[1] The following abbreviations are used: RNA, ribonucleic acid; DNA, deoxyribonucleic acid; ADP, GDP, UDP, CDP, and IDP, 5′-diphosphates (pyrophosphates) of adenosine, guanosine, uridine, cytidine, and inosine, respectively; AMP, GMP, UMP, CMP, and IMP, 5′-monophosphates of the same nucleosides; ATP, 5′-adenosine triphosphate; DPNH, reduced diphosphopyridine nucleotide; DAMP, DCMP, and TMP, 5′-monophosphates of deoxyadenosine, deoxycytidine, and thymidine, respectively; DADP and DATP, 5′-deoxyadenosine di- and triphosphate; Tris, tris(hydroxymethyl)-aminomethane; c.p.m., counts per minute.

rides, reversible phosphorolysis may be a major mechanism in the biological synthesis and breakdown of polynucleotide chains. For this reason, the name polynucleotide phosphorylase was proposed (16) for the new enzyme. Evidence has been presented (17, 20a, 32) that this enzyme brings about the synthesis of RNA-like polynucleotides.

The discovery of polynucleotide phosphorylase has provided definite answers to certain questions but, as is often the case, has raised a number of new ones. The main questions can be grouped in two categories: (a) the structure and nature of the synthetic ribopolynucleotides, and (b) the mechanism, specificity, and generality of the phosphorylase reaction. The mode of synthesis of deoxyribopolynucleotides raises a further question of obvious interest.

The answer to question (a) can be summarized by the statement that the polynucleotides synthesized by polynucleotide phosphorylase show the structural pattern of RNA. The enzyme has been found to be widely distributed in bacteria (1, 6, 24). The questions of group (b) remain largely unanswered.

The isolation, partial purification, and properties of the *Azotobacter* polynucleotide phosphorylase, as well as the preparation and isolation of polynucleotides, have already been described (18). The enzyme has also been partially purified from extracts of *Escherichia coli* (24) and *Micrococcus lysodeikticus* (2) and *Alcaligenes faecalis* (6a). Much of the experimental evidence bearing on the structure of the synthetic polynucleotides has also been presented (16, 17, 32). This paper will, therefore, deal only briefly with these aspects of the problem while considering in more detail some of the more recent work on structure along with some of the unanswered questions mentioned above.

POLYNUCLEOTIDE PHOSPHORYLASE

The reaction catalyzed by polynucleotide phosphorylase can be represented as in Equation 1, where R stands for ribose, P-P for pyrophosphate, P for orthophosphate and X for one or more of the following bases: adenine, hypoxanthine, guanine, uracil or cytosine.

$$n \text{ X-R-P-P} \rightleftarrows (\text{X-R-P}) \, n + n \, \text{P} \qquad (1)$$

In the direction to the right, the reaction leads to the formation of a polynucleotide from 5′-ribonucleoside diphosphates, with liberation of a stoichiometric amount of orthophosphate. Under suitable conditions the rate of liberation of phosphate is proportional to the concentration of enzyme and can be used for assay of the phosphorylase (18). Beers (2) has utilized the rate of formation of acid-insoluble nucleotides or the rate of disappearance of acid-soluble nucleotides to determine the activity of the enzyme obtained from *M. lysodeikticus.* The reversibility of the reaction leads to the incorporation of labelled phosphate in the terminal phosphate group of nucleoside diphosphates (16, 18). The rate of this incorporation or "exchange" provides a sensitive and convenient assay for the enzyme. The activity of the enzyme can also be determined by measuring the rate of reaction (*1*) in the direction to the left, i.e., in the direction of the phosphorolysis of polynucleotides. With the use of P^{32}-labelled orthophosphate this provides a very sensitive and a specific method of assay. The rate of phosphorolysis of the biosynthetic AMP polynucleotide can also be used in an assay method where the rate of production of ADP from the polynucleotide is measured enzymatically in the presence of phosphopyruvate, pyruvic kinase, DPNH, and lactic dehydrogenase. Under these conditions, pyruvate is formed through the transfer of phosphate from phosphopyruvate to ADP, and is reduced to lactate by DPNH with a decrease of the optical density of the solution at wave-length 340 mμ. As shown in Fig. 1, the reaction is dependent on the presence of polynucleotide phosphorylase, AMP polynucleotide, and orthophosphate, and its rate is proportional to the concentration of phosphorylase. Unfortunately, this assay can only be used with relatively highly purified preparations of the phosphorylase because of the development of turbidity with crude preparations.

Thermodynamically, the reaction catalyzed by polynucleotide phosphorylase utilizes the energy of the pyrophosphate bond in 5′-nucleoside diphosphates to form the diester bonds of a polynucleotide chain. On incubation of purified polynucleotide phosphorylase with nucleoside diphosphates singly or in combination, in the presence of Mg^{++}, there is liberation of orthophosphate. The reaction reaches equilibrium and comes to a standstill when 60 to 80 per cent of the acid-labile phosphate has been released as orthophosphate. No accurate data have yet been obtained on the position of the equilibrium but, as is the case with polysaccharide phosphorylase, it seems to be influenced mainly by the ratio of the concentration of orthophosphate to that of nucleoside diphosphate. Preliminary experiments with ADP or IDP as substrate indicate that equilibrium is reached when the orthophosphate/nucleoside diphosphate ratio is from 1.5 to 2. Thus, the reaction

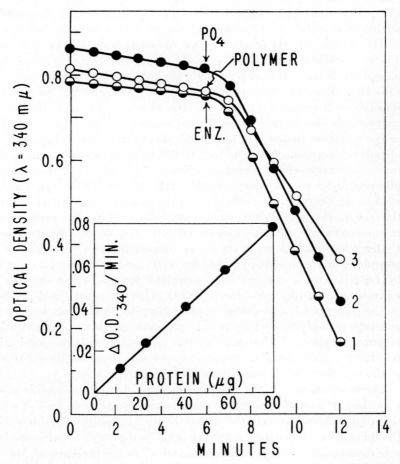

FIG. 1. Phosphorolysis of A polymer. 1.0 ml. of reaction mixture containing: Tris buffer, *p*H 8.1, 100 μmoles; MgCl₂, 5.0 μmoles; KH₂PO₄, 10.0 μmoles; DPNH, 0.15 μmole; A polymer, 0.085 mg. (0.25 μmole); phosphopyruvate, 1.6 μmoles; pyruvic kinase, 3 units; lactic dehydrogenase, 7 units; *Azotobacter* polynucleotide phosphorylase (Enz.), specific activity 8, 0.069 mg. Last addition (indicated by arrows): Curve 1, *Azotobacter* enzyme; Curve 2, phosphate; Curve 3, A polymer. Inset. Rate of phosphorolysis as a function of *Azotobacter* enzyme concentration. Rate (Δ optical density at wavelength 340 mμ) calculated from the period between the 3rd and 7th minute after start of reaction. Temperature, 25° C.

appears to favor polynucleotide synthesis and to indicate that the free energy of hydrolysis of the phosphodiester bonds in polynucleotides is lower than that of the pyrophosphate bonds of nucleoside disphosphates. However, the ready reversibility of the reaction suggests that it proceeds with a relatively small change in free energy and that there cannot be much difference in the free energy of hydrolysis of the two kinds of bonds. The ready reversibility of the reaction has also been observed by Beers (1, 2) and by Littauer (24).

The isolation of enzymes which utilize 5′-nucleoside diphosphates as immediate precursors of ribopolynucleotides raises the question whether these precursors are present in the cell. Potter and his collaborators (36) have in fact demonstrated the occurrence in tissues of the 5′-mono-, di-, and triphosphates of guanosine, uridine, and cytosine besides those of adenosine. The mechanism of formation of the 5′-polyphosphates has been elucidated through the discovery (11, 23, 23a, 30, 37, 38) of nucleoside monophosphokinases which catalyze the transfer of phosphate from ATP to GMP, UMP, or CMP, and from ADP to GDP, UDP, CDP, or IDP.

A number of polynucleotides have been prepared by incubation of partially purified preparations of polynucleotide phosphorylase from *A. vinelandii* with 5′-nucleoside diphosphates singly or in mixtures, in the presence of Mg^{++}. "Single" polymers have been prepared from ADP, IDP, GDP, UDP, or CDP and will be referred to as the A, I, G, U, or C polymers, respectively. Each of them consists of only one kind of monomeric unit. To date, two "mixed" polymers, i.e., polynucleotides containing two or more different monomeric units, have been prepared, one from approximately equimolar mixtures of ADP and UDP and one from mixtures of ADP, GDP, UDP, and CDP, in approximately molar proportions 1:0.5:1:1, as well as equimolar; these will be referred to as the AU and the AGUC polymers, respectively. The polynucleotides are usually isolated by precipitation with cold ethanol and purified by solution in a small volume of water, reprecipitation with ethanol, solution, and exhaustive dialysis against distilled water. They are then recovered from the dialyzed solution by lyophilization and are obtained in the form of white powders. The preparation of an A polymer with enzyme from *M. lysodeikticus* has been described by Beers (2). Another A polymer has been prepared by Littauer (24) with enzyme from *E. coli*. A and I polymers have recently been prepared with *A. faecalis* enzyme (6a).

STRUCTURE AND NATURE OF RIBOPOLYNUCLEOTIDES

The biosynthetic polynucleotides consist of 5'-nucleoside monophosphate residues linked to one another through 3'-phosphoribose ester bonds; therefore, they have 3'-, 5'-phosphodiester linkages just as natural RNA does (4). The chains are terminated by phosphate groups monoesterified at carbon 5' of the nucleoside moiety. On treatment with alkali or with specific phosphodiesterases these polynucleotides yield products in accordance with the action of the same agents on RNA. Thus, snake venom phosphodiesterase (7) hydrolyzes the polynucleotides to 5'-nucleoside monophosphates, while spleen phosphodiesterase (20) yields the corresponding 3'-nucleoside monophosphates. Hydrolysis by alkali cleaves polynucleotide chains at the same points attacked by spleen phosphodiesterase but, according to Brown and Todd (5), alkaline hydrolysis proceeds with the liberation of 2'-3'-nucleoside monophosphates (cyclic mononucleotides) which are further cleaved to give mixtures of the 2'- and 3'-nucleoside monophosphates. This was experimentally demonstrated by Markham and Smith (26).

On digestion with pancreatic ribonuclease, the biosynthetic polynucleotides also yield the same hydrolysis products as RNA. Pancreatic ribonuclease is a phosphodiesterase with characteristic specificity; it cleaves pyrimidine nucleoside phosphodiester bonds distal to a 3'-linkage. As expected from what is known about the specificity of pancreatic ribonuclease, this enzyme does not act on the A or I polymer (the G polymer has not yet been tried), but it cleaves the U, C, AU, and AGUC polymers. With the U polymer, which is the "single" polymer that has been more extensively investigated thus far, pancreatic ribonuclease gives 3'-UMP after exhaustive digestion. With shorter periods of hydrolysis, 80 per cent of the polymer may be converted to cyclic uridylic acid (uridine 2'-, 3'-monophosphate). This compound was first obtained from RNA hydrolysates by Markham and Smith (26). Very brief digestion with ribonuclease converts the U polymer largely to a mixture of cyclic di-, tri-, and tetranucleotides. Similar results have been obtained with the C polymer. Some noncyclic oligonucleotides also appear.

Structure of AU.

Some of the evidence bearing on the structure of the AU polymer has been presented in previous publications (17, 32). More recent experiments with a radioactive AU polymer prepared from a mixture of ADP labelled with P^{32} in the two phosphate groups and non-labelled UDP will be described here. Data on the preparation of this polynucleotide are summarized in Table 1. The quantitative analysis of the products obtained from this polynucleotide after exhaustive digestion with pancreatic ribonuclease is shown in Table 2. The structure of the polynucleotide chains is represented diagramatically in Fig. 2. Since the polymer was prepared with ADP labelled with P^{32}

TABLE 1

BIOSYNTHESIS OF RADIOACTIVE AU POLYMER

66.5 μmoles of ADP with P^{32} in both phosphates
62.5 μmoles of UDP (no label)
Ratio ADP/UDP = 1.06
Tris buffer, pH 8.0, 0.05 M.
$MgCl_2$, 0.01 M.
Azotobacter enzyme, specific activity, 14, 0.9 mg. of protein, total volume, 1.16 ml.

Obtained 11.0 mg. of AU polymer containing 15.7 μmoles of AMP and 15.1 μmoles of UMP (Ratio AMP/UMP in polymer = 1.03).

TABLE 2

RIBONUCLEASE DIGESTION PRODUCTS OF AU POLYMER

Mononucleotide (U)	38.0%	of the units	
Dinucleotide (AU)	35.0%	" "	"
Trinucleotide (AAU)	20.0%	" "	"
Tetranucleotide (AAAU)	4.9%	" "	"
Pentanucleotide (AAAAU)	2.1%	" "	"

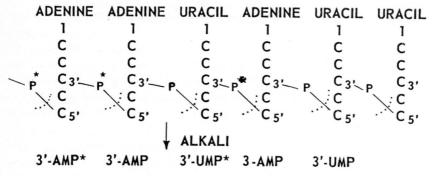

FIG. 2. Scheme of cleavage of A*U polymer by alkali.

in the acid-stable phosphate and non-labelled UDP, adenosine-5′-phosphoryl residues with P^{32} have been polymerized with non-radioactive uridine-5′-phosphoryl groups. If this polymer is hydrolyzed with alkali, splitting occurs as shown by the dotted lines in Fig. 2, and P^{32} originally linked to adenosine becomes transferred to a uridine residue if the diester bond happened to connect at carbon 3′ of a ribose moiety with the pyrimidine nucleoside. Accordingly, measurement of radioactivity appearing in the UMP liberated by alkaline hydrolysis gives an estimate of cross-linking between adenylic and uridylic acid residues. Such determinations gave 53 per cent cross-linking for the AU polynucleotide described here. This means that 53 per cent of the adenylic acid residues were preceded by uridylic acid in the polynucleotide chain.

Some information on the nucleotide sequence in this polynucleotide has been gained by hydrolyzing the labelled AU polymer with pancreatic ribonuclease and examining the separated oligonucleotides for radioactivity. An example of the method is shown in Fig. 3 for the case of the dinucleotide adenylic-uridylic acid (AU). This dinucleotide is released by ribonuclease whenever the sequence AU is preceded by uridylic acid; cleavage occurs at the points indicated by the dotted lines. In the upper half of the figure is shown the sequence UAUA. It will be noticed that in this case the dinucleotide split off by ribonuclease will have radioactivity (indicated by an asterisk) in the uridylic acid moiety but, in the sequence shown in the lower half of the figure, namely UAUU, the AU dinucleotide split off will be non-radioactive. Determination of the specific radioactivity of the dinucleotide AU released by digestion of the polymer with pancreatic ribonuclease will give information on the relative frequency of the above two sequences of nucleotide units, namely, UAUA and UAUU. Further information can be obtained by determining the specific radioactivity of the tri-, tetra-, and pentanucleotides liberated by ribonuclease digestion. Combination of these measurements with the determination of chain length by end-group assay (25) gave the data shown in Table 3. This table shows the number of units occurring in certain sequences, such as UUA, UUU, UAU, UAUA, etc., for an average chain length of 46 nucleotide units determined for this polynucleotide.

The preliminary data given above show that the adenylic and uridylic acid residues were rather freely interspersed in the AU polynucleotide studied. The average length of uridylic acid sequences was 2.35,

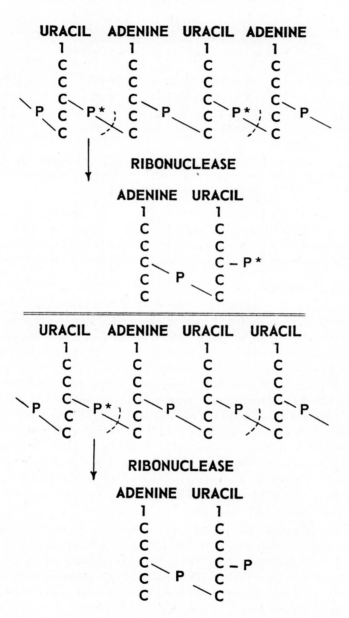

FIG. 3. Scheme of cleavage of A*U polymer by pancreatic ribonuclease.

TABLE 3

NUCLEOTIDE SEQUENCES IN AU POLYMER
Average chain-length, 46 nucleotide residues.

Sequence	Number of residues occurring as		Total
UU	UUA, 7.00;	UUU, 9.00	16.0
UAU	UAUA, 8.10;	UAUU, 7.10	15.2
UAAU	UAAUA, 4.60;	UAAUU, 4.10	8.7
UAAAU	UAAAUA, 1.07;	UAAAUU, 1.03	2.1
		Total residues accounted for	42.0[1]

[1] The remaining residues are derived from chain ends and include uridine-3',5'-diphosphate, adenosine-3'-5'-diphosphate, uridine, adenosine, adenosine-3':adenosine-5'-phosphate, etc.

that of adenylic acid sequences was 2.0. More experiments of this kind with different batches of polymers and a detailed analysis of the data obtained will be required to decide whether the distribution of mononucleotide residues in these chains is random or otherwise.

Structure of AGUC.

When RNA is exhaustively digested with ribonuclease and the reaction mixture is dialyzed against distilled water, there remains a non-dialyzable residue or "core" which consists of a mixture of oligonucleotides with relatively high proportions of purine mononucleotides. Ribonuclease hydrolysis of a sample of AGUC polymer and yeast RNA (17) showed that in both cases there remained a non-dialyzable core amounting to about 20 per cent of the total nucleotides. Analysis of the ribonuclease digestion products of the AGUC polymer by the technique of Markham and Smith (27) showed that the biosynthetic polymer yields the same products that would be obtained from natural RNA. Ribonuclease released 3'-CMP and 3'-UMP from this polymer, along with a number of oligonucleotides of which the following have so far been identified: the dinucleotides AU, AC, GU, and GC, and the trinucleotides AAU and AAC.

Smellie (unpub.) has recently determined the nucleotide composition of two samples of the AGUC polymer and of samples of RNA isolated from *Azotobacter* and other bacteria. The analyses were carried out on perchloric acid hydrolysates of the polynucleotides (29); the purine and pyrimidine bases were separated by paper chromatography in the isopropanol-hydrochloric acid solvent system (39) and determined from the ultraviolet absorption of the eluates of the corresponding spots (cf. also 9). The results, shown in Table 4, are the averages of a number of closely agreeing experiments. The first AGUC polymer in Table 4 was prepared as previously described (18) with *Azotobacter* polynucleotide phosphorylase of specific activity 18, from a mixture of about equimolar amounts of ADP, UDP, and CDP, but only half the molar amount of GDP. The reasons for this have been previously explained (18). This polynucleotide, on the basis of sedimentation data, had a molecular weight around 70,000 (32). It is apparent that the proportions of adenylic, uridylic, and cytidylic acids were essentially the same in this polymer and in *Azotobacter* RNA, whereas the proportion of guanylic acid in the biosynthetic polynucleotide was about half that in *Azotobacter* RNA. Another sample of AGUC polymer prepared later from an approximately equimolar mixture of the four 5'-nucleoside diphosphates (the second polynucleotide shown in Table 4) showed a proportion of adenylic and guanylic acid identical to that in *Azotobacter* RNA. Unfortunately, this polymer was prepared with a crude fraction of the *Azotobacter* enzyme and appeared to have undergone degradation, possibly by contaminating nucleases. This was indicated by the loss of some 70 per cent of the alcohol-precipitable polynucleotide upon dialysis. Degradation by a ribonuclease-like nuclease might account for the low value for uracil. Further work is required to determine the proportion of nucleoside diphosphates that would result in the same nucleotide ratios for biosynthetic AGUC and *Azotobacter* RNA. It appears possible that the isolated enzyme may bring about the synthesis of a polynucleotide of the same composition as the RNA from the same cells, when the four nucleoside diphosphates are present in approximately equimolar concentrations.[2]

The ribonucleic acids from the other three organisms listed in Table 4, namely *Staphylococcus aureus*, *Mycobacterium phlei,* and *Alcaligenes faecalis,* all of which are rich in polynucleotide phosphorylase, were isolated and analyzed to see if any of them would show significant differences in nucleotide composition from *Azotobacter* RNA. It may be seen that while the ratios of adenylic to cytidylic acid are rather constant, that is not the case for those of guanylic to uridylic acid. *Mycobact. phlei* and *Alc. faecalis* RNA showed sig-

[2] Smellie (unpub.) has recently analyzed such a polymer. Its average nucleotide composition was, adenine, 10.0; guanine, 14.4; uracil, 8.5; cytosine, 12.0.

TABLE 4

NUCLEOTIDE COMPOSITION

Polynucleotide	Adenine	Guanine	Uracil	Cytosine
AGUC (1:0.5:1:1)	10.0	5.9	7.1	9.9
AGUC (1:1:1:1)*	10.0	12.7	4.2	11.1
Azotobacter RNA**	10.0	13.0	7.3	9.0
Staph. aureus RNA	10.0	11.5	6.6	8.2
Mycobact. phlei RNA	10.0	15.0	7.4	8.7
Alcaligenes faecalis RNA	10.0	11.4	5.1	8.9

* Prepared with crude enzyme; polymer partially degraded by nuclease action.
** Cf. ref.

nificant deviations in nucleotide composition from *Azotobacter* and *Staphylococcus* RNA with regard to guanylic and uridylic acid, respectively. It would be of interest to purify the phosphorylase from these microorganisms to see whether these enzymes could bring about the synthesis of AGUC polymers of the same nucleotide composition as the corresponding RNA from equal mixtures of the four nucleoside diphosphates.

Molecular Weight and Chain Length.

The molecular weights of the polynucleotides synthesized by polynucleotide phosphorylase fall in the range of molecular weights determined for a variety of natural ribonucleic acids by several investigators. The data in Table 5 are shown for comparison. The sedimentation molecular weights for the polynucleotides prepared by synthesis with *Azotobacter* enzyme and for *Azotobacter* RNA are based on preliminary data (R. C. Warner, unpub.) and can be considered only as rough approximations. This may account for the discrepancy between the sedimentation and light-scattering values for the same preparation of the A polymer. The much higher values obtained by light-scattering for two samples of the A and I polymers may be due to the fact that, contrary to our usual practice of isolating the polynucleotides when the reaction reaches equilibrium following a single addition of nucleoside diphosphates, these samples were prepared by shifting the equilibrium at various times with supplementary additions of nucleoside diphosphates in order to promote further synthesis. It is possible that polymers of larger size are obtained by multiple additions of substrate. It should be noted that the sedimentation molecular weights of the AGUC polynucleotide and *Azotobacter*

TABLE 5

MOLECULAR WEIGHT OF RIBOPOLYNUCLEOTIDES

Polynucleotide	Method	Molecular Wght.	Reference
A* (Azotobacter enzyme)	Sedimentation	7×10^4	R. C. Warner, unpub.
U	"	7×10^4	" " " "
AU	"	3×10^5	" " " "
AGUC	"	7×10^4	" " " "
A*	Light-scattering	1.48×10^5	P. Doty, pers. commun.
A**	"	5.7×10^5	L. F. Cavalieri and M. Rosoff, pers commun.
I**	"	8×10^5	L. F. Cavalieri and M. Rosoff, pers. commun.
A (M. lysodeikticus enzyme)	"	1.86×10^6	2
Azotobacter RNA	Sedimentation	6×10^4	R. C. Warner, unpub.
E. coli RNA	Diffusion and sedimentation	1.75×10^4	21
Yeast RNA	Diffusion	$1—3.5 \times 10^4$	21
Yeast RNA	Dielectric	$6—7 \times 10^4$	21
Rat liver RNA	Sedimentation	2.64×10^5	15
Tobacco mosaic virus RNA	Diffusion and sedimentation	$1.5—2.9 \times 10^5$	8
Tobacco mosaic virus RNA	Light-scattering	$2—2.2 \times 10^6$	31

* Samples from same batch of A polymer.

** Reaction equilibrium shifted by multiple additions of ADP or IDP during preparation of these polymers.

RNA were of the same order of magnitude. This emphasizes further the analogy between the synthetic and the natural compound.

Some of the low values recorded for samples of RNA from natural sources (*E. coli,* yeast) are most likely due to degradation during isolation and may be far below the molecular weight of the native RNA in the cell. Studies of ribonucleic acids from plant viruses have emphasized the marked instability of the native compounds which, following isolation, undergo spontaneous depolymerization to fragments of smaller molecular weight than the original material. Thus, the tobacco mosaic virus RNA investigated by Cohen and Stanley (8), of molecular weight around 300,000, was depolymerized to fragments of molecular weight between 60,000 and 70,000. Further degradation to fragments of molecular weight 15,000 took place when the RNA was treated with alkali. More recent measurements (31) gave much higher molecular weights for what would appear to be essentially undegraded tobacco mosaic virus RNA, of the order of 2×10^6. It should be noted (Table 5) that the A polymer prepared by Beers (2) had a molecular weight close to 2×10^6. It can therefore be concluded that the molecular weight of the ribopolynucleotides synthesized by polynucleotide phosphorylase approaches the values obtained for relatively undegraded ribonucleic acids isolated from natural sources.

The average chain lengths of some of the polynucleotides prepared with *Azotobacter* enzyme have been determined by end-group assays (25). The fact that, with the possible exception of the A polymer, the molecular weights calculated from chain length were much smaller than those obtained from sedimentation data has been previously discussed (32), and evidence presented for the view that the larger molecular weights obtained by physical methods are caused by aggregation of polynucleotide chains. Of interest for our present discussion is the fact that the average chain length of a sample of AGUC was found to be 30 residues and that here again this value falls in the range of values previously obtained for RNA from natural sources. Thus, Markham and Smith (28) found the average chain length of two samples of yeast and turnip yellow mosaic virus RNA to be 12 and 53 residues, respectively. The molecular weights calculated from these values, roughly 4,000 and 16,000, respectively, are on the whole also much lower than the values obtained by physical measurements.

The question may now be asked whether in the light of present

evidence polynucleotide phosphorylase can be assumed to be responsible for the intracellular synthesis of RNA. The close structural
analogy between the ribopolynucleotides synthesized by polynucleotide phosphorylase and RNA and, in particular, the close analogy
between the AGUC polynucleotide and the RNA isolated from *Azotobacter* with regard to nucleotide composition and molecular weight,
would appear to favor this view. It must be pointed out, however,
that as far as has been determined the affinity of 5'-nucleoside diphosphates for the *Azotobacter* polynucleotide phosphorylase is very low.
Thus, the saturating concentrations of ADP and IDP were found to
be of the order of 10^{-1} M and 5×10^{-2} M, the half saturating concentrations being 2.7×10^{-2} M and 10^{-2} M, respectively (18). To
overcome the difficulty created by this fact one would have to assume
that high local concentrations of nucleoside diphosphates might be
available to the phosphorylase in the cell.

Problems Raised

As mentioned in the introduction, the discovery of polynucleotide
phosphorylase has raised more questions than it has answered. While
there is little doubt that the enzyme can bring about the synthesis of
polynucleotides like ribonucleic acid and may even be responsible for
the synthesis of RNA in the cell, a number of other questions have
only been partially answered or have as yet not been answered at all.
It is appropriate in a symposium of this nature to consider some of
these questions in detail.

Reaction Mechanism.

Little is as yet known of the mechanism of action of polynucleotide
phosphorylase. Studies aimed at elucidating this point may have to
await further purification of the enzyme. The question of whether
the enzyme, in analogy with muscle phosphorylase, can only add
nucleotide units to a preexisting polynucleotide chain, i.e., whether
the enzyme requires a primer, or whether it can build a polynucleotide
chain starting only from a mixture of nucleoside diphosphates, cannot
as yet be answered. Most of the enzyme preparations so far obtained
in our laboratory contain some nucleotide or polynucleotide, which
may represent merely a contamination, as judged from the ratios of
light absorption at 280 mμ to 260 mμ. To judge by the radioactive
phosphate exchange assay with ADP as substrate, pancreatic ribo-

nuclease has no effect on the activity of the enzyme. However, this treatment, followed by dialysis, does not bring about complete removal of the nucleotides in the preparation, and it is possible that ribonuclease would not attack a polynucleotide which was firmly bound by the protein. If no polynucleotide primer were required for the synthesis of a polynucleotide chain, the question would arise whether reaction is initiated between two nucleoside diphosphate molecules. A polynucleotide so synthesized should have a pyrophosphate endgroup, but so far no evidence has been obtained that such is the case. Another possibility would be that the reaction is initiated between a nucleoside monophosphate and a nucleoside diphosphate, the former acting as primer to start the chain. This possibility has been eliminated by experiments in which UDP was incubated with the enzyme in the presence of AMP. This should lead to a polynucleotide containing AMP at one end of the chain. However, end-group assay of the polynucleotide synthesized under these conditions showed that it was terminated by uridine residues. It should be added that when the synthesis of polynucleotide is followed at brief intervals of time, no evidence is found for any accumulation of small polynucleotides.

Since polynucleotide phosphorylase has been only partially purified, the possibility remains that it represents a mixture of enzymes rather than a single one. The fact that purified preparations of the enzyme from *E. coli* (U. Z. Littauer, pers. commun.) and *M. lysodeikticus* (P. Olmsted, pers. commun.) do not appear to react with GDP would seem to support the view that different enzymes are involved in the reaction with each of the nucleoside diphosphates. As previously pointed out (18), we have found that partially purified preparations of *Azotobacter* polynucleotide phosphorylase react with difficulty with GDP, and we have so far been able to obtain but small amounts of a GMP polynucleotide. However, GDP does react in the presence of the other nucleoside diphosphates and is incorporated as GMP in the AGUC polynucleotide. While the unity or multiplicity of polynucleotide phosphorylase cannot be definitely settled until pure preparations of the enzyme or enzymes are available, there are some facts which speak in favor of a single enzyme. Thus, the incorporation of radioactive phosphate is always decreased when more than one nucleoside diphosphate is present. This fact, which is particularly evident when the incorporation of phosphate brought about by each of the nucleoside diphosphates ADP, GDP, UDP, and CDP, is compared with that produced by a mixture of all four (cf. 18, Table 5), suggests a competition of the various diphosphates for the same site.

Specificity.

The *Azotobacter* polynucleotide phosphorylase shows considerable lack of specificity, since it can act on single nucleoside diphosphates, or on mixtures of two or more of them. It also lacks specificity in the direction of phosphorolysis, as it can attack ribonucleic acids from various sources besides the biosynthetic polynucleotides. However, the enzyme is inactive on certain non-naturally-occurring nucleoside diphosphates such as dihydrouridine diphosphate and 5-bromouridine diphosphate; it is also inactive on ribose-5-pyrophosphate.[3] The P^{32} exchange assay (18) was used in all these cases. In spite of the apparent unspecificity of the enzyme the possibility remains that, in the presence of adequate concentrations of the four naturally occurring nucleoside diphosphates, the enzyme could synthesize a polynucleotide chain with a determined sequence of nucleotides, i.e., a specific RNA.

In view of the belief that ribonucleic acids are involved in protein synthesis and of the widely held idea that they may provide templates for the synthesis of specific proteins, the problem of the specificity or non-specificity of RNA and of the manner in which specific nucleic acids could be synthesized is of considerable importance. The biological activity and specificity of RNA has recently been clearly demonstrated by the work of Fraenkel-Conrat (10) and Gierer and Schramm (12) with tobacco mosaic virus. It is apparent from that work that the RNA in plant viruses is the carrier of genetic information, like the DNA in bacterial viruses and in plant and animal cells. The ribonucleic acids from different strains of tobacco mosaic virus possess biological specificity even though they show no significant differences in nucleotide composition (21a). Now that we know in a general way how RNA is synthesized, the question may be asked how a specific RNA is made.

Since we have some indications that variations in the relative concentrations of nucleoside diphosphates can affect the nucleotide composition of the polynucleotides synthesized by polynucleotide phos-

[3] Dihydrouridine diphosphate was kindly provided by Dr. S. S. Cohen, University of Pennsylvania, 5-bromouridine diphosphate by Dr. Reginald Webb, Chemical Laboratory, University of Cambridge, and ribose-5-pyrophosphate by Dr. B. L. Horecker, National Institutes of Health. We are indebted to Dr. Sanae Mii for these assays.

phorylase, it is possible that the cell could determine the composition of the RNA it manufactures by mechanisms regulating the relative concentrations of nucleoside diphosphates available at the sites of synthesis. It is difficult to see, however, how a certain sequence of nucleotides could be produced unless this were an inherent property of the enzyme concerned. This would mean that there would be as many RNA-synthesizing enzymes as there are different ribonucleic acids. The other alternative, which would perhaps appear more likely from the information obtained with polynucleotide phosphorylase, would be that even if no polynucleotide primer were required for the synthesis of RNA, a given RNA or DNA, possibly bound by the protein, might act as a template for the reproduction of its nucleotide pattern.

Generality of Phosphorylase Reaction.

It cannot yet be decided whether the reaction catalyzed by polynucleotide phosphorylase represents a general biological mechanism for the synthesis of RNA. Wide distribution of the enzyme would favor such a possibility. However, while the enzyme is widely distributed in microorganisms, there is so far no unequivocal evidence for its presence in animal tissues. As previously reported, polynucleotide phosphorylase has been found in extracts of a number of bacteria (6, 32) whether aerobic or anaerobic, gram positive or gram negative. The enzyme has also been found in yeast extracts (M. Grunberg-Manago, pers. commun.) and, in small amounts, in ammonium sulfate fractions of spinach leaves (6).

Indirect evidence for the presence of polynucleotide phosphorylase in liver may be provided by Goldwasser's finding (13, 14) that AMP (5′-adenosine monophosphate) is incorporated as such into the RNA of pigeon liver homogenates. Similar results have been obtained by Heidelberger et al. (19a) with rat liver homogenates. Although these experiments do not show that AMP is incorporated following its conversion to ADP, that would not appear to be unlikely, inasmuch as the experimental conditions favored the formation of adenosine polyphosphates by oxidative phosphorylation. It is possible that polynucleotide phosphorylase is present in all cells, although in widely different amounts, and that much more enzyme occurs in rapidly proliferating cells, such as those of microorganisms, than in the cells of animal tissues which do not multiply rapidly.

Deoxyribonucleotides.

Another aspect of the problem of the generality of the polynucleotide phosphorylase reaction is the question whether enzymes similar to polynucleotide phosphorylase are concerned with the synthesis of DNA. The problem is at present under investigation in several laboratories. The presence of 5'-deoxyribonucleoside polyphosphates in tissues and the existence of mechanisms for the formation of the polyphosphates from the monophosphates would lend support to the view that the deoxyribonucleoside polyphosphates may be precursors of DNA. The occurrence of the mono-, di-, and triphosphates of thymidine and deoxycytidine in thymus extracts has been recently reported (34), and it has been shown (19, 35) that the 5'-di- and triphosphates of deoxyadenosine, deoxycytidine, and thymidine are formed in liver homogenates by phosphorylation of the corresponding 5'-nucleoside monophosphates, apparently through reactions involving phosphate transfer from ATP. Kornberg et al. (22) have reported the phosphorylation of thymidine by ATP to 5'-thymidine monophosphate and of the latter of the 5'-deoxythymidine di- and triphosphates.

We have found (D. O. Brummond, R. M. S. Smellie, and S. Ochoa, unpub.) that ammonium sulfate and ethanol fractions from *A. vinelandii* contain enzymes catalyzing the transfer of phosphate from ATP or ITP to 5'-deoxyribonucleoside monophosphates, with formation of the corresponding di- and triphosphates. Since the *Azotobacter* preparations contain polynucleotide phosphorylase, the occurrence of these transfers can be readily detected through the "exchange" of radioactive phosphate which occurs when ADP or IDP are formed. Typical experiments are shown in Table 6. The "exchange" was determined as the radioactivity remaining in the reaction mixtures at the end of incubation after removal of the orthophosphate, as described (18) for the assay of polynucleotide phosphorylase. While there was some "exchange" in the control experiments with ATP or ITP as the only added nucleotide, it was markedly increased in the additional presence of the 5'-monophosphates of deoxyadenosine and deoxycytidine. Some increase was also observed with thymidylic acid (5'-thymidine monophosphate) plus ATP. The "exchange" in the controls was probably due to the presence of some ATPase and ITPase in the crude enzyme fractions used, as well as to the slight contamination of the triphosphates with the corresponding diphosphates. The results indicate the occurrence of phosphate transfer from ATP or ITP

TABLE 6

PHOSPHATE "EXCHANGE" WITH VARIOUS NUCLEOTIDES

Nucleotides	P incorporation	Nucleotides	P incorporation
ATP (control)	3,150	ITP (control)	3,000
ATP + AMP	61,160	ITP + IMP	0
ATP + DAMP	55,560	ITP + AMP	79,460
ATP + DCMP	43,400	ITP + DAMP	79,820
ATP + TMP	3,710	ITP + DCMP	8,580

Per ml. of reaction mixture: Tris buffer, pH 8.0, 100 μmoles; MgCl$_2$, 3.0 μmoles; potassium phosphate buffer, 2.5 μmoles with P^{32}-labelled orthophosphate (800,000 c.p.m.); nucleotides, each 2.5 μmoles; and enzyme (*Azotobacter* ethanol fraction) with 0.4 mg. of protein. Incubation, 15 minutes at 30° C. Results expressed as c.p.m. incorporated in excess of controls. Exchange with nucleoside monophosphates was negligible.

to the deoxyribose nucleoside monophosphates with formation of ADP or IDP and deoxyribose nucleoside polyphosphates. It will be noted that there was some phosphate transfer from ITP to AMP, a reaction previously described by Strominger et al. (38) and others (11, 23, 23a), and that there was no transfer from ITP to IMP.

The transfer of phosphate from ATP can also be followed spectro-photometrically in the presence of phosphopyruvate, pyruvic kinase, lactic dehydrogenase, and DPNH, since formation of ADP will lead to the transfer of phosphate from phosphopyruvate to ADP and oxidation of DPNH by the pyruvate thus formed. The experiments of Fig. 4 illustrate the phosphate transfer between ATP and deoxycytidine monophosphate (DCMP) followed in this way. There was essentially no reaction until the system was completed by the addition of DCMP or the *Azotobacter* enzyme.

The transfer of phosphate from ITP to 5'-deoxyribonucleoside mono-phosphates can also be conveniently followed when the reaction is carried out in the presence of IDPase (33). Under these conditions the IDP formed as a result of the transfer reaction is hydrolyzed by IDPase to IMP and orthophosphate, and the liberation of orthophosphate is a measure of the phosphate transfer. Furthermore, through the removal of IDP the equilibrium of the transfer reaction is shifted and it proceeds to completion. This affords a convenient method for the biosynthetic preparation of 5'-deoxyribonucleoside polyphosphates. The course of the reaction between ITP and DAMP or DCMP is shown in Fig. 5. It may be seen that the phosphate liberation from ITP in the absence of other nucleotides was negligible.

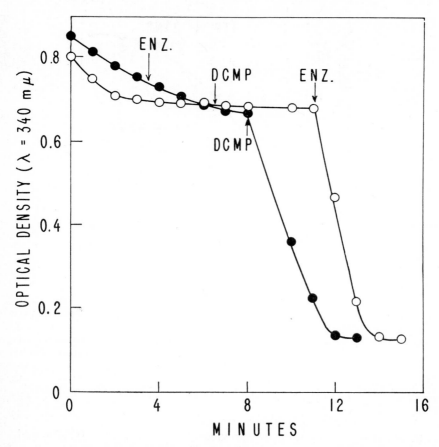

Fig. 4. Transfer of phosphate from ATP to DCMP. 1.0 ml. of reaction mixture containing: Tris buffer, pH 8.0, 50 μmoles; MgCl$_2$, 2.5 μmoles; DPNH, 0.15 μmole; phosphopyruvate, 1.6 μmoles; ATP, 0.5 μmole; DCMP, 1.0 μmole; pyruvic kinase, 3 units; lactic dehydrogenase, 7 units; *Azotobacter* ethanol fraction (Enz.), 0.1 mg. of protein. Temperature, 25° C. The two last additions to system are indicated by arrows.

The products of the transfer reactions with DAMP and DCMP, isolated by paper and ion-exchange chromatography, have proved to consist of the corresponding di- and tri-phosphates. The formation of di- and tri-phosphates probably occurs as illustrated by Reactions 2 and 3, for the transfer from ITP to DAMP and DADP.

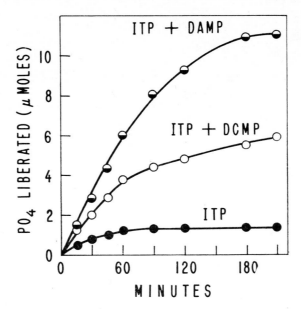

FIG. 5. Phosphate liberation during transfer of phosphate from ITP to DAMP or DCMP in the presence of IDPase. 1.0 ml. of reaction mixture containing: Tris buffer, pH 8.1, 100 μmoles; MgCl$_2$, 30 μmoles; *Azotobacter* ethanol fraction, 5.5 mg. of protein; IDPase, 0.9 unit; and nucleotides as indicated, each 10 μmoles. Temperature, 30° C.

$$\text{ITP} + \text{DAMP} \rightleftharpoons \text{IDP} + \text{DADP} \qquad (2)$$

$$\text{ITP} + \text{DADP} \rightleftharpoons \text{IDP} + \text{DATP} \qquad (3)$$

Reaction (2) is of the type previously described (37, 38) for ribonucleotides, and is catalyzed by nucleoside monophosphokinases. Reaction (3) is of the type catalyzed by nucleoside diphosphokinases, also described previously (3, 23) for ribonucleotides. Whether the enzymes involved here are the same or different from those concerned with the transfers between ribonucleotides remains to be determined. We have evidence (D. O. Brummond, R. M. S. Smellie, and S. Ochoa, unpub.) that Reaction (4), which could lead to the formation of DATP from IDP and DADP, does not occur; this is in line with the failure of Strominger et al. (38) to find enzymatic phosphate transfer between ATP and IMP (cf. Reaction 4, from right to left).

$$\text{IDP} + \text{DADP} \neq \text{IMP} + \text{DATP} \qquad (4)$$

While the existence of mechanisms in the cell for the phosphorylation of 5'-deoxyribonucleoside monophosphates suggests a function for these compounds, possibly as precursors of DNA, these and previously discussed (32) experiments of other investigators are no proof that the polyphosphates are really involved in DNA synthesis. More direct evidence for the participation of deoxyribonucleoside polyphosphates in the synthesis of deoxyribopolynucleotides has been recently presented by Kornberg et al. (22a) and is discussed by Kornberg in this symposium. With *Azotobacter* enzyme preparations (Brummond, Smellie, and Ochoa, unpub.) we have so far failed to obtain evidence for a net synthesis of deoxyribonucleotides upon incubation of DAMP or DCMP with ATP or ITP under conditions where the di- and triphosphates of deoxyadenosine and deoxycytidine are formed.

Summary

Polynucleotide phosphorylase, the enzyme which catalyzes the synthesis of highly polymerized ribopolynucleotides from 5'-ribonucleoside diphosphates with release of orthophosphate, is probably responsible for the intracellular synthesis of RNA in microorganisms. However, a number of questions related to the mechanism and generality of the reaction and to the mode of synthesis of specific ribonucleic acids remain unsolved. It is to be hoped that information on these various subjects will be rapidly forthcoming.

ACKNOWLEDGMENTS

The authors wish to acknowledge the collaboration of Drs. M. Grunberg-Manago, R. C. Warner, D. O. Brummond, R. M. S. Smellie, and Miss P. J. Ortiz in various phases of the investigations reported here. They are also indebted to Dr. M. Staehelin, Dr. S. Mii, and Mr. M. C. Schneider for help in some of this work.

REFERENCES

1. Beers, R. F., Jr., *Federation Proc.*, **15**, 13 (1956).
2. Beers, R. F., Jr., *Nature*, **177**, 790 (1956).
3. Berg, P., and Joklik, W. K., *J. Biol. Chem.*, **210**, 657 (1954).
4. Brown, D. M., and Todd, A. R., *Ann. Rev. Biochem.*, **24**, 311 (1955).
5. Brown, D. M., and Todd, A. R., in *The Nucleic Acids* (E. Chargaff and J. N. Davidson, eds.), **1**, 409, Academic Press, New York (1955).
6. Brummond, D. O., and Ochoa, S., *Federation Proc.*, **15**, 225 (1956).
6a. Brummond, D. O., Staehelin, M., and Ochoa, S., unpub.
7. Butler, G. C., in *Methods in Enzymology* (S. P. Colowick and N. O. Kaplan, eds.), **2**, 561, Academic Press, New York (1955).

8. Cohen, S. S., and Stanley, W. M., *J. Biol. Chem.,* **144**, 589 (1942).
9. Crosbie, G. W., Smellie, R. M. S., and Davidson, J. N., *Biochem. J. (London),* **54**, 287 (1953).
10. Fraenkel-Conrat, H., *J. Am. Chem. Soc.,* **78**, 882 (1956).
11. Gibson, D. M., Ayengar, P., and Sanadi, D. R., *Abstr. Am. Chem. Soc.,* (New York, Sept., 1954), 41c (1954).
12. Gierer, A., and Schramm, G., *Nature,* **177**, 702 (1956).
13. Goldwasser, E., *J. Am. Chem. Soc.,* **77**, 6083 (1955).
14. Goldwasser, E., *Federation Proc.,* **15**, 263, (1956).
15. Grinnan, E. L., and Mosher, W. A., *J. Biol. Chem.,* **191**, 719 (1951).
16. Grunberg-Manago, M., and Ochoa, S., *J. Am. Chem. Soc.,* **77**, 3165 (1955).
17. Grunberg-Manago, M., Ortiz, P. J., and Ochoa, S., *Science,* **122**, 907 (1955).
18. Grunberg-Manago, M., Ortiz, P. J., and Ochoa, S., *Biochim. et Biophys. Acta,* **20**, 269 (1956).
19. Hecht, L. I., Potter, V. R., and Herbert, E., *Biochim. et Biophys. Acta,* **15**, 134 (1954).
19a. Heidelberger, C., Harbers, E., Leibman, K. C., Tagaki, Y., and Potter, V. R., *Biochim. et Biophys. Acta,* **20**, 445 (1956).
20. Heppel, L. A., and Hilmoe, R. J., in *Methods in Enzymology* (S. P. Colowick and N. O. Kaplan, eds.), **2**, 565, Academic Press, New York (1955).
20a. Heppel, L. A., Smith, J. D., Ortiz, P. J., and Ochoa, S., *Federation Proc.,* **15**, 273 (1956).
21. Jordan, D. O., in *The Nucleic Acids* (E. Chargaff and J. N. Davidson, eds.), **1**, 447, Academic Press, New York (1955).
21a. Knight, C. A., *J. Biol. Chem.,* **197**, 241 (1952).
22. Kornberg, A., Lehman, I. R., and Simms, E. S., *Federation Proc.,* **15**, 291 (1956).
22a. Kornberg, A., Lehman, I. R., Bessman, M. J., and Simms, E. S., *Biochim. et Biophys. Acta,* **21**, 197 (1956).
23. Krebs, H. A., and Hems, R., *Biochim. et Biophys. Acta,* **12**, 172 (1953).
23a. Lieberman, I., Kornberg, A., and Simms, E. S., *J. Am. Chem. Soc.,* **76**, 3608 (1954)
24. Littauer, U. Z., *Federation Proc.,* **15**, 302 (1956).
24a. Lombard, A., and Chargaff, E., *Biochim. et Biophys. Acta,* **20**, 585 (1956).
25. Markham, R., Matthews, R. E. F., and Smith, J. D., *Nature,* **173**, 537 (1954).
26. Markham, R., and Smith, J. D., *Biochem. J. (London),* **52**, 552 (1952).
27. Markham, R., and Smith, J. D., *Biochem. J. (London),* **52**, 558 (1952).
28. Markham, R., and Smith, J. D., *Biochem. J. (London),* **52**, 565 (1952).
29. Marshak, A., and Vogel, H. J., *J. Biol. Chem.,* **189**, 597 (1951).
30. Münch-Peterson, A., *Acta Chem. Scand.,* **8**, 1102 (1954).
31. Northrop, T. G., and Sinsheimer, R. L., *J. Chem. Phys.,* **22**, 703 (1954).
32. Ochoa, S., *Federation Proc.,* **15**, 832 (1956).
33. Plaut, G. W. E., *J. Biol. Chem.,* **217**, 235 (1955).
34. Potter, R. S., and Schlesinger, S., *J. Am. Chem. Soc.,* **77**, 6714 (1955).
35. Sable, H. Z., Wilber, P. B., Cohen, A. E., and Kane, M. R., *Biochim. et Biophys. Acta,* **13**, 156 (1954).
36. Schmitz, H., Hurlbert, R. B., and Potter, V. R., *J. Biol. Chem.,* **209**, 41 (1954).
37. Strominger, J. L., Heppel, L. A., and Maxwell, E. S., *Arch. Biochem. and Biophys.,* **52**, 488 (1954).
38. Strominger, J. L., Heppel, L. A., and Maxwell, E. S., *Federation Proc.,* **14**, 288 (1955).
39. Wyatt, G. R., *Biochem. J. (London),* **48**, 584 (1951).

THE NATURE OF RNA LABELING IN HOMOGENATES *

Van R. Potter, John H. Schneider, and Liselotte I. Hecht

McArdle Memorial Laboratory, Medical School,
University of Wisconsin, Madison 6, Wisconsin

The incorporation of labeled ribonucleotides into RNA has been reported to occur in pigeon liver homogenates by Goldwasser (2), and in rat liver homogenates by Potter, Hecht, and Herbert (7). Cell-free homogenates and also nuclei-free homogenates that were simultaneously carrying out oxidative phosphorylation were able to convert added orotic-acid-6-C^{14} into all of the 5'-uridine nucleotides (7). Under these conditions the RNA native to the homogenate became labeled, and the acid-soluble fraction contained exclusively 5'-uridine nucleotides, in so far as we were able to determine. The RNA yielded only 2',3'-UMP upon alkaline hydrolysis (7), indicating that a typical RNA internucleotide bond had been formed, and that there was no contamination with acid-soluble nucleotides.

When the incorporation of label into RNA was studied as a function of time, it was found that after a period of active incorporation there was a period of progressive loss of label from the RNA, and moreover ATP was found to inhibit the incorporation (5).

When 5'-AMP^{32} was used to label the RNA in this test system, it entered the RNA and could be recovered as 5'-AMP^{32} in high yield by treating the labeled RNA with snake venom diesterase. However, when the labeled RNA was hydrolyzed with alkali, the P^{32} was recovered in high yield as CMP^{32} of the 2',3' variety (4). These observations raised several questions as to the nature of the incorporation being studied in the homogenate.

More recent studies have suggested a tentative explanation of these findings in terms of the lengthening of an existing RNA chain, which will be abbreviated as RNA-3'-OH, to indicate a postulated terminal riboside. If this reacts with a diphosphate as suggested by Ochoa (6), for example with U*DP (labeled with precursor orotic acid) the

* This work was supported in part by a grant (C–646) from the National Cancer Institute, National Institutes of Health, United States Public Health Service.

product would be RNA-U*R-3'-OH. However, the RNA-3'-OH might react with ATP to form RNA-3'-OH$_2$PO$_3$ (or pyrophosphate) (cf. Dounce, 1), which would presumably no longer be available for chain lengthening. These relationships are shown in Fig. 1, and the new experiments are described below.

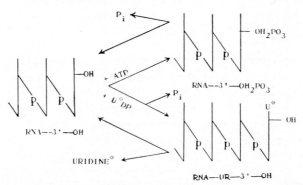

Fig. 1. Working hypothesis for studying the nature of RNA labeling in homogenates.

Effect of ATP on Incorporation

The above speculations suggest that the conditions for optimum incorporation require ATP to generate UDP and other diphosphates, but not too much, since UTP would be formed, and also the available end groups might all be phosphorylated. One way of achieving an optimum balance is to regulate the amount of reaction mixture per flask with a standardized rate of shaking. When this was tried it was found that there was indeed an optimum (Fig. 2). It is assumed that the degree of aeration was probably the chief variable in this experiment. Another approach was the addition of various amounts of ATP to the reaction mixture (5). It has now been shown that the inhibiting action of ATP on the system occurs very rapidly and that the effect disappears with time (Fig. 3). This result again suggests an optimum balance between the various phosphorylated compounds in the system, which includes both acid-soluble components and many kinds of RNA.

Loss of Label from RNA

Since the loss of label from RNA has been a constant feature of the system, it was decided to carry out experiments in which the

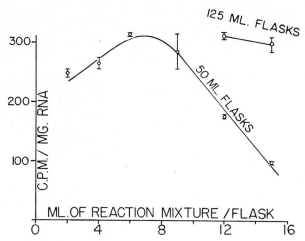

FIG. 2. Effect of varying the ratio of the volume of the reaction mixture to the volume of the flask on the labeling of RNA in rat liver homogenates. Conditions as in (7).

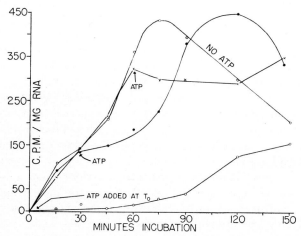

FIG. 3. Effect of additions of ATP (4 μmoles per ml.) on the labeling of RNA in rat liver homogenates.

microsomal RNA was labeled in one system and then reincubated in a fresh system with no additional radioactivity in the medium, and carried through the time period that would ordinarily result first in labeling and then in delabeling. When microsomal RNA was labeled in a homogenate system and the resulting homogenate-labeled microsomes were added to a fresh system, the delabeling began at once and continued until the end of the incubation (Fig. 4). It is important to

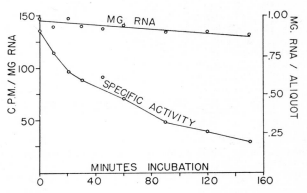

Fig. 4. Loss of C^{14} from rat liver microsomal RNA previously labeled by 45 minutes incubation as in Fig. 3, controls, when re-incubated in a similar but non-radioactive reaction mixture.

note that any increase or decrease in RNA was of questionable significance during this period, which included the time which would have resulted in an increase in the labeling had orotic acid-6-C^{14} been present. The conclusion seems inescapable that the labeling and delabeling involve some kind of an addition of labeled nucleotides to intact RNA molecules, and presumably at exposed positions or end-groups. If this conclusion is valid, then RNA labeled in positions farther from the exposed end-groups should be less rapidly delabeled. Accordingly microsomal RNA from whole animal labeling experiments (Fig. 5) were placed in similar reaction mixtures, and it was found that the RNA was not delabeled at all during the incubation. In this experiment the precursor orotic acid-6-C^{14} had been injected into the animals 24 hours before they were killed, and the peak of incorporation had been passed. Further experiments with shorter time periods for the labeling in vivo are obviously called for, but already the results suggest either different degrees of end-group labeling, or different

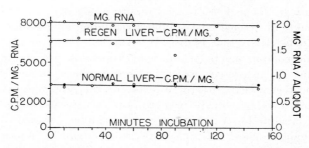

Fɪɢ. 5. Retention of C14 in rat liver microsomal RNA previously labeled in vivo during 24 hours following injection of orotic acid-6-C14 when incubated in reaction mixture that was non-radioactive as in Fig. 3. The upper line showing MG. RNA is an average, since the individual values were very similar. Individual values of the c.p.m. per mg. are plotted in this case.

classes of RNA molecules, each with different turnover rates and equilibrium constants.

The Role of the Nucleus in RNA Synthesis

The above experiments show that the homogenate still falls far short of being able to yield a net synthesis of RNA molecules in which delabeling is paralleled by a decrease in the absolute amount of RNA. Moreover, the question of whether the nuclei-free homogenates are actually free of nuclear enzymes cannot be answered unequivocally at this time.

These considerations led to the development of a different approach to this problem. The advantages of studying nucleic acid synthesis in the whole animal are many, but the main ones are the facts, first, that it occurs, and secondly, that it is subject to physiological controls. The disadvantages are that each animal can provide only one point on a time curve, and this fact coupled with the occurrence of biological variation, makes in vivo experiments somewhat difficult to interpret, especially in terms of a balance sheet of products accounted for along a time curve.

It appears that many of the advantages of the whole animal experiment can be retained and some of the disadvantages obviated if slices of tissue from a single animal are incubated in separate flasks for various periods of time to obtain points on a time curve. By injecting orotic acid-6-C14 into animals and killing them at times based on previous experience with labeling in vivo, it is possible to obtain slices that contain no labeled orotic acid or orotidylic acid but do contain large amounts of labeled acid-soluble pyrimidine nucleotides and also contain labeled RNA that is distributed between the nuclear and the cytoplasmic compartments in different proportions depending on the elapsed time. The present experiments have been carried out with normal and regenerating liver. By choosing the proper in vivo conditions, which have previously been worked out, tissue capable or incapable of labeling DNA in vitro (as slices) can be obtained (3). In all cases the balance sheet for isotope distribution can be determined for the tissue at the time of death, which then becomes the zero time point for the incubations in vitro. Such slice preparations can be homogenized after various periods of time to permit the separation of the nuclei from the cytoplasm, and it is thus possible to follow the distribution of label in the RNA of the separate cell fractions from a single animal at various time intervals and under varying conditions.

It has been found that at very early periods of time following the injection of orotic acid-6-C^{14} (when orotic and orotidylic acids are no longer available, nuclear RNA is relatively more radioactive than cytoplasmic RNA, and the acid-soluble pyrimidine nucleotides are still highly radioactive), the rate of further labeling of the total RNA in the slice is very low in comparison with what can be accomplished by the addition of more orotic acid-6-C^{14} to the flasks. The meaning of this observation and its further analysis in terms of the various cell compartments is under study.

REFERENCES

1. Dounce, A. L., and Kay, E. R. M., *Proc. Soc. Exptl. Biol. Med.*, **83**, 321 (1953).
2. Goldwasser, E., *J. Am. Chem. Soc.*, **77**, 6083 (1955).
3. Hecht, L. I., and Potter, V. R., *Federation Proc.*, **15**, 271 (1956); *Cancer Research*, in press.
4. Heidelberger, C., Harbers, E., Leibman, K. C., Takagi, Y., and Potter, V. R., *Biochim. et Biophys. Acta*, **20**, 445 (1956).
5. Herbert, E., Potter, V. R., and Hecht, L. I., *J. Biol. Chem.*, submitted.
6. Ochoa, S., *Federation Proc.*, **15**, 832 (1956).
7. Potter, V. R., Hecht, L. I., and Herbert, E., *Biochim. et Biophys. Acta*, **20**, 439 (1956).

DISCUSSION

DR. POTTER: I think there is an interesting question that appears from the work of the two preceding speakers. If these findings prove to have great generality, which they may well have, we see a situation in which triphosphates, etc., are used for DNA synthesis and diphosphates, etc., are used for RNA synthesis. This, of course, immediately forces the enzyme chemists to ask how these reactions may be oriented, and one may think that there are two possibilities: either there is a cyclic difference in the balance between these two factors in the cell, or there is a structural barrier between some of the reactants in the system. I think that both of these possibilities immediately suggest to you a number of ways in which these things can be answered, and I would just like to say that we have been studying these reactions in homogenates in which the total system can convert orotic acid to orotidylic acid—and incidentally it has not been previously shown that orotidylic is formed in animal tissue preparations, but we now have clear evidence for this—and this goes to UMP and then to UDP and then to UTP and then to UDPG, and then we have a reversible reaction between UDP and RNA, and finally an over-all irreversible conversion of uracil ribotides to DNA. In homogenates we have the reaction system from orotic acid up to and including RNA. In slices and whole animals we have the whole system, including the intermediate reactions to RNA and DNA. At the very outset we assumed that this balance between diphosphates and triphosphates was an important thing, and so we set up flasks with a fairly deep layer of the reaction mixture so that there would be oxidation but not too much oxidation. It is evident from the amount of a reaction mixture per flask that there is an optimal number of ml. per reaction mixture to give maximum incorporation of labelled orotic acid. Starting with labelled orotic acid and allowing it to label all these intermediates, we finally study the radioactivity in terms of counts per minute per mg. of RNA. Since the composition of the reaction mixture is constant, it is evident that degree of aeration is a controlling factor. Running the experiment under nitrogen prevents any labelling of RNA. It was found some time ago by Dr. E. Herbert in our laboratory that ATP at high levels inhibited the reaction. We were very worried about this, and we thought at first that there were metal contaminants in our reaction, but this was not the case. In the absence of ATP from our system it is seen that RNA is labelled for a while and then the label moves out of the RNA. On the other hand, if you put in 4 micromoles of ATP per ml. at zero time the reaction is inhibited and then incorporation begins. This shows that the ATP is not really contaminated with toxic material. If you add the ATP at some later point it stops the reaction; then it starts again still later and then goes through the normal course of events. We wanted to know why the RNA loses label in our system. Microsomal RNA which is labelled in vivo in the animal, when added to our reaction mixture is not delabelled. Using either normal liver or regenerating liver as a source of microsomes, there is neither net loss nor net synthesis of RNA in our system. If we add homogenate-labelled microsomes to our system, the mg. of RNA remain constant, but there is marked decrease in the specific activity of the RNA; so here we have a marked contrast in these two results, and I think this has a bearing on yesterday's discussion on the structure of RNA. I think we have to ask the question: What are the active forms of the end groups of RNA when it is undergoing synthesis? I think we have here an experimental system for possibly labelling the end groups. We think naturally occurring RNA may be in two forms in our system. The first one we would just write as RNA 3'OH, the other one represented as RNA with a phosphate on it; and we think it's possible to have pyrophosphates and cyclic phosphates, from the work of Markham and Smith and others, and we don't mean to specify what's on the other end yet. These are just some of the possible reactions in the system and the nature of the equilibrium reactions, and these systems may be thought of as competing with one another. The upshot of this is that, although ATP is needed for several of the reactions, a very strong production of ATP in this mitochondrial oxidative phosphorylation system pushes the equilibrium the other way and seems to operate against RNA synthesis. Although the deoxyribose triphosphate nucleotides are evidently required for DNA synthesis according to Dr. Kornberg's very conclusive data, these systems have a marked advantage, because they seem to be irreversible, whereas we think the reaction systems in RNA synthesis are reversible. We, of course, are asking the obvious question, since we are interested in control mechanisms in cancer tissue. As everyone knows, there is a good supply of hydrogen in the cancer cell, and so we are asking if the cancer cell, or any growing cell for that matter, is set up so it could have a suitable supply of diphosphates giving RNA plus a segregated supply of triphosphates and a segregated supply of reducing potential.

Dr. VOLKIN: I would like to ask Dr. Ochoa if he feels from his data that the mononucleotide composition of RNA seems to be mainly a function of the relative pool sizes of the diphosphates.

Dr. OCHOA: It appears to be so. I think this is probably due to the fact that the K_m values of the diphosphates are very high, so presumably the system is not saturated with diphosphates under the conditions in which the polynucleotides are made. If you have a low concentration of one of the diphosphates you can get a low concentration of the corresponding nucleotide in the polynucleotide. When you have equal concentrations of nucleotide diphosphates initially, the concentrations of mononucleotides in the polymers are very roughly 1:1:1:1, so it appears to depend very much on the starting concentrations.

Dr. SPIEGELMAN: I would like to ask Dr. Kornberg if he tried to run the reaction backwards by putting in pyrophosphate and, second, if there is any suggestion of an equilibrium in DNA synthesis.

Dr. KORNBERG: I would like to make a table to contrast RNA and DNA-synthesizing systems, which may answer your question and others.

Dr. KORNBERG: First, as to the question of reversibility: In the case of DNA synthesis, if we use inorganic pyrophosphate in concentrations which exceed the concentrations of the substrate by 1000-fold we get

	RNA	DNA
Reversibility	+	−
K_m	$>10^{-2}\,M$	$<10^{-5}\,M$
Number of nucleotides required	1	4
Primer requirement	No clear evidence	+
Extent of reaction relative to initial polynucleotide	Almost infinite	$1\frac{1}{2}$ times
Specificity	Complex (cf. Ochoa)	Some specificity (i.e. ATP fails to replace deoxy ATP)

only about 20% inhibition, whereas low concentrations of inorganic phosphate ($10^{-3}M$) will completely inhibit RNA synthesis or reverse it. The K_m value for the nucleoside diphosphates required for RNA synthesis is much higher than that for DNA. As to number of nucleotides required, RNA synthesis requires one and DNA synthesis at least 4. As to primer, we confirm Dr. Ochoa that there is no clear evidence for primer for RNA, but there is in DNA an obligate need for "primer." Concerning the extent of reaction, the kinetic values are not good, but let's say the best we have done in the case of DNA synthesis is a $1\frac{1}{2}$-fold increase. Maybe there is meaning to this. DNA synthesis reaches a limit; in the case of RNA the extent of reaction is almost infinite, considering that you start with essentially no RNA. As to specificity in the RNA-synthesizing system, Dr. Ochoa has discussed this; but in the case of the DNA system the little we have done indicates some specificity. If you substitute ATP for deoxy-ATP the system is totally inert; it cannot replace deoxy-ATP in any way.

Dr. Chargaff: I have one question for Dr. Kornberg. Is the primer replaceable? I understand your primer is *E. coli* DNA. Is it replaceable by other deoxynucleotides, or is it a specific primer?

Dr. Kornberg: Yes, let's say at the outset that in the routine assay experiments we are measuring an increment not of $1\frac{1}{2}$-fold but of 1.1-fold, so we are now dealing with only a 10% increment. In this sort of assay, *E. coli* DNA and thymus DNA are about equally effective, using equal amounts of DNA nucleotide; phage T2 DNA is about half as effective.

Dr. Chargaff: I have a question for Dr. Ochoa. I notice he hasn't said anything about animal cells. Is there any evidence for the existence of polynucleotide phosphorylase in animal tissues? The second question has to do with a statement that I remember from his paper where he states that the ribonuclease-resistant portion of an RNA is not split by his enzyme. Now, since the ribonuclease-resistant portion of the nucleic acid is very rich in guanylic acid, this fits in with his difficulty of putting in guanylic acid. If there are really several specific enzymes then one could be lacking or inhibited, and it is the one that handles guanylic acid. The next question is with regard to sequence—Dr. Heppel has done excellent sequence work—is the sequence more or less constant in parallel preparations? Could one get the same distribution of di- and trinucleotides in two preparations made from AU, or does it vary all over the lot? A factual statement from our own work has to do with the pentose in *Azotobacter*. We were interested in what pentose could actually be demonstrated in the naturally occurring RNA of *Azotobacter*, because we thought it would be funny if it turned out to be another pentose than ribose. Actually, we have looked at preparations of mononucleotides prepared by alkali hydrolysis of RNA of *Azotobacter*, and the main sugar is ribose.

DR. OCHOA: That is indeed reassuring, Dr. Chargaff. Concerning your question about constant sequence, I did point out that one would have to do more experiments of this kind on several batches of AU before one could conclude anything about the randomness of the sequence or otherwise. The experiment has been done only once, and I think Dr. Heppel plans to repeat it this next fall on another batch of AU; so until we have data on several batches we cannot say much one way or the other. In regard to the question as to the presence of the enzyme in animal cells, so far we have not found the enzyme in them—at least, let's put it this way: we have no unequivocal proof for its presence in animal cells.

DR. SADANA: Any evidence of this enzyme in plant tissues?

DR. OCHOA: Yes. A small amount of the enzyme was found in ammonium sulfate fractions from spinach leaves, so it seems to be present in the tissues of higher plants, but not in the amounts which are found in bacteria. I should like to think that it is present in animal cells but in very small amounts, and it is very difficult to detect. It is not surprising that cells that are growing rapidly would contain fair amounts of the enzyme and cells that aren't growing rapidly wouldn't contain much. In regard to Dr. Chargaff's question about the "core," by reacting ribonuclease with the AGUC polymer one gets a "core" the composition of which has not been studied, but the polymer yields the same percentage of "core" as that yielded by yeast RNA on digestion with RNAase. Whether or not the amount of phosphorolysis of this core is related to guanylic acid, we could not answer. We have not yet thoroughly investigated the guanylic acid polynucleotide. Polynucleotide phosphorylase has difficulty in making this one. However, I did point out that when you have GDP present with the other diphosphates it does get incorporated very nicely into the high polymer molecule. As to the question of multiplicity of the enzymes, both Littauer and Beers and Olmsted find that purified preparations of the *E. coli* and *M. lysodeikticus* enzymes appear to be inactive with GDP—that is, with GDP alone, but no other laboratory has put together the four disphosphates to see whether GDP will then react. I think that multiplicity of the enzyme is not very likely from the competition we observe among the 4 diphosphates, presumably for the same site on the enzyme.

DR. P. BERG: I would just like to ask a question of Dr. Potter. In using the terms ATP and UTP in connection with DNA I was wondering whether he was referring to the deoxynucleotides or if he was implying that in these preparations he had converted the ribotides to the deoxyribotides. That's a very important distinction.

DR. POTTER: I know. I meant the level of phosphorylation. We have studied the transphosphorylations between the ATP and the pyrimidine deoxyribose monophosphates, and there is ready transphosphorylation; and so it is clear that if you have a higher level of phosphorylation of ribonucleotides the phosphates just move over to the deoxy form, though of course at a level as yet unspecified. I am glad you pointed that out.

DR. BERG: You are referring, then, just to the phosphate level, rather than to the nucleotides?

DR. POTTER: I should have just said TP and DP or else I should have indicated the intermediate steps.

DR. BERNHART: I would like to say a few words about the energetics of the RNA structure. The total of the inorganic phosphates liberated in the process of polymerization tends to a value of 80%. If we assume that every phosphate bond is equivalent, then we can write the equilibrium expression:

$$ADP + ADP \rightleftharpoons AMP — ADP + P_i.$$

Taking into account all of the pertinent ionization constants for the equilibrium as measured by Dr. Ochoa, we get a value of — 450 to — 1700 calories. Comparing that with the hydrolytic process $ADP + H_2O \rightleftharpoons AMP + P_i$, for which we now have reasonably good thermodynamic data, the calculation leads us to the answer that the formation of this bond in RNA has an energy of about 7 kilocalories; and this is indeed a very high energy value, since it turns out to be essentially identical to the splitting energy of the second and third phosphate bonds of ATP. I would like to point out just one more thing to Dr. Ochoa, and that is that the reaction yielding the formation of the RNA bond has been pushed toward bond synthesis by working at pH 8—that is, by ionizing the phosphoric acid. If one could lower the pH to see if one gets shorter chains or fewer chains, then one could get some idea as to whether all the bonds in the molecule are equivalent.

DR. OCHOA: We have not explored this very extensively as yet. We have found pH 8 to be the optimum of what we call the "exchange" reaction. We didn't find much difference between pH 7 and pH 9 for the rate of phosphate liberation. I would like to leave the audience with a little food for thought, if I may—namely, that the work on polynucleotide phosphorylase has disclosed that the diester bonds in the ribopolynucleotides can very well be called high-energy phosphate bonds, and therefore there is a possibility that they could be used by the cells as energy-yielding groups for other synthetic reactions. This is along the lines that Dr. Spiegelman has been following. The other thing is that I was wondering when talking with Dr. Kornberg why it was that all the reactions I study (P enzyme, propionyl CoA carboxylation, polynucleotide phosphorylase), turn out to involve nucleoside diphosphates, whereas the ones he studies always seem to involve the triphosphates!

DR. KORNBERG: This is one of those cases of induced substrate specificity. Since Dr. Soodak isn't here, I would like to say something on his behalf. If he were here, Dr. Soodak would say that, in addition to RNA being a reservoir of energy, it might also be a reservoir of nucleotides for coenzymes.

THE BIOSYNTHESIS OF NUCLEIC ACIDS
IN SOME MICROBIAL SYSTEMS

Seymour S. Cohen

*The Children's Hospital of Philadelphia (Department of Pediatrics) and
the Department of Biochemistry of the University of Pennsylvania
School of Medicine*

Introduction

This paper will be concerned with the few studies of nucleic acid metabolism in the systems which have been used to dissect the chemical basis of inheritance. Detailed studies of nucleic acid metabolism have barely begun with organisms classically employed in cytogenetics such as *Drosophila* or maize. In some fungal systems used for the study of physiological genetics, e.g., *Neurospora,* a satisfactory measurement of deoxyribose nucleic acid (DNA) content has not yet been made, nor have the metabolic properties of the nucleic acids been examined in these organisms. In yeast it is not customary to fractionate the nucleic acids into their two main chemical groups because of the relative preponderance of ribose nucleic acid (RNA) and the presence of other fractions such as the metaphosphates. Finally, we can say virtually nothing about nucleic acid metabolism in transformable systems wherein the genetic determinants have been demonstrated to consist of DNA. In the latter instances we have not solved the problem of infecting a significant proportion of cells with the new genetic determinant in order to follow the consequent intracellular metabolic events. Also inhibitor and isotopic techniques have barely begun to be applied in these systems.

The questions which we would like to answer in a study of the chemical basis of inheritance include the following (33): What is the nature of the genetic material, how is its specificity determined by its structure, how does it multiply, and how does it produce its primary physiological action?

At the present time only a single system has begun to provide answers to all of these questions; this is the well-known case of

Escherichia coli infected by the T-even viruses. With this system we shall be concerned primarily with the inheritance and multiplication of the virus rather than of the bacterium.[1] This brief survey of our present experimental position appears to stress the limited character of the data which can contribute to the discussion of such an important topic. On the other hand, it is not accidental that the greatest progress has been made with the phage system. With this system a rigorous separation can be made of genetic material which is produced in isolable virus and the innumerable enzymatic systems present in bacteria which provide the metabolites used for the duplication of this genetic material.

This paper will consider data available on three major aspects of this phage system: (1) the complexity of the T-even viruses and the chemical structure of their DNA; (2) the interrelations of protein, DNA, and RNA synthesis in infected cells; and (3) the intermediary metabolism of the nucleic acids.

Finally I wish to present some data on thymine-requiring bacteria, in which an experimental separation of nuclear and cytoplasmic synthesis appears feasible. To the extent that this is so, it may become possible to obtain chemical information comparable to that to be presented in connection with studies on virus multiplication. In addition, recent data on these bacterial systems suggest some new approaches to the chemical study of mutagenesis.

It is my purpose in this paper to point to some current problems rather than to stress our successes in obtaining partial answers. To my mind, the major advances which have been obtained from the studies to be considered are not those of specific results, but rather the increasing precision with which the critical biological problems of our special systems can be posed in chemical terms.

CHEMICAL EVENTS IN PHAGE INVASION AND MULTIPLICATION

Introductory Remarks on Phage.

Before presenting the biochemical data on the T-even viruses, i.e., T2, T4, or T6, three comments may be made:

---

[1] In all other cases of bacterial viruses examined, including virulent viruses such as T3 (37), it appears that a structural homology may exist between their genetic materials and those of their hosts. In these instances, then, we may be able to reach some conclusions concerning the properties and behavior of the bacterial genetic apparatuses from the observed properties of their viruses.

(1) The T-even viruses are chemically unique and the extreme pathology which they produce in infected bacteria appears to be causally related to their unique chemical properties. Therefore many of the events observed may have no counterpart in any other system. Although it is probable that the genetic material of these viruses is DNA, it is too early to be able to separate all the properties derived from the special chemical features of T-even virus DNA from the more general attributes of DNA, or to be able to say to what extent these general attributes have been modified by the special properties. Although it can be hoped that the biochemical and genetic problems and solutions which will be examined in the light of experience with the T-even viruses will be comparable in other systems, it is probably wiser to begin with the clear understanding that extrapolation to other systems is a dangerous business at best, and a most unsatisfactory substitute for observation of the other systems.

(2) We should note that a feature of cells infected by these viruses is the apparent cessation of enzyme synthesis.[2] Thus the genetic determinants of the virus do not appear to control the synthesis of specific enzymes but produce their effects in some other manner. The solution of the mode of action of these viral genes may then be a simpler problem than that posed by cellular genes, many of which appear to control enzyme production or specificity. The problem of the mode of action of viral genes probably permits us to bypass the general problem of enzyme synthesis. By the same token, of course, the answers we can obtain with these viruses are that much more limited.

(3) It is known that a very large proportion of the metabolism of the infected cell is directly concerned with virus synthesis. The cellular responses due to these viruses which, in other systems, may appear to be a fairly distant effect of the gene mediated via some enzyme-forming system, may in this instance prove to be a direct concomitant of the multiplication of genetic material.

The Nature of the Genetic Material of T2.

The most recent data on the structure of the phage particle T2 are summarized in Fig. 1, A. The virus particle is seen to be hollow, consisting of a protein outer coat surrounding the compressed threadlike

---

[2] The result of Joklik (39), purporting to indicate an increase in formic acid hydrogenlyase in infected cells, could not be confirmed by Dr. D. B. M. Scott in our laboratory. The apparent enzyme increase was caused by lysis from without.

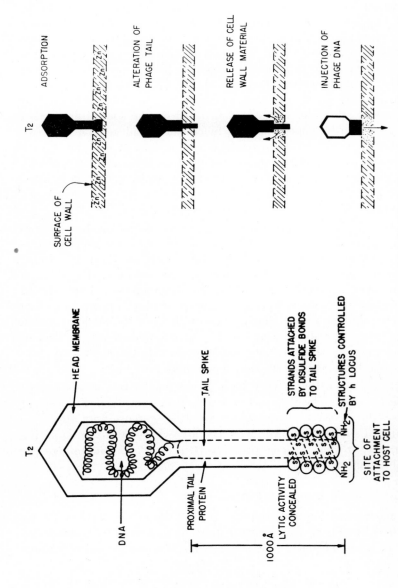

FIG. 1. A, A diagrammatic representation of the structure of T2. B, Adsorption and penetration of viral genetic material. These details have been postulated by Dr. L. Kozloff, who kindly lent the diagrams to the author.

DNA. This is the only type of nucleic acid in the virus (14). The outer coat is a complex differentiated structure consisting of a hexagonally shaped head and a tail, the tip of which is somewhat splayed. Several different proteins and antigens have been detected in the outer coat of the particle, and indeed the structure of the virus has been separated into a number of fragments. Empty heads, as well as bits of tail, have been isolated from infected cells treated with proflavin (51), a phenomenon which will be mentioned again below. The tip of the tail is essential for adsorption and may be unraveled by treatment with H_2O_2 (42) or split off with cyanide complexes of metals of the Zn group (45). Kozloff has suggested that a comparable cleavage of tail structure may occur to adsorbed virus at the surface of the cell, pointing to the presence of Zn at concentrations sufficient for this function (Fig. 1, B).

The virus particle, after removal of the tip, has a stubby tail containing a thin protein plug or spike which may be released by a number of compounds containing amino groups, of which glucosamine is an example. Upon the loss of the plug, DNA is discharged. It has been suggested by Kozloff that these events do occur at and then through the cell surface, as in Fig. 1, B. It appears that a hole is chewed through the cell wall, perhaps by enzymes within one or another of these virus structures. Such holes have been seen on direct examination of cell walls treated with virus (69) and a release of cell-wall nitrogen has been observed from such treated walls (4).

The existence of a head and several bits of tail consisting of structurally and functionally distinct proteins organized into the phage outer shell and constituting the attachment and penetration equipment of the phage outlines one major group of synthetic problems in infected cells. It has been shown that these complex protein substances do not constitute the genetic material of the phage and in fact do not supply the models for their own duplication. As Hershey and Chase have shown in their classic experiment (35), this outer shell of protein, with the possible exception of structures associated with the tail tip and plug (amounting to 3 per cent of the total protein), remains outside the infected bacteria. On the other hand, almost pure DNA enters the cell. The DNA may be accompanied by an amount of acid-soluble peptide equal at most to 1 - 2 per cent of total viral protein (33). Virus multiplication requires only the insertion of this genetic charge, since the outer coat of the infecting virus, which is left behind on the bacterial wall, may even be shaken off into the medium during the latent period without affecting virus production.[3] Thus the DNA not only supplies the information essential to its own duplication but also that necessary to encase the DNA in the differentiated proteins of the outer coat and tail.

Extruded virus DNA has been observed to exist in very long fibers of 20 to 25 Å diameter (38). The total charge of DNA per phage particle consists of about 2×10^{-16} g. of nucleic acid. If this were present in a single molecule, the DNA would have a molecular weight of about 120,000,000 and contain approximately 400,000 nucleotides. Molecular weights of virus DNA as great as this have not yet been observed. In physical studies conducted in conjunction with Dr. H. K. Schachman, the DNA of T4r, isolated by the urea method (8), was estimated from sedimentation and viscosity data obtained at very low concentrations (15 μg. per ml.). The molecular weight appeared to be about 25,000,000. Although this value is greater than others reported in the literature and was obtained with a product of exceptionally high intrinsic viscosity, it should be noted that the physical analysis of the preparation and properties of virus DNA has barely begun. It is conceivable that still higher values will be obtained.[4]

The isolated nucleic acids of three mutant pairs of T-even viruses, T2r[+] and T2r, T4r[+] and T4r, T6r[+] and T6r, have been found to possess identical base ratios (71). When these results were first obtained, it appeared necessary to infer that, if the structure of the DNA controlled the genetic bases of mutational difference among these phages, the mutational differences arose either from quantitative

---

[3] To explain the transfer of DNA from phage to bacterium it might be postulated that release of a plug permits a tightly coiled DNA within the phage to be extended by virtue of its self-contained electrostatic repulsive forces. Although this mechanism would extrude the DNA from the phage, we are then confronted with the problem of how the spring was coiled. We are far from a position in which we can hope to answer this question, but we already have data on the intracellular organization of virus DNA and protein which pose this problem sharply. These data will be considered somewhat later.

[4] Levinthal (50) has used an ingenious autoradiographic technique for estimating the size of virus DNA polymers containing radioactive P^{32}. He reports that following osmotic shock, virus DNA is liberated in a large fragment which is about 40 per cent of the size of the total phage DNA, as well as many smaller fragments of less than 7 to 8 million molecular weight. Our physical studies with DNA isolated by the urea method have not revealed two grossly different classes of this polymer.

differences too small to be detected by existing analytical methods or from differences in the sequential order of the nucleotides. As we shall see, the bases are not the only elements of the DNA molecule which may vary in amount.

Unique Chemical Features of Phage DNA.

In the course of the analytical study mentioned above, Dr. G. R. Wyatt and I discovered and identified a new pyrimidine base, 5-hydroxymethyl cytosine (HMC), which completely replaced cytosine in the virus DNA. Cytosine is the normal component of bacterial DNA and RNA, and at present it has been found in all other cellular nucleic acids studied. The possible metabolic role of HMC will be considered a little later; at this point let us examine some structural relations of this base in virus nucleic acid.

The HMC deoxyriboside was isolated following acid hydrolysis of DNA and subsequent treatment with phosphatase (12). It had been discovered that successive treatments with DNAase and phosphatase could not release significant amounts of HMC nucleosides, although most of the adenine, guanine, and thymine deoxyribosides were readily released in this way. It was suggested at that time that the structural relations of HMC in some manner protected the phosphodiester linkages of the HMC nucleotide and perhaps facilitated the survival of virus DNA within the bacterium. Our concern with the problem of the survival of phage DNA stems from the observation that infection with T-even virus rapidly activates a bacterial DNAase which appears to degrade the bacterial DNA (44, 53). The survival of injected viral DNA must then arise either from its special structural resistance to DNAase or from its separation within the cell from the DNAase.

The molecular basis of the resistance of virus DNA to enzymes was discovered by Volkin, working with T4r^+-DNA (64) and by Sinsheimer in studies on T2r^+-DNA (58). The hydroxymethyl group of HMC was found to be glucosylated and the presence of glucose was shown to protect the phosphate of the HMC nucleotide from enzymatic cleavage (58). The structures of these compounds are presented in Fig. 2.

Although the HMC of the DNA of T4r^+ was fully glucosylated (64), only 77 per cent of the HMC nucleotides in the DNA of T2r^+ contained glucose (58). We have recently confirmed these results (13). Thus although analyses of the base composition have not yet revealed

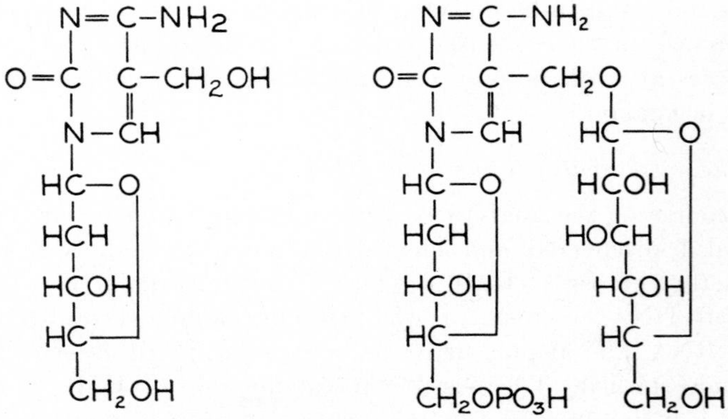

5-Hydroxymethyl cytosine
deoxyriboside

5-Glucosyl hydroxymethyl cytosine
deoxynucleotide

Fig. 2. A deoxyriboside and nucleotide of hydroxymethyl cytosine.

significant differences between the DNA of T2 and T4, such differences were revealed in the glucose content of the DNA of these viruses.

That these structural differences revealed within the structure of DNA do in fact relate to phage DNA survival appears to have been shown recently in a study of recombinants of T2 and T4 by Streisinger and Weigle (62). The parent T2 stock which they studied was characterized by a poor efficiency of plating (ability to produce a plaque) with certain host bacteria and the DNA of the virus was characterized by a low glucose content. This was in contrast to the T4 stock studied, which had a high glucose content and a high efficiency of plating. Most T2 progeny of T2 × T4 crosses possessed the high efficiency of plating characteristic of T4. These derived T2 strains also then possessed sufficient glucose to glucosylate all of the HMC of the DNA (62). In brief, then, the inheritable differences between T2 and T4 are not solely a matter of glucose content, but the glucose content does control certain other heritable properties of the viruses.

These authors have also suggested that the less glucosylated DNA would be more prone to a breakdown mechanism. This lowered resistance to breakdown of the T2-DNA could also account for the observed exclusion by T4 of inheritable markers derived from the parent T2 stock in certain T2 × T4 crosses.

In our comparisons of various r^+ and r pairs of T2, T4, and T6 DNA we have consistently observed more glucose in preparations of the r phages than of the r^+ strains (13). Mindful of the problem of purifying r phages, which because of their lytic properties are more prone to be contaminated by bacterial debris, numerous DNA preparations were also isolated from the r viruses. These also possessed high hexose contents, and all of the hexose has been identified as glucose. It appears that these DNA's may contain HMC polyglucosides but these have not yet been isolated.

In recent studies of the sensitivities of virus DNA to disruption by pancreatic DNAase, Miss H. Barner and I have observed that the $T2r^+$ DNA loses its integrity only slightly less slowly than does thymus DNA. $T4r^+$ and $T6r^+$ are cleaved more slowly than is $T2r^+$. Although the DNA's of $T4r^+$ and $T4r$ were cleaved at comparable rates, three different samples of the DNA of $T6r$ were degraded less rapidly than three samples of the DNA of $T6r^+$ (Fig. 3). The DNA of $T2r$ also seemed to be cleaved less rapidly than that of $T2r^+$. In general, then, the resistance of virus DNA to DNAase correlates fairly well (in all but one case) with their glucose contents. However, when the terminal products of DNAase degradation were studied in the ultracentrifuge, the phage nucleic acids did not contain fragments much larger than the products of degradation of thymus DNA.

Thus the nucleic acids of these viruses possess new and unique chemical configurations. The presence or absence of glucosylated HMC nucleotides appears to be important in determining the survival of virus DNA in certain bacterial hosts. Both the configuration and this property are heritable, which means in this instance that in compelling the synthesis of DNA like that of the parent, it is not only necessary at least to decide the position of the bases but also whether to put glucose on one of them or to select one of two types of HMC nucleotide. It must be admitted that no theory of DNA structure has yet proposed a mechanism for this addition or withholding of glucose from HMC or for the selection of one or the other HMC nucleotide.

From the point of view of the enzymologist, the glucose should not be present in the first place. If, in the glucosylated HMC nucleotide, the presence of glucose inhibits the action of phosphatase, it might be expected that the presence of phosphate would inhibit the addition of glucose, if this addition occurs at the nucleotide level. Conversely, the addition of glucose at the nucleoside level ought to inhibit a sub-

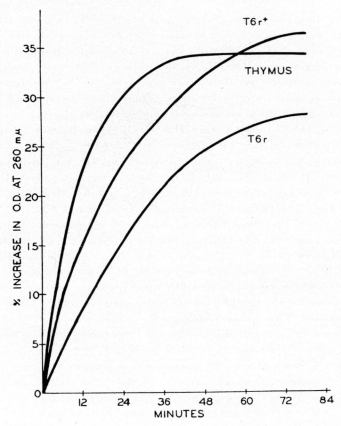

FIG. 3. The action of deoxyribonuclease on $r+$ and r nucleic acids.

sequent phosphorylation. However, since the compounds exist and one of these reactions must proceed, it will be interesting to see which one is permitted in virus-infected *E. coli.*

THE TRANSFER OF GENETIC INFORMATION

After the DNA is inserted into the bacterium it is necessary to follow its initial steps and those essential to multiplication. By means of a very sensitive radioautographic technique Levinthal (50) has followed the P^{32}-labelled DNA of individual phage particles through three infectious cycles involving phage adsorption, multiplication, and liberation. Since he could detect significantly labelled DNA in the progeny despite the formation of more than 1000 virus particles, he was able to conclude that a fairly large fragment of virus DNA was maintained intact. Furthermore, he determined that in the first transfer this unit possessed a molecular weight equal to 40 per cent of the size of the parental DNA, and that in the second generation derived from the progeny of the first cycle, a phage was obtained containing 20 per cent of the original parental radioactivity. In this step, the 40 per cent fragment was cut in half; however, in subsequent generations the 20 per cent fragment was maintained as a unit. Levinthal has suggested that this unit is the viral "chromosome" and the bearer of genetic information.

Stent, Jerne, and Sato (61) have also followed the initial steps in the transfer of DNA labelled with P^{32} sufficiently radioactive to produce destruction of the genetic material at a rate proportional to radioactive decay. As will be discussed later in this symposium, they have also observed a non-random transfer of some large DNA fragments, without however concluding that the big piece rather than the small pieces is necessarily the basis of the continuing replication.

Indeed the work of Stent and Fuerst (60), who used highly radioactive phage to study the transfer of the information necessary for phage synthesis, has suggested that immediately after insertion of the DNA, the genetic information is transferred to a non-DNA moiety. P^{32}-labelled cells were infected in P^{32} medium with P^{32}-phage and on immediate storage at —197° C. the ability of the infected cells to produce phage could be shown to decrease as a function of radioactive decay. After a few minutes of intracellular phage development, however, the ability of these cells to produce phage became independent of radioactive decay. One hypothesis to explain this result states that the code for phage production was transferred to moieties free of P, perhaps to protein.

SOME RELATIONS OF PROTEIN SYNTHESIS AND DNA SYNTHESIS

It was shown almost 10 years ago that the infected cell continues to make protein from the moment of infection (8). This result was confirmed by following the incorporation of S^{35} from inorganic sulfate into the acid-precipitable fraction of infected cells (37). However, it was found that only about 10 per cent of the sulfur incorporated by the cells during the first 5 minutes after infection appeared in the mature phage, whereas 50-60 per cent of the sulfur incorporated at later times appeared in phage. These results implied the synthesis of at least two kinds of protein in the infected cell, and it was even suggested that early protein synthesis was not directly related to phage multiplication, perhaps being concerned with the repair of the cell wall, which has been observed to be degraded during virus penetration. However, it had been shown in 1947 that the early protein synthesis was essential to the production of phage DNA. Thus it had been demonstrated that the amino acid analogue, 5-methyl tryptophan, which inhibits protein synthesis, can prevent the development of bacteriophage T2 and the net synthesis of DNA in infected *E. coli*, both observations indicating that the synthesis of DNA was dependent on the synthesis of protein (8, 18). The action of the analogue was reversed by tryptophan, and it was also demonstrated by means of reversal experiments that the requirement for tryptophan existed throughout the latent period (18, 54).

These results have recently been confirmed and extended by Burton (7), who has also shown by means of 5-methyl tryptophan, as well as with amino-acid–requiring mutants, that if the initial protein synthesis is permitted to occur and subsequently is inhibited, the synthesis of phage DNA (containing HMC) can proceed in the absence of continuing protein synthesis. The further processing of this DNA into intact phage requires the additional synthesis of protein. Comparable results have also been obtained by Melechen and Hershey (34) and by Tomizawa and Sunakawa (63), who used chloramphenicol as an inhibitor of protein synthesis. In uninfected bacteria, chloramphenicol also inhibits the synthesis of bacterial protein without inhibiting the synthesis of bacterial nucleic acid (27, 70).

The possibilities that genetic specificity initially embodied in DNA is transferred to protein before nucleic acid synthesis can begin and that the proteins are the models for subsequent DNA synthesis are clearly at odds with the Watson-Crick replication scheme. It is also conceivable that the early inhibition of protein synthesis introduces a nonspecific metabolic block, unrelated to the question of genetic specificity.[5] In this sense, then, the problems of the genetic nature of the early protein synthesis and the isolation and identification of the newly formed peptides are crucial questions in developing our understanding of the mechanisms of specific DNA synthesis.

Early studies of the net synthesis of DNA in T-even infected cells had revealed that after cessation of DNA synthesis for 7 to 8 minutes

(8) a markedly stimulated constant rate of DNA synthesis occurred.[6] Most of the newly formed DNA was actually incorporated into virus. These results were then subjected to a most careful scrutiny, as the following history will indicate:

The group at the University of Chicago demonstrated that in infected cells, bacterial DNA was degraded to the nucleoside level, at least in part, and that these fragments were then converted into virus DNA (46). Weed and I subsequently found that most of the degraded bacterial DNA appeared in the first quarter of phage particles produced in an r^+ system (68). We also showed that the cytosine of host DNA was converted to virus HMC (20). It was then asked whether the observed pattern of net synthesis did not obscure the true pattern of virus DNA synthesis, which may actually have begun from the moment of infection, even as protein synthesis did.

An examination of the rates of disappearance of cytosine and of appearance of HMC in the DNA of infected cells revealed an apparently reciprocal pattern (36). These results of Hershey et al. have occasionally been interpreted to suggest that the synthesis of DNA containing HMC starts with infection. A careful examination of the published data, however, reveals the existence of a short lag in synthesis even in these experiments (36). The time of appearance of HMC-containing DNA in infected cells has been carefully reexamined by Vidaver and Kozloff (pers. commun.) by following the incorporation of isotope of a C^{14}-labelled carbon source into the HMC and thymine of DNA in infected cells. This study has clearly revealed a lag of 5 to 9 minutes in the synthesis of this DNA. A complete analytical equality was obtained between the formation of virus DNA and

[5] That the early protein synthesis is directly involved in the multiplication process has been indicated by experiments with ultraviolet radiation. Irradiation of phage-infected cells reduces the number of cells which can yield phage. The radiation sensitivity of these systems decreases in the early stages of the latent period, prior to the formation of intact phage. Burton (7) has also shown that this decrease in sensitivity in early stages of multiplication, prior to the formation of intact phage, requires protein synthesis, while Tomizawa and Sunakawa (63) have demonstrated that the nucleic acid synthesis in the absence of protein synthesis does not then increase the radiation sensitivity of infected cells.

[6] The linear kinetics of DNA synthesis and of phage formation may merely reflect the existence of some rate-limiting step, such as the supply of DNA precursors, rather than a basic characteristic of viral multiplication. On the other hand, the rate of DNA synthesis might be determined by the number of genetically specific protein templates elaborated prior to the inception of DNA synthesis, as has been suggested by the results of the chloramphenicol experiments (63).

net DNA synthesis in their system. The observed lag in virus DNA synthesis is of course consistent with the requirement for a prior protein synthesis.

ON RNA SYNTHESIS IN INFECTED BACTERIA

Approximately a decade ago it was shown that the RNA content of infected cells did not increase (42). The incorporation of P^{32} into the nucleic acids of infected cells was also studied in order to test the hypothesis that RNA was or was not converted to DNA (9). Our data showed that after an hour the RNA fraction contained about 2 per cent of the activity of the DNA. However, it was thought, in that era before the ion exchange, ionophoresis, and chromatography of nucleotides, that this small amount of radioactivity probably arose from contamination of the RNA fraction by other P^{32}-containing materials. Although the possibility was considered, it was believed unlikely that, if the RNA was indeed labelled, a turnover of this small fraction could account for the large amount of DNA produced. Several years ago, Hershey obtained evidence to suggest the incorporation of P^{32} in RNA (32). It remained for Volkin and Astrachan (65) to prove recently that the P^{32} was indeed incorporated into RNA nucleotides, including that of cytosine. However, the extent of incorporation, in contrast to that into DNA, was as small as that described earlier. Although this result does not demonstrate a functional role of RNA synthesis in virus production, the distribution of radioactivity in the RNA nucleotides is most suggestive, i.e., the P^{32} contents of adenine and uracil nucleotides are equal and about $1\frac{1}{2}$ to 2 times those of the equivalent guanine and cytosine nucleotides. These ratios more nearly resemble the ratios of adenine and thymine and of guanine and HMC nucleotides in virus DNA than the ratios of the RNA bases of the host bacterium. Evidently a study of the turnover rate of these newly synthesized RNA nucleotides and measurement of the extent of the conversion to virus DNA would be very important at the present time.

ON THE FORMATION OF INTACT VIRUS

In an early experiment carried out in conjunction with Dr. A. Doermann, it was observed that the net synthesis of DNA (now known to be equivalent to phage DNA) preceded any detectable formation of intracellular phage by several minutes. The formation of both materials paralleled each other in the infected cell (36). Hershey has since shown, by means of a "pulse" experiment using P^{32}, that this DNA is indeed incorporated into phage, and he has estimated the size of this precursor pool of DNA (32). The final organizing steps to complete the virus are not clear, but some interesting experiments bear on this point.

If infected cells are treated with proflavin, protein and DNA synthesis proceed, as does lysis. However, the lysate in that case does not contain intact virus but instead contains bits of tail protein, soluble HMC-containing DNA, and empty phage heads. This picture is also observed when infected cells are disrupted at certain stages of the latent period (51). The questions which are posed by these results include the following: Was the soluble DNA contained in the phage head and did it subsequently leak out? If so, was DNA or outer skin an organizer for the other or were both made separately?

Studies of the sizes of the DNA and protein-precursor pools have revealed that the former is considerably greater (37), a ratio suggesting that the DNA need not be formed within an intact phage skin. An elegant experiment of Melechen and Hershey (33) has revealed that the very large pool of virus DNA which can be made in the presence of chloramphenicol can subsequently be encased by the protein which the infected cells make when the chloramphenicol is removed from the system. However, as Hershey pointed out, this experiment does not exclude the possibility that nucleic acid was initially made in a very thin protein membrane or that such a protein was removed prior to the next steps leading to the final enclosure of DNA in protein. Although such possibilities may appear unlikely, the alternatives are also unlikely. If one conceives of the formation of the precursor pool in solution, it seems reasonable to expect that this polymer will be formed as extended molecules. The manner of their subsequent compression to fit within the phage head, the synthesis of whose proteins they have presumably directed, then becomes the next question, unless it is postulated that the DNA is indeed made within a very thin protein skin. It is easy to see that compared to these problems of model building, the molecular models of the Watson-Crick era can be considered to be child's play. It should certainly be possible to distinguish between a free or enclosed DNA, if it proves possible to disrupt the cells without introducing artifacts. Perhaps a modification of Behren's technique of disruption and fractionation in anhydrous solvents will help to solve this problem.

I wish to comment briefly on the well-known inertness of DNA, revealed in an apparent lack of turnover of DNA phosphorus, since this inertness bears on the problem of organizing protein synthesis. In view of the schema now being promulgated for the formation of nucleotide anhydrides of the amino acids, it is a very simple matter to draw a picture in which the DNA or RNA nucleotides are held in position by hydrogen-bonding of their bases to another nucleic acid or protein. The internucleotide diester linkages could then be cleaved to produce diphosphates which might form the desired amino acid anhydrides. The base-catalysed condensation of the latter to peptides can presumably free the nucleotides for the regeneration of the phosphodiesters in the same position as they previously existed and with the same phosphorus atom bridging the internucleotide gap. In brief, then, if such a picture approximates reality an apparent lack of turnover of P^{32} in the nucleic acids need mean very little concerning their potentially high metabolic and organizing activity.

Intermediary Metabolism of the Nucleic Acids

We have been interested in the controlling mechanisms which permit the T-even viruses to compel the host bacteria to redirect their activities to support the multiplication of virus. Accordingly we have been exploring some aspects of the intermediary metabolism of the nucleic acids as our major interest since about 1948. The particular areas in which we have concentrated were determined by a few working hypotheses concerning the nature of the controlling mechanisms. The validity of these hypotheses is by no means unequivocally demonstrated.

In our limited experience the most difficult problems in this field do not arise from a dearth of demonstrable enzymatic reactions; on the contrary, the main difficulty seems to be that there are too many such reactions to be found in cell-free systems or which can otherwise be demonstrated. Having observed a number of alternative pathways which form or depart from whatever compound is conceived to be interesting, the problem which must be faced is whether those reactions actually operate in the biological situation under investigation, and if so, to what extent. It is in this sense that enzymology constitutes only a small basic fragment of the discipline of biochemistry.

Our first efforts to understand the apparent cessation of RNA synthesis and the stimulation of viral DNA synthesis were directed toward an exploration of the utilization or nonutilization of different pathways of glucose metabolism which could be expected to produce ribose phosphate and deoxyribose phosphate. Evidence was obtained to show that, in the intact cell, infection did reduce the degree of utilization of the oxidative phosphogluconate pathway (11), a pathway mainly responsible for ribose production in growing *E. coli* (47). However, it was also possible to show that virus infection did not directly inhibit the enzymes of the phosphogluconate pathway (19). As interesting as the problems of glucose metabolism in *E. coli* have proved to be, and despite the esthetic pleasures afforded by discovering new isomerases and kinases at every turn, it has seemed necessary to look elsewhere for the site of control of the pathways.

Before discussing our present working hypotheses, I call attention to our additional observation that, in growing bacteria, deoxyribose may well be formed from ribose derived from phosphogluconate, whereas the over-all pathway for deoxyribose formation from glucose in infected cells is evidently different (48). When glucose-1-C^{14} is fed to growing cells, the specific activities of the ribose of RNA and the deoxyribose of DNA are comparable (0.23-0.25 of the radioactivity of the exogenous glucose). When glucose-1-C^{14} is consumed by infected cells, the specific activity of the deoxyribose is at least doubled, to about 0.5. A new pathway for the formation of deoxyribose phosphate formation is operating, e.g., by means of a condensation of acetaldehyde and triose phosphate, or newly formed ribose no longer stems from the phosphogluconate pathway to the same relative degree prior to conversion to deoxyribose. In the former instance, the amount of radioactivity in deoxyribose might also suggest that the deoxyribose of pyrimidine deoxynucleotides may arise by a route different from that of the purine deoxynucleotides. This possibility is being tested at the present time.

That virus infection possibly opens a new pathway for DNA formation is also suggested by the observations of Herriott (31). When *E. coli* treated with mustard gas to block DNA synthesis is infected with phage T2, DNA synthesis is reactivated.

PYRIMIDINE BIOSYNTHESIS IN INFECTED CELLS

The discovery of HMC has led to another hypothesis of the mechanism of controlling RNA and DNA synthesis, and one which appears to be consistent with the existing data. Since virus DNA does not contain cytosine and the infected cell converts the cytosine of host DNA into viral HMC, it is suggested that the hydroxymethylation of the deoxyriboside of cytosine or of a cytosine derivative is an irreversible trap for this pyrimidine (12). The entrapment and resulting deficiency of cytosine derivatives could account for the failure of cytosine-containing nucleic acids (host RNA and DNA) to accumulate in virus infection. Consistent with this idea is the finding that hydroxymethyl pyrimidines and their deoxyribosides cannot fulfill the pyrimidine requirements of pyrimidineless strains of *E. coli* (12), i.e., the hydroxymethyl group cannot be released so as to form the required pyrimidines.

It is a consequence of this hypothesis that HMC formation cannot occur in normal cells in significant amounts, or else the cell would be compelled into a pathological path of synthesis. The formation of HMC or an appropriate derivative is then conceived to arise in infected cells in a reaction normally inhibited in growth or induced by infection, either as a result of the virus supplying an inducing agent, a coenzyme, or the enzyme itself. In any case it will not be possible to determine just what happens until the enzymatic steps necessary to form HMC can be unravelled as a preliminary to a test of these hypotheses. As will be seen, the solution of this problem also appears to be tied to the problem of the origin of thymine.

In *E. coli*, free uracil or cytosine or their nucleosides readily enter the uracil and cytosine of bacterial RNA and the thymine and cytosine of bacterial DNA (37, 57). Since free thymine and thymidine are not utilized significantly by *E. coli* strain B, the common host in our metabolic experiments on DNA synthesis (57), it was concluded that formation of the thymine deoxyribotide occurs in normal cells at the nucleotide level. However, in the conversion of labeled bacterial DNA to viral DNA, the presence of exogenous thymidine markedly diminishes (by about two-thirds) the conversion of preformed thymine in bacterial DNA into viral thymine (37). Reactions at the nucleoside level are evidently more capable of being handled in the economy of the infected cell than in that of growing cells.

This result might ensue if the hydroxymethylation to HMC and the methylation to thymine now occurred mainly at the nucleoside level. This could produce a shift of metabolism to mechanisms favoring the formation of deoxyribose-1-phosphate, essential for deoxyriboside formation. Thus uracil would condense with deoxyribose-1-phosphate to form deoxyuridine, which can presumably be aminated to form deoxy-cytidine. One or the other deoxyriboside, it is proposed, is a primary precursor of HMC deoxyriboside and of thymidine in infected cells. The deoxyribose-1-phosphate would be generated from deoxyribose-5-phosphate, the condensation product of acetaldehyde and triose phosphate. The latter would arise with greater ease from the Embden-Meyerhof scheme rather than from the phosphogluconate pathway, and would possess a higher labeling as a consequence of being derived from glucose-1-C^{14} via the Embden-Meyerhof scheme.

Our concern with the deoxyriboside level is dictated by two other facts. Free HMC is not appreciably incorporated by infected cells (12). *E. coli* will not incorporate nucleotides without prior dephosphorylation (49). The latter point does not exclude the pyrimidine deoxyribotides as the major level at which hydroxymethylation and methylation occur but only suggests that it might be easier to attack the nucleoside level first. Finally, since these critical events might actually occur at this level, as the previous discussion has indicated, we are exploring these pathways first.

It might be thought that this elimination of two of the three possible levels of base metabolism is a great simplifying factor. It is so, of course, but our choices for study are still rather extensive, as indicated in Fig 4. In addition, the following observations condition our thinking: Cytosine contained in bacterial DNA will serve as precursor for both viral HMC and thymine, while bacterial thymine will not be

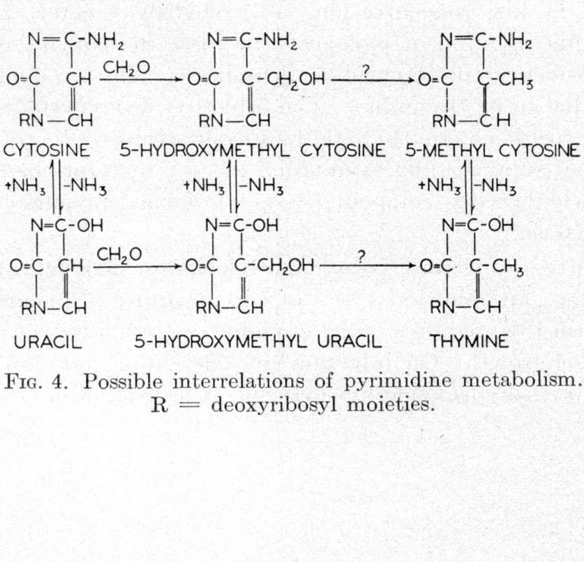

Fig. 4. Possible interrelations of pyrimidine metabolism.
R = deoxyribosyl moieties.

transformed to HMC (68). The β-carbon of serine can form both the hydroxymethyl group of HMC and the methyl group of thymine (20).

When methyl-labeled methionine was fed to a methionine-requiring organism during growth and virus-infection, the methyl group of thymine was not derived from the methionine although the amino acid was incorporated into bacterium and virus, respectively (M. Green and S. S. Cohen, in press). It was also shown that the hydroxymethyl-carbon of S-hydroxymethyl homocysteine did not enter HMC or thymine. In view of the above the following possibilities can be considered:

(1) deoxycytidine may be converted directly to HMC deoxyriboside;

(2) deoxycytidine can be deaminated to deoxyuridine by the active pyrimidine nucleoside deaminase of *E. coli*, then hydroxymethylated to hydroxymethyluracil deoxyriboside, which may finally be aminated to HMC deoxyriboside;

(3) hydroxymethyluracil deoxyriboside may then be converted to thymidine, a possibility which appears to have been excluded recently by several workers;

(4) HMC deoxyriboside may be converted to 5-methyl cytosine deoxyriboside, which is then converted to thymidine.

We have recently obtained some data which bear on the last possibility. 5-Methyl cytosine has never been observed in bacterial DNA. This situation might occur either if it were not formed or if the compound or its derivatives were metabolized and not permitted to accumulate. Miss H. Barner and I have isolated 5-methyl cytosine deoxyriboside. The compound is deaminated by the deoxycytidine deaminase of *E. coli* at low concentrations at a slightly greater rate than is deoxycytidine. Indeed, it is conceivable that the enzyme ought to be called a 5-methyl deoxycytidine deaminase. The product has been demonstrated to be thymidine. The 5-methyl deoxycytidine does promote the growth of our thymine-requiring strain of *E. coli* at a rate equal to that supported by thymidine. It may therefore be asked quite seriously whether this compound is not a normal precursor of thymidine in bacteria.

Before attempting the hydroxymethylation of deoxycytidine and of deoxyuridine, an additional set of circumstances appears relevant. *E. coli* strain 15_T- requires either thymine or thymidine, or a precursor of these, for growth. On infection by T2r^+, the very low ability of 15_T- to make a hydroxymethyl cytosine (the pyrimidine of thiamine) and thymine (about 2 to 4 per cent of its normal requirement) is enormously expanded to permit the synthesis of HMC and thymine for virus synthesis (2). Since this ability to open other metabolic blocks has not been observed after infection by any other mutant, it has seemed possible that in this instance virus infection has opened some reaction leading to a common precursor of both compounds.

Our system of hypotheses has accordingly been expanded to propose that the conversion of the hydroxymethyl group to the methyl group occurs on a pyrimidine deoxyriboside. To facilitate the removal of oxygen as H_2O, in keeping with other biochemical deoxygenations, the existence of dihydropyrimidine nucleosides is suggested. Additional reactions then become possible, as elaborated in Fig. 5.

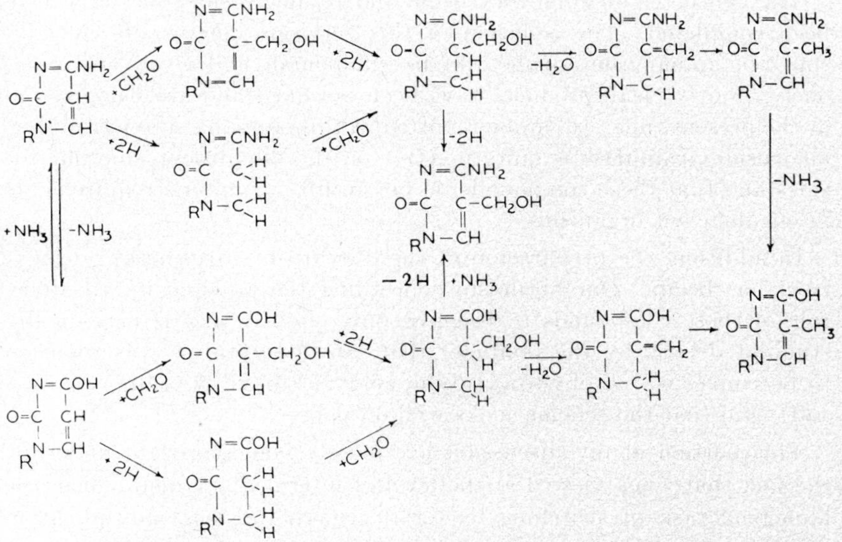

FIG. 5. Postulated steps in the formation of HMC and thymine deoxyribosides.

Even with this simplifying guess, at least two series of compounds are possible, one at the aminopyrimidine level and the other at the hydroxypyrimidine level. Dr. M. Green and I elected to work at first with the dihydrouracil compounds primarily because it was reported that deoxyuridine could be converted to thymidine (25). In any case dihydrouracil derivatives have proven to be easier to prepare than the cytosine derivatives. Crystalline dihydrodeoxyuridine and dihydrothymidine have been made as well as dihydrouridine (29).

None of these compounds has yet revealed any significant biological activity. Dihydrodeoxyuridine is not cleaved by pyrimidine nucleoside phosphorylase, although the glucosyl linkage is far more labile than in deoxyuridine. The compound does not fulfill the uracil requirements of several uracil-requiring strains of *E. coli* nor the thymine requirement of strain 15$_{T-}$. Radioactive dihydrodeoxyuridine, prepared by exchange of uracil-2-C^{14} and deoxyuridine followed by subsequent hydrogenation and crystallization of the nucleoside, was not converted to thymine by any of 6 systems, which have included growing bacteria or virus-infected organisms. The compound was metabolized to the nucleotide level by strain 15$_{T-}$, but its metabolism apparently stopped there.

The syntheses of dihydrocytosine and its nucleosides have recently been completed. The isolation of this series is much more difficult, since the amino group of the dihydro compounds hydrolyses spontaneously. Fairly clean products have been obtained and are being tested at the present time. It can be reported at this time that the pyrimidine nucleoside deaminase is quite inactive on the dihydrocytosine nucleosides and that these compounds do not fulfill pyrimidine requirements in our deficient organisms.

In addition, the preparation of the dihydro-hydroxymethyl derivatives has begun. Our optimism concerning the possible intermediary role of these compounds is dragging only slightly and is periodically stimulated both by the reminder that labelled cytidine was reported to be converted to dihydrocytidylic acid via dihydrocytidine in liver (30), and that the schema looks well on paper.

This portion of my discussion has merely endeavored to underline the fact that when viewed at the level of intermediary metabolism the biological task of switching bacterial growth to virus multiplication poses many still unsolved biochemical problems. These include such important subjects as the control of the metabolism of glucose, pentose, and deoxypentose, the routes and mechanisms of nucleotide formation, the nature of amination, hydroxymethylation, of methylation in the pyrimidine series, etc. Furthermore, these problems must be solved in terms which will describe a single organism in a defined biological state. It should be noted that solutions to these problems are essential to an understanding of the chemical basis of parasitism and inheritance in the one system we know most about.

Nucleic Acid Synthesis in a Thymine-Requiring Bacterium

Problems of the localization of the sites of synthesis of nucleic acid have been considered in detail elsewhere in this symposium. Some of these data may be summarized as follows. Enucleated cells may produce RNA, containing new nucleotides, as evidenced by the incorporation of radioactive orotic acid into RNA (5). However, net synthesis has not yet been observed in enucleated systems. Certainly, intact cells make far more RNA than do enucleated systems. The production of this material in the nucleus and the subsequent transfer of nucleotides in some as yet undetermined state from nucleus to cytoplasm has been described (28).

The beautiful results obtained in the laboratories of Brachet and Mazia stem from their application of ultra-micro-methods to very small numbers of carefully selected cells, such as amoebae or *Acetabularia*. Most biological systems used for studying the possible interrelations of RNA and DNA synthesis present difficulties of interpretation. On the other hand, the material exploited by the schools of Brachet and Mazia are not easily adapted to an analysis of genetic change.

In recent years, Barner and I have studied the nucleic acid metabolism and some physiological properties of pyrimidine-requiring strains of *E. coli*. These strains were collected to facilitate the study of HMC. It appears that some pyrimidine-requiring organisms possess certain attributes which can permit both the separate control of DNA and RNA synthesis and also some measure of analysis of genetic change. Our work in this direction began with *E. coli*, strain 15_T-, a thymine-requiring strain. The organism had originally been isolated by Roepke after a painstaking testing of the survivors of an ultraviolet irradiation of strain 15. The organism has only the single deficiency and grows well in a glucose-ammonium-salts medium supplemented by thymine. At first the organism was used to test possible thymine precursors and it is still being used in this way. A more intensive interest began when it was observed that T2 infection released the block in thymine synthesis (2).

In contrast to most auxotrophs (e.g., amino acid-, purine-, or uracil-deficient strains) which merely stop dividing but remain viable in the absence of their requirement, this organism lost the ability to multiply, or "died" in the absence of thymine in an otherwise complete medium. The omission of other elements of the complete synthetic medium prevented death; in other words, the metabolism of glucose, nitrogen, and phosphate was essential to the killing process. Omission of thymine alone produced a lag of 25 to 30 minutes, during which the viable count remained constant. This was followed by a decrease in viable count at the rate of about 90 per cent division time (2), as presented in Fig. 6. The loss of the ability to multiply was irreversible, as determined by plating on both simple and complex media containing thymine.

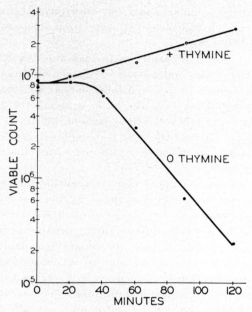

Fig. 6. The death of *E. coli*, strain 15$_T$– as a result of thymine deficiency.

Cells which had lost the power to multiply had increased in length and diameter. They had at least doubled their protein and RNA content while their DNA content had increased at the most by a few percent. We have used the term "unbalanced growth" to describe this pathological synthetic pattern.

In media containing labelled glucose and lacking thymine, strain 15$_T$– made uracil, orotic acid, and hypoxanthine, which appeared in the medium among very small amounts of other compounds. Uracil was the major product excreted, to the extent of several micrograms per ml. in 2 hrs. by 10^9 bacteria. It was shown that the deficient bacteria could make 2 to 4 per cent of their normal thymine requirement; the newly made thymine appeared in the nucleic acid fraction.

We and numerous other workers have found the thymineless bacteria useful in studying a number of different problems. For example, it could be shown that the induced biosynthesis of a number of enzymes, e.g., xylose isomerase (16), beta-galactosidase (59), and nitrate reductase (66), could occur under conditions of thymine deficiency. These results suggest that such enzyme synthesis is independent of DNA synthesis and presumably occurs in the cytoplasm.

When thymineless bacteria are deprived of thymine for the period in which the viable count does not change, the cells have greatly increased their cytoplasmic constituents, e.g., RNA and protein, and have achieved a state in which a critical cellular event is either prevented from occurring or occurs in a pathological way. If thymine is added at this point, the cells do not die. The viable count remains constant for an additional 30 min., during which time the DNA approximately doubles. At this point 70 to 100 per cent of the cells rapidly divide; during division, DNA synthesis stopped. A second cycle of DNA synthesis and division quickly follows on the first cycle, as if to catch up with the excess cytoplasm which has been formed in the initial 60 minutes without division. Although synchrony is obscured in the second division, it has been observed to be more pronounced in the third and fourth cycles. No phasing of RNA synthesis has been observed in this system, although the phasing of both nucleic acids was obtained by Lark and Maaløe in bacteria synchronized by temperature shocks (6).

A duplication of DNA before the onset of division has been observed in many other systems, and it can be seen that in this respect these bacteria resemble plant and animal systems.

It is a very simple matter to establish this situation in this organism for purposes of correlating chemical and genetic events, since large cultures may be deprived of thymine and started instantly merely by the addition of the pyrimidine. At the present time we have used this system in two unrelated studies, and these are mentioned only to indicate some of the opportunities for study made available by such synchronized cultures. Synchronized cultures of 15_T- have been infected with T2 at several stages of division. The course of multiplication of the virus appeared to be independent of the stage of division of the host cells.

In study of the sedimentation behavior of extracts of bacteria at different stages of division, it was observed that a characteristic central component ($S_{20} = 22\text{-}24$) of the schlieren pattern disappears during division and is replaced by a new component ($S_{20} = 14$). The latter has not been observed under any other condition. Following division the new component disappeared, to be replaced by the familiar large polymer.

Fuerst and Stent (26) have used 15_T- for the specific incorporation of highly radioactive P^{32} in the presence and absence of thymine. The incorporation of P^{32} into both nucleic acids in the former case produced a high degree of lethality as a function of radioactive decay. In the latter case, only slightly less P^{32} entered the organisms and very little entered the DNA. In the latter case, radioactive decay was only about one quarter as effective in killing the organism.

Amino acid auxotrophs of strain 15_T- have also been isolated, and experiments have been begun on the separation of protein and DNA synthesis in these double mutants. For example, if bacteria possessing phenylalanine and thymine requirements are grown on a complete medium, it is possible to compare the effects of removing one or the other requirement, or of determining the effects of preincubation on the system. Some results of this type are summarized in Table 1.

TABLE 1

PERCENTAGE INCREMENT IN 60 MINUTES

	DNA	RNA	Protein
Normal growth	+137	+144	+133
$+T-\phi A$	+ 49	0	2
$-T+\phi A$	0	+116	+100
Preincubation with ϕA			
$+T-\phi A$	+ 77	0	+ 24
$-T+\phi A$	+ 11	+ 68	+ 44
$-T-\phi A$	0	0	+ 13
Preincubation with T			
$+T-\phi A$	+ 21	+ 20	+ 16
$-T+\phi A$	+ 18	+175	+ 90
$-T-\phi A$	+ 18	+ 17	+ 15

T = thymine; ΦA = phenylalanine.

It can be seen that in the presence of thymine and in the absence of amino acid the net synthesis of DNA may occur without any apparent synthesis of RNA. In such a system it is evidently important to reexamine this question from the point of view of the possible turnover of RNA. It is of interest that a 30-minute preincubation with phenylalanine permits an increased synthesis of DNA in the presence of thymine alone. In the absence of thymine, the presence of amino acid produces a joint synthesis of RNA and of protein, the synthesis of RNA always being disproportionately larger than that of protein.

It is difficult to say how much further we can go in separating the syntheses of DNA, protein, and RNA.[7] The easy manipulability of the specific nutritional deficiencies of these mutant organisms and the availability of various inhibitors such as chloramphenicol or 5-OH uridine suggest many obvious experiments. The performance of these experiments with synchronized cultures in specific stages of the division cycle will undoubtedly provide much new information on problems of integrated function and on the control of particular functions.

The Induction of Thymine Deficiency.

Bacteria, normally capable of synthesizing thymine, can be made incapable of this and other syntheses by cultivation in the presence of sulfanilamide (55) or of folic acid analogues such as Amethopterin (67). The folic acid deficiency of *E. coli* strain B, produced by sulfanilamide, can be partially replaced by a group of compounds containing essential one-carbon fragments. These compounds include methionine, serine, histidine, a purine derivative, several vitamins, such as pantothenate, and thymine. As shown in Fig. 7, the elimination of thymine from the fortified medium results in death, whereas elimination of the other compounds inhibits growth but does not kill (15, 17). In this manner, a bacteriostatic compound such as sulfanilamide can be converted into a bactericidal compound by limiting the specificity of the inhibition of synthesis to that of DNA synthesis, and thereby provoking unbalanced growth.

Having induced thymine deficiency and death as a consequence of unbalanced growth in organisms other than strain 15$_T-$, it seems reasonable to suppose that these organisms may similarly have their divisions synchronized and be converted to experimental material suitable for making correlations of various synthetic processes and biological function.

Thymine Analogues and the Synthesis of Abnormal DNA.

Another approach to the control of DNA synthesis has involved the use of thymine analogues. A fairly extensive literature on plant sys-

---

[7] A recent study of a methionine-requiring mutant of *E. coli* by Borek et al. (*J. Bacteriol.*, **71**, 318, 1956) has revealed that in the absence of methionine the organism will accumulate large amounts of RNA without synthesizing DNA or protein, and without leading to the death of the cell.

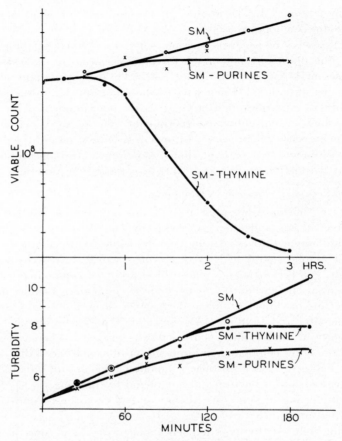

FIG. 7. Thymineless death in *E. coli* strain B, grown in sulfanilamide + essential nutrients.

tems has indicated that analogues such as 5-aminouracil, or even uracil itself, can induce chromosome breaks in onion root tips. When applied to bacteria several different types of effect of analogues have been observed. For example the inhibitor, 5-aminouracil, which is a thymine analogue, does not replace thymine in DNA. However, Dunn and Smith (23) have shown that, in the presence of aminouracil, a purine normally existing in very small amounts in the DNA of *E. coli* (6-methylamino purine) can be produced in considerable amounts and does replace thymine in the DNA structure. This phenomenon would also not appear to be explicable in terms of the Watson-Crick scheme of DNA synthesis.

If one of several 5-halogenated uracils, e.g., 5-bromouracil, is added to a medium in the presence of small amounts of thymine, growth and multiplication of the organism can occur in some cases. However, the bromouracil can now be built into the DNA up to a maximum of about 50 per cent of the thymine present, as shown by Dunn and Smith (22) and by Zamenhof (72).

In our studies of the effect of 5-bromouracil on strain 15_T-, the addition of bromouracil and thymine at a ratio of greater than 3 to 1 permits only a single division before the cells lose the power to multiply. In the absence of exogenous thymine, bromouracil inhibits killing slightly. Very long filaments are produced in which have been synthesized considerable RNA and a DNA containing bromouracil. Thus the use of thymine analogues leads frequently to the formation of pathological DNA, i.e., of DNA incapable of supporting chromosomal continuity or of fulfilling the role of a tape in the recording or transmission of genetic information.

The killing of 15_T- by bromouracil is more readily inhibited by thymidine than by thymine, although the growth rate of 15_T- is the same in the presence of thymine or of thymidine. In addition, the activity of thymidine in supporting growth is much more readily overcome by bromouracil deoxyriboside than by bromouracil. In this organism it would therefore appear that thymine is converted to the nucleoside level, thymidine, before formation of the nucleotide. Other strains of E. coli B, W, and 15, which do not appear to insert exogenous thymine into DNA, are not affected by even very large amounts of bromouracil deoxyriboside. Thus the inhibitor technique also appears to demonstrate the existence of alternative routes for the formation of thymine nucleotides, as discussed earlier.

Mode of Action of Some Bactericidal Treatments.

It is useful to scan a number of bactericidal treatments in terms of the observation that either the specific inhibition of DNA synthesis or the production of pathological DNA may lead to an irreversible damage to cell division. Such a survey is presented in Table 2. It can be seen that treatment with ultraviolet light, the nitrogen mustards, and penicillin alike produces a pathological pattern superficially very similar to that induced by thymine deficiency. Kanazir (40) has

TABLE 2

PROPERTIES OF BACTERIA UNDER CONDITIONS PRODUCING DEATH

Agent	Cell Size	Ribosenucleic Acid Synthesis	Deoxyribose-nucleic Acid Synthesis	Accumulated Products in Medium	Bacterial Activity
Thymineless death	Enlarged	Active	Inhibited	Uracil, orotic acid, hypoxanthine	Must metabolize and grow
Ultraviolet irradiation	Filamentous	Active	Inhibited	Deoxyribonucleotides, thymidylic acid	Must metabolize and grow
Nitrogen mustard	Filamentous	Active	Inhibited	?	?
Penicillin	Filamentous	Somewhat inhibited	?	Uracil nucleotides	Must metabolize and grow

observed that thymidylic acid is a major accumulated product in *E. coli* after low doses of ultraviolet irradiation which specifically inhibit DNA synthesis (41). Barner and I have shown that metabolism and growth must follow quickly on ultraviolet irradiation to reveal the potentially lethal lesion (3). Otherwise the absence of growth permits repair. The effects of nitrogen mustard on nucleic acid synthesis in *E. coli* have been described by Herriott (31); reactions of the nitrogen mustards with DNA have also been recorded. It must be acknowledged that the literature is quite obscure on the question of the specific effect of penicillin on nucleic acid synthesis. However, it is of considerable interest that penicillin (and streptomycin as well) kills only under conditions in which cell growth occurs. It may be suggested as a working hypothesis that each of these bactericidal treatments creates blocks specifically in the metabolic chain leading to DNA synthesis and that death in each instance is a consequence of unbalanced growth.

Inhibition of DNA Synthesis and Mutagenesis.

One view of mutagenesis postulates that mutations arise as an error in the duplication process. This fitted the findings that mutations could not be induced in isolated and inert virus preparations, as well as the view that nucleic acids and particularly DNA are inert in non-dividing cells. However, several workers have obtained the perplexing result that under certain conditions the mutation rate in *E. coli* is independent of the division time of the bacteria (24, 52). Spontaneous mutations have also been observed to occur in many types of non-dividing organisms (56).

In the study of Novick and Szilard (52) it was also shown that certain normal metabolites, such as adenosine, might act as anti-mutagens. Koch (43) has postulated that compounds, such as theophylline, which inhibit nucleoside phosphorylases, produce their mutagenic effect by affecting the intracellular concentrations of metabolites of nucleic acid metabolism. Fox (24) has elaborated the studies of Novick and Szilard, and has shown that mutation rates tend to be higher in complex media than in simple synthetic media. So-called spontaneous mutations are thus seen to be dependent on the nutrition and hence on the metabolic activity of the organism.

Two recent findings seem to bear most significantly on this problem. Zamenhof et al. (73) have found that bromouracil and thymine nucleotides can exchange in non-dividing bacteria, a finding which shows clearly that DNA can be metabolically active in the systems studied.

Coughlin and Adelberg (21) have found that the survivors of thymineless death (99% killing) in a thymineless-histidineless organism have a 100-fold increase in mutation rate, i.e., mutation may be induced in cells which cannot multiply because of the specific inhibition of DNA synthesis induced by a thymine deficiency. The increased number of reversions from histidineless to independence was shown not to be a selection process. Several pieces of evidence had previously seemed to suggest that the DNA of the bacterium was inert during unbalanced growth. The DNA did not change significantly in amount during thymine deficiency. Furthermore, analytical ultra-centrifugation of extracts of organisms killed by thymineless death revealed polymeric DNA in its usual position in the schlieren sedimentation pattern, and so indicated the absence of extensive degradation. Nevertheless, the genetic material of these thymine-deficient, non-dividing, growing cells is clearly not inert. Indeed one might imagine that the same kind of disruptive event which was lethal to 90 per cent of the cells per division time was also occurring to the DNA of the remainder of the cells. However, in the small surviving fraction the position of the lesion or repair permitted the organisms a non-lethal division.

Barner and I have observed that killing stops after the thymineless death of 10^5 cells in a population of 10^8 cells per ml. Only 1 to 2 per cent of the survivors are reversions to thymine independence. The remainder are predominantly slow-growing organisms. It may be asked to what extent these leaky mutations are induced by thymine deficiency.

This question is possibly of considerable practical significance. The folic acid analogue, Amethopterin, has been shown to inhibit the synthesis of DNA, and particularly that of thymine, in leukemic spleen to a much greater extent than the synthesis of RNA (1). The continuing treatment of leukemia and other tumors with Amethopterin usually fails with the appearance of Amethopterin-resistant cells. In the light of the mutagenesis induced by thymine deficiency, it must be asked if these resistant cells have arisen as a consequence of the selection of spontaneous mutations, or as a result of mutagenesis induced by the treatment itself. It should be noted that there is a considerable similarity in the chemotherapeutic effects of Amethopterin and that of radiation or of the nitrogen mustards which are known to be mutagens.

The implication that the stability of inheritance or the occurrence of mutations may be determined to some extent by nutritional techniques and more particularly by metabolic reactions concerned with nucleic acid synthesis is an additional incentive for the exploration of mechanisms of the synthesis and degradation of the nucleic acids. Of all known areas of biochemistry, that of nucleic acid structure and biosynthesis seems to hold the greatest possibilities in determining the present and future of cells. It appears likely that pragmatic achievements in the area of chemotherapy and mutagenesis have occurred by affecting one parameter or another of nucleic acid structure or biosynthesis. We shall undoubtedly see a considerable increase in our efforts to convert pragmatic achievement to a more consciously directed control of the nucleic acids and the cells which they influence. Although at the present time some people believe that our urgent problems are more likely to be aided by reserpine and phenobarbital than by thymine, we seem to be approaching a position wherein research on the nucleic acids will possess a significance for the future of Man greater than merely that of improving the lot of a few biochemists.

REFERENCES

 1. Balis, E., and Dancis, J., *Cancer Research,* **15**, 603 (1955).
 2. Barner, H., and Cohen, S. S., *J. Bacteriol.,* **68**, 80 (1954).
 3. Barner, H. D., and Cohen, S. S., *J. Bacteriol.,* **71**, 149 (1945).
 4. Barrington, L. F., and Kozloff, L. M., *Science,* **120**, 110 (1954).
 5. Brachet, J., and Szsfars, D., *Biochim. et Biophys. Acta,* **12**, 588 (1953).
 6. Bruce, V. G., Lark, G., and Maaløe, D., *Nature,* **176**, 563 (1955).
 7. Burton, K., *Biochem. J. (London),* **61**, 473 (1955).
 8. Cohen, S. S., *Cold Spring Harbor Symposia Quant. Biol.,* **12**, 35 (1947).
 9. Cohen, S. S., *J. Biol. Chem.,* **174**, 295 (1948).
10. Cohen, S. S., *Bacteriol. Revs.,* **13**, 1 (1949).
11. Cohen, S. S., *Nature,* **168**, 746 (1951).
12. Cohen, S. S., *Cold Spring Harbor Symposia Quant. Biol.,* **18**, 221 (1953).
13. Cohen, S. S., *Science,* **123**, 653 (1956).
14. Cohen, S. S., and Arbogast, R., *J. Exptl. Med.,* **91**, 607 (1950).
15. Cohen, S. S., and Barner, H. D., *Proc. Natl. Acad. Sci. U. S.,* **40**, 885 (1954).
16. Cohen, S. S., and Barner, H. D., *J. Bacteriol.,* **69**, 59 (1955).
17. Cohen, S. S., and Barner, H. D., *J. Bacteriol.,* in press.
18. Cohen, S. S., and Fowler, C. B., *J. Exptl. Med.,* **85**, 771 (1947).
19. Cohen, S. S., and Roth, L., *J. Bacteriol.,* **65**, 490, (1953).
20. Cohen, S. S., and Weed, L. L., *J. Biol. Chem.,* **209**, 789 (1954).
21. Coughlin, C., and Adelberg, E., *Nature,* in press.
22. Dunn, D. B., and Smith, J. D., *Nature,* **174**, 305 (1954).

23. Dunn, D. B., and Smith, J. D., *Nature,* **175**, 336 (1955).
24. Fox, M. S., *J. Gen. Physiol.,* **39**, 261 (1955).
25. Friedkin, M., and Roberts, D., *Federation Proc.,* **14**, 215 (1955).
26. Fuerst, C. R., and Stent, G. S., *J. Gen. Physiol.,* in press.
27. Gale, E. F., and Folkes, J. P., *Biochem. J. (London),* **53**, 493 (1953).
28. Goldstein, L., and Plaut, W., *Proc. Natl. Acad. Sci. U. S.,* **41**, 874 (1955).
29. Green, M., Lichtenstein, J., Barner, H., and Cohen, S. S., *Federation Proc.,* **15**, 265 (1956).
30. Grossman, L., and Visser, D., *J. Biol. Chem.,* **216**, 775 (1955).
31. Herriott, R., *J. Gen. Physiol.,* **34**, 761 (1951).
32. Hershey, A. D., *J. Gen. Physiol.,* **37**, 1 (1953).
33. Hershey, A. D., *Brookhaven Symposia Biol.,* **8**, 6 (1956).
34. Hershey, A. D., Burgi, E., Garen, A., and Melechen, N., *Carnegie Inst. Wash. Yearbook,* **54**, 216 (1955).
35. Hershey, A. D., and Chase, M., *J. Gen. Physiol.,* **36**, 39 (1952).
36. Hershey, A. D., Dixon, J., and Chase, M., *J. Gen. Physiol.,* **36**, 777 (1953).
37. Hershey, A. D., Garen, A., Frazer, D., and Hudis, J. D., *Carnegie Inst. Wash. Yearbook,* **53**, 210 (1954).
38. Jesaitis, M., and Goebel, W., *Cold Spring Harbor Symposia Quant. Biol.,* **18**, 205 (1953).
39. Joklik, W. K., *Brit. J. Exptl. Pathol.,* **33**, 368 (1952).
40. Kanazir, D., *Biochim. et Biophys. Acta,* **13**, 587 (1954).
41. Kanazir, D., and Errera, M., *Biochim. et Biophys. Acta,* **14**, 62 (1954).
42. Kellenberger, E., and Arber W., *Z. Naturforsch.,* **10 B**, 698 (1955).
43. Koch, A. L., and Lamont, W. A., *J. Biol. Chem.,* **219**, 189 (1956).
44. Kozloff, L. M., *Cold Spring Harbor Symposia Quant. Biol.,* **18**, 209 (1953).
45. Kozloff, L., and Henderson, K., *Nature,* **176**, 1169 (1955).
46. Kozloff, L. M., Knowlton, K., Putnam, F. W., and Evans, E. A., Jr., *J. Biol. Chem.,* **188**, 101 (1951).
47. Lanning, M., and Cohen, S. S., *J. Biol. Chem.,* **207**, 193 (1954).
48. Lanning, M., and Cohen, S. S., *J. Biol. Chem.,* **216**, 413 (1955).
49. Lesley, S. M., and Graham, A. F., *Can. J. Microbiol.,* **2**, 17 (1956).
50. Levinthal, C., *Rend. ist. lombardo sci., Pt. I,* **89**, 192 (1955).
51. Levinthal, C., and Fisher, H., *Biochim. et Biophys. Acta,* **9**, 419 (1952).
52. Novick, A., and Szilard, L., *Cold Spring Harbor Symposia Quant. Biol.,* **16**, 337 (1951).
53. Pardee, A. B., and Williams, I., *Arch. Biochem. and Biophys.,* **40**, 222 (1952).
54. Raff, R. N., and Cohen, S. S., *J. Bacteriol.,* **60**, 69 (1950).
55. Rutten, F. J., Winkler, K. C., and DeHaan, P. G., *Brit. J. Exptl. Pathol.,* **31**, 369 (1950).
56. Ryan, F. J., *Genetics,* **40**, 726 (1955).
57. Siminovitch, L., and Graham, A. F., *Can. J. Microbiol.,* **1**, 721 (1955).
58. Sinsheimer, R. L., *Science,* **120**, 551 (1954).
59. Spiegelman, S., Halvorson, H. O., and Ben-Ishae, R., in *Amino Acid Metabolism* (W. D. McElroy and B. Glass, eds.), p. 124, Johns Hopkins Press, Baltimore (1955).
60. Stent, G. S., and Fuerst, C. R., *J. Gen. Physiol.,* **38**, 441 (1955).
61. Stent, G. S., Jerne, N. K., and Sato, in press.
62. Streisinger, G., and Weigle, J., *Proc. Natl. Acad. Sci. U. S.,* in press; Sinsheimer, R., *Proc. Natl. Acad. Sci. U. S.,* in press.
63. Tomizawa, J., and Sunakawa, S., *J. Gen. Physiol.,* **39**, 553 (1956).
64. Volkin, E., *J. Am. Chem. Soc.,* **76**, 5892 (1954).

65. Volkin, E., and Astrachan, L., *Virology,* **2**, 149 (1956).
66. Wainwright, S., and Nevill, A., *J. Bacteriol.,* **71**, 254 (1956).
67. Webb, M., and Nickerson, W. J., *J. Bacteriol.,* **71**, 140 (1956).
68. Weed, L. L., and Cohen, S. S., *J. Biol. Chem.,* **192**, 693 (1951).
69. Weidel, W., *Z. Naturforsch.,* **6b**, 251 (1951).
70. Wisseman, C. L., Smadel, J. E., Hahn, F. E., and Hopps, H. E., *J. Bacteriol.,* **67**, 662 (1952).
71. Wyatt, G. R., and Cohen, S. S., *Biochem. J. (London),* **55**, 774 (1953).
72. Zamenhof, S., and Griboff, G., *Nature,* **174**, 306, 307 (1954).
73. Zamenhof, S., Reiner, B., DeGiovanni, R., and Rich, K., *J. Biol. Chem.,* **219**, 165 (1956).

RNA METABOLISM IN T2-INFECTED *ESCHERICHIA COLI* *

Elliot Volkin and L. Astrachan

Biology Division, Oak Ridge National Laboratory

A RECENT report (3) describes the ability of T2-infected *Escherichia coli* to incorporate labeled inorganic phosphate into ribonucleic acid (RNA). It was demonstrated that in this system, where DNA and protein synthesis proceed at a vigorous rate, some metabolic activity of RNA does occur despite the absence of RNA net synthesis. By the virtual elimination of uninfected bacteria before the addition of isotopic phosphate, and by the unambiguous identification of isotopically labeled RNA mononucleotides, we feel that these experiments are more conclusive than those reported previously and interpreted both for (1) and against (2) the concept of a metabolically active RNA in the host cell.

Three points of interest were evident from the data in this report (3). First, it was observed that whereas the increase in RNA-P^{32} content was approximately linear with time in synthetic medium, in peptone broth culture the extent of isotope incorporated into RNA leveled off very quickly. Second, it was noted that at very short time intervals after the addition of $P^{32}O_4$, the amount of isotope accumulated into RNA was at least as great as that found in DNA, the DNA representing the sole end-product of nucleic acid synthesis in this system. Finally, as a result of the analyses of alkali-produced RNA mononucleotides, it became evident that the isotope incorporation could not have resulted from a uniform activity of the host's total RNA. Thus significantly higher specific activities were found associated with adenylic and uridylic acids than those found in cytidylic and guanylic acids (Table 1).

Though other mechanisms may account for this last phenomenon, we have adopted the working hypothesis that a uniform synthesis of a minor species of RNA occurs, and the percentage of total radioactivity associated with each of the mononucleotides therefore reflects

* Work performed under USAEC Contract No. W–7405–eng–26.

TABLE 1

SPECIFIC ACTIVITIES OF RNA MONONUCLEOTIDES

Time after Infection (min.)	Peptone Broth Experiment				Synthetic Medium Experiment			
	Cytidylic Acid	Adenylic Acid	Uridylic Acid	Guanylic Acid	Cytidylic Acid	Adenylic Acid	Uridylic Acid	Guanylic Acid
10	6.1	9.5	12.3	5.9	2.2	3.5	4.1	2.3
15	5.8	9.3	11.3	6.3	3.7	7.4	7.0	4.3
30	5.5	8.0	8.5	5.0	7.8	11.6	12.9	7.7
60	5.8	8.3	9.7	5.8	13.0	20.1	22.6	11.9
120								

Values are (cts./sec.)/μg. of P. Bacteria in logarithmic growth were infected with an 11:1 input ratio of T2r⁺ in the peptone broth experiment, 22:1 in the synthetic medium experiment. Five minutes later, neutralized inorganic P³²O₄ was added. At this time the uninfected bacterial population had deceased from over 10⁸/ml. to well under 10⁴/ml. Aliquots of the cultures were removed at the times indicated, chemically fractionated, and the RNA mononucleotides produced by alkaline hydrolysis isolated by ion-exchange chromatography (3).

the base composition of this species. This concept has been borne out, at least qualitatively, by the results of an approach designed at direct isolation of the host cell's RNA-containing subcellular constituents (4). When enough time had elapsed for $P^{32}O_4$ to become incorporated into the infected cell, the bacteria were first fragmented by alumina grinding, and then two particulate components and a soluble portion of the extract were separated. The results of these experiments are shown in Table 2, whence it is evident that, in spite of quantitative uncertainties resulting from possible cross-contamination among fractions, labeling of the various RNA's in the host cell had occurred in a heterogeneous manner. In addition, it should be noted that the specific activity of the P_1 fraction, because of probable contamination with relatively less active P_2 and S fractions, must be a minimal value, and may, in fact, be many times as high.

The question arises as to the functional nature of the active RNA, since the T2 virus contains no RNA, and therefore no requirement exists for the net synthesis of this nucleic acid. The results in Table 1 might fall in line with the notion that some RNA-phosphorus may serve as a precursor to DNA-phosphorus. It can be seen that the specific activities of adenylic and uridylic acids are about $1\frac{1}{2}$ to 2 times as high as those of the cytidylic and guanylic acids and are therefore roughly in the same proportion to one another as the analogous mononucleotides of T2 DNA—18 cytidylic: 32 adenylic: 32 thymidylic: 18 guanylic acids (5). Although no definite conclusions can yet be made about a possible RNA to DNA precursoral relation, evidence shows that some of the host's RNA exhibits a biological turnover, i.e., synthesis and utilization (or degradation). If only a brief interval of P^{32} incorporation was allowed shortly after infection, it was observed that at the early time intervals the RNA quickly reached high levels of radioactivity, greatly exceeding the amounts entering the DNA. About 6 minutes after dilution of the isotope, the RNA isotopic content began a steady decrease, whereas the isotope continued to accumulate in the DNA. These observations are illustrated in Fig. 1, and the corresponding specific activity data of one such experiment are shown in Fig. 2. It should be mentioned that any conclusions based on a comparison of the specific activities of total RNA with DNA are probably useless, since the most active RNA of the host (P_1-RNA, described) contributes only a very small fraction of the cell total RNA-phosphorus. These experiments have revealed still

TABLE 2

P³² Incorporation in RNA of Subcellular Fractions

Fraction	Radioact. (tot. c./s.)	Percentage of Total Radioactivity	Phosphorus (tot. μg.)	Percentage of Total Phosphorus	Specific Activity
Peptone broth experiment (30 min.)					
P_1	3,950	21	25	3	158
P_2	5,350	27	550	72	10
S	9,990	52	188	25	56
DNA	(337,600)		(348)		(970)
Synthetic medium experiment (60 min.)					
P_1	3,450	12	12	4	286
P_2	5,570	18	173	59	32
S	20,900	70	107	37	196
DNA	(1,330,000)		(671)		(1990)

These experiments were carried out similarly to those described in Table 1, except that at the times indicated, the infected bacteria were collected by centrifugation, washed once with the corresponding isotope-free medium, then ground with alumina (4). Fraction P_1 represents the pellet collected from the extract by centrifuging at 20,000 g for 15 minutes, P_2 the pellet collected at 140,000 g for 90 minutes, and S the supernate remaining. The three fractions were then subjected to fractionation and mononucleotide separation as indicated previously. The values of the total DNA at these times are shown for comparison.

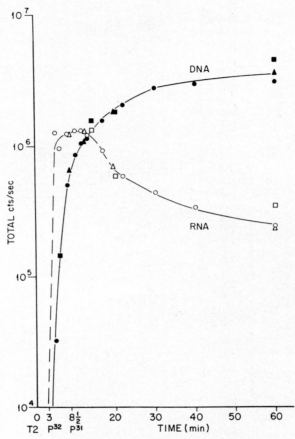

FIG. 1. *Isotope Content of RNA and DNA after Short P³²O₄ Pulse*

The figure represents data collected from three separate experiments, corresponding to the three different symbols. In order to reduce the initial phosphate concentration to a low level, peptone broth was largely depleted of inorganic phosphate by NH_4MgPO_4 precipitation. Tris(hydroxymethyl)aminomethane was added for buffering, and the medium adjusted to pH 8.0. The final inorganic phosphate concentration was about 6 μg./ml., the total phosphorus concentration about 10 μg./ml. Bacterial growth and killing by phage infection (input ratio about 10/1) proceeded normally in this medium. Isotopic phosphate was added at 3 minutes, and at 8½ minutes a 200-fold excess of phosphate buffer was added to virtually dilute out the P³². Analysis of aliquots was carried out in the usual fashion for total DNA and RNA mononucleotides.

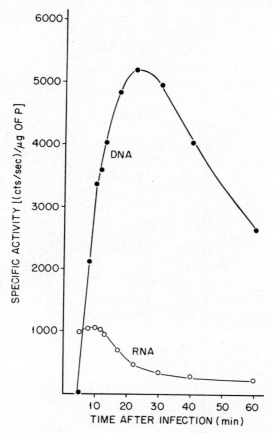

Fɪɢ. 2. *Specific Activities of RNA and DNA after a Short P³²O₄ Pulse*

The data are taken from one of the experiments illustrated in Fig. 1.

another aspect of the mode of isotope incorporation into, and loss from, the RNA mononucleotides. A comparison (Table 3) of the relative total radioactivities in the four RNA mononucleotides at various time intervals shows that such values gradually change during the period of isotopic loss from initial proportions of roughly 18 cytidylic: 30 adenylic: 30 uridylic: 22 guanylic, to values approaching those of the mononucleotide composition of bacterial RNA itself. Generally, the nature of the radioactive RNA disappearing between any adjacent time intervals corresponds to that of the species at the prior time.

TABLE 3

RNA Mononucleotide Ratio Variations with Time.

Ratios Based Solely on Total Radioactivity in Each Mononucleotide

	Experiment No.							
	1		2				3	
	Sampling Time (min.)							
	12.5	60	10	17	30	60	14	60
Cytidylic	18	21	18	18	22	25	18	24
Adenylic	29	27	33	30	27	25	30	25
Uridylic	29	27	29	29	27	22	30	24
Guanylic	24	25	20	23	24	28	22	27

Sample times selected from three experiments illustrated in Fig. 1. These values may be compared with the mononucleotide composition of *E. coli* total RNA—23 cytidylic:23 adenylic:23 uridylic:31 kuanylic (3).

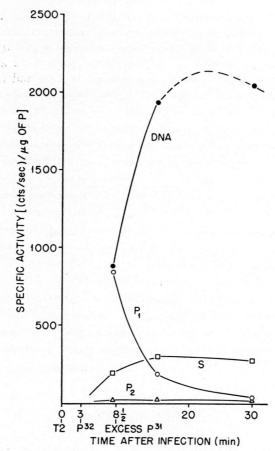

Fɪɢ. 3. *Rate of Depletion of Isotope from RNA Contained in Bacterial Subcellular Constituents. Short $P^{32}O_4$ Pulse Experiment*

Experiments were carried out in phosphate-depleted peptone broth as described in Fig. 1. The sample taken at 8 min. preceded by a half minute the 200-fold addition of excess phosphate buffer; the other two samples were taken at indicated times after dilution of P^{32} by phosphate buffer. Collection of the pellets and supernatant fraction (P_1, P_2, and S, respectively) was similar to that described in Table 2.

It is implicit in these findings that the isotopic turnover of the host's total RNA may be a summation of at least two types of RNA turnover: a more active type, similar to phage DNA in mononucleotide composition, and a relatively slower species, similar in composition to whole bacterial RNA. This concept was confirmed in part by an experiment in which the RNA's of the subcellular parts were analyzed, as described, at a period of short-term isotope feeding and twice subsequent to dilution of the isotope with excess phosphate buffer. Although the method was beset with some difficulties owing to rather extensive rupture and loss of infected cells during centrifugal collection, and as a consequence material balance data were of questionable value, the data, shown in Fig. 3, could be compared with regard to specific activities of the three RNA's. It is seen that only the P_1-RNA loses radioactivity at a rapid rate, the loss from S fraction being considerably slower, while the P_2-RNA remains relatively inert.

As a result of these studies, it can be stated that biological turnover of some part of the host cells' RNA indeed exists. As yet, however, these findings are too incomplete to establish whether the RNA is directly concerned in the pathway of phage DNA synthesis. Whatever its function, the fact that phosphate incorporation into the RNA appears to precede that entering the DNA raises the question of whether the infecting phage particle exerts genetic influence not only on viral DNA synthesis, but on host RNA synthetic processes, as well.

It is a pleasure to acknowledge the technical assistance of Miss Martha H. Jones.

REFERENCES

1. Hershey, A. D. Nucleic acid economy in bacteria infected with bacteriophage T2. II. Phage precursor nucleic acid. *J. Gen. Physiol.*, **37**, 1-23 (1953).

2. Manson, L. A. The metabolism of ribonucleic acid in normal and bacteriophage-infected *Escherichia coli*. *J. Bacteriol.*, **66**, 703-711 (1953).

3. Volkin, E., and Astrachan, L. Phosphorus incorporation in *Escherichia coli* ribonucleic acid after infection with bacteriophage T2. *Virology*, **2**, 149-161 (1956).

4. Volkin, E., and Astrachan, L. Intracellular distribution of labeled RNA after phage infection of *E. coli*. *Virology*, **2**, 433-437 (1956).

5. Wyatt, G. R. The quantitative composition of deoxypentose nucleic acids as related to the newly proposed structure. *Cold Spring Harbor Symposia Quant. Biol.*, **18**, 133-134 (1953).

Discussion

Dr. Kornberg: I would like to ask one question with respect to Dr. Volkin's presentation. In calculating the base composition of the RNA, isn't there an alkaline hydrolysis, so that the phosphate of a nucleotide in the hydrolyzate doesn't necessarily belong to the nucleotide from which it would originate, assuming that 5'-nucleotides are the originating groups?

Dr. Volkin: That is correct. We assumed, however, that the labeled RNA in this system might originate by de novo synthesis of a single RNA molecular species from a single pool of $P^{32}O_4$, whereby all the phosphorus in this "active" molecule would have the same specific activity. If this assumption is correct, it seems to me that the base composition of this RNA can be calculated from the relative total activities of the resultant mononucleotides, whether these are produced by alkaline hydrolysis or as 5'-nucleotides by enzymatic hydrolysis.

Dr. Potter: Aren't you just saying that the RNA is converted into DNA without breaking up?

Dr. Volkin: No. We don't really have any evidence for that. The only thing we can say is that, if our calculated base composition of the "active" RNA is valid, it is rather close to the composition of the analogous nucleotides in phage DNA.

Part VII

MECHANISM OF DUPLICATION

ON THE MECHANISM OF DNA REPLICATION

Max Delbruck

California Institute of Technology, Pasadena

and

Gunther S. Stent *

Virus Laboratory, University of California, Berkeley

Our discussion of the mechanism of DNA replication will center on bacteriophages, which have been the object of most of the very few experimental attacks on this problem. We believe it to be not unlikely, furthermore, that experiments on DNA replication more decisive than those which we can discuss at this time will likewise be carried out with bacteriophages.

The double-stranded, helical DNA molecules of an infecting bacteriophage particle enter the bacterial host cell and generate several hundred replicas identical to themselves to furnish the DNA duplexes with which the progeny virus particles are to be endowed. We ask: How are different deoxyribose nucleotide building blocks copolymerized into macromolecules in an order identical to the specific nucleotide sequence of the DNA introduced by the parent virus? The complementary arrangement of the purine and pyrimidine bases of the two polynucleotide chains of DNA suggested to Watson and Crick (41) that the DNA macromolecule replicates itself directly by having each chain serve as a template for the formation of its complement. The two strands of the original duplex were thought to separate and each base to attract a complementary free nucleotide already available for polymerization within the cell. These free nucleotides, whose phosphate groups probably already possess the free energy necessary for polyesterification, would then link up with one another after being held in place by the parental template chain to form a new polynucleotide molecule of the required nucleotide sequence.

* Research supported by grants from the National Cancer Institute of the National Institutes of Health, U. S. Public Health Service, and from The Rockefeller Foundation.

Topology of the DNA Duplex

The intertwining of the two polynucleotide chains of the DNA duplex, however, presents an obstacle to their separation which must be overcome if such a macromolecule is to act as a template for replication in the manner proposed by Watson and Crick, or in fact, for replication by any other mechanism in which the "information" contained by the original DNA is "read off" through growth of a second macromolecule making contact with the purine-pyrimidine base pairs of the duplex. We propose to discuss first the problems posed by this fact and to begin by a definition of what is meant by the "winding" of the duplex.

We imagine a finite length of the duplex (Fig. 1, a). The upper ends

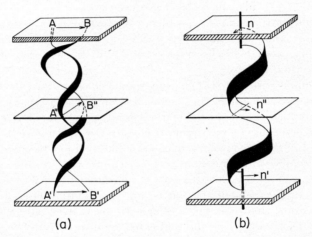

(a)   (b)

FIG. 1. *Definition of the "winding number."*

(a) Point A is fixed exactly above point A', and B above B'. The vector A"B" connects the intersection points of the two chains with a plane which moves down from the upper to the lower board. During this travel the vector executes an integral number of turns which is invariant under any distortion of the chains which leaves the ends fixed. This number is the "winding number."

(b) The vector n is the projection of the normal to the strip onto the moving plane. Its number of turns is the invariant "winding number" of the strip.

of the chains are tied to a board and the lower ends to another board precisely under the upper end. We will further assume without loss of generality that the duplex lies between the two fixed boards in such a manner that any horizontal plane between the two boards intersects each chain only once. We will then draw in each of these planes the vector from the intersection point of chain A to the intersection point of chain B. This vector has in no plane length zero. As we travel down the duplex, the vector will rotate, generally in a clockwise direction (as viewed from above), and its end position will coincide with the initial position. Its total travel will correspond to a *finite* and *integral* number of turns. This number is an *invariant under any distortion of the chains which leaves the ends fixed* and this invariant we define as the *winding number* of the particular length of duplex. It amounts to 150 per million molecular weight of DNA. For any winding number greater than zero, the "braid" consisting of the two chains cannot be "combed," and the chains cannot be separated laterally from each other without breaks (1).

If we imagine that replication does not involve any separation of the two chains of the duplex but rather that the daughter duplex is synthesized *de novo*, using the whole parental DNA duplex as a template for the formation of either the daughter duplex directly or of a non-DNA intermediary which later synthesizes the daughter duplex, the topological situation remains unchanged. In this case we note that the parental template can be represented as a twisted strip, i.e., a surface bounded by two closely adjacent lines (Fig. 1, b). As we travel down along the strip, the projection of the normal to this surface onto a horizontal plane will rotate similarly to the vector connecting the two chains in the preceding analysis, and the winding number of the strip is the same as the winding number of the two chains defined above. If we now postulate that the daughter duplex or the hypothetical intermediary is synthesized always on the same side of the parent strip, then the parent and daughter duplex, or the parent duplex and the intermediary, will have a winding number relative to each other identical to that of the two chains of the parent duplex, and the separation of the parent from the daughter duplex or from the intermediary will run into the same topological difficulty as the separation of the two chains of the parent duplex.

Watson and Crick (41) enumerated, and to some extent discussed the possible ways of meeting this difficulty:

(1) The Watson-Crick structure of DNA is wrong, specifically with respect to the winding number.

(a) The duplex consists of short sections of alternating positive and negative winding numbers. This possibility has been rejected by

Watson and Crick on the grounds that, for stereochemical reasons, they found it impossible to construct a model involving left-handed helices.

(b) DNA occurs in reality not as a very long duplex but in the form of short sections built according to Watson and Crick, alternating with short sections of non-DNA material twisted in a complementary fashion. This seems to be completely ruled out by chemical evidence.

(c) The Watson-Crick structure is completely wrong, in the sense that the real winding number is zero for even the shortest section. It is indeed possible to wind two chains approximately helically around the same axis and at the same time wind them around each other in a compensating fashion. The resulting configuration has been called a "paranemic coil" (because the chains will be parallel to each other when stretched) (19) in contrast to the "plectonemic" coil of the Watson-Crick structure (involving "plexi" or knots). This alternative was discussed by Watson and Crick (41), and completely ruled out on the basis of the x-ray diffraction evidence. We may, therefore, ignore the revival of this idea in a later paper (14) which makes no reference to this discussion and to the arguments against this structure.

(2) The separation of the chains occurs by pulling them past each other longitudinally. If this is to be done without a continuous twisting motion, it implies an inconceivable internal flexibility and presents many mechanical difficulties.

(3) The separation of the chains occurs by unwinding. The chief reason for hesitating to accept the topologically simple solution of unwinding the two threads is that it involves a very large number of turns, and that *for each turn to be unwound, essentially the whole mass of the duplex has to be rotated one complete turn around its axis.* To resolve a difficulty which seems to be a local one involving only the immediate neighborhood of the point where the interlock takes place, the whole mass of the duplex, involving many thousand chain links, has to be moved through distances at least comparable to the diameter of the duplex. In the limit of an infinitely long duplex this would clearly lend to excessive energy requirements *per turn.* It is therefore of interest that Levinthal and Crane (pers. commun.) have made calculations of the mechanical aspects of unwinding and have arrived at encouraging answers. They derive a formula for the energy needed to rotate one full turn a cylinder of length L, radius R, with an angular speed of n turns per second, in a medium of viscosity η.

This energy is

$$E/\text{turn} = 16\pi^3 L R^2 \eta n$$

If we substitute here $L = .006$ cm., $R = 10^{-7}$ cm., $n = 200$ sec.$^{-1}$, values corresponding to the whole length of the DNA of a large phage and of its likely speed of replication, and take $\eta = 4$ cp., we obtain a value of 2×10^{-13} erg, or 150 cal. per mole of replicated chain link, still small compared to the total energy required for the formation of the phosphate diester linkage of the polynucleotide chain. This calculation refers to a straight rod. The actual shape of the DNA will of course not be straight, but bent, folded, and coiled to fit into the volume in which it has to operate (the length of the DNA of phage T2 straightened out is about 60 times the diameter of the bacterium in which it replicates). How will such a snake react to a twisting torque applied at one end, when it is moving in a viscous medium? Levinthal and Crane argue very plausibly that it will rotate like a speedometer cable, that is, without flopping, since any off-axis motions would enormously increase the viscous drag. They calculate further that the torque needed to produce this twist at the needed speed would produce only a negligible stretch in the chemical bonds to which it would be applied. Let us now look at this hypothetical untwisting mechanism a little more closely. Levinthal and Crane, like most other authors, assume that the untwisting which leads to separation of the two chains goes hand-in-hand with the replication process, so that we would have at a certain moment in this process a "Y"-shaped configuration (Fig. 2). As untwisting and replication proceed downwards all three arms of the Y have to rotate in a clockwise direction as seen from the foot of the Y, at a rate of, say 200 turns per second. Presumably the motor keeping this maneuver in motion would be located in the "working section" of the system, where the synthesis takes place, in the crotch of the Y. It is likely that a torque would be present tending to twist the two upper arms of the Y around each other, but without a much more detailed picture of the processes in the working section it would be difficult to predict how many relational twists between the two arms would result.

The calculations for the "speedometer-cable" rotation of the DNA duplex can also be applied to those replication schemes in which the chains do not separate at all and in which the *intact* duplex serves as a template. As we have seen, in this case parent and daughter duplex or parent duplex and intermediary become intertwined in the course

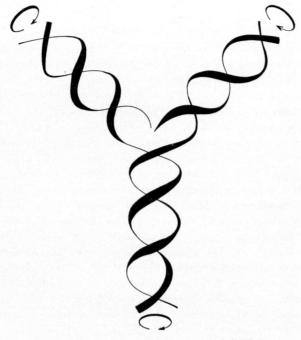

Fig. 2. *The scheme of Watson and Crick.*
Unwinding and replication proceed *pari passu*. All three arms of the Y rotate as indicated.

of replication and must finally be unwound to achieve their separation. The mechanical considerations and energy requirements of such unwinding would be very similar to those made by Levinthal and Crane.

Platt (30) has proposed a different mechanism of unwinding. In this scheme, unwinding of the chains of the parental duplex and replication are separate and alternating events. The untwisting is imagined to occur as a "transfer twist" (Fig. 3) by assuming that the original duplex has an inversion point in the middle such that the two halves of *each* chain to the right and left of this point are complementary to each other. If this is the case, then the chains of the original duplex can be separated by pulling sideways at the inversion point and twisting each chain upon itself. Replication is then imagined as a process in which this self-winding is reversed, involving two Y-shaped configurations and a process identical to that described in Fig. 2. Both during the untwisting and during the replication each arm of the four-

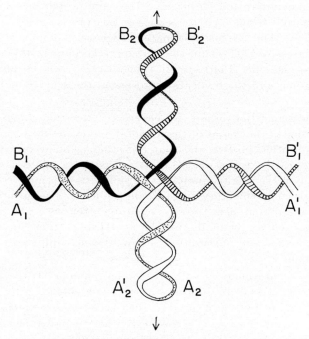

Fig. 3. *(a) The scheme of Platt, involving "transfer-twist."*

Untwisting of the parental duplex and replication are alternate events. Only the untwisting of the parental duplex is shown here. Replication occurs exactly as in Fig. 2.

The parental duplex consists of two chains, $A_1A_2A_2'A_1'$ and $B_1B_2B_2'B_1'$. The section A_1A_2 is complementary to $A_1'A_2'$, and similarly for the other chain. The original chains are separated by "transfer-twist," involving rotations of the four arms of the star-shaped figure in the directions indicated.

(b) The scheme of Butler.

The parental duplex consists of the two chains B_1B_2 and $B_1'B_2'$. The contraction of histone molecules attached to B_1 and B_2 pulling to left and right respectively, causes the duplex to unwind. Daughter chains A_1A_2 and $A_1'A_2'$ complementary to B_1B_2 and $B_1'B_2'$ respectively are then formed. Upon completion of replication, histone molecules attached to B_2B_2' and A_2A_2' contract in the direction of the arrows, causing the parental chains B_1B_2 and $B_1'B_2'$ as well as the daughter chains A_1A_2 and $A_1'A_2'$ to rewind about each other to generate one entirely old and one entirely new duplex.

armed or three-armed star will continually rotate, similarly to the model of Levinthal and Crane, and the same arguments concerning the energy and torque requirements for this process apply as in the other model. The ad hoc assumption of a self-complementarity of the two halves of each chain thus produces no gain in the simplicity of the process, since Platt's replication process alone is identical to the unwinding *and* the replication process in the scheme of Levinthal and Crane.

(4) The separation occurs by enzymatic digestion. It is possible that only one of the chains of the parental duplex actually participates in the replication process and that the other chain is digested away before replication takes place. In that case, the single chain could conceivably serve as a template for the synthesis of a number of either identical or complementary single-chain replicas not necessarily intertwined with it and hence easily separable from it. These replicas would later act as templates for the synthesis of their own complementary chains for "maturation" into "resting" duplexes (Watson, pers. commun.).

(5) The separation occurs by breaks and reunions. If the interlocks are to be resolved not by rotations of the whole duplex or by digestion of one chain, but by a local process, then breaks and reunions must be invoked. An interlock can be resolved either by breaking one of the chains, passing the other one through, and rejoining the original break, or by breaking both chains and rejoining them crosswise (Fig. 4). The first process is unattractive because it introduces an asymmetry between the two chains; the second process is impossible in the present case because it would involve rejoins between chains of opposite polarity. A more reasonable process has been envisaged by Delbrück (10) by imagining the breaks and rejoins to occur pari passu with replication (Fig. 5). One may imagine that both chains of the parental duplex break approximately at the same time and that their lower terminals rejoin with the free terminals of the replicate chains of equal polarity. The upper terminals of the broken chains now become the free terminals at which replication continues. It has to be postulated that this maneuver occurs on the average once every half turn of the parental duplex, i.e., every five links. The principal implication of such a scheme is that the parental material is very uniformly distributed at each replication. Each chain in each daughter duplex consists of very short alternate sections of old and new material.

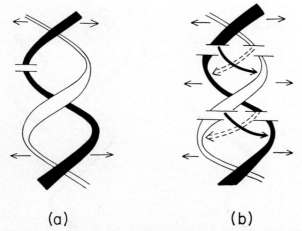

(a)   **(b)**

FIG. 4. *Two methods of resolving an interlock between two chains by breaks and reunions.*

(a) By breaking one chain and passing the other through the gap. One break per interlock. The process is asymmetric.

(b) By breaking both chains at each overlap (each half turn:) and rejoining them crosswise. Four breaks are needed to resolve one interlock. Chains of opposite polarity are joined.

The schemes here discussed probably exhaust the simple alternatives for resolving the intertwining of the plectonemic DNA duplex. On a priori grounds we have little reason to choose between them.

DISTRIBUTION OF PARENTAL ATOMS

An important operational distinction between different DNA replication mechanisms is their prediction concerning the distribution of the atoms of the parental molecule over the replica duplexes. The considerable number of proposed schemes may be divided into three general classes as *conservative, semi-conservative,* and *dispersive* replication (Fig. 6).

(a) *Conservative* mechanisms are those which do not destroy the integrity of the entire parental DNA duplex in the course of the replication process, so that among the daughter duplexes produced by one or more replications there is one which is entirely parental and the rest entirely new. This would be true, for instance, if DNA were replicated indirectly through the intermediary of another substance (33), e.g., protein or RNA, which is first synthesized on the surface of the intact

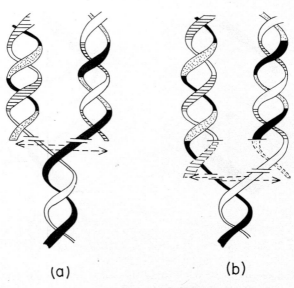

FIG. 5. *The scheme of Delbrück.*

Separation is accomplished by breaks and rejoins. Separation and replication occur pari passu. The process proceeds from the top down. At each half turn of progress the old chains break and the lower terminals of the breaks are joined to the free ends of the new chains of equal polarity. Two such moments of changing connections are shown (a, b). Between these moments replication has progressed one half turn. The old chains are black and white, respectively. The new sections complementary to black are striped, those complementary to white are dotted.

parental duplex and then serves as a template for the synthesis of daughter DNA duplexes. The mechanisms proposed by Bloch (3) and by Butler (9), in which the parental duplex as a whole serves as a direct template for the production of a daughter duplex, likewise fall into this class. Bloch imagines that the parental duplex undergoes a change of structure, in which the bases of the parental chains rotate approximately through an angle of 180° around their glycosidic bonds, while the backbones are held rigidly in position by their attachment to a histone (Fig. 7). The bases then face in such a way as to form a template in the shape of a twisted strip on which a complementary duplex structure might form. The replication of the histone, of course, would have to go hand-in-hand with the replication of DNA. Bloch's scheme implies, therefore, an obligatory parallel synthesis of histone and DNA. Butler proposes (see Fig. 3) that the two chains of the

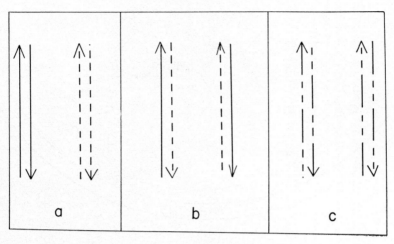

Fɪɢ. 6. *The distribution of parental material between the daughter duplexes.*

(a) Conservative: One daughter duplex old, one new.

(b) Semi-conservative: In each daughter duplex one chain is old and one is new.

(c) Dispersive: The distribution of parental material is uniform through the four chains of the two daughter duplexes.

duplex are first separated by unwinding through a contractile action of histone molecules attached to one of their ends. The single chains then form complementary chains, after which the two parental chains and the two daughter chains are rewound about each other by the counter-contraction of other histone molecules to form one parental and one daughter duplex.

(b) *Semi-Conservative* mechanisms are those which conserve the atomic identity of *single chains* of the parental DNA duplex, although effecting a permanent separation of the two chains from each other in the course of replication. This is the original suggestion of Watson and Crick and certainly the one most obviously suggested by their structure. One imagines that the chains are separated and that each serves as a template for the formation of a complementary chain. This scheme unites the chemically most reasonable process of complement formation and the biologically most fundamental process of replication in an appealing manner. If we imagine a population of duplexes originating in one duplex and replicating in a synchronized manner through n steps, we will have in the end 2^{n+1} duplexes. According to the scheme now under discussion, in each duplex of the final genera-

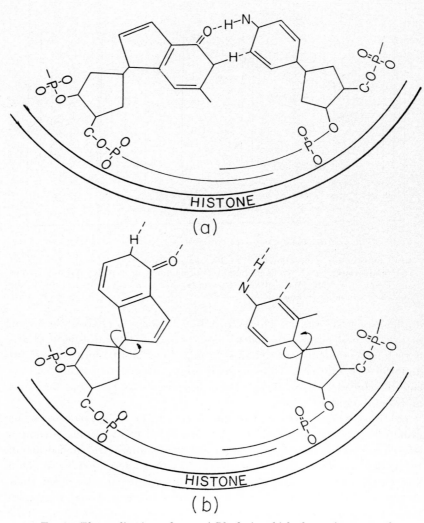

FIG. 7. *The replication scheme of Bloch, in which the entire parental*
duplex is used as a template.

(a) Cross-section through the parental duplex in its standard configuration.

(b) The bases have rotated 180° around the indicated bonds and the whole structure now forms a template in the form of a twisted strip. The template is held in shape by a backbone histone.

tion one chain will be of age zero. Of the complementary chains one half will be of age one, one quarter of age two, and so on. If it were possible to label differently the new material synthesized in each generation, then one could read off in each duplex the ages of the two chains. One of them must be age zero, and the other any age m with probability 2^{-m}.

(c) *Dispersive* mechanisms are those which do not conserve the atomic integrity of the chains of the parental duplex but result in the dispersion of its atoms among the replica duplexes. The scheme proposed by Delbrück (10), which involves numerous breaks in the original chains, falls into this class. Each chain in every daughter duplex consists of alternating sections of old and new material, all the old material in any one chain deriving from the parental chain of equal polarity. Under this scheme, it is meaningless to identify parental and daughter chains: each chain is partly old and partly new.

Any schemes, furthermore, which envision that the parental DNA duplex is broken down into low molecular weight substances as it is being replicated and that allow the breakdown products to be re-utilized in the synthesis of daughter duplexes can likewise be classified as dispersive.

Unambiguous experimental tests of the actual distribution of the atoms of the parental DNA molecule could thus eliminate a considerable fraction of potential replication mechanisms, and would permit us to focus our attention on a more restricted class.

GENETIC RECOMBINATION AND DISTRIBUTION OF PARENTAL ATOMS

Before considering the evidence relevant to the distribution of parental DNA atoms after replication gathered from experiments with bacteriophage, it is necessary to discuss genetic recombination, a phenomenon associated with replication whose possible effects on this distribution may be superimposed on those inherent in replication. If two related bacteriophage particles differing in some genetic markers infect the same bacterial cell, recombinant virus progeny issue whose genome is derived in part from one and in part from the other parent. These recombinants appear to arise in successive rounds of random *matings* between vegetative, i.e., actively multiplying, phages. In the case of the coli bacteriophages T2 and T4, it can be estimated that the *number* of such rounds of mating is about equal to the number of successive rounds of replication which must occur in order to produce the requisite number of progeny DNA units (39). In other words, the vegetative phages appear to mate as often as they replicate. If now that part of the vegetative phages which is involved in the genetic recombination process is DNA, a notion for which there is actually as yet no experimental proof, it is apparent that the frequent recombinations could affect the final distribution of the parental DNA atoms and must be reckoned with when one desires to conclude from experimental observations whether replication is conservative, semi-conservative, or dispersive. Two circumstances make it unlikely that replication of the DNA of bacteriophage T2 can ever be observed in the absence of recombination. One of these is that even in single infection "incestuous" matings may occur between the parental phage and its own vegetative descendants and the other is that at the end of the eclipse phase, at the earliest time when any progeny phages can be examined, two to three rounds of mating have already taken place.

If mating and replication are independent processes, then recombinants would have to be produced by mating of already formed vegetative phages through breaks and crossover rejoins (Fig. 8, a). Such recombination would lead to the destruction of the atomic identity of the parental DNA, which would become progressively more *fragmented* the more matings it has experienced with other vegetative phages.

The results of more detailed genetic studies of the phage recombination mechanism, however, favor the view that there *is* a connection between recombination and replication (24, 20, 4) and that recombinants arise through what has been called "partial replicas" (16) or, more appropriately "copying choice" (22) (Fig. 8, b). The copying choice hypothesis envisions that a recombinant vegetative phage is formed *incidentally* to its replication, if a partially synthesized replica growing along one parental template switches over and continues its growth along another, nearby parental template. In order for such switching to produce the observed genetic results, the two templates must enter into a specific union, i.e., they must *mate* during the replication act so that homologous genetic regions are in perfect molecular apposition. The principal genetic support for this view is derived from the finding that opposite recombinants, though produced with equal frequency, do not appear to arise from the same elementary recombination act.

In contrast to simple crossing-over, which necessarily demands fragmentation of the parental DNA during recombination, a copying-

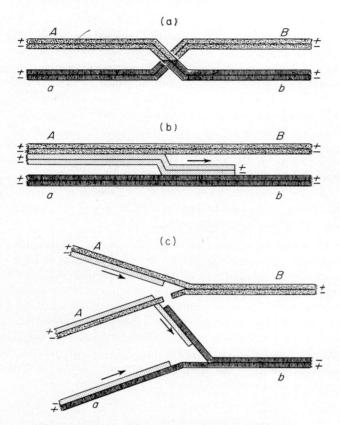

FIG. 8. *Three mechanisms of genetic recombination.*

A and B represent two genetic loci and a and b their alleles. $(+)$ and $(-)$ signify the opposite polarity of the two chains of the DNA duplex.

(a) Fragmenting crossing-over. Two parental duplexes synapse, break between A and B and between a and b, and heterologous pieces rejoin.

(b) Non-fragmenting copy-choice. Conservative replication (in the direction of arrow) generates entire daughter duplex, using first one and then the other of two mated duplexes as template. The switchover occurs between A and B.

(c) Fragmenting copy-choice. Semi-conservative replication (in the direction of the arrows) by complement formation to single strands as parent duplexes unwind. Single daughter chain grows complementary to single parent chain of one of two mated duplexes, then switches over between A and B to continue growth complementary to single chain of second duplex. Parent chains break near switchover point to permit daughter duplexes to separate.

choice mechanism may be non-fragmenting, since the integrity of the template could conceivably remain undisturbed whether a replica being copied along it has switched over to another template or not (Fig. 8, b). There are also copying-choice mechanisms of recombination which *do* involve fragmentation of the parental DNA. For instance, it would appear that copying-choice recombination would produce fragmentation if replication occurs through the original Watson-Crick scheme of pari passu unwinding and complement formation to single chains. In this case, the structural deadlock produced by the switching of the growing replica chain from one duplex to the next could be resolved only by breakage of one of the parental chains in each of the mated duplexes (Fig. 8, c). It may be stated, therefore, that under the copying-choice hypothesis non-fragmenting *or* fragmenting recombination could occur.

The principal result of this discussion is the realization that the only experimental result capable of an unambiguous interpretation is one in which the integrity of either the entire parental DNA duplex, or of each of its polynucleotide chains separately, is found to have survived many successive rounds of replication and recombination. In that case, it may be inferred that replication proceeds by either a conservative or semi-conservative mechanism and that recombination, if it involves participation of DNA molecules, is due to non-fragmenting copying-choice. If the results are not this simple, it will be very much harder to draw conclusions.

Transfer Experiments with Bacteriophage

A great deal of effort has been spent during the last six years to obtain clues concerning replication through isotopic tracer experiments on the multiplication of bacteriophages. The principal advantage of this system resides in the small size and hence simplicity of the DNA unit whose replication is being studied, since one T2 phage particle contains only of the order of 10^{-13} mg. DNA, compared with 10^{-11} mg. of DNA per nucleus of its bacterial host or 10^{-10} mg. DNA per mammalian chromosome. A second advantage of phage T2 is the ease with which it lends itself to tracer experiments. Since nearly all of the phage phosphorus is in nucleic acid, one can be sure that if a phage particle is labeled with P^{32} the tracer resides exclusively in DNA. The experiments which we shall now consider are of the following sort:

A uniformly labeled phage population is prepared by infection of bacteria growing in labeled medium. This phage population, which has been freed from extraneous material by certain purification procedures, is the *parental* generation. The parental phage is then used to infect unlabeled bacteria growing in unlabeled medium to obtain a *first progeny* generation, which may be similarly purified and analysed for its label, or it may be used for infection and production of its own *second generation* progeny. The analysis concerns two distinct points, which are highly relevant to our discussion. First, the total amount of label *transferred* from the labeled parent to the progeny, second, the *distribution* of the transferred label among the progeny particles.

Efficiency of Transfer.

Putnam and Kozloff (32) were the first to study the transfer of P^{32} from parental DNA to the progeny DNA. Their experiments, as well as those of many subsequent workers, have given transfer values of 30-50 per cent. Kozloff (21) extended these findings to the transfer of isotopically labeled DNA *nitrogen,* and Watson and Maaløe (42) to the transfer of C^{14}-labeled adenine, with similar results. The non-transferred fraction of the parental DNA label is mostly released by the infected bacteria along with the progeny phages as either low molecular weight, i.e., "acid-soluble," material or as free DNA (12, 40).

The finding that the transfer is incomplete raises the possibility that it might be unspecific. It is conceivable that the replication mechanism as such involves no transfer at all, but that some of the input DNA is degraded and unspecifically reincorporated. That this type of transfer can occur was demonstrated by Watson and Maaløe (42), who performed experiments in which bacteria were mixedly infected with unlabeled T4 and labeled T3. Phage T3 is unrelated to T4, and in such mixed infections no T3 particles are produced. They found that some of the label of T3 was transferred to the T4 progeny. In this case the T3, which does not transfer its genetic information, is presumably degraded and its label unspecifically reincorporated. A similar breakdown of genetically non-contributing material occurs probably in most cases of multiple infection, particularly if the individual infections are spaced within a few minutes (23). In the case of single infection there is certainly less of this breakdown, but it cannot be excluded. Another conceivable interpretation of the incomplete transfer might be that the phage DNA consists of two portions, one of which is transferred intact, while the other is not transferred at all, or only slightly and unspecifically. If this were correct, then the label in the first generation progeny should be enriched in the specific part, and a second generation transfer experiment should give a higher transfer value. Maaløe and Watson (28) carried out such a second generation transfer experiment and obtained the result that the transfer is neither increased nor decreased. This experiment has been recently extended by Stent, Jerne, and Sato (unpub.) to a third-generation transfer, with similar results. These observations can be schematized as follows:

Parent (label = 100) → 1st progeny (label = 50) →
2nd progeny (label = 25) → 3rd progeny (label = 12).

They indicate that the DNA which is transferred neither originates from a preferentially transferable part which remains intact nor winds up preferentially in a part which is preferentially lost in the next infection. It would appear, rather (although the above experiments do not rigorously prove it), that the incomplete transfer of T2 DNA to its progeny is due to random losses experienced by the entire parental DNA in the course of the infection, replication, and maturation processes. The observation that the purine and pyrimidine base composition of the transferred DNA is identical to that of the infecting phage (17) supports this notion. Finally, the fact that in the case of the *Salmonella* phage P22 the DNA transfer from parent to progeny can be as high as 80 per cent (Garen, pers. commun.) suggests that the absolute magnitude of the percentage of transfer does not reflect some basic aspect of the DNA replication mechanism. We conclude, therefore, that the phage DNA does not consist of two portions differing with respect to their transferability.

Distribution of Transferred DNA.

We now turn to the experimental attempts to get at the *distribution* of the transferred label among the progeny particles. Early experiments (12, 42) utilized the fact that the early crop of progeny can be singled out from the phage particles produced in a single bacterium. Although the whole crop produced by any one bacterium is released at the moment of lysis, this lysis can be provoked prematurely, or it can be delayed beyond its normal term. The picture that we have of the intracellular events of phage growth is this: the phage multiplies in a state in which it is not infective, the vegetative state. After a certain amount of vegetative multiplication has taken place, and a "pool" of vegetative particles has been established, some vegetative particles mature to become infective particles, and the maturing particles are, it seems, drawn at random from the vegetative pool (37). The early experiments just referred to compared the transferred label in the crop which had matured early to the total transfer, and demonstrated that most of the transfer went to the early crop. In view of what has just been said about the over-all kinetics of replication and maturation, this result is perfectly reasonable. One must expect on any scheme for the elementary replication process that the label in the pool would be gradually diluted. This finding, therefore, although we can understand it, does not help us to clarify the elementary replication process.

The real distribution of the transferred parental DNA over the progeny can only be determined by some method which measures the amount of label contained in *individual* phage particles. The most direct way of doing this is the use of nuclear photographic emulsions and quantitative P^{32} β-track autoradiography. This method has been adapted with great success to the determination of the P^{32} content of single T2 phages by Levinthal (25), whose results we will now briefly summarize, in the hope that Dr. Levinthal will supplement this summary by an account of his recent experiments. Levinthal has found that among the progeny of a P^{32}-labeled parental generation there appear a few individuals, each possessing about 20 per cent of the label of its parent. The frequency of these highly labeled progeny is such that they account for about half of all the transferred P^{32}. The remaining half of the transferred DNA must have been fragmented into pieces too small to be detected by the nuclear plate technique. When bacteria were infected with this first generation progeny population, there could be recognized among the second generation progeny a number of individuals which still harbored 20 per cent of the P^{32} possessed by the original parental population. In addition, Levinthal inferred from experiments involving the release of the bacteriophage DNA from intact labeled parental or progeny particles by "osmotic shock" that there exists inside each T2 phage one DNA fraction non-dispersible by osmotic shock and amounting to 40 per cent of the entire nucleic acid content, and that the progeny harbor the transferred 20 per cent within that non-dispersible part.

A more indirect method of measuring the distribution of the transferred DNA makes use of the discovery of Hershey, Kamen, Kennedy, and Gest (18), that phage particles are sensitive to decay of P^{32} atoms incorporated into their DNA. Radioactive transmutation of P^{32} atoms into S^{32} atoms kills the phage, so that the rate of inactivation of a P^{32}-labeled phage population can be used as an accurate measure of its degree of label. In a mixed phage population consisting of subclasses labeled to various degrees, each class is inactivated at a rate proportional to its content of label. The whole population thus gives rise to a compound inactivation curve which starts out steeply, at the rate of inactivation of the most highly labeled fractions, and then flattens out as the population of survivors gets more and more depleted of highly labeled particles. Conversely, an accurate determination of the inactivation curve permits an estimate of the composition of the whole population with respect to its variously labeled fractions.

By means of this technique, Hershey, Kamen, Kennedy, and Gest (18) had already observed that among the progeny of *non*-labeled T2 particles grown on P^{32}-labeled host bacteria in P^{32}-labeled medium there was less than one phage in 10^4 which was not subject to P^{32} death. The 50 per cent transfer of DNA from parent to progeny generation can, therefore, not represent the occasional reappearance of an entire parental phage DNA complement within one progeny particle, for any such particle would have been unaffected by P^{32} decay in this experiment. On the other hand, in the reverse experiment with labeled parent phage multiplying in an unlabeled host, Stent and Jerne (36) observed that the majority of the progeny are inactivated by P^{32} decay at a rate less than 0.2 per cent of the rate of inactivation of their parent, although the progeny population studied contained an *average* of 2 per cent parental P^{32} per particle. Most of the transferred DNA cannot, therefore, be widely dispersed but must be confined to a few progeny individuals.

A further refinement of this technique consists in measuring, instead of the inactivation of the first generation progeny, the decrease of the fraction of the label that can be transferred in a second generation transfer experiment as a function of P^{32} decay. In this technique an excess of unlabeled, or very slightly labeled particles, which represent a very undesirable background for the determination of a simple inactivation curve, is automatically eliminated.

The result of such an experiment carried out by Stent, Jerne, and Sato (unpub.) utilizing this method is presented in Fig. 9. It is seen there that before P^{32} decay has occurred, about 50 per cent of the parental phosphorus transferred to the first generation progeny can again be transferred to the second generation progeny. As more and more radioactive decay takes place, less and less of the transferred phosphorus remains transferable to the second generation progeny until a plateau of 25 per cent is reached, when no further decrease in transferability is observed. This finding means that about half of the radioactive DNA transferred from parent to progeny is transferred in pieces big enough to make their carriers unstable and half is transferred in pieces so small that their carriers are stable. If the transferability curve of Fig. 9 is analyzed in terms of a two-component system (the simplest but by no means the only way of analyzing such a curve), then comparison with the rate of P^{32}-inactivation of the labeled parent indicates that the unstable particles each contain from 10-20 per cent of the P^{32} of the parent. In other words, among the first generation progeny there appear one or two particles per parental phage which have received a piece amounting to 10-20 per cent of the parental phage DNA. This method has also been extended to the study of the distribution of the DNA in *second* generation transfer by examining the effect of P^{32} decay on the transferability of the parental P^{32} harbored by the second generation progeny to third generation progeny. The result of this experiment is likewise presented in Fig. 9. It may be seen there that the kinetics of the loss of transferability from second to third generation progeny is very similar to that from first to second generation progeny, commencing near 50 per cent transfer and decreasing rapidly to an asymptote near 25 per cent transfer. This last finding would imply that a second growth cycle had not seriously altered the ratio of the amount of the parental label in big pieces to that in small pieces.

On first sight it might look, therefore, as if both autoradiography as well as P^{32}-inactivation experiments show that the DNA of the parent phage is distributed over its progeny more widely than could be reconciled with conservative or even semi-conservative replication in conjunction with non-fragmenting recombination. The observed distribution of the parental DNA among the *first* generation progeny could be explained in terms of dispersive replication with unequal "family tree" (Fig. 10) or in terms of conservative or semi-conserva-

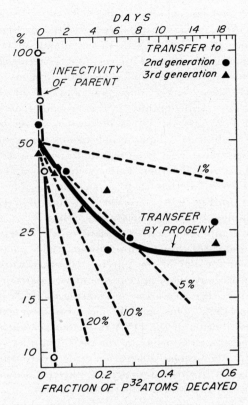

FIG. 9. *The transfer decay experiment of Stent, Jerne, and Sato.*

A population of highly P32-labeled T4 bacteriophage (parents) was allowed to produce in single infection a first generation progeny, containing about 50 per cent of the label of the parents. An aliquot of these first generation progeny was then allowed to produce in single infection a second progeny generation, containing about 50 per cent of the label of the first generation progeny, or 25 per cent of the label of the parents. First and second generation progeny were then stored at 4° C. On various subsequent days, after an amount of P32 decay indicated on the abscissa had taken place, first and second generation progeny were allowed to reproduce in single infection to generate their own second and third generation progeny *du jour*. The percentage of label transferred from the original first generation progeny to each second generation progeny *du jour* and from the original second generation progeny to each third generation progeny *du jour*, is indicated on the ordinate. The stippled lines indicate survival curves corresponding to rates of inactivation constituting various percentages of the rate of inactivation of the labeled parent.

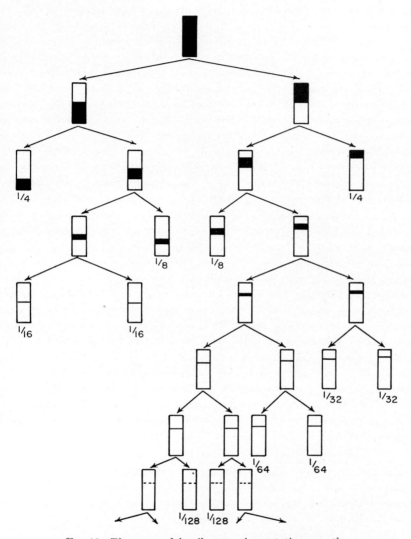

FIG. 10. *The unequal family tree of vegetative growth.*

If the label were partitioned equally at each replication but if replication were non-synchronous, then a very heterogeneous distribution of the parental label could be found among the descendants after numerous rounds of replication. The numbers indicate the fraction of the parental label harbored by progeny individuals at different levels of the tree.

tive replication followed by recombinational fragmentation in random matings. In both these cases, however, a further dispersion or fragmentation of those big DNA pieces which escaped the dispersive or fragmenting processes of the first generation transfer should have occurred in the *second* generation transfer. An exact estimation of the further dispersion or fragmentation of the parental DNA which unequal family trees or recombinational fragmentation *should* produce in second generation transfer is rather difficult, and a detailed discussion of this problem will not be attempted here. Rough calculations according to various models indicate that the accuracy of the second generation data now at hand suffices to exclude dispersive replication but still admits fragmentation as an explanation of the observed dispersion of the transferred DNA into pieces of different sizes.

Now, if the dispersion of the parental DNA among the progeny is *not* produced by a random fragmentation of the whole phage, then it would have to reflect some a priori partition of the parental DNA into sections which differ as to whether, when transferred at all, they will appear as big or small pieces. The notion of such a *bipartite* structure of the bacteriophage DNA would become very plausible if the inference (25) that the 20 per cent DNA piece transferred to the first generation progeny resides within a part of the progeny phages not dispersible by osmotic shock can actually be substantiated. Some detailed calculations would seem necessary, before it can be decided whether the available results are of sufficient statistical accuracy to eliminate the possibility that the labeled DNA which is not dispersed by osmotic shock of either parent or progeny populations has not simply escaped certain physical breakage forces operating on the phage DNA as a whole.

The realization, however, that the DNA of the parent phage may be bipartite introduces an entirely new element into all the foregoing arguments and very much complicates the interpretation of the distribution experiments. It would be tempting, of course, to infer from the persistence of the big pieces through repeated transfers that they replicate by a conservative or semi-conservative mechanism and that *their* recombination must be non-fragmenting. Unfortunately, however, that part of the DNA which is transferred in small pieces and about whose possible further dispersion in the second generation transfer we do not yet know anything, may also play an important part in the growth processes. It is by no means excluded that these two hypothetical parts of the parental DNA in fact perform *differenti-ated functions* in the infective processes, e.g., that only one of them is concerned with replication while the other serves, say, as a template for phage protein synthesis. If that part of the DNA which is the source of the big pieces replicates and recombines, then replication cannot be dispersive and recombination cannot be fragmenting; if, on the other hand, the source of the small pieces serves for the replication of the entire phage DNA, then these bacteriophage distribution experiments do not permit the definite exclusion of any of the replication mechanisms discussed above.

Linkage Between Material and Genetic Transfer.

Some hope exists, nevertheless, for unraveling the meaning of the transfer distribution experiments by combining such measurements with *genetic* observations. Garen (17) has carried out an experiment designed to answer the question whether the transferred DNA in a mixed infection from several genetically different parental particles is coupled to a particular genetic marker. For this purpose, he infected bacteria with *equal numbers* of P^{32}-labeled T4 and non-labeled T2 particles (i.e., two strains whose genomes differed at the *host-range* locus) and determined the fraction of the transferred label which appeared in progeny endowed with T2 host range by selective adsorption to bacteria sensitive to T2 but not to T4. Garen observed that about 40 per cent of the label transferred from the labeled T4 parents had been separated from the host-range locus with which it was introduced into the infected cell and was found to be incorporated into T2 particles. This experiment has been extended by Burgi (pers. commun.) by crossing T2 with labeled T2h (i.e., two strains differing genetically *only* at their host-range locus). Burgi, furthermore, reduced the relative input of labeled h to non-labeled h^+ parents from equality to 1 h for every 10 h^+ particles per bacterium, so that only 10 per cent of the progeny particles were endowed with the h locus. These 10 per cent now harbored 35 per cent of the label transferred from parents of the homologous h genotype, the remaining 65 per cent having "crossed over" to h^+ progeny.

These observations show that the parental DNA is dispersed in the course of replication, recombination, or both, so that it can reappear associated with genetic markers different from those with which it entered the cell. Such a change of genotype of the parental DNA could be due to unspecific transfer (e.g., to a complete breakdown similar to that known to occur under certain conditions of multiple infection (23) and resynthesis of part of the parental DNA) or to fragmenting recombination. The dispersion, on the other hand, is not so extensive that the parental DNA is *randomized* among the progeny, for in that case only 10 per cent instead of 35 per cent of the label introduced by the minority h parent in Burgi's experiment should have been found among the h progeny. The results suggest, rather, that in a phage cross from 20 to 30 per cent of the parental DNA remains "true" to a given genetic marker and the remainder is distributed to the progeny particles at random with respect to genotype. The "true" fraction of the parental DNA could reflect: (a) in case of non-specific transfer, an average portion of the parental DNA which happens not to be broken down; or (b) in case of fragmenting recombination, an average length of DNA surrounding the marker which is not fragmented by random recombinational events; or (c) in the case of a bipartite phage structure, a sector in each parental particle which remains true to *all* the genetic markers and probably identical with the sector which is transferred as a big piece (complemented by a second sector which is dispersed over the progeny).

It has been attempted (Sato and Stent, unpub.) to test the last possibility, i.e., to see whether that 10 to 20 per cent piece of transferred DNA which has been detected by the transfer decay experiments of Fig. 9 carries with it all the genetic loci of its parent. Under conditions similar to those employed by Burgi, one highly P^{32}-labeled T2h r_1 r_7^+ m^+ (minority parent) was crossed with 10 non-labeled T2h^+ r_1^+ r_7 m particles per bacterium (the markers r_1, r_7, and m concern plaque morphology and are only distantly linked to each other and to h). Among the progeny, there appeared less than one half of a minority parental type per infected bacterium, as is to be expected in such a four-factor cross (39). Now if there existed a piece of transferred DNA inseparably linked to all genetic markers, then, *nolens volens*, almost all of the few minority parental types appearing among the progeny of this four-factor cross would have to possess this piece. If this piece, furthermore, were identical to that responsible for transfer decay, then the bulk of the minority parental types among the progeny should have been inactivated by P^{32} decay at a rate from 10 to 20 per cent of that of their parent. No P^{32}-inactivation of the minority parental types could, however, be detected. It appears, therefore, that the portion of the parental DNA which appears to be linked to the *h* locus in Burgi's experiments is either not equally linked to other genetic loci or is not identical with the portion which is transferred as a big piece.

Transfer from Ultraviolet Irradiated Parental Phages.

UV-irradiated phage particles which are unable to produce progeny in single infection are able to contribute genetic markers to the progeny if they are accompanied into the bacterial host cell by live particles. This phenomenon is called "cross-reactivation" or "marker rescue" (26, 8). The latter name is preferable, for the reason that if the UV-irradiated parent carries several unlinked genetic markers, then it can be shown that these markers are "rescued" independently of each other. Thus, we are not dealing with a reactivation of the whole UV-treated parent particle, but only with the rescue of undamaged segments of its genetic material by recombination. When Kozloff (21) studied the transfer from labeled UV-treated parents to progeny under conditions of marker rescue in mixed infection with live, non-labeled parents, he observed that the transfer is nearly the same as from live, i.e., non-UV-irradiated parents. These experiments, however, did not permit a decision as to whether this transfer is specific or unspecific, i.e., whether the transferred label is imbedded in the genetic segments which are rescued, or whether, in addition to this genetic rescue which may not be accompanied by transfer of label, there is some breakdown and reincorporation of parental label.

Hershey (pers. commun.) has recently extended these studies, and has made the remarkable discovery that a large part of the transferred label from the UV-treated parent is not in live progeny, but in progeny particles which are dead in the same sense in which the UV-treated parent is dead, i.e., particles which are unable to produce a progeny when they are used in single infection, but are able to transfer their label to a second generation progeny when they are accompanied into the bacterium by live particles. Hershey examined the dependence on UV dose of the fate of the transferred label and observed that even at extremely high doses only about 45 per cent of the transferred label is in dead particles, and the rest is in live progeny.

How did the parental label get into *dead* progeny? Since it can be shown that the *number* of such dead progeny is not very much greater than the number of UV-treated parental phages, we can say, to a first approximation, that the dead parents do not replicate as dead particles. Hence part of the UV-treated DNA must have remained intact throughout replication and recombination to achieve maturation within a progeny particle rendered non-viable by its UV-lesions. How did any label then get into *live* progeny? The possibilities here are analogous to those which may account for the separation of the parental DNA from the *h* locus in Garen's and Burgi's experiments: (a) a fraction of the UV-treated parental DNA may be broken down and unspecifically incorporated into live progeny; or (b) marker rescue may imply a concomitant rescue of material elements from the UV-treated parents, i.e., genetic recombination may be fragmenting; or, finally, (c) the phage DNA may be bipartite, consisting of two portions, one of which, transferred inviolate, carries along any of the original UV lesions and may be identical with the transferred big pieces, and the other which is transferred specifically in such a way that any UV lesions are somehow erased during transfer with marker rescue.

Some support for either of the last two interpretations may be derived from Hershey's "reverse" cross, in which the live parent is labeled and the UV-treated parent is unlabeled. The result here is that some 10 to 20 per cent of the label transferred from the live parent is incorporated into dead progeny. Since we concluded above that the dead parent does not replicate and carries UV lesions to the progeny, we must now conclude that part of the DNA of the live parent can wind up in a progeny particle which also harbors DNA with UV lesions either because live and dead DNA become mixed by fragmenting genetic recombination or because a few of the bipartite progeny particles have drawn the UV-treated big piece for their "genetic" portion and some small pieces for their "non-genetic" portion from the randomly distributed "non-genetic" portion of the live parent.

These experiments of Hershey's are of a preliminary nature and are susceptible to refinement in various directions. At present their most significant aspect would appear to be the finding of a tie-up between material transfer, recognized by the P^{32} label, and a specific transfer, recognized by the specific properties of UV lesions.

DISTRIBUTION EXPERIMENT WITH BACTERIAL NUCLEI

Decay of P^{32} atoms incorporated in the DNA, i.e., in the "nuclei," of *Escherichia coli* bacteria destroys the ability of the cells to give rise to colonies, the rate of inactivation being proportional to the specific P^{32} content of the DNA (13). If now in the course of bacterial reproduction the atomic identity of the parental nuclei is conserved, i.e., if newly assimilated phosphorus atoms are introduced only into the daughter DNA, then the stable nuclei of a non-radioactive culture of cells inoculated into a medium containing P^{32} would never acquire any radioactivity, and hence would remain stable. After growth in the radioactive medium the culture would still possess its initial number of non-radioactive nuclei and the colony-forming ability of cells harboring these nuclei could not be eliminated by radioactive decay. Conversely, when a radioactive culture, homogeneously subject to loss of colony-forming ability by radioactive decay, is inoculated into a medium containing no P^{32} and if the nuclei subsequently synthesized contain only *de novo* material, then very quickly a class of cells would arise which would contain entirely non-radioactive, i.e., stable, nuclei immune from inactivation by decay. On the other hand, if the atomic identity of the bacterial nucleus is destroyed during its replication and the parental atoms are dispersed among daughter nuclei, then in the two experiments just considered stable nuclei of non-radioactive cells will quickly become radioactive upon growth in the presence of P^{32} and radioactive nuclei will still give rise to radioactive, albeit *less* radioactive nuclei upon growth in the absence of P^{32}.

When experiments of this sort were carried out (13), it was observed that more than 99.9 per cent of the cells of an initially unlabeled culture which had assimilated P^{32} for only slightly more than one generation were subject to P^{32}-death in a manner indicating that duplication had dispersed the DNA atoms of each bacterial nucleus equally over its daughters. Similarly, when a P^{32}-labeled culture of bacteria was allowed to grow for slightly more than one division in non-radioactive medium, the rate of P^{32}-inactivation of the culture was reduced in a manner as if an equipartition of the radioactive atoms between the daughter nuclei had taken place. Upon further divisions in non-radioactive medium, however, a minority of cells began to appear in the culture which were less P^{32}-sensitive than if equipartition of the original P^{32} atoms had continued, although even after nearly four divisions no completely P^{32}-refractory bacteria had yet appeared. This result is compatible with semi-conservative replication, which would predict equipartition of the original P^{32} atoms in the first, but conservation in subsequent nuclear divisions, provided that the failure to observe P^{32}-stable cells after several divisions is attributed to random segregation of different "chromosomes." These results, however, are also compatible with either conservative replication followed by post-replication fragmentation, or with dispersive replication, either of which would explain the equipartition of nuclear substance at the first division. The slowly dying cell minority appearing after further divisions could then reflect a heterogeneity in growth rate of the bacterial population. For the descendants of rapidly growing cells which have made more than the average number of divisions would have reduced their specific P^{32}-content more than anticipated on the basis of equipartition calculations. The only possibility definitely eliminated by this experiment is that the DNA of the *E. coli* nucleus replicates by a conservative mechanism without being subject to post-replication fragmentation.

Distribution Experiment with Chromosomes

Plaut and Mazia (31) permitted root tissue of hawk's beard *(Crepis capillaris)* to incorporate the C^{14}-labeled DNA precursor thymidine for a time long enough to allow some cells to pass from early interphase to telophase. The radioactivity contained in the six chromosomes of each of the two sister nuclei of a number of telophase figures was then measured by autoradiography, and certain significant inequalities in C^{14} content observed between pairs. The frequency distribution of the magnitude of these inequalities was of such a nature that it could be accounted for by synthesis de novo of the six daughter chromosomes, followed by a random selection of either the (non-radioactive) mother or the (radioactive) daughter chromosome for migration to each pole. If these observed inequalities in C^{14}-content between telophase nuclei were not due to heterogeneities inherent in either the autoradiographic technique or the metabolism of the thymidine, then it would seem that the DNA of one of the daughter chromosomes contains very few of the atoms of the progenitor. Dispersive or semi-conservative replication mechanisms would thus, at first sight, be ruled out, and conservative replication indicated. A single chromosome, however, may contain a large number of DNA molecules, and it is here even less certain than in the case of the much smaller bacteriophage that every DNA molecule actually participates equally in the replication processes of the interphase. In the extreme case, it is conceivable that only one of n identical DNA molecules of an n-fold chromosome has given rise to n duplicates of itself through repeated replication cycles to supply the substance of the daughter chromosome while the remaining $n - 1$ molecules have remained inactive. In that case, the average "age" of the atoms of the daughter chromosome would be less than that of the mother chromosome atoms, whether the elementary replication act involved conservation or dispersion of the atoms of the duplicating DNA molecule. As Mazia and Plaut have pointed out, their experiment excludes the possibility that all the DNA molecules of the chromosome participate equally in replication and do so by either semi-conservative or dispersive mechanisms.

Summarizing the attempts carried out up until the present time to discover the distribution of the parental atoms in the course of replication, we may state that two fundamental difficulties have so far prevented us from drawing any unambiguous conclusions concerning the question whether DNA replication is conservative, semi-conservative, or dispersive. An observed *unequal* distribution of the parental atoms may be due to an unequal role in the duplication process of various fractions of the total DNA contained in the self-duplicating structure, while an observed *equal* distribution may only reflect the randomizing effect of some post-replication event like fragmentation by genetic recombination.

Interruptions of the Polynucleotide Chain

We may now discuss some other experimental results relevant to the mechanism of DNA replication. It has been noted that the resting DNA duplex appears to be able to sustain numerous interruptions of its two polynucleotide chains without thereby losing the capacity to reproduce itself. The mechanism by which bacteriophages and bacterial nuclei are inactivated by decay of P^{32} atoms incorporated into their DNA indicates that as little as one in every twenty to thirty breakages of the phosphate diester bonds responsible for the continuity of the sugar-phosphate backbone may actually be lethal (13, 18, 34). The increased heat-sensitivity of *Hemophilus* transforming principle partially digested by DNAase likewise suggests that the biological activity of DNA molecules may survive enzymatic hydrolysis of a number of their phosphate ester bonds (45). While it is easy to see how the great number of intra-chain hydrogen bonds can preserve the structural integrity of the DNA duplex in spite of numerous interruptions in each single polynucleotide chain (11), it is more difficult to understand how the replication of such an interrupted DNA duplex could be successful if it required unwinding and separation of the two strands. The interrupted chains would present no difficulty, on the other hand, if the resting DNA duplex is replicated by a conservative mechanism not requiring any unwinding of the parental molecule.

INFORMATION TRANSFER

Two sets of observations have recently been made which lend themselves to the interpretation that the DNA introduced into the bacterial cell by the infecting bacteriophage does not replicate itself directly but rather through an intermediary substance to which the genetic information is temporarily transferred in the course of the replication act. Neither one of these observations *proves* such a notion, but in view of the unexpected nature of these findings it would be unwise not to give some currency to "information transfer" as a possible replication mechanism.

In the first of these experiments, P^{32}-labeled bacteria were infected with P^{32}-labeled T2 particles and the inactivation by P^{32} decay of the infective center was studied at various stages of phage development (33). It was discovered that soon after phage development has got under way, the ability of the infected cell to liberate infective phage progeny can no longer be suppressed by radioactive decay, even though the parental DNA and all of its vegetative replicas are highly radioactive and ought, therefore, to be subject to destruction. If now at the outset of the infection the "information" of the infecting DNA is transferred to some substance not sensitive to inactivation by P^{32}-decay, either because it contains no phosphorus (protein?) or because it possesses a structure of greater stability than the free DNA duplex (nucleoprotein?), then this intermediate could always generate more infective progeny DNA even if P^{32}-decay had destroyed the parental DNA and all of the replica duplexes formed prior to decay. Alternative explanations of this observation not involving the notion of information transfer are, however, not excluded.

Some studies on the relation of protein synthesis to the replication of bacteriophage DNA have revealed that replication of phage DNA does not commence in T2-infected bacteria in which protein synthesis has been inhibited either by the presence of an amino acid analogue, or by the absence of a required amino acid or by the presence of chloramphenicol (7, 6, 29, 38). However, if the required amino acid is removed or chloramphenicol is added only some time after the start of phage development, phage DNA synthesis does proceed in the absence of any further formation of protein, the *rate* of DNA synthesis being the greater the later protein synthesis was arrested. It seems, therefore, that the formation of a protein is required before replication of the bacteriophage DNA commences; once some of this protein has been made, DNA replication can proceed. One might suppose that this protein is an inducible enzyme required for the synthesis of some building block of the phage DNA, e.g., the pyrimidine 5-hydroxy-methylcytosine, were it not for the observation of Tomizawa and Sunakawa (38) that the UV-resistance of T2-infected bacteria does not increase further after the addition of chloramphenicol even though more and more phage DNA accumulates within the cells. Tomizawa and Sunakawa's findings fit better with the idea that the high UV-resistance of T2-infected bacteria late in their eclipse (2, 27) is due to the appearance of a protein or nucleoprotein capable of directing the synthesis of progeny DNA after ultraviolet light has damaged the parental DNA and any of its replicates formed prior to irradiation.

GENETIC RECOMBINATION AND REPLICATION

It is clear that if "copying choice" is actually the mechanism under-lying genetic recombination in bacteriophage, no proposed DNA repli-cation scheme can be considered satisfactory unless it also brings some structural insight into how the "mating" of templates and switching of growing replicas can be accomplished. What molecular forces make it possible for these highly specific matings to be so frequent during the multiplication of T2 and T4 bacteriophages that virtually every replication appears to proceed along a "mated" template? Under the Watson-Crick replication mechanism in its *conservative* (Bloch, Butler), *semi-conservative* (Levinthal-Crane, Platt), or *dispersive* (Delbrück) guises the mated templates would be two entire parental DNA duplexes which have come into point-by-point alignment. The structure of the intact DNA duplex, however, does not suggest any obvious way as to how two such molecules could manage to pair in such a way that regions of identical base sequence are in exact apposition.

Perhaps some fresh approach to the molecular mechanism of DNA replication could be made by considering that mating of templates is not a facultative but rather an *obligatory* feature of the replication process, in contrast to all the replication schemes so far discussed, which have assumed implicitly that only one parental template is involved in each replication act. It is conceivable that there exists some fundamental reason why replication along a single template cannot get under way unless the template is "mated" with one of its opposite numbers. A consequence of this hypothesis is naturally an equivalence of rounds of replication and mating, which, as we have already mentioned, does, in fact, obtain in the multiplication of T2 and T4 phages.

Unlike the case of T2 and T4, the number of observed rounds of mating and replication is actually not at all equal during the growth of two other phage strains whose recombination mechanism has been studied in detail. Coli-phages lambda and T1 appear to experience very few rounds of mating in the course of their normal latent period, while undergoing roughly the same number of rounds of replication as T2 and T4 (5, 44). This fact, which on first sight appears to rule out the hypothesis just advanced, can actually be reconciled with an obligatory mating-replication relation when some of the growth characteristics of these strains are compared with those of T2 and T4. Phage lambda is a *temperate* bacteriophage, i.e., one which is capable of being carried as a prophage in the nucleus of a lysogenic bacterial cell; strain T1 has never been observed in the prophage state and is, therefore, strictly speaking not temperate. It is possible, however, that T1 shares with temperate phages the characteristic which is important for the present considerations, viz., that it can mate with the nucleus of the bacterial host cell (15). There exist a number of genetic and radiogenetic observations which make it appear that temperate phages mate with the nucleus of the host cell not only during their lysogenic response, in which the genome of the infective phage particles becomes integrated with the genome of the host cell, but also during their vegetative development following induction or infection in the lytic response (15, 35, 43). If temperate vegetative phages, therefore, choose host templates as mating partners in the replication process, most of the matings during the latent period may not produce any detectable recombinants and would hence go unnoticed. That is, since the number of rounds of mating is necessarily measured by the frequency of recombination between markers introduced by two or more *infecting* particles, only a fraction of the total rounds of mating taking place during the lytic growth of temperate bacteriophages would be scored in any cross. The apparent discrepancy between rounds of replication and mating in the case of temperate phages thus does not eliminate the notion that mating is required for replication.

It would not seem too profitable, however, to speculate much further about the chemical nature of the molecular species representing the mating structure and serving as the template in the synthesis of daughter DNA molecules. Such a proposal should incorporate the fundamental notion of replication by complementary pairing of purines and pyrimidines or substitute for it an idea at least as plausible as the mechanism of Watson and Crick, the only specific molecular mechanism of replication conceived until this day.

Summary and Conclusion

Let us now briefly recapitulate. We first discussed the topological difficulty in the replication of DNA arising from the fact that the two strands of the Watson-Crick structure are wound around each other in many turns. We pointed out a number of ways by which this difficulty cannot be overcome and some ways in which it can be.

We then attempted a general classification of replication schemes according to the manner in which a parental label is distributed during replication. This distribution may be *conservative, semi-conservative,* or *dispersive.*

Next we considered the fact that in phage, at least, replication and genetic recombination appear to be events which are experimentally not separable. In a discussion of experiments relating to the distribution of a parental label, therefore, genetic recombination cannot be ignored. In view of our ignorance of the real nature of the mechanism of genetic recombination, we can as yet do no better than to classify the various recombination schemes, and a useful classification would appear to be again one which makes reference to the fate of a parental label. Thus we were led to the classification of the schemes into *fragmenting* and *non-fragmenting* recombination.

We reviewed the findings concerning the transfer of DNA from a labeled bacteriophage parent to its progeny from the point of view of the distribution of the parental DNA in the course of replication and recombination. The fact that the transfer is incomplete, i.e., of the order of 35-50 per cent, was seen not to reflect an a priori division of the phage into transferable and non-transferable DNA. On the contrary, the indications are that the label which fails to be transferred represents a random section of the parental DNA. With respect to the distribution among the progeny particles of the transferred parental label, both autoradiographic as well as P^{32}-inactivation experiments show that about half of the transferred parental DNA is transferred in big pieces and that the remainder of the transferred parental label is more widely distributed. What shall we make of this odd distribution? One might be inclined to conclude that the DNA of the bacteriophage is *bipartite*, one portion being of such a nature that it is transferred in small pieces. In support of this conclusion one may point to the results of second generation experiments, which, as can be inferred from both autoradiographic as well as P^{32}-inactivation measurements, suggest that the big pieces do not suffer appreciable further fragmentation during a second transfer. It would remain to be seen, however, whether this lack of further fragmentation of big pieces has been proven with sufficient rigor to exclude their origin in fragmentation processes operating on an unipartite phage DNA.

The possibility of a bipartite structure of the phage DNA now brings a further complication into the interpretation of the distribution results as to whether replication is conservative, semi-conservative, or dispersive. It is possible that the two hypothetical parts do not play equivalent roles in the replication drama, and hence it must be established that the big pieces are, in fact, replicating, before their persistence through repeated growth cycles can testify against dispersive replication or fragmenting recombination schemes. It is by no means excluded that the small pieces could be responsible for the replication of the *entire* phage DNA. Thus if the bipartite structure should turn out to be real, then it appears to us that the function of the two parts must be clarified before any valid conclusion can be drawn regarding the replication mechanism.

Further support for the bipartite structure of the phage DNA may be derived from the fact that experiments in which the transfer of label from parent to progeny is linked to a genetic marker or to UV lesions can likewise be interpreted in these terms. Explanation of these results by means of replication and recombination schemes not involving bipartite structure is, however, equally possible, and at least one experiment showed that the fraction of the parental DNA which stayed "true" to a genetic locus either was not identical with the fraction transferred as a big piece or was not linked equally to all loci.

Finally, we have discussed several groups of experiments which suggest the involvement of complications of another sort. There exists suggestive experimental evidence that protein synthesis may be an essential part of DNA replication, that information transfer occurs to some unknown molecular structure, that mating may be an integral part of replication.

It appears to us that no definite conclusions regarding replication can be drawn at the present moment. Our review can do no more than delineate the problem and assess the evidence. We hope that it will help to clarify the issues and to speed the answers. We are confident, in fact, that the whole issue will be resolved before many a day. Who knows, perhaps even before this goes to press?

REFERENCES

1. Artin, E., *Ann. Math.*, **48** (1947).
2. Benzer, S., *J. Bacteriol.*, **63**, 59 (1952).
3. Bloch, D. P., *Proc. Natl. Acad. Sci. U. S.*, **41**, 1058 (1955).
4. Bresch, C., *Z. Naturforsch.*, **10b**, 545 (1955).
5. Bresch, C., and Mennigmann, H. D., unpub.
6. Burton, K., *Biochem. J. (London)*, **61**, 473 (1955).
7. Cohen, S. S., *Cold Spring Harbor Symposia Quant. Biol.*, **12**, 35 (1947).
8. Doermann, A. H., Chase, M., and Stahl, F. W., *J. Cell. Comp. Physiol.*, **45**, Supp. 2, 51 (1955).
9. Butler, J. A. V., *Radiation Research*, **4**, 20 (1956).
10. Delbrück, M., *Proc. Natl. Acad. Sci. U. S.*, **40**, 783 (1955).
11. Dekker, C. A., and Schachman, H. K., *Proc. Natl. Acad. Sci. U. S.*, **40**, 894 (1954).
12. French, R. C., Graham, A. F., Lesley, S. M., and van Rooyen, C. E., *J. Bacteriol.*, **64**, 597 (1952).
13. Fuerst, C. R., and Stent, G. S., *J. Gen. Physiol.*, in press.
14. Gamow, G., *Proc. Natl. Acad. Sci. U. S.*, **41**, 7 (1955).
15. Garen, A., and Zinder, N. D., *Virology*, **1**, 347 (1955).
16. Hershey, A. D., *Intern. Rev. Cytol.*, Vol. I, p. 119, Academic Press, New York (1952).
17. Hershey, A. D., Garen, A., Fraser, D., and Hudis, J. D., *Carnegie Inst. Washington Yr. Bk.*, **53**, 210 (1954).
18. Hershey, A. D., Kamen, M. D., Kennedy, J. W., and Gest, H., *J. Gen. Physiol.*, **34**, 305 (1951).
19. Huskins, C. L., *Cold Spring Harbor Symposia Quant. Biol.*, **9**, 13 (1941).
20. Jacob, F., and Wollman, E. L., *Ann. Inst. Pasteur*, **88**, 724 (1955).
21. Kozloff, L. M., *J. Biol. Chem.*, **194**, 95 (1952).
22. Lederberg, J., *J. Cell. Comp. Physiol.*, **45**, Supp. 2, 75 (1955).
23. Lesley, S. M., French, R. C., Graham, A. F., and van Rooyen, C. E., *Can. J. Med. Sci.*, **29**, 128 (1951).
24. Levinthal, C., *Genetics*, **39**, 169 (1954).
25. Levinthal, C., *Rend. ist. lombardo sci.*, Pt. I, **89**, 192 (1955).
26. Luria, S. E., and Dulbecco, R., *Genetics*, **34**, 93 (1949).

27. Luria, S. E., and Latarjet, R., *J. Bacteriol.,* **53**, 149 (1947).
28. Maaløe, O., and Watson, J. D., *Proc. Natl. Acad. Sci. U. S.,* **37**, 507 (1951).
29. Melechen, N., *Genetics,* **40**, 584 (1955).
30. Platt, J. R., *Proc. Natl. Acad. Sci. U. S.,* **41**, 181 (1955).
31. Plaut, W., and Mazia, D., in press.
32. Putnam, F. W., and Kozloff, L. M., *J. Biol. Chem.,* **182**, 243 (1950).
33. Stent, G. S., *J. Gen. Physiol.,* **38**, 853 (1955).
34. Stent, G. S., and Fuerst, C. R., *J. Gen. Physiol.,* **38**, 441 (1955).
35. Stent, G. S., and Fuerst, C. R., unpub.
36. Stent, G. S., and Jerne, N. K., *Proc. Natl. Acad. Sci. U. S.,* **41**, 704 (1955).
37. Stent, G. S., and Maaløe, O., *Biochim. et Biophys. Acta,* **8**, 260 (1952).
38. Tomizawa, J., and Sunakawa, S., *J. Gen. Physiol.,* **39**, 553 (1956).
39. Visconti, N., and Delbrück, M., *Genetics,* **38**, 5 (1953).
40. Watanabe, I., Stent, G. S., and Schachman, H. K., *Biochim. et Biophys. Acta,* **15**, 46 (1954).
41. Watson, J. D., and Crick, F. H. C., *Cold Spring Harbor Symposia Quant. Biol.,* **18**, 123 (1953).
42. Watson, J. D., and Maaløe, O., *Biochim. et Biophys. Acta,* **10**, 432 (1953).
43. Weigle, J. J., *Proc. Natl. Acad. Sci. U. S.,* **39**, 628 (1953).
44. Wollman, E. L., and Jacob, F., *Ann. Inst. Pasteur,* **87**, 1 (1954).
45. Zamenhof, S., Leidy, G., and Hahn, E., *Records Genetics Soc. Am.,* No. 23 (1954).

THE MOLECULAR BASIS OF GENETIC
RECOMBINATION IN PHAGE

C. Levinthal and C. A. Thomas, Jr.*

*Physics Department, University of Michigan,
Ann Arbor, Michigan*

Molecular autoradiography allows one to carry out tracer experiments on single DNA molecules and single virus particles. It also makes possible the determination of the size or molecular weight of individual particles. The details of the method and most of the preliminary results obtained with phage have been reported elsewhere, or are in press (3), and have been partially included in the review by Delbrück and Stent (see their review in this volume for full references on the transfer studies with phage). In this paper we will give a brief summary of the previous work and indicate the status of some of the current experiments. We will also discuss briefly some of the theoretical and experimental problems which are raised by these results.

The method of molecular autoradiography consists of surrounding the radioactive particle with an electron-sensitive nuclear emulsion (Ilford, Ltd. G-5 emulsion) in which the passage of a fast electron produces a track composed of exposed silver grains. If a single particle has several radioactive atoms which decay during the exposure time, then, on development, one can observe a star in the emulsion, that is, a point from which there emanate several electron tracks (Fig. 1). The observable quantities are the number of tracks per star, which we designate r, and the number of stars per unit volume of emulsion. When used with P^{32}, the detection of the β emission is approximately 100 per cent efficient, as has been demonstrated by counting the mean number of tracks per star produced by virus particles of a known P^{32}-content. Using radioactive phosphorus as the label, the activity of a particle can be determined if it is as high as about 15 disintegrations per month. Thus the method is about 10^5 times more sensitive than a Geiger counter for measurement of localized radioactive label.

Obviously, the number of tracks observed in any one star is affected

* NRC Fellow in Medical Sciences for which funds were provided by the Rockefeller Foundation (1955-56).

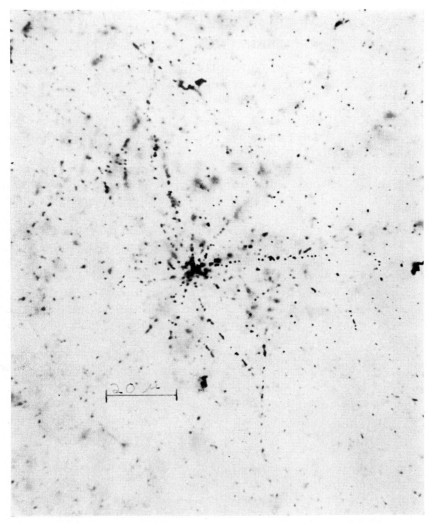

Fɪɢ. 1. This photomicrograph was taken with an objective of N.A. 1.32. Only a small fraction of the tracks can be seen at one focal setting. For counting purposes individual tracks must be followed by changing the fine focus control.

by the random incorporation of the radioactive isotope, as well as the laws of radioactive decay. In all cases to be discussed here, the observed distribution for r is consistent with a single Poisson distribution with a mean designated $\bar{r}$. Thus $\bar{r}$ is the only number which can be meaningfully used to describe the size of the stars from a given plate. In general, enough stars have been counted so that the probable error in $\bar{r}$ due to sampling alone is approximately 10 per cent. The inherent uncertainties in the count of any one star due to overlapping tracks produce an error which is smaller than this.

TABLE 1

	Intact Phage	After Osmotic Shock
Uniformly Labeled Parental Phage	100	40 ± 4
First Generation Progeny	24 ± 3	23 ± 3
Second Generation Progeny	26 ± 3	Too dilute for study

This table gives the number of P^{32} atoms in the star-forming particles of the various fractions normalized to 100 for the original uniformly labeled phage.

The results previously reported are summarized in Table 1. They indicate (a) that there is a large piece of DNA in the phage T2 which has a molecular weight of approximately 45 million, if we take the total phosphorus content of the phage as 2×10^{-11} μg. Recent measurements show that there is, on the average, one large piece liberated from each phage by osmotic shock, and this measurement has an error of less than 10 per cent. Osmotic shock of the phage T4 also liberates a large piece of DNA of the same size as that found in T2. Dr. Geoffrey Brown will present in the following discussion his evidence that this piece of DNA is not associated with the protein coat. (b) The table shows that when radioactive phages are allowed to go through one cycle of growth in non-radioactive bacteria, there are among the progeny a few phage particles in which this large piece of DNA has approximately half the P^{32} atoms of the corresponding piece in the parental virus particles. And (c) if these first progeny viruses are allowed to go through a second growth cycle in unlabeled bacteria, then the mean value of the star size $\bar{r}$ does not change. Measurements of the number of stars indicate that the P^{32} in the large piece has roughly the same probability of being transferred to the progeny as does that in the smaller fragments.

The most appealing interpretation of these data is that this large piece of DNA in phage is the chromosome, that is, the physical structure containing the genetic information of the phage. Since it is known that the "half-hot big piece"[1] of DNA appears in an active phage particle, it now becomes of primary importance to learn whether or not its presence has conferred on this particle a particular set of genetic characters. To examine this question, crosses are being carried out to test the correlation between the presence of stars and various genetic markers of the phage. The cross $T2P^{32}h^{+}r_1 \times T2P^{31}hr_{13}$ has been studied in detail. The rapid lysis marker r, which produces a modified plaque morphology, is used so that one has an independent marker to follow genetic recombination. Phage particles with the host range mutant h can be separated from the wild type h^{+} by absorption on a bacterial cell resistant to the phage T2. However, it has been shown (Novick and Szilard, 6) that from a cross of this type one obtains particles whose phenotype, as judged by the ability to absorb, does not conform to the genotype of the particle as judged by the phenotype of the progeny it produces. It is therefore necessary to allow the progeny of the cross to grow in bacteria which are singly infected in order to remove this confusion of phenotype and genotype. When this is done, we find that at least 90 per cent of the particles able to form stars have the absorption characteristics of the h^{+} parent. This result indicates that the large piece of DNA which entered the cross in the h^{+} parent is not distributed at random among the progeny, but remains closely associated with the presence of at least one gene. It will obviously be necessary to carry out this type of cross with other genetic markers before one can be sure that the large piece of DNA is the chromosome of the phage, but this does seem to be a useful hypothesis with our present knowledge.

These crosses can demonstrate that the genetic information of the phage is carried into the infected cell in the large piece of DNA. However, we cannot by this method hope to demonstrate that the information is not then transferred to some other cellular component before replication and mating occur. The only basis for assuming that this does not occur is the requirement of simplicity. There is at the moment no convincing evidence to the contrary, and it seems most profitable to explore the simpler explanations before considering the more complex ones.

[1] One of the aims of this work is to replace the phrase, "the big piece," by the word "chromosome."

We will adopt as working hypotheses both that the genetic information enters the infected cell in the 45 million piece of DNA, and that it remains in structures of this type throughout the phage growth cycle. We can then conclude that half of the atoms of this piece of DNA remain together in one particle in spite of many successive acts of recombinant production and replication. This suggests that the phosphate-ester linkages in one chain of the double helix of DNA are not broken either by replication or by recombination. It is not possible to conclude that the two chains are separated, with one going to each of the two daughters at every act of replication. All that is suggested by the current experiments is that at least once in each growth cycle the two strands which were originally together in one molecule become separated. This would account for the drop in the star size associated with the large piece of DNA from 40 per cent of the P^{32} of the original phage to 20 per cent in the progeny of the first generation of growth.

In order to consider specific ways in which recombinants might be formed, it is necessary to recall the genetic data indicating that the heterozygotes act as intermediates in the production of recombinants. Hershey and Chase (1) discovered the heterozygous phage particles and showed that on infection they give rise to two kinds of progeny which differ with respect to the markers in a short region of the genetic map. Further genetic analysis (2) indicated that the progeny of the heterozygotes were usually recombinants for markers on opposite sides of this duplicated region. It has also been shown that there are enough heterozygous particles observed so that they could account for all of the recombinants formed. Therefore, it seems likely that these structures are the direct product of the mating act and that their further intracellular growth produces most of the observed recombinants.

This genetic evidence would be satisfied if the heterozygotes contained a single DNA molecule with the order of the nucleotides in the heterozygous region not being strictly complementary, but determined by the sequence from the two different parents of the cross. The nucleotides on either side of this special region would show exact complementarity, but the sequence on one side would be determined by one of the parents, while that on the other side would be determined by the other parent. The lack of complementarity in the heterozygous region would not be expected to have any significant structural consequences, since it would involve only a few nucleotide pairs in a region of several thousand pairs.

It is, unfortunately, very difficult on the basis of present knowledge to decide whether or not a plausible dynamic scheme can be constructed to account for the formation of such a particle by the interaction of two DNA molecules during the course of their replication. However, a preliminary study of the mechanics of this process with very crude models indicates that it is possible to find a sequence of plausible operations which will lead to the production of the required type of heterozygous particles. Each of the two chains would be partially copied on one parent, and partly on the other, and the heterozygous regions would arise if the template switch occurred at a different point on each chain. Although such speculation does not prove a positive point at this stage of our knowledge, it does serve to show that there is no compelling reason to believe that recombination cannot take place between essentially free DNA molecules under appropriate conditions.

The static model of DNA given to us by the crystallographer cannot easily account for recombination or even for specific pairing of the structures preparatory to recombination. It is, however, clear that even if only a small fraction of the hydrogen bonds which are normally responsible for intramolecular pairing were available for intermolecular pairing, sufficient specificity could be obtained for precise pairing. These speculations require much more knowledge of the physical chemistry of the DNA molecule. One would have to know how the base pair hydrogen-bond energy compares to the energy involved in forming hydrogen bonds with water before one could calculate the fraction of the bases which will be unpaired in the equilibrium situation. And one would also have to know the activation energies in order to estimate the probability of the equilibrium situation being achieved.

Since mating does not seem to involve breaks in the phosphate ester links, we can rule out breakage and reunion of already formed DNA molecules, i.e., crossing-over, as being responsible for recombinant formation. However, further detailed model building and more information on the energetics of base pairing will be necessary before it will be possible to see if one can construct a simple scheme involving de novo synthesis of recombinants by minor modifications of the Watson-Crick ideas of complementary replication of DNA.

REFERENCES

1. Hershey, A. D., and Chase, M., Genetic Recombination and Heterozygotes in Bacteriophage, *Cold Spring Harbor Symposia Quant. Biol.*, **16**, 471-479 (1951).
2. Levinthal, C., Recombination in Phage T_2; Its Relationship to Heterozygosis and Growth, *Genetics*, **39**, 169-184 (1954).
3. Levinthal, C., The Mechanism of DNA Replication and Genetic Recombination in Phage, preliminary report at Pallanza Conference, *Rend. ist. lombardo sci., Pt. I*, **89**, 192-199 (1955).
4. Levinthal, C., The Mechanism of DNA Replication and Genetic Recombination in Phage, *Proc. Natl. Acad. Sci. U. S.*, **42**, 394 (1956).
5. Levinthal, C., and Thomas, C. A., Jr., Molecular Autoradiography—The β-Ray Counting of Single Virus and DNA Particles in Nuclear Emulsions, in press.
6. Novick, A., and Szilard, L., Virus Strains of Identical Phenotype but Different Genotype, *Science*, **113**, 34-35 (1951).

DISCUSSION

DR. BROWN: By combining these astronomical methods of Dr. Levinthal with the more plebeian methods of fractionation we have been able to get some chemical information about these big pieces in the bacteriophage DNA. Our original fractionation method was that by combining fractionated histone with cellulose by diazotization and then by adsorbing the nucleic acid on the cellulose histone and then eluting with sodium chloride we obtained elution patterns showing two large peaks. We determined the base ratios in the elution diagram. The ratio was $\frac{\text{adenine} + \text{thymine}}{\text{guanine} + \text{5-hydroxymethyl cytosine}}$. The base ratios in the different fractions turned out to be slightly different. In one case fraction A was 1.9 and fraction B was 2.1. Then we measured the glucose content by reacting these fractions with anthrone, and we found the amount of glucose in fraction A to be molecularly equivalent to about 65% of the 5-hydroxymethyl cytosine. In the case of fraction B we found a 100% equivalence of glucose to 5-hydroxymethyl cytosine. With Dr. Neville Simons we have examined these. We put osmotically shocked hot phage on these columns and then examined the number of stars in each fraction. Most of the P^{32} label appeared in fraction A. We measured nucleic acid and P^{32} in these fractions. It appears that fraction A contains about 35% to 40% of the total DNA on the large-scale fractionation, and we assume that small-scale fractionation is the same as the large-scale one. This was done by shocking 10^9 hot phages and then running them and counting P^{32} as stars. It appears that fraction A, which had the low glucose content and the low base ratio, is Dr. Levinthal's large piece.

DR. LEDERBERG: Dr. Stent mentioned an experiment which involved the inactivation of *Escherichia coli*. He made the very interesting statement that the bacterial nucleus apparently does not replicate by a nondispersive mechanism. I think he was careful to say nucleus rather than chromosome or DNA. What bacteria were you using? *E. coli* B?

Dr. Stent: No, strain B/r.

Dr. Lederberg: Well, we know as little about B/r and its detailed genetical constitution with regard to how many chromosomes there are, etc., as we do about B. In addition, I think there would be the question of what the mechanism of killing in bacteria would be. If there were one hit in several of the nuclei in the bacterium, it is far from clear that that would not kill the cell; so it might be worthwhile to consider experiments with uninucleate bacteria, which *E. coli* is not.

Dr. Stent: We have.

Dr. Lederberg: Would you like to comment on that?

Dr. Stent: These experiments were carried out by Dr. Clarence Fuerst in Berkeley. One labels the bacteria, with a high level of P^{32}, freezes the system at —200°C., lets P^{32} decay proceed and then from day to day thaws samples and plates them for colony counts. One then obtains a 3- to 4-hit survival curve. The number of hits, I believe, corresponds to the number of nuclei which Witkin has identified by cytological techniques in the same strain under the same condition. We believe that the number of hits of the survival curve is a reflection of the number of nuclei. If the final slope of the inactivation curve, which reflects the rate at which the last nucleus is killed, is compared with the rate with which bacteriophages, which of course are entirely different in size and properties, are killed by P^{32} decay, practically the same efficiency of killing per P^{32} disintegration is found. So we believe that the same P^{32} killing mechanism is at work in phage and in bacterial nuclei. If these P^{32}-labelled bacteria are starved for phosphorus, so that they get very small, then the number of hits of the survival curve is reduced although the final slope is unchanged, indicating then that if the number of nuclei per cell is reduced the survival curve becomes more nearly exponential. Finally, it is necessary to make control experiments to see that indeed it is the DNA decay that is lethal, because most of the P^{32} is in RNA or in other cellular fractions. We had the good fortune that Dr. Seymour Cohen happened to be in Berkeley and he gave us *E. coli* 15T⁻, the thymineless strain which doesn't synthesize DNA unless it is given thymine. We grew two cultures of 15T⁻ and then placed both cultures in P^{32}, one with thymine and one without thymine. Both cultures took up practically the same amounts of P^{32}, because DNA synthesis is only a minor contributor to the total phosphorus assimilation. After 30 minutes both cultures contained practically the same amount of intracellular P^{32} except that one of them didn't have any P^{32} in its DNA. We then froze aliquots of the two cultures, let P^{32} decay take place, and thawed and plated samples from day to day to see what is the survival. The cells which had assimilated their P^{32} in the presence of thymine showed a much faster death rate than those which had taken up their P^{32} in the absence of thymine, indicating that the principal lethal effect was due to decay of P^{32} atoms in the nuclear material.

DR. JACOB: I just wanted to add a comment to Dr. Stent's about killing the bacteria by P^{32} decay in the DNA. It is possible to mate bacteria in which the donor Hfr was labelled with P^{32}, and the F— recipient was not labelled with P^{32}. The cross can be performed under conditions where no synthesis of DNA occurs. It is therefore possible to have zygotes in which the part of the F— cell is non-radioactive, whereas the part issued from the Hfr is labelled with P^{32}. Now, we know a certain number of markers here, and we can follow the inactivation of various types of recombinants as a function of P^{32} decay. We then select for recombinants having one given length of genetic material inherited from the Hfr parent or another length. Such experiments performed in collaboration with Dr. C. Fuerst and Dr. E. Wollman have shown that the decay is roughly proportional to the length of the piece that is acquired, so it seems likely that the killing of the bacteria in this instance is due to P^{32} inactivation in the DNA.

DR. LEDERBERG: Would you care to comment on the hint that you dropped about the dissociation of genetic markers from big pieces?

DR. STENT: This experiment is described in the written version of our discussion and concerns a four-factor cross of a P^{32}-labeled parental phage in minority against a non-radioactive parent in majority. The conclusion of this experiment was that there doesn't seem to be a phage chromosome which survives the mixed infection and reappears intact among the progeny. This conclusion, however, must be considered as rather tentative since it is possible that the genetic markers which we employed may have had some physiological effect on the course of phage development and produced an abnormal behaviour not otherwise encountered. This four-factor cross is now being repeated in Ann Arbor by Dr. Levinthal and his collaborators with different markers.

DR. LEVINTHAL: Dr. Martha Baylor and I have been repeating the 4-factor cross, reported by Stent and Sato, using a series of host-range markers which she has been studying for the past two years. At present the results are preliminary, and a good deal more work will be necessary before we have precise data. However, it is clear from our present work that about half of the single bursts which show any genes of the minority parent also show at least one copy of the minority parental type itself.

This result, of course, is in serious contradiction to that reported by Stent and Sato. We believe that the reason for this difference lies in the fact that they used the so-called "minute" marker and had a burst size which is approximately 1/5 to 1/10 of the normal. It seems very likely that this reduction in burst size represents some kind of faulty maturation of the phage and, therefore, is responsible for an incomplete sampling of the genetic units which are actually produced. This incomplete sampling would mean that the lack of suicide observed by Stent and Sato would be expected on any model of recombination. Any copies of the minority parent produced by growth would be expected to contain non-radioactive phosphorus atoms, and therefore not show the suicide effect.

We believe that they were looking primarily at those single bursts in which there had in fact been replication, and in which, therefore, most of the parental type copies were non-radioactive. I do not believe that any controls have been done to test this point in the minute system. One does not, for example, know in this case whether or not the P^{32} transferred is normal. If our explanation is correct, we would predict that this transfer would be very much lower than normal in the system used by Stent and Sato.

DR. CHARGAFF: I would like to ask Dr. Stent a question. When you label the nucleic acid with P^{32} and the phosphorus explodes you create a sulfuric acid ester at this point. There is little known about the sulfuric acid diesters and their stability. However, you assume, I suppose, that the chain breaks at the point where the P^{32} has gone to pieces. Is any chemical work known on sufficiently strongly labelled DNA to show that actually such breaks do occur—for instance, change in viscosity or sedimentation constants? Furthermore, I would think it would make a difference whether you have a large number of such phosphate bridges throughout the length of the molecule whether you break the molecule in half, if the phosphorus happens to be in the middle of the chain. I was just wondering whether anything has been done chemically on this.

DR. STENT: The difficulty is that the quantities of DNA which we have available for work, because of the extremely high level of label, are so small that direct viscosity measurement of breakage of DNA molecules is not possible. It would be possible to measure the decrease in molecular weight after P^{32} decay by diffusion techniques, in which the diffusion is followed by the radioactivity itself. This hasn't been done. The physiological and genetic properties of the P^{32}-activated phage particle fit nicely with the notion that the DNA molecule is actually cut by the radioactive decay.

DR. LEVINTHAL: We are testing this point experimentally, using the star method, but the plates are still in the icebox and we won't have any results for several weeks.

DR. CRICK: As essentially a new structure has been proposed by Dr. Stent, I feel that I should comment on it. The base pairing suggested is like-with-like pairing; adenine goes with adenine, cytosine with cytosine, and so on. You may perhaps wonder why this wasn't pointed out by Donohue, who published a paper recently on all the possible base pairs. The reason is that Dr. Stent has turned over two of the base pairs with respect to the other two. This makes the position of the glycosidic bonds of the four pairs much more similar than they would be otherwise, and thus makes it easier to fit the base pairs onto a regular backbone.

Although each particular structure has to be examined separately, it seems unlikely to ask, from looking at models, that the pyrimidines can be inverted without getting bad van der Waal contacts. Adenine can usually be turned over. Whether one can turn guanine over depends upon where its NH_2 group ends up, and this may vary from one structure to another.

The proposed structure, then, is certainly not an impossible one, but I should like to have the details of it from Dr. Stent and Dr. Donohue before commenting further. In order to get guanine to pair with guanine the authors have had to invoke a tautomeric shift of a hydrogen atom. This means that guanine could also pair with adenine, so that really the pairing rules are purine with purine, cytosine with cytosine, and uracil with uracil. If the pyrimidines also are allowed tautomeric shifts, the rules would be purine with purine and pyrimidine with pyrimidine. However, Dr. Stent's idea is that this is not a replicating structure but a *mating* structure. In a replicating structure one expects the bases to pair rather accurately, so that mistakes are rare. In a mating structure, however, you want bases to go together which are similar but not necessarily identical. So the fact that guanine can pair with either guanine or adenine, which would be surprising for a structure used for replication, does not matter for a mating structure.

I suppose I should point out that this idea of a structure for RNA is not too dissimilar from our own recent ideas, which Dr. Watson explained, that perhaps RNA consists of two parallel intertwined helical chains, with occasional base pairing. However, we shall have to do a lot more x-ray work before this very tentative model can be taken seriously. The present x-ray data certainly do not prove that such a structure exists, and the quality of the pictures suggests a more disordered model than Dr. Stent has described, but that may be due to the way our RNA specimens have been treated. In short, there is an interesting coincidence here between the idea of a mating structure for RNA and the ideas derived from the x-ray data, but this coincidence should be treated with great caution for the moment.

Finally, it's clear that if we are to judge models of the nucleic acids as they may exist in the cell—that is, without having the x-ray data to guide us—we shall have to collect a lot more physico-chemical data on which to base our judgments. One of the results of this meeting, as far as I'm concerned, is to convince me that we shall have to obtain much more of this background information; for example, measurements on base pairing, tautomeric forms, van der Waal's contacts, preferred orientations, and so forth.

DR. LEDERBERG: I would think it more plausible not to require pairing between similar structures—in fact, at points of pairing the two structures would have to be precisely alike, but at points of difference they simply don't pair.

DR. CRICK: That is certainly a possibility. I think it's a matter of the intimacy with which such regions are interspersed in such a structure. We don't know whether you can pair for two bases and then have a bit which doesn't pair, or whether you have to pair for 10 bases and after that have a bit that doesn't pair.

DR. LEVINTHAL: I think it would be impossible to judge this by any x-ray method. You know that if you do a genetic experiment you may put in 4 markers, or if you are Lederberg, several more than that, but mis-matching at this level could certainly not be detected crystallographically.

DR. CRICK: This is true if we are handling the actual genetic material, but we might be able to study an analogous situation using special synthetic polymers; for example, one in which we have a repeating sequence consisting of three paired bases followed by three non-paired bases. This may seem a little ambitious, but perhaps in another five years we might get such a polymer.

DR. LEDERBERG: I wonder if the nucleoprotein molecule couldn't be considered as a model system for considering the problem of winding and unwinding. Evidently one can make nucleoprotein from nucleic acid and protamine, and once you have studied the conditions of dissociation you might be able to get some idea of the energetics of uncoiling from that type of system.

DR. RICH: An interesting and perhaps useful model system for studying the energetics of forming a two-stranded helix is the polyadenylic acid plus polyuridylic acid system which I described previously. These two linear molecules meet in solution and then form systematic hydrogen bonds between the bases, similar to those in DNA. I should note, however, that if these two chains are parallel, then there is an additional hydrogen bond between the two backbones, from the hydroxyl group on carbon 2, to the phosphate oxygen of the opposite chain. At the present time, I cannot give you any data on the energies of this combination, except to say that it does not dissociate even under extreme dilution. By working with a series of polymers of gradually increasing length, it should be possible to learn a great deal about the cumulative effect of both systematic hydrogen bonding and the stacking of flat bases in a two-stranded helical nucleic acid molecule.

DR. BARBARA LOW: I should like to make a further comment on Dr. Levinthal's structure, if I understood him correctly. It seems to me that, if you carry this argument to the limit, you are saying that it is the regions which are not paired and not integrated in a regular configuration which are carrying the information. Isn't that so?

DR. LEVINTHAL: No. I am not suggesting that there are any large regions in which the bases are not paired. All I am suggesting is that the bonds have a finite energy. Therefore, there will be a finite number of them which are open at any one time. It seems that since we are in the very unfortunate position of knowing little about this binding energy, we cannot make any sensible comment on the fraction of them which is likely to be open at any one time. Therefore I am suggesting that in trying to consider mating interaction between molecules, one must worry about this physico-chemical problem. As far as mutations are concerned, I am suggesting only that if you make a mating— that is, a cross—involving several different markers, between hetero-parents each of which differs with respect to 4 markers, the pairing will be exact with respect to 160,000 bases less 4 times the length of a muton, which Benzer tells us is only a handful of nucleotides.

DR. BARBARA LOW: It seems unlikely on thermodynamic grounds that you would get quite random openings. It appears to me that here you may be beginning to get a structure with some kind of relationship to a protein, where we feel that the backbone structure is probably the helical chain, whereas at the reactive sites the molecular configuration may be irregular.

DR. LEDERBERG: I think that Dr. Levinthal was emphasizing that the hydrogen bond strengths of the individual base pairs are not well known and that at any particular point on the double helix you might have an opening out, which doesn't require a great deal of energy. It might be as much a function of time as of place.

DR. CRICK: Don't the experiments where you break one chain to see if it comes apart really involve 2 breaks?

DR. LEVINTHAL: I haven't been able to see from any thermodynamic arguments why these things should run up and down. There are 2 problems to worry about. One is the energy difference which will determine Boltzmann's distribution factor; the other is the activation energy. Now, we know very little about the Boltzmann's energy, and we know virtually nothing about the activation energy. This will determine the speed of running.

DR. CRICK: Don't the experiments in which you break one chain to see how the molecule comes apart suggest that any unpaired regions are not running up and down?

DR. LEVINTHAL: Yes, but this evidence is not nearly enough. There are two problems to worry about. One is the energy difference which will determine Boltzmann's distribution factor; the other is the activation energy. Now we know very little about the Boltzmann's energy, and we know virtually nothing about the activation energy. This will determine the speed with which equilibrium is established.

DR. DEMARS: I just want to propose a simple extension of the transfer experiments of Stent, and also of Brown's fractionation, which might give us some interesting results as to the function of hydroxymethyl cytosine in DNA, perhaps suggesting in a crude way what the hydroxymethyl cytosine is doing in the DNA. This is very peculiar DNA, because glucose is on the hydroxymethyl cytosine, and most of the hydroxymethyl cytosine is associated with diester bonds, which are not split by the diesterase which splits all the other DNA's which have been tested. That is, 30% of the diester bonds of this DNA cannot be split with venom diesterase or by the combined actions of coli and pancreatic DNAase and venom diesterase. One of the implications of the transfer experiments is that P^{32} of the infected particles is distributed more or less at random—that is, in the third generation transfers. If the transfers are indeed at random, then you should have a more or less random distribution of the resistant and labile diester linkages. This can be tested at each generation by obtaining the DNA by osmotic shock and seeing what fraction of the phosphorus from the initially labelled parental stock is localized in resistant linkages and labile ones. It would also be interesting to take Brown's fractions and see where the resistant linkages are localized, if they are localized.

DR. FRAENKEL-CONRAT: About the imperfections of the proposed RNA model as pointed out by Dr. Crick, I should like to draw attention to the fact that RNA seems to be somewhat more chemically imperfect than DNA. The bases are unreactive, the hyperchromic effect is small, and you never quite get the structure as suggested by the remarkable polymer of the mixture polyadenine and polyuracil. In other words, RNA is apparently not a very firmly and stably constructed double strand, if it is a double strand.

DR. BUTLER: I was just going to comment on Dr. Levinthal's suggestion that some of the hydrogen bonds are broken. That can be determined by titration, and in fact it's found that very few of them are broken.

DR. SINSHEIMER: I was just going to say that, in large RNA molecules, the hyperchromic effect is not small. It is about 30%, less than DNA, but comparable to the synthetic polymers.

DR. CARLSON: With regard to Dr. Levinthal's suggestion that some of the hydrogen bonds might be broken, there doesn't seem to be enough data to get any accurate estimate, but possibly Dr. Schachman or Dr. Doty from their viscosity and sedimentation studies have formulated a picture as to how flexible these molecules are. This might indicate how many hydrogen bonds were open.

DR. SCHACHMAN: I would just say that Thomas in Levinthal's laboratory has just published results which are identical with ours and which are both rather surprising. If you treat the kinetics of the enzyme digestion, the results show that if the enzymatic attacks in the two strands are staggered by only a few nucleotides apart, which means only a few pairs of hydrogen bonds, then the two pieces still remain held together. This would imply that just a few hydrogen bonds can hold two long pieces together. That is the result of the kinetic treatment, and it is all based on a mathematical analysis and our guess as to how DNAase is attacking DNA. This indicates that the hydrogen bonding is very strong, but there is no good reason to believe that these hydrogen bonds are that strong. I would guess, for example, that they would not be as good as the hydrogen bonds presumably holding polypeptide chains in a folded configuration.

DR. CARLSON: You are talking about breaking the backbone, aren't you?

DR. SCHACHMAN: No, I am referring to the hydrogen bonds. We allow the enzyme to break bonds in the backbone and from the data calculate how many pairs of hydrogen bonds are needed to prevent the two strands from separating. I should point out here that Dekker and I much earlier had inferred that the strands come apart when the molecular weight of the enzymatically degraded material approaches 50,000 to 100,000. This implies rather weak hydrogen bonding. It seems to me that this, too, is an unsettled problem.

DR. ALLFREY: I would just like to ask Dr. Crick a question of fact. I know nothing about x-ray crystallography procedure. I would like to know, if a large part of the DNA was rather randomly uncoiled and if a small portion was coiled, whether it would still give a regular diffraction pattern.

DR. CRICK: This was one of the points I was talking about yesterday. X-ray diffraction is a poor method for telling how much of a material is in a regular structure. I should be surprised if the regular part was less than 50% of the total, but this is only a guess.

DR. WATSON: Infrared analysis of DNA solutions suggests that a large majority, if not all, of the DNA molecules have the double helical configuration. This technique measures the properties of all the molecules in solution, not just the oriented fraction which the x-rays detect. Blout et al. found that native DNA in solution gives two very characteristic peaks. When denaturation occurs, these peaks move to slightly different frequencies. It is very unlikely that these changes would be so clear if a sizable fraction of the DNA possessed a configuration other than the double helix.

DR. CRICK: The answer is to try different techniques, as suggested by Watson. The x-ray technique is a bad one.

DR. CARLSON: A possible technique is based on the study of the mechanical properties of the fibers. Can you tell us something about the mechanical properties of these fibers? Are they like a hair, or are they softer and more flexible? Such information might be used to obtain an estimate of the amount of crystalline material present.

DR. RICH: DNA fibers are very brittle except when the humidity is quite high. At over 90% relative humidity they begin to soften and can be pulled.

DR. LEDERBERG: An optimistic report of this symposium might indicate a new era in genetic study, where factorial descriptions are (about to be) replaced by chemical ones. The details of the speculations which have been put forward here may all prove to be wrong, but we are at a stage in the development of chemical genetics where we need stepping stones as well as foundation blocks. Furthermore, most of the experimental reports have been designedly tentative, and their authors assure us they are aware of the gaps which have to be filled. It may therefore be inappropriate to question them too closely in critique.

Some of the residual issues are so obvious that they perhaps ought to be stated. On the chemical side:

1. What is the detailed structure of DNA? No one appears to have taken serious exception to the Watson-Crick model for the basic plan, but many microscopic deviations have been suggested, and may be needed to explain singularities of genetic behavior such as variable mutation rates. Is pairing always perfect? Are there interactions between adjacent nucleotides in the same chain? Are there segmental interruptions in the chains? Are there linkages other than phosphate-3-5-diester bonds? Having achieved the general plan, what are the prospects of a complete analysis of sequence of bases? We lack precise methods of end-group analysis of polynucleotides, and more work in sugar chemistry and enzymology may be needed to find them. And if we had the chemical methods, what would we analyze? Levinthal gave us the only plausible answer here, the large "piece" in the phage nucleus: any other material now evident, and perhaps this too, would certainly be hopelessly heterogeneous. Until we have real information along these lines, we cannot pretend to know the chemical basis of genetic differences, however plausible the guesses of the moment may appear.

2. How is DNA synthesized? Kornberg and his associates have made such startling progress in the elaboration of an in vitro system that one is tempted to call a moratorium on other speculation. They have emphasized the urgency of knowing whether the polymer is a biologically specific product. The requirement for a DNA primer and for all four deoxynucleoside triphosphates hints that it is, but we must still learn whether the synthesis is a replication or a random lengthening of the polynucleotide primer.

3. Tests of biological specificity of nucleic acids. These are sadly rare. For RNA we have hardly more than the infectivity of tobacco mosaic virus, either as the native RNA, or reconstituted with a protective protein. For DNA we have the pneumococcal and Hemophilus transforming systems. The problems involved in quantitative assay for biological activity with the pneumococcus have been amplified by Hotchkiss and Ephrussi-Taylor. Goodgal's report suggests that the Hemophilus system may be in some respects easier, but this also needs to be studied more extensively. At the present time we have no method

of assaying the biological activity, hence specificity, of extracted DNA from phage or from other sources. A number of other claims of DNA-mediated transduction (transformation) may be found in the literature, but none of them has yet stood up well enough to serve the purpose. It would be highly desirable to work out a DNA-transductional system in an enteric bacterium (e.g., Salmonella or *E. coli*) because of the technical facility and background knowledge of genetic work with these organisms. The reports of Boivin, which are often quoted, unfortunately cannot be verified owing to the loss of his cultures at the time of his death. Perhaps the protoplast systems mentioned by Spiegelman may serve as analytical tools for the specificity both of DNA in heredity) and RNA (in functional development).

Until such systems are further refined, we may have to call our symposia "Chemistry and Heredity" rather than "Chemistry of Heredity."

Dr. Chargaff indicated the very real language barrier, and the trouble it can raise at a symposium of genetics, chemists and crystallographers. He may have been interested to learn that this is a problem even among the geneticists, to the point where 'gene' is no longer a useful term in exact discourse. It should not be surprising that (some) geneticists are remarkably preoccupied with semantic problems. The series of constructs involved in genetic analysis are not necessarily more abstract than those used, e.g., in structural analysis of organic compounds, but they are usually expressed verbally rather than mathematically. Because the words are part (I hope not all) of the tools of the trade, the geneticist has to try to keep them sharp. One of the outstanding grinding wheels here was Benzer, who with "muton," "recon" and "cistron" has fabricated some euphonious and utilitarian contributions to our language. I don't know whether he meant them any more seriously than the Anglo-Saxonized "mit," "rit" and "pfit," but whether he did or not, we are going to find it difficult to avoid talking about cistrons from now on. Unfortunately, as I eavesdropped to catch notes for this discussion, I heard variant uses, and we can only beg that our colleagues adhere scrupulously to the new dictionary: a distron is not defined in respect to any enzyme or other purported gene product, but is a group of mutants whose functional relationship is inferred from their common membership in a cis-trans position-effect group.

One danger in postulational terminology is to confuse the word for a fact. An important contribution from Benzer was his demonstration that his mutants could be grouped into *unique* cistrons. No other case of position effect has been so intensively studied, and it would be premature to hold that this is a general description of patterns of position effect, and therefore that position effect must be interpreted in terms of common primary function. The well-known effect of transposed heterochromatin in Drosophila, and McClintock's findings (reviewed by Rhoades at this symposium) in maize, speak for another mechanism of position effect: disturbances at one point of a chromosome may spread some distance down its length. Depending on the overlap of these spreading effects, of three mutants, *a*, *b*, and *c*, *a* and *b* might be found to show position-effect, as well as *b* and *c*, but *a* and *c* might not. The *a-b* and *b-c* cistrons are therefore not unique, but overlap on *b*. This mechanism makes no demand of functional identity of the mutants. Only further study can tell how generally position effects may be understood from these two, or from other, viewpoints.

The term *gene* represented the hope that the chromosome could be considered as an array of discrete units, whose irreducibility would be confirmed by mutational, recombinational, and functional tests. Finer analysis and current theories of DNA structure, if translatable to the chromosome, suggest a more monotonous continuum which is not segmented into natural unit "genes." A mutation is therefore a local change on a chromosome, not necessarily in a "gene." Rhoades showed that many mutations are disqualified as "point mutations." Their existence is not a semantic fancy. A point mutation is most concretely defined as one which results from the substitution or deletion of a single nucleotide. It remains to be seen whether any mutations actually arise in this way. One helpful criterion might come from the prediction that at any (recombinational) point, no more than four (or including deletion, five) alternative configurations would be possible, one for each base. Benzer's studies represent the most encouraging approach to this kind of demonstration. Until the finer structure is cleared up, there is bound to be nomenclatural confusion. I had hoped that such terms as *locus* and *allele* might be reserved to the traditional and (to my own mind) more objective concept of recombinational units, but there is no agreement on this point today. Perhaps we should adopt Levinthal's suggestion that all discussion of terminology be proscribed, but that each author prescribe his own use of the terms. The topic is belabored only because of the discordance in current literature.

Language problems are not confined to genetics. I was struck by several references to "*mere* exchange reactions"; I thought I understood what "exchange reaction" meant, but I didn't understand the "*mere.*" Is it true that a macromolecule can exchange an interstitial monomer and keep its biological specificity? If so, it might help to understand the incorporation step of transductional genetics, wherein a fragment presumably must exchange with an organized chromosome.

DR. SPIEGELMAN: I should like to say a few words about the exchange problem. It seems to me unwise to accept without caution conclusions about the protein synthesizing mechanism which are derived solely from incorporation data. I think it unlikely that a labeled amino acid can be inserted in the middle of a fully-formed protein molecule in solution. The act of incorporation is therefore probably not trivial and related to the protein-synthesizing mechanism

There remains, however, an element of uncertainty which makes it difficult to interpret incorporation data unambiguously. I have already noted in my discussion the experiments of Gale and Folkes and their relation to the interpretation of unequal labeling of a protein molecule.

There are three types of auxiliary experiments, the performance of which could help in assaying the significance of incorporation experiments:

(1) The effect of homologous and heterologous amino acid analogues on the extent and rate of incorporation.

(2) A comparison of incorporation in the presence and absence of supplementation by a complete mixture of amino acids.

(3) Evidence that the labeled amino acid is being inserted all along the protein molecule in α-peptide linkages.

DR. HOAGLAND: Let me add to Dr. Spiegelman's discussion the following comments in clarification of the meaning of so-called amino acid "exchange" reactions and their significance in protein synthesis, since much work has been done in our and other laboratories on the assumption that the incorporation of C^{14} labelled amino acids into protein is indicative of protein biosynthesis. It would appear to be highly unlikely that an amino acid could exchange with an already formed and completed protein, and Gale has suggested that the anomalous exchange he observes may be due to interaction of the amino acid with some pre-protein on a template. Furthermore, the possibility of glutathione synthesis as an explanation for glutamic acid "exchange" in Gale's system must be considered.

We have used the word "incorporation" to describe the *irreversible* incorporation of C^{14} amino acids into protein which we and others are studying in mammalian tissues. In these reactions, both in vivo and in vitro, the addition of C^{12} amino acids after an initial incorporation of C^{14} amino acids results in no loss of previously incorporated amino acid. Furthermore, this process is dependent, in vitro, upon ATP for energy, a soluble protein fraction containing amino acid activating enzymes, small amounts of GDP or GTP, and intact ribonucleoprotein particles. When the protein so labelled is isolated and subjected to all procedures known to remove any non-peptide bound amino acids, the radioactivity remains. The radioactive amino acids are released from the protein on hydrolysis at the same rate as the corresponding C^{12} amino acid. Small peptides which contain the labelled amino acid have been isolated from the hydrolysate and identified. The labelled amino acid is found throughout the protein and not just in terminal positions. We believe for these reasons that incorporation is very likely a measure of protein biosynthesis.

A SUMMARY OF THE SYMPOSIUM ON THE CHEMICAL BASIS OF HEREDITY

Bentley Glass

Department of Biology,
The Johns Hopkins University

Cellular Units of Heredity

The Role of the Nucleus in Heredity.

In the introductory paper of the Symposium on the Chemical Basis of Heredity, Beadle has summarized current points of view in genetics together with a vast amount of recent information that has led to modifications, often very radical ones, of the views of yesteryear. His survey even included much information from papers presented scarcely a week previously, at the 1956 Cold Spring Harbor Symposium on "Genetic Mechanisms," and still unpublished.

In spite of the reluctance of a number of geneticists to abandon the once universal view that the primary coding of genetic information in chromosomes resided in the protein portion of the nucleoproteins, the evidence from the transformations of genetic type in pneumococci and from phage infection and transmission of genetic traits has compelled most persons now to accept the view that the primary genetic material is deoxyribonucleic acid (DNA), except in some plant viruses, such as tobacco mosaic virus, where ribonucleic acid (RNA) must take its place. If this be accepted, the genetic information would almost certainly have to be coded in the form of specific sequences of purine and pyrimidine bases. Assuming the validity of the Watson-Crick model of DNA structure as a double helix of two complementary polynucleotide chains opposite in polarity and held together by hydrogen bonds between the opposed bases (adenine-thymine; guanine-cytosine), it would seem that the "gene" is to be conceived as "a localized unit of nucleic acid with a specific function . . . presumed to consist in the determination of the specificity of a nongenic molecule such as a protein." Gene replication is then to be analyzed in terms of a replication of the DNA double helix, gene mutation in terms of an alteration of nucleic acid structure at sites within a gene, and gene function in terms of the translation of DNA specificity into protein specificity, probably via an RNA template mechanism.

757

The problem as to the mechanism of replication may be seen at its simplest in the bacterial viruses, the genetic material of which appears to be comprised of a single continuous Watson-Crick double helix of DNA made up of some 200,000 pairs of nucleotides. The simplest proposed mechanism for replication envisions a separation of the complementary polynucleotide chains, each of which may then serve as a template for the synthesis of a new complementary chain as partner. The replication of the RNA of tobacco mosaic virus and related viruses poses special problems. It is not known whether the replication occurs directly, or indirectly through the intermediation of the DNA, and possibly the protein, of the host cell.

Gene mutation might occur through substitution of bases at one or more levels, through rearrangement of base-pair sequences, through duplication of one or more base-pairs, or through deletion of base-pairs. The three last-named intragenic types of change would correspond in nature to the chromosomal aberrations of higher organisms which transcend the limits of a single gene.

Genetic recombination in the higher organisms occurs by means of crossing over, a process in which two homologous chromosomes, each in a subdivided or 4-strand stage, pair intimately and exactly locus by locus, and then two random non-sister strands exchange exactly equivalent segments of chromosome. There is no evidence at present to rule out the supposition that this process is always *inter*genic. In fact, the evidence that chelating agents cause the dissociation of chromosomes into units about 4000 Å long and that they also increase the frequency of crossing over supports the view that the chromosomes may consist of segments of DNA and protein held together by Ca^{++} ions, and that crossing over normally occurs in the chelated regions.

In the genetic recombination of the genes in the DNA of phages, reciprocal recombinant strands are not formed simultaneously. The fact that only one recombinant is formed suggests that the mechanism is quite different from that occurring in conventional crossing over in plants and animals, where reciprocal recombinants are regularly formed by the same event. Phage recombination is often intragenic, but may be intergenic as well, although there is no saying whether or not the successive genes are contiguous or have "spacer" segments of DNA between them. In *Neurospora, Aspergillus,* and yeast, in all of which conventional crossing over between genes occurs, intragenic recombination may be brought about by a shift in copying small segments of genetic material from one chromosome model to its homologue. [This event, termed "conversion" by Lindegren and "transmutation" by Beadle, might better be called by some entirely new name, such as "transreplication," rather than by terms which have already acquired some other significance in the genetic literature.] The feature of this process that distinguishes it from crossing over is that the single event does not give rise to reciprocal products and does not necessarily lead to a recombination of genetic markers on either side of the "trans-replicated" segment. Nevertheless, in spite of the distinctness of this process from crossing over, the two processes are positively correlated in occurence, probably because they each depend upon a close contact of the homologous chromosomes. The discovery in microorganisms of this process, so similar to genetic recombination in phages and to transformation and transduction processes in bacteria, serves to relate the genetic recombination of the latter to that of higher organisms, otherwise so different.

The fine structure of the gene is now being worked out by the study of genetic recombination of these various types, not only in the bacteriophages, but also in bacteria such as *Salmonella* and in yeast. Thus two types of alleles may be distinguished, (1) *homoalleles* which are presumably identical in site as well as function, since no reversions or recombinations occur in an organism carrying a combination of two homoalleles; and (2) *heteroalleles,* between which recombination does occur, and which are therefore presumably not at the same location within the over-all boundaries of the functional unit. Studies of the functional relations of homoalleles and heteroalleles may be expected to yield insight into the nature of gene functioning in general. Beadle calls attention to the illuminating studies of Bonner, Yanofsky, and Suskind on the *Neurospora* mutants at a locus (*td*) that affects the enzyme, tryptophan synthetase, which is responsible for coupling indole and serine to produce the amino acid tryptophan. Of 25 independently arising mutants of this type, all proved to be at the same locus. Some were homoallelic, others heteroallelic, to judge from reversions occurring with some rarety in the latter combinations. Suppressor genes at other loci act specifically on particular heteroalleles, although there may be several different non-allelic suppressors of the same *td* allele. The *td* mutants lack the active enzyme, but some possess a serologically closely related protein. Hence it is suggested that the mutations may result in enzyme inactivation by so modifying the protein structure that some normally present metabolite may react with it and serve as an inhibitor of the synthesis of tryptophan. Different suppressors could interfere with the formation of different inhibiting metabolites, or with the formation of a single inhibitor in various ways.

The template hypothesis of gene action, according to Beadle, still accounts quite adequately for the significant observation that numerous mutants which affect the same protein, e.g., hemoglobin, are found to be alleles, i.e. to have occurred at a single locus. Possibly RNA may serve as an intermediate template between DNA and the genetically modified macromolecule. No structure of RNA which would imply that it replicates like DNA has yet been postulated; but the constitution of the core of the tobacco mosaic virus out of RNA implies either that RNA can replicate itself, or else that its information is somehow transferred to the DNA of the bacterial host, and that this DNA is then replicated and the information transferred back to RNA.

The localized regions of specific function recently found in bacteriophages and bacteria "quite clearly correspond to the units that geneticists have long called genes," says Beadle. He proceeds to draw an analogy between the use of the term "gene" in genetics and the term "enzyme" in biochemistry. In spite of the discovery that some enzymes are made up of dissociable subunits and that some are functional only when associated in a particular organized way with certain other enzymes, the concept of the "enzyme" remains of everyday use. The "gene" concept will stay so too, in spite of subdivisibility and position effects. As in the case of the enzyme, a complete definition of the gene will have to await the full analysis of its chemical structure and its macromolecular products. Meanwhile, it is useful to be able to say that many genes act so as to confer specificity on particular enzymes, and that sometimes the total specificity of an enzyme is attributable to a single gene.

Chromosome Structure.

Ris has distinguished four successive phases in the study of chromosome structure and its relation to genetic function. In the pioneer period, up to 1920, the basic problems were outlined: the number of strands in a chromosome and the nature of the elementary strand, or chromonema; the nature of its longitudinal differentiation, that is, the relation of chromosome structure and chemistry to the "reproductive" and "metabolic" activities of genes; the significance of the coiling cycle in mitosis; and the processes underlying chromosome duplication. The next period involved a more detailed analysis of the structure, coiling cycle, and reproduction of chromosomes, with an identification of heterochromatin and euchromatin, of chromomeres, spindle attachment organs, nucleolar organizers, etc. The major achievement of this period was the analysis of the coiling cycle of the chromosomes during mitosis and meiosis. The chromosome helix was observed to originate in prophase and to relax during telophase. The third period, commencing about 20 years ago, witnessed a revival of interest in chromosome chemistry. The principal discoveries then made were that the absolute amount of DNA per chromosome is remarkably constant from cell to cell within individuals of the same species and that DNA is metabolically rather inert except for its doubling in amount with each cell generation, an increase in which it is closely paralleled by the histones; whereas RNA and the non-histone protein part of the chromosomes are metabolically very active and vary considerably in amount from cell to cell depending on the level of metabolic rate in the tissue. The fourth and current period of cytogenetic study must relate the findings of chromosome chemistry to the outcome of the cytological studies. It is commencing with an investigation of chromosome organization on the macromolecular level, by means of polarizing microscopy, x-ray analysis, and electron microscopy. Still, much work must yet be done to fill the gap between the macromolecular level and that of chromosome strands visible in the ordinary light microscope.

In general discussion, Lewis clarified the significance of F. O. Schmitt's analogy between chromosomes and such other macromolecular structures as myosin, fibrinogen, and keratin. What has impressed Schmitt most about these systems is that it is not from the precise chemical composition of the units, but rather from the particular organization and integration of the macromolecules into the system as a whole that its properties derive. Secondly, this integration of the component macromolecular units is extremely sensitive to certain environmental conditions. It is definable in physical-chemical terms, such as thermal agitation, van der Waals forces, hydrogen bonds, and electrostatic links affected by ionic strength, pH, etc. Chromosomes are obviously much more complex systems than those of collagen, but the same principles of physical-chemical organization may likewise apply to them.

From many electron-microscope studies of the lampbrush chromosomes of amphibian oocytes, the giant salivary gland chromosomes of *Drosophila* and other Diptera, and the beautiful coiled chromosomes of lilies, *Tradescantia*, and other plants, Ris draws the conclusion that the basic morphological unit of all chromosomes is a fibril some **200 Å** thick, commonly found in pairs of sister-fibrils with an interspace between them, so that the unit of next larger size is a double fibril of approximately **500 Å** diameter. By comparison and analogy with the tobacco mosaic virus particle, which like the ultimate chromosome fibril in cross section in electron micrographs resembles a tiny doughnut, Ris formulates a model of the ultimate chromosome fibril as having a core of nucleic acid enveloped by a protein sheath.

Chromosomes, then, are multistranded bundles of these ultimate fibrils, but exactly how many cannot be said at present, except that it should be some power of 2. The number probably varies in different organisms and in different cells of the same organism; if so, that would account for the variation in the DNA content of chromosomes. There are, for example, probably 1000 times as many fibrils in the salivary gland chromosomes of a fruitfly as there are in its ordinary somatic chromosomes.

The question of greatest genetical interest, of course, relates to the longitudinal differentiation of the chromosomes. What is the significance of the chromomeres, those beadlike swellings of characteristic size and position which Belling once took to be the sites of the genes, but which are too few in number for any such correspondence? Ris strongly argues for a continuous structure of the chromosome strands, and against the view that chromomeres are interruptions of the linear continuity of the fibers. Like a number of other cytologists, Ris holds that the ultimate visible chromomeres of the most fully extended (leptotene) chromosomes are no more than tight gyres of the new coil which makes its appearance in prophase. In electron micrographs chromomeres can be seen to contain the same fibrils as the interchromomeric segments. What, then, are the sharply staining bands and the unstainable interbands of the dipteran salivary gland chromosomes? Ris and Crouse once put forward the view that the bands are homologous with chromomeres of the usual sort, and the result of a specific coiling pattern of a bundle of chromonemata. The electron micrographs support this view; for although the salivary gland chromosome may be separated into thinner strands which still retain the banded pattern, electron micrographs show that the bands do consist of microfibrils like those of the interband segments but greatly twisted and closely packed together.

The term *heterochromatin* generally refers to chromosome material that remains densely stainable when the rest of the genetic material (*euchromatin*) loses its stainability. Heterochromatin may remain persistently stainable, or may vary in stainability but be out of phase with the euchromatin. As to organization, it differs from euchromatin notably in the degree of spiralization of the chromonema (relative width of gyres, degree of packing, presence of a double helix). But in good preparations it can readily be seen that the chromonema is continuous from euchromatin to heterochromatin, and that a basic fibril of the same 200 Å diameter is found in both. No clear chemical difference between the two forms has been established. The so-called matrix, formerly thought to be a sheath surrounding the euchromatic chromonema during mitosis, is now demonstrated by cytochemical tests to be nothing except a shrinkage space left around the chromosome after certain types of chemical fixation—in other words, to be pure artifact. It is never observable in electron micrographs of sections through chromosomes. There is also no evidence that the chromosome has a definite membrane of its own. The functional, organizational, and chemical distinctions between euchromatin and heterochromatin remain among the greatest riddles for present-day cytologists, geneticists, and cytochemists to solve.

Ris dicusses without commitment the evidence for the organization of the chromosome fibril by end-to-end aggregation of rod-like particles. Under conditions that remove calcium and magnesium from the chromosomes, native nucleoprotein from sea urchin sperm forms rods about 4000 Å long and 200 Å wide (Berstein and Mazia). Agents that break hydrogen bonds dissolve salivary gland chromosomes (Ambrose). Spontaneous chromosome breakage in plants is greatly increased when they are grown in media deficient in calcium or magnesium (Steffensen). *Drosophila* larvae fed excess calcium yield a diminished amount of crossing over; if they are fed a chelating agent, ethylenediamine tetraacetic acid (EDTA), the crossing over is increased above normal (Levine). A similar result with EDTA was demonstrated in the unicellular plant *Chlamydomonas:* a lowering of the Ca^{++} and Mg^{++} concentrations in the cells increased crossing over considerably, and this effect could be reversed by treatment with Ca^{++} and Mg^{++} (Eversole and Tatum). These are very stimulating discoveries, but it remains hard to relate such generalized effects to the very exact pattern of breakage at precisely the same level which takes place in two chromosomes undergoing genetic recombination.

The study of the structural and chemical variations in the chromosomes which take place in relation to their functioning promises insight into the nature of gene action. Electron microscope studies suggest the existence of considerable activity on the nuclear-cytoplasmic boundary, and some transfer of material through gaps in the nuclear membrane. Two types of specially favorable chromosomes for these studies are the lampbrush chromosomes of amphibian oocytes and the polytene (multistranded) giant chromosomes of the dipteran salivary glands. Ris presented evidence from the studies of a number of cytologists to demonstrate that the loops of the lampbrush chromosomes are continuous parts of the chromonemata and that the chromomeres between them are places where the fibrils are tightly coiled and heterochromatic. The evidence is convincing that the loops bridge discrete gaps between one chromomere and the next. In the chromomeres submicroscopic fibrils (500 Å diam. and each composed of two subunits of 200 Å diam.) are coiled in a helix. Chemically, the loops themselves seem to contain mainly RNA and protein; only the chromomeres stain Feulgen-positive, i.e., are composed of DNA. Treatment with EDTA disperses the loops quickly but does not affect the chromomeres.

In the salivary gland chromosomes, at certain definite stages in development, particular bands enlarge greatly into structures which have been called "puffs" or "Balbiani rings." The puffs seem to be produced by a great lengthening of the strands of the chromosome, which separate from one another and form loops projecting laterally from the chromosome like the loops of lampbrush chromosomes. The puffing is associated with an accumulation of basophilic but Feulgen-negative material (Pavan and Breuer). As in the lampbrush chromosomes, the chromonemata must have increased greatly in length to make these loops or puffs—as Beerman and Bahr estimate, up to 5 times the normal length of the salivary chromosome band and up to 50 times the length of the unit in a common (pachytene) chromosome. Each of these very elongated segments still corresponds to a single gene locus, and appears to involve only an increase in RNA and non-histone protein, not an increase of DNA. Do the fibrils of the loops have a core of RNA and a sheath of protein? Are they particulate like the tobacco mosaic virus particles? It is suggestive that the relative proportion of RNA to protein in tobacco mosaic virus, namely, 6 per cent, is like that of the chromosomes, 7-14 per cent. Maybe the growth in length occurs by an intercalation of ribonucleoprotein particles in the fibrils— in lampbrush chromosomes at many loci, in salivary gland chromosomes at a restricted number. When the loops later diminish in size, material must be released from them, and perhaps in this way RNA units synthesized in the chromosome are released to enter the cytoplasm. Information might thus be transferred from specific genes to regions of protein synthesis in the cytoplasm, the ergastoplasmic particles.

The coiling of the chromosomes is not simple but involves a hierarchy of helical systems, of minor coils superimposed upon major coils. Even so, it is a long step from the microscopically visible coils of smallest size to the coiling of the elementary fibrils and of the nucleic acid and protein macromolecules. Some electron micrographs have shown a rod-like core around which prophase chromosomes are coiled; but it is not known how common this may be or whether it is essential to the coiling. A major problem for the future will certainly be that of the relationship of the different orders of coiling to one another. There is evidence that the microfibrils are twisted around one another. If so, their ultimate separation must involve a change into a coiling system that will permit separation. By coiling a twisted pair of strands into a helix with one gyre for each relational twist, the helices can be separated. Perhaps this is the significance of the tightening helical coiling seen in every prophase.

Chromosome reproduction may be considered, as Ris points out, on three levels: "the synthesis of nucleic acids and proteins; the replication of the elementary chromosome fibril; and the splitting of the bundle of fibrils into units of higher order such as chromatids, half-chromatids, and quarter-chromatids." It is particularly important to realize the distinction between the last two levels, for it implies that daughter chromosomes at anaphase of a mitotic division are not one new, one old, but rather both new and both old, because each contains both old and new fibrils. Depending on the number of hierarchical sub-units between the chromosome and the unit of replication, the fibril, it will take several to many cell generations before newly formed micro-fibrils separate as fully grown daughter chromosomes.

The Fine Structure of the Gene.

Benzer's work on the linear sequence of genetic units in the *E. coli* bacteriophages, and his studies of the finer structure which can be elaborated within each unit of genetic function by studies of recombina-tion, have shown with graphic clarity what other workers with other organisms have likewise pointed out: the "gene" is not an operationally properly defined concept, inasmuch as at least three distinct opera-tions—mutation, recombination, and function—can be used to define the gene; and the units so defined are not the same in the three cases. Benzer suggests a new terminology so apt as to be certain of widespread adoption. The smallest element in the unidimensional array of genetic units that is interchangeable, but not divisible, by genetic recombina-tion is to be called the *recon*. The smallest element that, when altered, can give rise to a mutant form of organism is to be called the *muton*. The functional unit is to be defined by the *cis-trans* test. If the two mutants in the trans configuration (heterozygous; heterocaryotic; or host doubly infected with virus) yield a defective or mutant pheno-type, it may be concluded that they are defective in the same function; whereas the cis arrangement of the same mutants is usually fully nor-mal. The mutants are thus identified as belonging to the same func-tional genetic unit, or *cistron*. [This test will apply readily only to recessive genes, for dominant genes will give a mutant phenotype even when they are at entirely different genetic loci.]

The studies Benzer reported to the Symposium represented an en-deavor to place limits on the sizes of these three types of genetic units in the case of a specific genetic region of the bacterial virus T4, the segment containing the *rII* mutants. Two mutants are crossed by in-fecting a susceptible bacterium with both types and then examining the phage progeny for recombinant types. Phage T4 has already been fairly well mapped and behaves as a haploid organism with a single linkage group. It should be noted, however, that the portion of the genetic map which can be studied varies according to the bacterial strain utilized as host. The *rII* mutants form small wild-type plaques on *E. coli* strain S, and large *r*-type plaques on strain B; while on strain K some, but not all, *rII* mutants grow slightly, that is, produce minute plaques. The map of the *rII* region which would be derived from the use of strain B as host would differ significantly, according to Benzer, from the map derived from using strain K.

To determine the length of the recon, mutants in a limited region must be mapped to so high a linear density that their distances apart diminish to the magnitude of their own individual sizes. Only an upper limit of size can be set, equal to or smaller than the smallest observed recombination interval greater than zero. The muton can be calculated from the discrepancy in a 3-point test between the recombination interval A–C and the sum of the intervals A–B and B–C. The difference will presumably be the size of the muton B. Only an upper limit can be set to the size of the muton by the smallest observed discrepancy found by this method; and the size of the muton would appear to be zero if it were equal to or smaller than the recon. A second method for estimating muton size would be to determine the maximum number of mutations separable by recombination which could be placed within a definite length of the genetic map. Finally, the length of the cistron must be at least as large as the distance between the most distant mutons within it. Only a lower limit of size can be set for it, unless studies are made of recombination between mutons of adjacent cistrons, right and left.

Benzer has also made use of the method of using "deletions," stable mutations which do not recombine with any of a number of mutants which do recombine. These mutations, like demonstrable deletions in higher organisms, never revert to normal. [In the phage chromosome they might, of course, be inversions.] The mutations of any single cistron can first be classified into subgroups according to their inclusion within the segment covered by one of these "deletions." Without elaborating on the procedures used, it may be said that subclassification after the initial identification of a mutant as belonging to one of the two *rII* cistrons involved spot testing on *E. coli* strain K, as well as on a mixture of B and K cells, preliminary crosses, standard crosses, and determination of reversion rates and of the "leakiness" of the mutants. A series of 923 *r* mutants was thus classified hierarchically into six levels. Any mutants belonging to the same subclass which showed recombination of less than 0.001% of recombination were assigned to the same "species." For example, within one subclass of the *rII*–A cistron there turned out to be 11 "species," very unequally represented, since 123 of the 149 mutants in the subclass belonged to a single "species." The upper limit found for the recon, by the crosses between these 11 "species," was approximately 0.02 per cent. Eight cases of 3-point crosses could be utilized for the estimation of the size of the muton. The discrepancies found ranged from —0.03 to +0.14, with an average of +0.01; but because of the magnitude of the experimental error the upper limit could not be set at less than 0.05 per cent recombination. From the number of "species" within a given length of map an upper limit of 0.09 per cent was obtained (9 "species" in a map length of 0.8%); but again the factor of uncertainty is relatively large.

The stable *r* mutants ("deletions"), of which 72 were found, have also been crossed by Benzer in all possible pairs. One mutant was found that failed to complement mutants of either the A or B cistrons of the *rII* segment; in other words, it belongs to both. Another represented a deletion of the entire B cistron, in spite of which the mutant form can still grow normally on *E. coli* strains B and S. Stable mutants tend to occur all over the map, but some localities seem to be favored.

Benzer has daringly made the attempt to relate the above estimates of genetic size to the genetic material of the virus. Assuming that the total DNA content of a virus particle is 4×10^5 nucleotides, of which 40 per cent is the genetic material (calculated from Levinthal's experiment, q.v.), and assuming further that there is only one copy of the genetic material and that the Watson-Crick double-helix affords a satisfactory model, the total length of genetic material in phage T4 should be 8×10^4 nucleotide pairs. The genetic map is roughly estimated to comprise at least 200 recombination units, and by simple summation of small segments would contain about 800 recombination units. If, finally, the recombination per unit length of chromosome is assumed to be uniform, one arrives at an estimate of 0.01 recombination units per nucleotide pair. In other words, if two mutants, when crossed, do not give more than 0.01% of recombination, then the locations of those mutations are probably not separated by more than one nucleotide pair.

The upper limit of size of the recon, estimated to be 0.02% recombination, would on the above basis include no more than two nucleotide pairs. The muton would involve no more than 5 nucleotide pairs. The cistron is more complex. Among 241 *r* mutants there were 33 "species" in the A cistron. This number will probably be doubled when the 923 mutants now available have all been analyzed; and ultimately perhaps 100 sites may be found to lie within this one cistron. Although these estimates are acknowledged to be very rough, it is challenging to have them at all. If the testing of time shows that the techniques and methods used by Benzer are sound, the work he has done will unquestionably assume classical importance in the development of genetics.

Genetic Recombination in Neurospora.

Crossing over in classical form has been analyzed in *Neurospora* in great detail. The possibility of recovering all four haploid products of each cell that enters meiosis has greatly aided those studies. It has also made possible the identification of occasional instances of recombination where the conventional process has not been involved, since instead of getting the two reciprocal types of recombinants in each ascus only one of them is found to be present. As already stated in the discussion of Beadle's introductory paper, such events have been found in a number of microorganisms. A particularly thorough and careful study has been made of this phenomenon in *Neurospora,* however, by Mary B. Mitchell; and the Symposium paper by H. K. Mitchell treated the further analysis of this newly discovered phenomenon quite fully because of the light it may possibly throw on the mechanisms of mutation and genetic replication.

The genes involved were the pyrimidine-3 (*pyr, pyra, pyrd*) and pyridoxine (*pdx, pdxp, pdxq*) loci. At each of these loci several alleles were available for study, and nearby marker loci could be utilized in addition. In the first cross, *co pyrd* $\times$ *+ pyra,* 31 recombinants either *+ +* or *co +* were recovered among **32,080** progeny in approximately equal proportions. Either one of these classes might be expected to arise by conventional crossing over if the two *pyr* mutants were not at identical sites but could undergo recombination. However, conventional crossing over could account only for one class and not both, since to get the one recombinant *pyra* would have to lie to the left of *pyrd,* but to get the other it would have to lie to the right. In a second cross, recombination between *pdx* and *pdxp* was tested, one chromosome carrying a marker to the left and the other a marker to the right of the *pdx* locus. Again the unexpected type of recombination was found. The parent types when self-fertilized yielded no recombinations, but the heterozygote from the cross between them yielded **103** recombinants between *pdx* and *pdxp* in a total of **66,959** progeny. Tetrad analysis confirmed the finding; **585** asci yielded 4 asci which contained recombinants. In two of these, for example, two pairs of ascospores were parental in type, one pair in each ascus had reverted from pyridoxine-requiring to normal, and one pair was *pyr pdx* or *pyr pdxp.* Crosses showed that neither of these was a double mutant, i.e., carried both *pdx* and *pdxp.* Whatever relative position of *pdx* and *pdxp* on the chromosome might be assumed, no single arrangement can consistently account on the basis of conventional crossing over for the types of recombinants found in these two asci.

Mitchell points out that the conditions which favor crossing over are likewise favorable for the occurrence of transreplication ("gene conversion"). Heat shock is one of these. Since short heat treatments at 60° C. had been found to increase the mutation rate, the effect of heat shocks was tested simultaneously on crossing over and transreplication involving the *pyr* and *pdxp* loci. No significant change was found in ordinary crossing over between these loci after 30- or 60-second heat shock administered either to protoperithecia or to conidia, but the frequency of the extraordinary recombinants not attributable to crossing over fell to almost zero. Since the heat treatments were given before fertilization, whereas transreplication occurs during meiosis some hours or even days later, a delayed effect appears to be involved.

After some speculation about the possible roles of enzymes in transferring a functional group from one gene to another within the nucleus or from metabolic pool to gene, and further as to the reason why in the latter instance this can occur only in the heterozygous state and not when both genes are identical, Mitchell stresses that the significance of "gene conversion" will not become clear until ways other than tetrad analysis, which is limited to so few organisms, can be found to recognize its occurrence. It may, for instance, occur in maize (Laughnan's A^d cases) and in *Drosophila* (Demerec's reversions of reddish)—although remaining unidentified. In studies of very closely linked genes, and especially of the pseudoallelic clusters of genes which seem to function in so highly organized a way in the determination of the phenotype, this new phenomenon must be taken into account.

St. Lawrence and Bonner, in their paper, discuss other cases in *Neurospora* in which "gene conversion" may be suspected. Giles has found reversions to inositol-independence in crosses between different inositol-dependent mutants, which when selfed yield no reversions; and in some of these cases crossing over failed to supply an adequate explanation. Adenine-requiring mutants behaved similarly (de Serres); and in *Aspergillus* the same phenomenon was encountered (Pritchard). St. Lawrence has herself made a fuller study of a similar phenomenon encountered at the *q* (niacin-requiring) locus of *Neurospora*. There is evidence that these *q* mutants block the same metabolic reaction, and none of them, when self-fertilized, yields any recombinations. Yet in crosses between different pairs of these four mutants, rare non-mutant progeny appeared in frequencies and combinations of marker genes that depended on which two particular mutants had been crossed together. In some crosses a single recombinant type appeared in high frequency along with either one (but not both) of the parental types. These results once again seemingly cannot be accounted for by conventional crossing over. The suggestion that in such instances a large amount of multiple crossing over occurs within a very short chromosome segment ("negative interference") may meet certain formal requirements, but appears wanting as new instances of transreplication are discovered.

The brief report by Suskind describes the study of an extensive series of alleles at a single locus in *Neurospora*, the *td* locus already referred to. The interactions of these genes and their specific suppressors at other loci illuminate in almost unparalleled fashion the nature of gene function and enzyme formation. All 25 of the independently occurring *td* mutants affect the activity of tryptophan synthetase. The suppressors of these mutants show great specificity; thus, 5 occurrences of Su_2 all suppress only td_2, and not td_1, td_3, td_6, or td_{24}; Su_3 suppresses td_3 and td_{24} but not the three other *td* mutants tested; Su_6 suppresses only td_2 and td_6 among the five; Su_{24} resembles Su_3 in specificity. By using partially purified *Neurospora* tryptophan synthetase as an antigen injected into rabbits, an antiserum was produced that reacted quantitatively with the enzyme, and completely inactivated it. Upon testing the reaction of this antiserum with extracts of various *td* mutants, it was found that although none of the mutants possess active enzyme, several of them (e.g., td_2) possessed a cross-reacting substance (CRM) very similar in properties to the enzyme, while others (e.g., td_1) did not. Here, then, are alleles which fail to recombine with each other by crossing over and which in heterocaryons fail to complement one another, yet are subject to the action of different suppressor genes and are distinguished by the ability of the one and the inability of the other to form a protein serologically very similar to the active enzyme whose specificity depends on the *td* locus. (Enzyme neutralization curves obtained with anti-CRM serum are indistinguishable from those obtained with the homologous antiserum. Only by the stability of the inactive protein during dialysis and the inactivation of the enzyme serologically, as well as enzymatically upon dialysis, can the two proteins at present be distinguished.)

The wild-type strain contains not only active tryptophan synthetase, but a small amount (about 10% as much) of the cross-reacting protein. A temperature-sensitive member of the allelic series, td_{24}, which at 25° C. forms no enzyme but does form CRM, forms both enzyme and the related protein at 30° C. Mutants in the presence of their specific suppressor genes form both active enzyme and cross-reacting protein; but td_1, unsuppressible by any known suppressor gene, forms neither enzyme nor the related protein, even when one of the suppressor genes is present. It is indeed tempting to speculate on the role of the cross-reacting protein. Is it a precursor of the enzyme? A byproduct of the blocked reaction? An enzyme active in some closely related metabolic step? It is too early to say, but the experimental pathway here lies open. As to the functioning of specific suppressor genes, it is becoming clear that it can hardly relate to major aspects of enzyme specificity, but may be concerned with the removal of inhibitors from the enzyme (Beadle), or with repair of minor damage to the enzyme (Suskind), or with the inhibition of other reactions competing for the same substrate utilized by a basically "leaky" mutant (Glass).

The Role of the Cytoplasm in Heredity.

Avoiding the attempt to review the various types of cytoplasmic heredity in plants, animals, and microorganisms, Nanney has instead prepared a thought-provoking consideration of mechanisms of interaction between genes and cytoplasm. He starts by contrasting two widespread conceptions of this interaction: the "Master Molecule" concept and the "Steady State" concept. The first partakes of the character of a totalitarian regime, with the gene as dictator of organic specificity—although hard facts force holders of this view to admit the existence of some "master molecules" in the cytoplasm as well. "The steady state government is a more democratic organization, composed of interacting cellular fractions operating in self-perpetuating patterns." The dynamic self-perpetuating character of this kind of organization owes its specific properties not to any one kind of molecule, but "to the functional interrelationships of these molecular species." Of course, the distinction is not really so sharp; the two concepts are not mutually exclusive, and the real truth may embody both.

According to Nanney, the best understood examples of cytoplasmic transmission in sexual organisms are those involving "master molecules," that is, particulate bodies such as *sigma* (the CO_2-sensitivity factor in *Drosophila*), *kappa* (the killer factor in *Paramecium*), "plastogenes" responsible for some plastid characteristics in plants, enzymatic particles in yeast, etc. Clearly the existence of a class of such cytoplasmic particulates controlling certain hereditary traits, and very diverse in structure, function, and probable origin, is fully established. The question remains: how widely are they distributed and what is their general significance? The problem is that of the relative roles of the nucleus and the cytoplasm in heredity.

Nanney would discount the argument which presumes a relative inefficiency of cytoplasmic in contrast to chromosomal mechanisms, and he points out that the relative scarcity of described cytoplasmic mechanisms of this sort may arise more from the biases of workers and the difficulties of detecting essential cytoplasmic elements than from their actual rarity. The chief reason for believing that the great majority of particulate determiners of heredity reside in the nucleus rather than the cytoplasm has anomalously become the fact that all the DNA is in the nucleus—anomalously because that very fact was formerly the chief piece of evidence for assigning a hereditary role of major importance to DNA. Yet if the evidence that most hereditary determinants in sexual organisms are particulate in nature and also that most of them are carried in the nucleus is compelling, there is also evidence for a class of cytoplasmically controlled traits the inheritance of which does not at present appear to depend upon discrete units: the "barrage" phenomenon in *Podospora*, serotypes in *Paramecium*, streptomycin resistance in *Chlamydomonas*, "pokey" in *Neurospora*, and the plasmon characteristics of *Epilobium* and other green plants.

Cellular differentiation during the growth and development of multi-cellular organisms has for a long time been supposed to be entirely cytoplasmic in character—to result from the segregation of cytoplasmic materials and the action on the differentiated substrates of nuclei which remained equivalent. The classical work of experimental embryologists sufficiently demonstrated the totipotency of the nuclei in the cells of embryos in early cleavage. More recently, however, the implantation of nuclei from considerably later stages of development into enucleated eggs (King and Briggs) has disclosed that some permanent nuclear differentiation must eventually occur. There is also evidence from bacteria that long-enduring modifications of serotype have a basis in changes brought about in the bacterial chromosome itself. We must now think in terms of nuclear-cytoplasmic interactions that bring about permanent differentiations in both components of the cell. Nanney has considered examples of these interrelationships and has attempted to explain them in terms of antagonistic biochemical pathways.

The serotype system in *Paramecium aurelia* and the mating type systems in Group A and in Group B of the same species offer three examples which, in spite of their differences, are alike in the following respects: (1) the initial genotype of a clone determines its capacity to develop any one of a spectrum of alternative phenotypes, but does not dictate which one of these will become expressed; (2) the differentiation of one of the alternative phenotypes excludes the development of any other; and (3) when a particular phenotype does become established, it constitutes a hereditary characteristic of the clone. The essential differences between the three systems lie in the location of the mechanisms for perpetuating the characteristic. In the case of the serotypes, the mechanism is entirely cytoplasmic; the mating types of Group B depend upon a dual system in cytoplasm and nucleus; the mating types of Group A depend entirely upon the nucleus. In the serotypes the cytoplasm alone exercises the choice of phenotypes among the several potentialities made available by the nuclear constitution.

In the Group A mating types genes presumably exert the choice as well as determine the potentialities. [This is like the situation in the differentiation of sex in the higher animals, where each individual is sexually bipotential but the XY or XX chromosome constitution determines primarily which sex organs and characteristics will actually develop.] In the Group B mating types there is an interesting feedback, for the cytoplasmic mechanism is under the control of the mature nucleus. The primary determination of the mating-type character of each "new" nucleus (following conjugation or autogamy) is exercised by the cytoplasm; but once determined by it, the nucleus is thereafter autonomous in perpetuating the mating-type character. A mature nucleus cannot be altered by the cytoplasm in respect to mating type.

To interpret these relationships, Nanney visualizes certain self-perpetuating metabolic patterns—certain interrelated biochemical systems leading to the phenotype and potentiated both by the genetic constitution and the environment. Establishment of a particular biochemical pathway is considered to inhibit all alternative pathways. In the Group A system the essential reaction sequences are then limited to the nucleus, in the Group B system they reside in the nucleus, but produce inhibitory agents spilling over into the cytoplasm, and in the serotype system they are uniformly distributed, or at least the inhibitors are freely diffusible throughout the cell. The serotype system might alternatively be interpreted in terms of plasmagenes, but the foregoing interpretation seems more harmonious with the nature of the systems governing the two groups of mating-type systems. The plasmagene hypothesis is supererogatory. The mating-type systems, on the other hand, could doubtless be explained by some special shifting back and forth of master molecules; but this would leave them quite unrelated in nature to the determination of the serotypes. The attractiveness of the proposed theory is that it embraces all of these phenomena in the same biochemical context.

Nanney's recent studies on mating-type determination in *Tetrahymena pyriformis* extend the analysis of nuclear-cytoplasmic interactions to include a fourth type. Here, to begin with, each new somatic nucleus by virtue of its genotype possesses a spectrum of potentialities as to mating type; after a short time these are narrowed down to two; then, depending upon which particular two potentialities remain, one or the other is rapidly or slowly excluded; in some instances an intermediate condition can be fairly stably maintained over a long period.

The hereditary variations which arise in the above ways contrast with mutations in the gradualness with which they arise, but they need not differ altogether in kind. The genes may, as master molecules, impose constitutional limitations on the capacities of the protoplasm to differentiate. Biochemical antagonisms provide mechanisms for selecting between the alternative possibilities of differentiation. Such antagonisms, if located within the chromosomes, are represented by the alternative forms of genes, that is to say, by alleles produced from one another by mutation. Other antagonisms, less localized, may diffuse into the cytoplasm and bring about cytoplasmic differentiation. It is conceivable that some may even pass beyond the cell boundaries and become the agents which create those embryonic fields that cause associated cells to differentiate under a common influence into similar patterns. In such a conceptual framework as this, the genetic and biochemical matrix of the nucleus and cytoplasm becomes an all-pervading homeostatic mechanism relating life to its environment. Such a mechanism is hereditary and in its entirety is a part of the physical basis of inheritance.

Mutation and the Nature of the Gene.

In an illuminating discussion of the nature of mutation in maize (unfortunately not submitted for publication), Rhoades pointed out that the studies of Stadler, Laughnan, and McClintock of the *A* and *R* genes and the *Ds-Ac* complex, respectively, force one to the conclusion that at least in this genetically best-known plant there is no assurance that mutations are ever strictly intragenic in nature. Those mutations which have been critically analyzed turn out to be either deficiencies or consequences of alterations of position, and this conclusion applies equally to the x-ray-induced and the spontaneous mutations. Stadler's *A* mutations, when gross chromosomal aberrations were excluded, were all traceable to small deficiencies. Laughnan's are resolved into recombinations between pseudoalleles. McClintock's remarkable analysis has disclosed a dissociation locus (*Ds*) that can shift its position within a given chromosome or from chromosome to chromosome, when potentiated by another locus (*Ac*—"activator"). *Ds* causes chromosome breakage to occur in its vicinity, with a consequent loss of genetic material; or it suppresses the normal genetic action of adjacent loci; or it may act in a variety of other ways. A second system of this kind, originally studied by Rhoades, is that of the Dotted locus, which when properly activated causes a specific gene (*a*) controlling anthocyanin pigmentation to mutate with very high frequency during a definite stage in the development of the seed.

The discussion (also necessarily remaining unpublished) which followed Rhoades' presentation of the view that mutation of a true intragenic type cannot be demonstrated in maize was animated. The question of the generality of "controlling elements" like the *Ds-Ac* system as an explanation of mutation in other organisms came up. So far there is no definite evidence for them outside of *Zea,* but this may be simply the consequence of lack of analysis. There are numerous instances of unstable genes and variegated patterns which suggest their presence. Zamenhof argued strongly for the occurrence of intragenic changes in bacterial transformations. Ravin expressed serious doubt regarding this, on the basis of "allogenic transformations" in which a genetic agent different from that which has caused the transformation is recoverable in the progeny; and Austrian described a pneumococcal genetic unit possessed of high reverse mutability irrespective of the host cell into which it was introduced. On the other hand, Benzer expressed the opinion that it is possible to distinguish among his phage mutants between (a) those that are definitely deficiencies, by the criterion of their "stability," that is, their inability to revert, and (b) the 10 times more numerous mutants, presumably intragenic, that can undergo reversion to normal. And Glass referred to experiments in *Drosophila melanogaster* in which, by comparing sex-linked lethal mutations induced in the male germ line with those induced in the female germ line, it seems possible to discriminate between mutations that result from small deficiencies and those that are true "point mutations"—inasmuch as in the female germ line, at least at certain stages, chromosome rearrangements, including small deficiencies, appear to be non-inducible although mutations continue to occur at a low frequency.

Without doubt the analysis of the nature of mutation will continue to be most provocative and will eventually be clarified in terms of the basic chemical structure and organization of the genetic material. Yet at present it is impossible to be sure whether the mutations studied by geneticists ever descend to the level of simple alterations in nucleotide sequence or molecular structures. Even Benzer's estimates of the size of the muton in phage, if correct, do not prove crucial in this respect, since one might still be dealing with minute losses; while the argument from the reversibility of mutants, on the other hand, proves a weak reed in view of the demonstrable reversibility of such extragenic changes as chromosomal position effects and the modifications of gene function imposed by "controlling elements."

Role of the Nucleus, Nucleic Acids, and Associated Structures in Cell Division and Protein Synthesis

The Chemistry of Mitosis.

According to Mazia, virtually nothing is yet known about the chemistry of the most significant parts of the mitotic apparatus, namely, those which relate to the movements of the chromosome, such as the spindle attachment points (kinetochores or centromeres) and the division centers (asters and centrioles, when the centers are definable at all). Nor has there yet been enlightenment as to the nature of the processes that coordinate chromosome duplication with the formation of the mitotic apparatus, or that coordinate the dissolution of the spindle with the reversion of the chromosomes to the interphase state. One important advance in understanding relates to the spindle's elongation, which can be brought about artificially in glycerin-extracted cells by means of ATP (Hoffman-Berling). There is good evidence, to be sure, that during the mitotic process the genetic material itself is passive, and that the principal changes which bring about its ordered distribution to the two daughter nuclei are chiefly cytoplasmic.

Mazia has investigated the composition of the mitotic apparatus (spindle, chromosomes, centrioles, and asters), as seen in cleaving sea urchin eggs. Satisfactory methods of dispersing the enveloping cytoplasm and of leaving the mitotic apparatus intact were found: at first, subzero temperatures in 30 per cent ethanol followed by a dispersing agent, digitonin, which does not denature proteins; and later, an even better preservation of the native spindle mechanism by using ATP (0.01 M) instead of digitonin. Only the chromosomes tend to be dissolved. The isolated mitotic apparatus proves to be very sensitive to its ionic environment. It swells greatly in water and contracts reversibly when returned to an electrolyte.

The chemical analysis of the isolated mitotic apparatus revealed that it can be dissolved by agents that split the disulfide bond, and that it consists of a protein relatively homogeneous and completely precipitable at pH 4.5, with two electrophoretic components. When the isolation is carried out with digitonin, a nucleotide component amounting to 2-3 per cent of the total mass of the apparatus is obtainable. It is probably not, as was once thought, RNA itself, but has a single nucleotide component that might be ADP, or cytosine or uridine monophosphate. In view of the well-known relation of ATP to contractile proteins, its possible presence in the mitotic apparatus is of particular interest.

The protein content of the mitotic apparatus constitutes in the sea urchin egg 11.6 per cent of the total cell protein—a considerable proportion. This amount is far more than could be contained in the nucleus even if it were solid protein, and the observation thus excludes the possibility that more than a small portion of the spindle can be derived directly from the nucleus. There is no *net* synthesis of protein in the cell during the formation of the apparatus, so the question arises where it does come from. The protein might exist in a pool from which it is simply assembled; or structures of the interphase state of the cell might be dissolved and reassembled; or previously existing protein might be broken down to amino acids or polypeptides and the products used for a total synthesis of the protein of the apparatus. Experiments demonstrated that a protein like that of the apparatus, soluble and precipitable at pH 4.5, does exist in the unfertilized egg. Extracted and subjected to analytical ultracentrifugation, this protein exhibited two components, one of which could be shown to disappear during mitosis and reappear during interphase. This parallel behavior to the formation and dissolution of the spindle does not prove but certainly makes it plausible that the mitotic apparatus is formed by means of an assembly of preexisting material. There is, however, no change during mitosis in the proportional amount of soluble (or insoluble) protein in the cell. It must therefore be concluded that the formation of the spindle is at the expense of the dissolution of some other insoluble protein, and is not drawn simply from a pool of soluble protein. The effort to isolate the presumed precursor of the spindle protein from the unfertilized egg has succeeded to the extent of obtaining by precipitation with $CaCl_2$ a very fibrous protein with the expected sedimentation constant, containing 2 per cent of bound nucleotide, and amounting to some 10 to 12 per cent of the total protein of the cytoplasm. The protein readily redissolves when calcium ions are removed. The hope that this may indeed be the protein precursor of the mitotic apparatus and that it may now be subjected to study like that which has illuminated muscle contraction seems justified. Ultimately, such investigations should lead back to an illumination of the mechanism for the distribution of chromosomes and of certain aspects of the chemical basis of heredity.

Alfert's comments are directed to the hypothesis of the constancy of DNA and the chemical properties of the nucleoprotein complexes of the nucleus. As to the first, he points out that quantitative cytochemical methods—in particular the microspectrophotometric measuring technique developed by Swift—have provided data which clearly show that the DNA contents of various cells (within the same species or closely related ones) fall into a simple series of integers corresponding to the number of chromosome sets observable in them through the microscope. The nuclear DNA content doubles prior to mitotic division and increases by powers of 2 when polyploidy or polyteny occurs; but in the absence of chromosome duplication, the DNA content of the nucleus remains relatively unaltered. The quantitative constancy of the DNA is not sufficient to prove its genetic role; that must of course be adduced from other evidence. The constancy of DNA does make it possible, however, to estimate the extent of chromosome replication in cells where chromosome counts cannot be made, to distinguish between polyploid and polytenic conditions where these too cannot be observed

dialyzable products of the digestion of DNA by deoxyribonuclease proved to be just as effective in restoring the checked protein synthesis. The role of DNA in amino acid uptake could also be filled by DNA from calf liver or yeast, and even by RNA from those same sources. Mononucleotides, certain dinucleotides, mixtures of purine and pyrimidine bases, and AMP, ADP, and ATP were however not effective. The effectiveness of RNA in restoring the protein synthesis of these nuclei from which DNA had been removed is particularly remarkable in view of the fact that treatment of the nuclei of the original preparation with ribonuclease was without effect—although it is true that only a little over half of the RNA could be removed by this means. The activity of DNA in the incorporation of amino acids was shown not to depend greatly upon the presence of free phosphate groups on the molecule.

The proteins of the isolated nuclei were fractionated and tested to determine which ones carried most of the activity of the incorporated isotopes. Very little was found in the histones. A fraction soluble in phosphate buffer at pH 7.1 had most activity, except for a fraction closely associated with the DNA of the nucleus. The fraction containing most of the RNA also had a high activity. It was also shown in these experiments that the isolated thymus nuclei can incorporate labeled glycine into nucleic acids, and that the nuclei have the capacity to generate ATP from AMP. The synthesis of ATP in the nucleus could be inhibited by a large number of well-known inhibitors of oxidative phosphorylation.

It follows from these studies that at least certain cells are able to synthesize protein in the nucleus as well as in the cytoplasm. These nuclei themselves possess the oxidative systems which generate the high-energy phosphate bonds presumably required for the synthesis of protein.

The Nucleic Acids and Protein Synthesis.

As Spiegelman points out, it has become virtually a biological dogma within the past decade to attribute the specificity of biological syntheses to the trinity, RNA, DNA, and protein. The nature of the interrelations between these three, despite all the theorizing, remains veiled in a mystic aura. Inasmuch as the immediate agents of specificity, the enzymes, are proteins, the problem may be framed in another way: is there a stepwise synthesis of polypeptides of increasing length and complexity, or is a single template responsible for the fabrication of each particular kind of protein molecule? ". . . The first mechanism implies that at each step contact between the appropriate catalyst and the molecule being formed is limited to relatively small proportions of the molecular structure of either. Consequently, each of the many catalysts can have but limited information of what has gone before. In the template mechanism, on the other hand, contact between the molecule being synthesized and the single guiding catalyst is comprehensive. The template can therefore in principle possess complete knowledge of geometrical detail at all stages in the synthesis of the protein molecule." It is because of an appreciation of this distinction, here so well put, that most biologists have felt that the "poly-enzyme theory," as Spiegelman terms the former theory, runs into such inherent complications and difficulties that it must be abandoned in favor of the "template theory." "Consider," says Spiegelman, "the situation in which 50 out of 100 residues of a particular protein molecule have been put together. To make the proper choice, the catalyst presumed by the poly-enzyme mechanism to mediate the addition of the 51st amino acid would have to possess detailed information on the succession of the existing 50 amino acids. The difficulty of transmitting the required information would appear to pyramid for the stepwise mechanism as the synthesis progresses."

In addition to the theoretical difficulty, there is some evidence bearing on the matter. To block the utilization of a single amino acid is enough to block the utilization of any and all of them. Amino acids are the only identifiable precursors of the proteins in specific syntheses of enzymes and antibodies, whatever the experimental method used and whether in single cells or in entire organisms. There is no convincing evidence of the existence of any peptide intermediates. Unequal labeling, such as Anfinsen and his coworkers have found in the synthesis of ovalbumen, insulin, and ribonuclease, may result from an incorporation of amino acids into proteins by exchange reactions and may have no real bearing on complete protein synthesis, as Gale's studies show.

In the quest for a suitable template, we note first that it must be at least as large as the molecule being synthesized and that it must contain within its own structure the information prescribing the sequence of residues in the product. We can also deduce that it must have at least three elements, e.g., different nucelotides, in its makeup and ought to be universally distributed among organisms, since so "centrally necessary [a] mechanism as protein synthesis would [scarcely] be mediated in some forms by one type of chemical template, and by a completely different sort in others." We are looking, then, for a macromolecule that is universally distributed, composed of at least three elements in roughly equivalent proportions, and itself synthesized by a mechanism that insures an accurate sequence, since it cannot function effectively as a template if its own order is inconstant. This brings us back to the trinity, RNA, DNA, and protein.

Spiegelman excludes protein by itself as a suitable template because, even if that capacity were limited to certain proteins and not possessed by all, the template proteins would have to possess the ability, not only to control the synthesis of their products, but also to catalyze their own synthesis. There is, he asserts, no cogent reasoning or experimental evidence to support such a view. At any rate, one can proceed to consider which of the two nucleic acids is most likely a component of the protein-synthesizing mechanism.

The work with the transforming principles of *Pneumococcus* and *Hemophilus* shows that genetic information can be stored in DNA and be transmitted by it. But there are also a lot of experiments that demonstrate a dissociation of DNA metabolism from the synthesis of protein. X-ray inactivation and photoreactivation after ultraviolet inactivation will eliminate DNA synthesis while leaving that of RNA and protein. Especially convincing is the capacity of a thymine-requiring mutant of *E. coli* to synthesize several enzymes in the absence of thymine, and therefore while DNA synthesis is in abeyance. Allfrey's observation that isolated thymocyte nuclei treated with deoxyribo-nuclease lose the ability to incorporate labeled amino acids into protein and regain it upon the addition of fresh DNA, represents a puzzling exception.

On the other hand, while in general RNA synthesis can proceed in the absence of protein synthesis, the converse does not hold. There are some apparent exceptions, and the exceptions are often the test of a theory. Sometimes it may be a matter of the superiority of a tracer: labeled glycine, which produced the exception, is probably not as good a detector of RNA synthesis as P^{32}, which did not. Another seeming exception was the synthesis of protein in phage-infected bacteria in the apparent absence of RNA synthesis; but recently Volkin has shown that actually there is an active turnover going on in a fraction of the RNA under these conditions. Not all of the RNA need be functioning at one time or in respect to one synthesis.

Evidence that RNA is closely tied to protein synthesis came from the studies of the synthesis of induced enzymes in yeast. The ultra-violet dose required to stop enzyme synthesis was far higher than that necessary to inhibit DNA synthesis, although the action spectrum was that of the absorption spectrum of nucleic acid (Swenson and Giese); whereas a dose that inhibited RNA metabolism by 22 per cent suppressed enzyme formation by 95 per cent (Halvorson and Jackson). Minute amounts of the analogue 5-OH-uridine, which inhibits the utilization of uracil in the synthesis of RNA, inhibit induced enzyme formation (β-galactosidase in *E. coli*), even after its onset. In other words, synthesis of RNA is required for the continued uninterrupted production of the enzyme. The synthesis of other proteins was not so sensitive to variations in RNA metabolism, however; and it may be that an active synthesis of RNA is a requirement unique to the formation of induced enzymes, and not of constitutive enzymes. (An exception to this is the constitutive formation of β-galactosidase in certain mutants of *E. coli*. It is just as sensitive to RNA inhibition as when inducible.) All of these, and numerous other experimental findings, provide only interesting correlations of RNA activity and protein synthesis. RNA is in some way implicated in protein synthesis; but this is no proof that it serves as a template. We want "an unequivocal demonstration that a specific RNA functions as a guide in the formation of a specific protein," or an equivalent disproof of it.

Spiegelman next proceeded to examine experiments performed with fractions of cells. Anucleate systems, such as reticulocytes, enucleated eggs, and enucleated amoebae, provide convincing evidence of the ability of protoplasm to synthesize protein in the absence of DNA, although interpretation is somewhat complicated by the limited metabolism, results of damage, or starvation of the various systems. Experiments on *Acetabularia* by Brachet and his coworkers are more satisfactory because the enucleated portions retain their photosynthetic capacity. In all these cases the performance of DNA as a template would seem to be ruled out.

Work with cytoplasmic particles, such as microsome fractions of rat liver cells, has also demonstrated that amino acids can be incorporated in the absence of DNA, provided ATP and guanosine triphosphate are supplied to activate the carboxyl groups of the amino acids (Zamecnik, Hoagland, DeMoss and Novelli, and others). Although no net protein was synthesized in these systems, the labeled amino acids were irreversibly incorporated into protein by means of peptide linkages. From Straub's laboratory has come a report of even a net synthesis of protein (amylase) in a cell-free system obtained from pigeon pancreas. ATP was required, and ribonuclease stopped the synthesis of amylase.

Working with microsomal particles derived from pea seedlings, Webster has found that amino acids are rapidly incorporated into protein and that a small *net* synthesis of protein can be obtained. The requirements for this to occur are complex. Unlike the results of Gale and Folkes with a bacterial system, in the present case intact RNA is not needed but a mixture of the four ribonucleosides or ribonucleotides will serve, if supplemented with ATP, Mg^{++} and K^+ ions, and the mixture of 17 or 18 amino acids which was used. The deoxyribonucleosides are considerably less effective in promoting the incorporation of amino acids into protein by these particles. A mixture of the four 5'-ribonucleotides surpassed a mixture of the four ribonucleosides in effect. Polynucleotides released by enzymatic digestion from yeast proved ineffective, and in some cases even inhibited the incorporation of amino acids. The interdependence of protein and nucleic acid syntheses in these particles was shown by the effects of inhibitors. In every case an inhibitor of nucleic acid synthesis also inhibited amino acid incorporation, and conversely. Webster consequently holds that the nucleotides act by becoming incorporated into RNA, which is essential to the protein synthesis. Hoagland, too, reported (in discussion) on the firm association of one or more nucleotides with enzymes that activate amino acids preparatory to their incorporation into the protein of microsomes obtained from liver.

The work with sonically ruptured bacterial cells by Gale and his colleagues has excited wide interest since the announcement in an earlier McCollum-Pratt Symposium that protein synthesis was demonstrable in them. These preparations can be selectively rid of DNA, RNA, or both, by the appropriate nuclease or by 1 M salt solution. The incorporation of labeled glutamic acid from a complete amino acid mixture proceeds linearly during the experiment, is markedly reduced when nucleic acid is removed, and is resumed when staphylococcal DNA or RNA is restored. DNA is in this instance more effective. The synthesis of complete enzymes (glucozymase, catalase, and β-galactosidase), as judged by an increase in the specific enzymatic activities, is not checked by removal of even 85% of the nucleic acids. But when 93% of the RNA and about 90% of the DNA have been removed, synthesis stops. The synthesis of catalase is thereafter strongly stimulated by an addition of RNA, the synthesis of β-galactosidase not by RNA but by a mixture of purine and pyrimidine bases. DNA possesses little or no reactivating effect, but in a preparation even more thoroughly depleted of its nucleic acids, neither RNA nor the mixture of bases is of avail, but DNA markedly stimulates the synthesis. The results seem to fall in line best with the supposition that DNA is required for RNA synthesis, and that RNA in turn synthesizes protein.

Spiegelman himself has turned to studies of protein synthesis in "protoplasts," subcellular fractions of bacterial cells produced by the action of lysozyme under hypertonic conditions. Bacteriophages will multiply in protoplasts, and they retain a high respiratory activity and a major portion of the synthetic potentialities of the entire cells. They will even form spores, but have a limited capacity for division. C^{14}-labeled glycine was demonstrated to become incorporated within them both into protein and into the purines of nucleic acid (McQuillen). Arabinokinase was synthesized by protoplasts of *B. subtilis* (Wiame et al.) and β-galactosidase by protoplasts of *B. megaterium* (McQuillen; Landman and Spiegelman). The ability to synthesize enzymes can be abolished in the protoplasts by treatment with either lipase or trypsin, to which intact cells are quite insensitive; but this is because of the general destruction of the protoplasts by the enzymes and is not a specific inhibition of synthetic activity. The nucleases, which also do not affect intact cells, strikingly modify the synthetic capacity of the protoplasts. Considerable amounts of DNA can be removed, up to 99%, without a loss in the enzyme-forming ability; in fact, the latter may even be stimulated. But when the removal of RNA exceeded 35%, drastic inhibitions of enzyme synthesis occurred. The only element of uncertainty appeared to lie in the fact that the degraded DNA is not removed from the protoplasts by the treatment, and if fragments of it are active or can be reconverted into active material, the elimination of DNA from direct participation in the synthesis of protein would not be assured. Great difficulty in restoring the nucleic acids to the protoplasts after the initial removal made it clear that these systems were unsuited for a final demonstration.

Osmotically shocked protoplasts were the next resort. By carefully controlling the osmotic shock produced by suddenly adding water, by means of a stabilizing medium such as 0.5 M succinate solution, "shockates" of the same size and shape as protoplasts but of a lower optical density can be produced. The "shockates" are much more sensitive to ribonuclease and deoxyribonuclease and to various other treatments than are protoplasts. Extraction with 1 M sodium chloride removes both RNA and DNA from them; and empirically a special "resolving mixture" was hit upon that performs a highly selective and efficient removal of DNA without greatly modifying RNA or protein content. The experiments were expected to be crucial. When all DNA was removed, enzyme synthesis was unabated. Treatment with ribonuclease or 1 M salt solution effectively decreased the enzyme formation. Spiegelman, however, then did the one experiment he might have considered unnecessary. He tested the shockates from which DNA had been wholly removed for the possible resynthesis of DNA during the course of the experiment. Extensive resyntheses had in fact occurred, and at a rate exceeding by 10-fold the maximal rate of DNA synthesis in a growing bacterial culture. The capacity of the shockates to synthesize RNA and protein is scarcely a quarter of their capacity to synthesize DNA. In this they contrast strikingly with protoplasts, which synthesize DNA, RNA, and protein in equivalent proportions.

The quest for the template consequently seems no nearer its goal today than a year or two ago—perhaps it *seems* farther away. Nonetheless, the use of these subcellular systems offers many avenues of attack; and by shifting from *B. megaterium* to *E. coli*, the rich genetic knowledge of that organism can be made a potent tool. Spiegelman reports that his preliminary tests show that it is feasible to produce shockates of *E. coli*.

The study by Vogel of the "adaptive" formation of acetylornithinase throws a novel light on the formation of enzymes. Acetylornithinase removes the acetyl group from N^α-acetylornithine, so making ornithine which is fed into the arginine-ornithine-citrulline cycle. The enzyme is constitutive, and yet an adaptive mechanism is involved in the synthesis of the enzyme by means of a feedback. The phenomenon is as follows: a mutant in *E. coli* that is blocked in the formation of acetylornithine will grow when supplied either with that compound or any one of the three amino acids of the cycle. Since no acetylornithine is formed endogenously by the mutant, the effect of exogenous acetylornithine on the induction of the enzyme could be tested. On arginine, the strain grows exponentially; on a limited amount of arginine plus acetylornithine, it grows at the typical rate on arginine until the supply is exhausted, then at a slower exponential rate as it utilizes the acetylornithine. The longer it grows on arginine, the slower becomes the rate of growth observed when the shift to acetylornithine is made. There is evidence that this is because of a reduced enzymatic capacity to convert acetylornithine to ornithine. The presence of arginine thus itself inhibits the synthesis of the acetylornithinase. The presence of exogenous acetylornithine in proportionately large amounts (100:1) is quite unable to overcome this regulatory action of arginine. The amount of acetylornithinase formed is controlled by the amount of arginine present and is quite independent of the amount of the enzyme's own substrate in the system. The same phenomenon was found in wild-type *E. coli* as well.

Vogel calls this feedback control over the formation of an enzyme by the term, "enzyme repression." Although the possibility that the formation of acetylornithinase is also induced by its substrate has not been excluded, that hypothesis appears quite unnecessary. The repressibility of acetylornithinase formation by arginine serves to limit the formation of the enzyme when plenty of arginine is present and thus to economize on the formation of the enzyme except when necessary. Repressibility and inducibility of an enzyme are thus both of positive selective advantage to an organism and may be expected to arise in the course of evolution. As to which mechanism of control over enzyme formation is more efficient and as to which is commoner, only the future can tell.

Nucleic Acids as Transforming Agents

The great interest of the studies with the transforming principles of *Pneumococcus* and *Hemophilus* lies in the fact that an extracted and purified DNA can be reintroduced into the living system. The DNA can furthermore be modified by chemical means in vitro and then returned to the living cells, and thus the relationship between change in structure and change in function may be determined.

The transformations, as is now so well known, in general transfer genetic units singly from the donor strain to the recipient. It is particularly significant, as Hotchkiss points out, that in the case of an inducible enzyme the genetic potentiality may be transferred without regard to the current state of the donor. For example, the capacity to dehydrogenate mannitol adaptively may be transferred to a non-fermenting strain irrespective of the adapted or nonadapted enzymatic state of the donor cells. Thus the transferred units of DNA may be regarded as equivalent to bacterial genes which act upon the recipient cells at short range and either modify the DNA of the latter or substitute themselves for it at the time of replication. The transfer is not reciprocal. In this it resembles other kinds of bacterial and phage recombination and transduction, and differs from the better-known genetic recombination of higher organisms.

The special interest of these transformations lies in the possibility of analyzing the interaction between a cell and a cellular component, that is to say, between a reactive, or competent, bacterium and a DNA particle endowed with transforming activity. Here exists a real possibility of determining whatever quantitative relationships exist, but there are also many pitfalls. The original transformations, those of capsule character in *Pneumococcus*, soon proved to be unsuitable for such studies either because of the loss of many transformed cells which were sedimented with the unencapsulated bacteria upon exposure to antibody against the latter, or because sedimentation started too late and the transformed cells were subjected to competition in growth with untransformed cells. It was possible to demonstrate that the antibody plays only a selective role, not a formative one, in producing the transformations; but it also became clear that the transformed cells only slowly acquire their new character and even more slowly become able to compete in growth with the excess of untransformed cells present.

For the above reasons, workers turned to drug-resistance transformations as more suitable for quantitative studies. In this type of experiment, the untransformed cells are killed by the drug, which acts as a screening agent. By precisely regulating the exposure of the reactive cells to the transforming DNA by destroying it after a precise interval with deoxyribonuclease, it became evident that there is always a two-phase increase in the number of transformed cells. After a lag of about one division period, there is an extremely rapid increase. An interval of 1 or 2 hours follows with no further increase. Then a slower, logarithmic increase begins. The first rise represents the actual transformation; the plateau may be described as a maturation period, and occurs while the total culture of untransformed cells is still growing; the final phase is that of the division of the transformed cells. Both streptomycin-resistance (S^r) and penicillin-resistance in *Pneumococcus*, and streptomycin-resistance in *Hemophilus*, have been shown to behave in this way.

Pneumococci grow in broth in single clone-clusters which settle to the bottom. By shaking the tubes vigorously, the clusters can be broken up, and Hotchkiss has used this observation as a basis for determining the time at which the transformed cell starts to multiply. In replicate tubes shaken after 1 hour and then treated with streptomycin, the transformed cells are distributed at random, according to a Poisson distribution, and expression of the character is complete. As incubation is prolonged before shaking and addition of the streptomycin, the same number of empty tubes is found, but many more transformed cells are present in those tubes which contain any transformed cells at all. In other words, the new portion of transformed cells comes from the division of the original ones and there is no subsequent transformation. The onset of division among the transformed cells is irregular, coming within the second hour for about half of them, not until the fourth hour for some. Clearly, the frequency of transformation must be the ratio of the original transformed cells to the total present at the time of transformation; and this can only be determined prior to the onset of replication, yet after the full development of the transformed character. Hotchkiss consequently uses a very brief exposure of the cells to the transforming agent, viz., 5-10 minutes; and he regards more than 15 minutes as most unwise. The physiological sensitivity of the growing cells to be transformed is not constant but cyclical. It reaches a maximum late in the exponential growth phase of the population, and may last some hours or, under particular conditions, may be greatly shortened. These are additional reasons why the timing and duration of the exposure to DNA are so important. Hotchkiss believes the brief periods of sensitivity found by Thomas and Ephrussi-Taylor in their experiments (see below) are a consequence of the shortening and phasing of the physiological sensitivity of the cells.

Higher concentrations of DNA yield more transformed cells, but again certain precautions must be observed. In assaying by dilution end-points, it is the number of test populations containing transformed cells that is observed, and not the number of individual transformed cells. Statistical error combines with the uncertainties of selection to becloud the result. Yet concentration-response curves have been obtained for penicillin resistance, for mannitol dehydrogenation, for streptomycin resistance (in *Hemophilus* as well as *Pneumococcus*), and for capsule character. All of these show an exponential relation of DNA concentration to number of transformed cells over about a 1000-fold concentration range. There is no detectable competition between different DNA transforming agents within this range, according to Hotchkiss' elegant experiment using known mixtures of streptomycin-resistance and sulfanilamide-resistance DNA's. At high concentrations, competition becomes evident. When the number of cells transformed is plotted against the S'-bearing DNA concentration, each curve flattens to a horizontal plateau; that is, saturation is reached at a level which is characteristic for each mixture of different DNA's and which is proportional to its content of the DNA being assayed. The saturation level is thus a direct measure of the potency ("quality") of any transforming DNA, i.e., of its capacity to transform relative to the total DNA content; and the relative activities of different DNA's at saturation can be compared without a knowledge of the actual DNA concentrations.

Harriett Ephrussi-Taylor has used x-ray inactivation of the transforming factors in the hope of arriving at the dimensions of the biologically active particle. She concludes that in so far as the streptomycin-resistance factor is concerned, no simple form of the target theory is applicable. Like Hotchkiss, she is much concerned with the difficulties of quantitation, in particular with the problem posed by the briefness of the period during which the reacting bacteria remain competent. In her cultures this period lasts, on the average, some 15 minutes per bacterium, and all the bacteria pass through the phase almost synchronously, in contrast to the longer phase of physiological sensitivity recorded by Hotchkiss under his own experimental conditions. Because of the brevity of the reactive state, Ephrussi-Taylor mixed the bacteria and the transforming DNA in the culture medium at the outset, and let them go through one or more cycles of competence before assaying on medium containing streptomycin for selection of the transformed cells. At high DNA concentrations the yield of transformed cells departs from the logarithmic linearity observed at lower concentrations. A plateau is reached, or there is even a slight decrease, followed by a second, roughly linear log rise until a second plateau is attained. Suspecting heterogeneity of the DNA, Ephrussi-Taylor, like Hotchkiss, carried out an experiment with known mixtures of the streptomycin-resistance and unmarked DNA's. The levels of both plateaus were lowered roughly in proportion to the relative amounts of unmarked DNA present; and the first plateau emerged at lower concentrations of the streptomycin-resistance factor. Ephrussi-Taylor postulates that the first break in the curve occurs because bacteria which have reacted with one unit of DNA, generally an unmarked one, are inhibited from reacting with another and so from being transformed, that this inhibition is later reversed as the concentration of the marked DNA is increased; and that finally a second plateau occurs for some other reason, such as a limit to the number of DNA units a bacterium can absorb. Support for the hypothesis was seen in the absence of any doubly transformed bacteria until DNA concentrations were reached at the level of the first plateau for singles. Doubles at this level are about as frequent as expected if the factors are unlinked. Ephrussi-Taylor suggests that a sort of fatal genic imbalance may arise when a single cell acquires more and more molecules of a single sort of DNA, but that balance (and consequently viability and transformability) would tend to be restored when enough of different sorts were taken up.

When the S^r-bearing DNA is heavily x-rayed, so as to retain only 3 per cent of its original activity, the exponential proportionality of activity to concentration is maintained at low concentrations and the first plateau occurs as usual. Further experiments were done in the linear region of the curve. Calculation of the radiation-sensitive volume, which is rendered difficult by the sensitivity of the S^r-DNA to free radicals, was gauged by comparing the effects of irradiating in the liquid state with those of irradiating in the frozen state.

Activity as a function of x-ray dose diminishes exponentially, but with a sharp break at a level between 5 and 10 per cent of residual activity. The activity remaining below that level is much more resistant to ionizing radiation. From the first portion of the curve comes an estimate that the molecular weight of S^r-DNA is perhaps 0.7×10^6, or about one-tenth of the estimated molecular weight of pneumococcal DNA in general. The S^r particle may be smaller than average or only a part of it may comprise the radiation-sensitive volume.

The residual resistance at high doses above the break in the curve is very puzzling. Any protective effect upon untransformed particles by those already transformed, or the presence of a second distinct S^r factor of higher resistance, can be excluded. Neither of the two remaining hypotheses which have been suggested, namely, (a) two sorts of particles associated with the activity and of different sensitivity, or (b) the presence of aggregates, has been supported by experimental evidence. As to the former, two fractions of transforming DNA differing in guanine content proved to behave alike in respect to x-ray inactivation. As to the latter, treatment with 5 M urea to dissolve any aggregates, if present, failed to affect the inactivation characteristics, although another preparation which showed marked resistance to x-rays up to a dose of 8×10^5 r units proved to be more typically sensitive after treatment with urea. In other words, aggregation of particles, when present, does increase resistance and is readily detectable. It therefore cannot be the cause of the residual resistance, which is not affected by urea.

Another enigma appeared when a S^r-DNA preparation was fractionated into a supernatant portion which was of typical behavior, and a second fraction (pellet and lower portion of solution) which was far more sensitive to x-rays, was inactivated at about 2.5×10^5 r, was altered by treatment with urea, and upon long standing (10 months) acquired the typical inactivation behavior. It seems that there can exist some aggregates which are more resistant to x-rays and others which are more sensitive.

The urea-stable units may be considered the more fundamental particles of S^r-DNA. Because there seem to be two units differing in calculated size by an order of magnitude, and because even the larger is an order of magnitude smaller than Doty's estimates of the average DNA molecule, Ephrussi-Taylor is led to suggest that the S^r-particle is a complex target. These conclusions must be evaluated in the light of the report by Goodgal and Herriott that their measurements of the sedimentation constants and diffusion data for the S^r-transforming factor of *Hemophilus* lead to an estimated molecular weight of 15 $\times 10^6$.

Goodgal and Herriott used S^r-transforming DNA derived from *Hemophilus influenzae* and tagged with P^{32}. They found that the DNA absorbed, which at dilute concentrations of DNA is proportional in amount to the DNA concentration, is taken up in two forms, a reversible state removable by washing with saline solution, and another state irreversible and, since it is inside the cell, resistant to DNAase and permanently transmitted during growth and division. The number of cells transformed was found to be directly proportional to the DNA taken up irreversibly, about 120 molecules of DNA being absorbed for each transformed cell. This irreversibly absorbed DNA can be liberated from the cell by lysing it, can be shown to correspond to the expected amount of transforming factor, and after liberation is susceptible to attack by deoxyribonuclease. The uptake of transforming factor is apparently not selective; that is to say, the cells will take up other DNA's along with the S^r variety, in proportion to their respective concentrations. One may then conclude that about 1 in every 120 particles of DNA in the donor cell carries the S^r factor, unless the efficiency of transformation is less than complete.

An especially interesting report was that made by the same two workers in collaboration with Rupert, in regard to the photoreactivation of the S^r-transforming factor from *Hemophilus* after it had been inactivated by ultraviolet light. Initial attempts to do this were unsuccessful until an *E. coli* extract was added to the system. A similar extract made from *Hemophilus influenzae* itself would not work. Heating the *E. coli* extract destroyed its effectiveness. The transforming activity of the ultraviolet-treated S^r factor which had subsequently been exposed to visible light was tenfold that of the same preparation kept in the dark. These results show that transforming DNA can be photoreactivated after ultraviolet inactivation, like bacteria and bacteriophage, *Neurospora* microconidia, etc., in which the genetic material is known to be involved. The conviction that the common element in all of these phenomena resides in the DNA of the various kinds of living systems is hereby greatly strengthened.

A phenomenon which was reported by Miss Leidy and which aroused much discussion related to the activity of S^r-transforming agents from different species (*Hemophilus influenzae, H. parainfluenzae,* and *H. suis*) on the character of cells of a single recipient strain, *H. influenzae* strain Rd. The homologous DNA proved to have a very much greater transforming power than the heterologous ones, the characteristic frequencies being of the order of 1 per 10^{-3} for the homologous DNA and 1 per 10^{-6} or 10^{-7} respectively for the heterologous DNA. A high degree of species-specificity is thus demonstrable for these types of transforming DNA, each of which modifies the same phenotypic character.

Zamenhof, in reviewing the properties of the transforming agents, first summarized the evidence that the transforming agents can be identified as DNA. Not only do the usual chemical analytical tests demonstrate the presence of DNA and of no other substance, but also serological methods have failed to reveal the presence of any antigenic substances in the transforming agent. Of a variety of enzymes only deoxyribonuclease destroys its biological activity. Zamenhof himself has purified the transforming agent of *Hemophilus influenzae* to a protein impurity level of less than 0.4% of the amount of DNA present; and Hotchkiss has purified the transforming agent of *Pneumococcus* to the 0.02% level of protein contamination, which would correspond to about 12 molecules of molecular weight 10^5, or about one molecule of weight 10^6, in the amount of DNA required to transform one cell. Critical tests with inactivation by heat or pH provide convincing evidence of the loss of transforming activity at the same temperatures where the viscosity of the preparation begins to decrease. It indeed requires a hypertrophied skepticism to set aside the evidence that DNA is actually the genetic transforming material which is derived from one strain of bacteria and becomes incorporated into the hereditary material of a recipient.

The molar ratios of the purine and pyrimidine bases of the transforming factors of *Pneumococcus* and *Hemophilus* resemble those of human DNA (1.6A:1.7T:1G:1C), but the DNA of *E. coli* is quite different (close to 1:1:1:1). The native composition may be altered, however, either by incorporating in place of thymine a halogenated uracil provided in the medium, or by merely changing the thymine content of the medium [the content of 6-methylaminopurine in an *E. coli* thymine-requiring strain can be modified 10-fold]. If the DNA molecules in the organism from which the transforming agent is derived are heterogeneous, the measured ratios of the bases would of course be mere averages of the individual kinds. Evidence does exist that the DNA molecules may differ in length as well as in the proportions of the respective purines and pyrimidines, for polydispersity is revealed by ultra-centrifugation; and DNA preparations can be fractionated into portions characterized by different ratios of the bases.

Bendich and his collaborators reported to the Symposium their studies of DNA fractionation by means of column chromatography on "ECTEOLA," a substituted cellulose derivative. Carbon-2-labeled 5-bromouracil was supplied to a thymine-requiring mutant of *E. coli*, strain I, and gradient elution from the column was used for the fractionation, first with increasing concentrations of NaCl at neutrality, then with increasing pH at constant salt concentration. The specific radioactivity of different fractions was found to vary greatly, even when derived from a single culture, and the shapes of the curves for the specific radioactivity and the optical density were not superimposable. The results signify that in *E. coli* varieties of DNA exist which have different capacities to incorporate thymine. By means of the same methods (see Discussion) they have also fractionated the DNA of the pneumococcus transforming principle, and find that the streptomycin-resistance transforming activity is widely distributed through the fractions, which differ in activity over a fifty-fold range. Some fractions were as much as five times as active as the original DNA preparation.

Using the retention of its transforming ability as a criterion of the "functional intactness" of extracted bacterial DNA, Zamenhof has surveyed its physical properties, molecular nature, and resistance to physical and chemical agents. Transforming DNA resembles calf thymus or human spleen DNA in electrophoretic mobility, viscosity, and x-ray diffraction. Its molecular weight was estimated to be 6×10^6, and the lowest amount of unfractionated DNA which will still transform a particular character is of the order of 10^{-8} μg. This is only five times as great as the estimated total amount of DNA in a single cell, and makes conceivable the assumption that each cell contains only a single DNA molecule of each kind. If that were so, the number of DNA molecules per cell (about 250) would seem to be too few to determine all the hereditary characteristics on a one-for-one basis. Zamenhof, on the basis of some association of characters in multiple transformations in *Pneumococcus,* suggests that a single molecule may determine more than one genetic marker.

The transforming DNA is rather stable to heat, and the temperature coefficients of heat inactivation are large and suggestive of high energies of activation. The transforming DNA is also stable over a wide pH range on either side of neutrality. Inactivation at low pH might depend upon destruction of the salt form, deoxyribonucleate, or upon removal of purines, since removal of less than 2 purines per thousand reduced the activity by 99 per cent. Exposure to a low ionic strength, such as distilled water, rapidly inactivates the transforming agent; and dehydration in any form is drastic in effect. Deamination even to the extent of 0.1 per cent reduces the activity to one-thousandth. It is interesting that inactivation may to a considerable extent precede any noticeable depolymerization (reduction in viscosity) in the response of the transforming DNA to crystalline pancreatic deoxyribonuclease.

The reaction of transforming DNA to mutagenic agents is naturally of great interest. Not all mutagens will inactivate it, but most of them do so. Inactivation itself may be compared to a lethal mutation; less extreme mutations, to a destabilization of the active transforming agent. The latter phenomenon has been observed after treatment by heat, acids, mustards, deoxyribonuclease, and ultraviolet irradiation. The inactivation curve produced by different doses of ultraviolet radiation is of a multi-hit type. Approximately the same dose (500 ergs/sq. mm.) produces inactivation to 0.1 per cent in both transforming principle and bacterial viruses. This dose is only 1/500 of that required to produce a detectable change in viscosity. X-rays and other ionizing radiations are of course also effective inactivators of the transforming DNA. Ferrous ions and hydrogen peroxide, which like ultraviolet radiation produce H• and OH• free radicals, inactivate—especially the ferrous ions, which at low concentrations inactivate without depolymerizing. Mustards, at concentrations below 10^{-4} M, likewise inactivate without depolymerizing. Formaldehyde, on the other hand, inactivates and depolymerizes simultaneously. The alkylating agents dimethyl sulfate, diethyl sulfate, methyl iodide, and β-propiolactone inactivate either by alkylating the amino groups of the bases—the purines, and especially guanine, being most susceptible—or by esterifying phosphate groups. Protein-denaturing agents, such as 4 M urea, some general mutagens, e.g., urethane, and some carcinogenic and carcinostatic agents, such as methylcholanthrene and azo dyes, fail to inactivate the transforming agent.

Particularly intriguing is the demonstration by Zamenhof and his coworkers of a difference in stability of *Hemophilus* transforming agents carrying different markers, such as streptomycin resistance and several types of capsule character. The differences in stability of transforming agents from organisms of capsule types b and d, as well as that of streptomycin resistance in those two strains, were most marked, and were demonstrable not only in response to ultraviolet radiation, but also to nitrogen mustard, ferrous ions, etc. Streptomycin resistance in capsular type b reaches a distinct plateau which is maintained to very high doses that completely inactivate, for example, streptomycin resistance in type d. It is thus rendered possible to separate the genetic mixture into certain pure components by inactivating the more sensitive types. Transforming-DNA from the strain with streptomycin resistance (capsule b) after exposure to 16,000 ergs/sq. mm. and a consequent reduction to 1 or 2 per cent of its original activity, yielded transformed cells the DNA from which was inactivated by only 900 ergs/sq. mm. It thus appears that the differences in stability are not transmitted but may reflect heterogeneity in particle size or other properties. There is therefore no evidence from these experiments that the single factor for streptomycin resistance can be separated into two types of permanently distinct stability.

The heterogeneity reported by Bendich, Pahl, and Brown is presumably of a different sort, although they have presented no evidence that it is heritable. They suggest that it may rest on differences between the cells in respect to growth. One would expect a complete synthesis of DNA in growing cells and merely an exchange of thymine for labeled 5-bromouracil, such as Zamenhof has demonstrated, in cells that are not dividing. If this were so, the DNA of the actively growing cells would possess the lowest amount of radioactive label. Since those fractions eluted in the alkaline region have the highest streptomycin-resistance transforming activity, as well as the nearest ratio to unity for the four bases and a relatively low specific radioactivity, Bendich thinks that these later fractions possibly represent the true genetic material.

Viruses as Bearers of Heritable Characteristics

The bacterial viruses appear to belong on an equally basic level of replication with the bacterial transforming factors. According to Herriott, who introduced this group of papers, the virulent, T-even-numbered phages which attack *E. coli* are particularly suited for such studies. The DNA of these tadpole-shaped phages resides in the head, surrounded by a protein coat continuous with the substance of the tail. By osmotic shock, the DNA can be released, leaving behind a "ghost" which cannot replicate within the host bacterium, although it possesses the host range specificity and the capacity to "infect" and "kill" it. It can also inhibit the synthesis of RNA and adaptive enzymes in the bacterium, and can lyse it. The bacterium so infected forms DNA and protein, but they are not proper phage components.

Upon adsorption of an entire phage particle to the host, the DNA, together with about 3 per cent of the protein, enters the cell. Most of the remainder of the protein may be stripped away from the host without altering the course of infection or the replication of the virus. During an "eclipse" period subsequent to entry of the phage, no mature or infective particles can be isolated from it. This is the period when new phage particles are being made. Fortunately, these events can be followed to some extent by the fact that phage DNA is unique in containing the pyrimidine 5-hydroxymethylcytosine; and viral and bacterial proteins can be distinguished serologically. The immediate metabolic changes observed are the following: the synthesis of RNA is reduced to 2 or 3 per cent; synthesis of phage DNA commences after a brief lag; and protein synthesis continues unabated. The latter is very significant. If protein synthesis is interrupted, then the synthesis of phage DNA cannot commence; but only a brief interval of protein synthesis is sufficient to start the DNA synthesis going, and then it will continue even if protein synthesis is blocked. This early-formed protein does not, however, enter the phage progeny in its entirety. Perhaps it represents the special enzymes needed to synthesize the phage's unique pyrimidine.

No appreciable proportion of isotopically labeled protein from the phage parent enters the progeny, but about half of P^{32}-labeled phosphate, nearly all of which is in the nucleic acid of the virus, is transmitted to the descendants. By freezing infected bacteria, Stent was able to follow the inactivation of the phage brought about by the radioactive decay of the P^{32}. One in every 12 disintegrations proved fatal to the phage particle, whence it is deduced that at least 8 per cent of the DNA is essential to the replication of the phage. Some of the genetic markers of the inactivated phage might, however, be rescued by becoming incorporated into the progeny of unlabeled phage introduced simultaneously into the host bacterium. Doermann and his coworkers showed that genetic markers can likewise be rescued from ultraviolet-inactivated phage particles; that the individual genetic units are only 4 per cent as sensitive as is the infectivity of the entire phage and hence are probably of that relative size in comparison to the entire amount of DNA; and that while unlinked genetic markers are inactivated independently by ultraviolet, linked ones are in general inactivated together. The evidence supplied by Stent and by Doermann's group is, according to Herriott, "the best existing evidence that the genetic structures are associated with the phage DNA."

It is somewhat puzzling that only 30-50 per cent of the labeled phosphorus of phage DNA gets into the progeny. The present tendency is to view this loss as a sum of the inefficiency of a number of steps. Of the several hundred progeny released from a single bacterium infected with labeled phage, only 5 to 25 carry the P^{32} label (Stent and Jerne), so that by no means all progeny receive a material contribution from the parent for every unit of DNA. It still seems most probable that, as Luria originally proposed, each infecting parental phage particle undergoes a geometrically progressive replication in producing its progeny.

Transduction.

Four years ago, in 1952, Zinder and Lederberg reported the discovery that phage may serve as a vector of genetic material from one host to a second. The bacterial species involved was *Salmonella typhimurium*. In a very comprehensive review Hartman has undertaken to compare the nature and effects of transduction, and the light it has thrown on the genetics of bacteria, with other processes that likewise lead to genetic recombination in bacteria. These include, besides transformation (discussed in the previous section), also sexual recombination and transfer of the capacity to produce bacteriocins,* both of which require conjugation of the participating cells.

Transductions are in general mediated by temperate, or lysogenizing, phages, although their virulent mutants can also transduce. Only a single genetic unit is generally transduced at one time, that is, into a single recipient cell, although all known genetic markers in *Salmonella*,

---

* Several unusual types of mutants have been reported in the gram-negative enteric bacteria. Bacteriocins or colicins are substances which become adsorbed to and which kill sensitive bacteria, usually without lysing them. They are produced by certain strains, more commonly in *E. coli* and *Shigella* than in *Salmonella*. The property of producing such substances is inherited, and resistance to them is also hereditary and may be acquired by mutation; but these loci have not yet been placed on the genetic map of the *E. coli* chromosome given by Hartman.

with the exception of a few in one particular strain, are separately transducible. Transducing phages have also been found for *E. coli*, and transduction may even occur between *E. coli* and *Shigella*. The phage, when supplied with sensitive cells which it lyses, apparently incorporates and transports into the recipient cell a fragment of DNA bearing a certain genetic factor. This transduction takes place for a particular unit only with a very low frequency, about 10^{-6}. If the recipient cell escapes lysis, the transduced element becomes separated from the phage DNA. It then either remains free in the cell, in which case it does not multiply and is segregated at each cell division, so as to form a unilinear "semiclone" (abortive transduction); or it synapses with homologous genetic material in the bacterial chromosome and can then replicate itself (transduction proper). In the latter event, it may become integrated into the chromosome, by replacing either a part or all of the original homologous material; or both new and old genetic elements may remain together and thereby produce an effectively diploid but unstable condition, segregating about once in every thousand divisions. About one-third of the transduction clones are of the former, stable variety; about two-thirds, of the diploid, unstable sort.

Much study has been devoted to the behavior of transduction in *E. coli* strain K12 and to its temperate phage lambda. In the lysogenizing bacteria, the capacity to produce the phage is located at a definite locus in the chromosome, the locus *ly*λ, which is closely linked to a galactose-fermenting locus, *gal*. The prophage, as the bacterial virus is called when it occupies a site in the bacterial chromosome, is characteristically specific in the locus it selects. In fact, lambda phage never occupies any other locus except the *ly*λ locus and it transduces only the *gal* and other markers closely linked with it. When diploidization occurs, mostly the *gal* locus behaves as if heterozygous, but sometimes the *ly*λ locus is heterozygous too. In so far as the prophage comprises a part of the bacterial genome and acts like other genetic units in modifying characters, such as conversion to toxigenicity, production of immunity to lysis by homologous phage, etc., the process of lysogenization which leads to the incorporation of the phage into the chromosome may be regarded as analogous to transduction, although there are not a few ways in which lysogenization and transduction differ. Notably, the phage may lose by mutation its ability to transduce without losing its ability to lysogenize.

Like Hotchkiss, Hartman emphasizes the significance of the fact that transformation and transduction, and probably also sexual recombination in bacteria (Lederberg; Jacob and Wollman, see below) are unidirectional, and not reciprocal, transfers of genetic material. In this respect they differ fundamentally from sexual recombination in the higher plants and animals. It is perhaps a consequence of the nature of the transduction process that the size of the piece which can be transferred is minimal; and it may well be that the puzzling phenomenon of "negative interference" (that is, the occurrence of double exchanges with a frequency greater than the product of the frequencies of single exchange in each of the regions involved), has no other meaning than this, and was puzzling only because we thought of what was to be expected in terms of the sexual processes in higher organisms, where crossing over between large, somewhat inflexible chromosomes is conventional.

There is no direct evidence that the genetic material of transduction is DNA, as there is in the case of the transforming agents. There is, however, a considerable body of indirect evidence to that effect. It is of the same nature as the evidence that DNA is involved in genetic recombination, evidence which is strengthened by demonstrations that in recombination P^{32} in labeled DNA follows the direction of genetic transfer, so that recombinants may be killed by decay of P^{32} transferred to them from a labeled donor strain.

There is also no direct evidence in regard to the absolute size of the transduced material. Sensitivity of phage infectivity to ionizing radiation is much greater than that of the ability to carry out a single transduction; accordingly, one might deduce that the transduced element is much smaller than the material in the phage which is required for a lytic or lysogenic infection. The transducible prophage may be equally small in relation to the infecting phage material. In *Salmonella*, the fragment is "at least several gene loci long." In *E. coli* the piece transduced by lambda phage carries not only the $ly\lambda$ locus but two adjacent *gal* loci.

It is a striking confirmation of the genetic linkage studies based on sexual recombination that loci transferred together in transduction are those known from sexual recombination to be very closely linked to one another. Transduction here offers a tool for finer analysis of the bacterial linkage map than does sexual recombination. By transduction, the *gal* locus of *E. coli*, and likewise the $ly\lambda$ locus, have been shown to be compound. Morse and the Lederbergs have studied 8 galactose-utilizing mutants, which are distinct (except for gal_1 and gal_4) and yet are closely linked. Gal_1 and gal_4 in the trans heterozygous configuration yield a negative phenotype; in the cis configuration they produce a positive phenotype. This very interesting example of the "position effect" phenomenon is differently interpreted than in *Drosophila*. There such an interaction occurs between non-alleles (pseudoalleles) which can crossover and recombine. Here in *E. coli* it is taken as evidence of the "allelism" of gal_1 and gal_4, which together yield a negative trans phenotype, and of the non-allelism of those two *gal* mutants with gal_8 and others, all of which yield a positive trans phenotype in such combinations as gal_4/gal_8.

Kalckar, from studies on human galactosemia, a congenital hereditary disorder in which the affected person is unable to invert galactose to glucose, presented an analysis that bears dramatically on the array of galactose-negative genes studied in *E. coli* by means of transduction with lambda phage (Morse and the Lederbergs). Four steps are involved in the utilization of galactose, mediated respectively by a galactokinase, responsible for galactose phosphorylation; a phosphogalactose-uridyl transferase; a galacto-waldenase, responsible for the actual inversion; and finally an enzyme responsible for the release of phosphoglucose from the uridyl compound and the regeneration of uridine triphosphate. The *E. coli* mutants so far found fall into two groups, those lacking the kinase, and those lacking the transferase (Kurahashi). A combination of extracts from mutants of different types restores the utilization of galactose; but combined extracts of mutants blocked in the same step fail to do so. Mutants 1, 4, 6, and 7, all blocked in the transferase step, are very closely linked in the transduction experiments; mutant 2, blocked in the kinase step, recombines with mutants of the first group rather more freely.

The lactose-fermenting mutants of *E. coli* K12 are also interesting. They occur at 7 different loci, two of which, lac_1 and lac_4, are closely linked with each other and with a third locus, *ind*, that governs the constitutive versus inducible character of the enzymes controlled by the two adjacent *lac* loci (lac_1 governs the production of a galactose permease which is necessary to permit lactose to enter the cell; and lac_4 governs the production of β-galactosidase). Other *lac* loci are not closely linked with each other or with the lac_1-lac_4 group.

It is in *Salmonella*, however, that such analyses have progressed farthest, through the work of Demerec, Hartman, and their coworkers. The clustering in *E. coli* of loci of a similar nature, viz., in addition to the *gal* and *lac* loci just mentioned, the close proximity of two other *ly* loci to *ly*λ, and of two methionine-requiring loci to each other forecast the discovery of a much more highly organized arrangement of metabolically related loci in *Salmonella*. For example, all mutants which require histidine for growth lie within one small region of the *Salmonella typhimurium* chromosome. This histidine region, studied by Hartman, is revealed as comprising four genetic loci arranged in the same linear order as the sequence of biochemical steps in the synthesis of histidine from a precursor of imidazole glycerol phosphate (Fig. 1). Within each of these four loci *A-D* (Benzer's cistrons) numerous independent mutations have occurred, which yield very few if any wild-

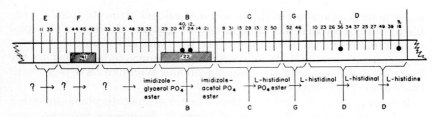

Fig. 1. *Linkage map of the histidine region of the*
Salmonella typhimurium *chromosome*
Probable relation of gene loci (A–G) with enzymatic reactions (A–G) in the
proposed primary pathway of L-histidine synthesis. (From Hartman.)

type recombinants with other mutations of the same group, but do recombine with mutants belonging to any of the three other groups. The mutants of any single group, all of which according to present evidence affect the same biological step, are nonetheless distinguishable either (a) because they yield some wild-type forms by genetic recombination, or (b) because they mutate to wild-type or to other mutant alleles at different rates, or (c) by virtue of "secondary" properties such as differences in response to specific suppressor genes, temperature sensitivity, or growth requirements. One mutant form of the *B* group, *hi-22*, does not recombine with any other mutant of that group, and is presumably, like certain of Benzer's phage mutants, the result of a deficiency for the entire region or some other kind of chromosomal rearrangement. In the entire series of 32 tentatively mapped histidine-requiring mutants, only two appear to be identical.

The tryptophan-requiring mutants of *Salmonella* likewise fall, according to the studies of Demerec et al., into several groups which are arranged in the same sequence as the biochemical steps in the synthesis of that amino acid. This is not true of all biochemical mutants studied in *Salmonella*, however; for example, the cystine-requiring loci are more scattered. [Still, the implication of such an arrangement, namely, that linked biochemical steps, either at the substrate or the enzymatic level, take place in sequence along the surface of the chromosome, offers a fascinating subject for speculation. Presumably, in organisms such as *Neurospora* where some closely related chemical steps are controlled by almost randomly distributed loci, the apparently superior efficiency of such an arrangement has been supplanted by advantages of some unknown sort.—B. G.]

Lysogenicity.

An outgrowth of transduction studies has led to a recent rapid development of our knowledge of the bacterial chromosome map and the genetic relations between the loci and subloci. It arose from a spectacular discovery that has brought new insight into the nature of sexual recombination in bacteria, a discovery that emerged from the study of lysogenizing virus and its conversion into prophage, attached to the bacterial chromosome of the host. Jacob and Wollman have dealt with these newest developments.

It is important to recognize that when a temperate phage infects a sensitive bacterium and, instead of lysing it, becomes a prophage, one cannot disrupt the lysogenic bacteria and find infectious particles within them. The lysogenic bacteria are, nevertheless, rendered immune to the strain of virus that has thus entered them, and to all its mutant forms as well, except one special class. Furthermore, the lysogenic bacteria possess also the capacity to lyse and release once more the same type of infectious phage. Spontaneously, such lysis occurs rather infrequently, but at a definite rate (10^{-2} to 10^{-5}) for a given strain under constant conditions. Nevertheless, the production of phage from lysogenic bacteria can be induced in virtually all individuals of certain strains, by exposing them to the action of an inducing agent such as ultraviolet light or certain mutagens. The induction process must in some way convert the prophage into phage which multiplies inside the bacterium before release, for it can be shown that the average number of prophages per cell is *one per nucleus,* yet many infectious virus particles are released upon lysis of the bacterium.

The prophage must, on the other hand, replicate in step with the bacterial nucleus, since a 1:1 prophage/nucleus ratio is maintained. It not only possesses genetic continuity, but can mutate, often so as to produce defective lysogenic strains which lyse upon induction with ultraviolet radiation but fail to form and liberate active phage (except in some 10^{-7} individuals which represent back mutations to regular prophage). Since the prophage can give rise to infectious phage particles of the original type, the prophage must also carry the store of genetic information of the original normal virus. Since, as has already been said, infectious virus particles inject their DNA and but very little protein into the host cell, it is highly probable that the prophage is a part or is all of the virus DNA. How then does it differ from the vegetative phase that normally intervenes between the infection of a bacterium by a virus and the lysis of the host cell with liberation of the replicated virus particles? The answer must lie in the coordination of the replication of the prophage with the replication of the bacterial chromosome, and in its failure to cause the host cell to manufacture virus protein until "induced." The coordination referred to is no doubt a consequence of the attachment of the prophage to a particular site on the bacterial chromosome. How this has been learned is one of the most fascinating stories in the entire development of bacterial and phage genetics.

In *E. coli* strain K12 there is a well-known lambda prophage, which has already been referred to. The genetic behavior of the lysogenic character could therefore be studied in crosses between lysogenic and non-lysogenic varieties of this strain, which for a long time was the only one in which sexual recombination could be demonstrated. It was discovered that the lysogenic character segregates like other bacterial genes and exhibits a very close linkage to a galactose-fermenting locus, *gal* (Lederbergs; Wollman). In crosses between two lysogenic types carrying different prophages, the prophage characters themselves showed this linkage to the *gal* marker (Appleyard).

When in 1952 Hayes and the Lederbergs discovered the F+ and F− mating types in *E. coli* K12, and the frequency of mating could thenceforward be controlled and greatly enhanced, it was learned that λ-lysogeny could not be transmitted from an F+ bacterium to an F− *ly−* mate, whereas the reciprocal transfer went very readily; that is, from an F+ *ly−* donor the non-lysogenic character could be transferred to the F− *ly+* recipient, replacing the lysogenic prophage of the latter. As Hayes noted, the bacterial recombination is a consequence of a partial transfer of genetic material from the donor to the recipient parent. Not all F+ bacteria can accomplish mating, but only certain rare Hfr mutants; and the isolation of the Hfr (for high frequency of mating) strain of F+ mating type has speeded up the analysis of genetic recombination in *E. coli* enormously. When it appeared that the Hfr strain could transfer to F− mates only a particular region of the bacterial chromosome, a segment *O-R*, Jacob and Wollman had the happy idea of interrupting the mating process at timed intervals after it had commenced by agitating the cells in a Waring blendor. They then discovered that the Hfr donor always contributes the genes of the segment transferred in a particular order, beginning with the *O* end of the segment. The longer the period of mating permitted, the longer the piece of chromosome transferred, up to a rupture point (*R*), beyond which the transfer did not go. Consequently it was readily possible to locate the genes on the transferred piece in their sequence from *O* to *R*. In this piece lies the *gal* locus, and 15 recombination units from it but nearer *R* lies the locus of the prophage lambda. Consequently *gal* might sometimes be transferred to the recipient strain without λ, but λ was never transferred without *gal*. The prophage λ is definitely situated in the bacterial linkage map, and along with the other genes in the transferred piece, is injected by the donor into the recipient. (In electron micrographs of mating Hfr and F− cells, a narrow bridge-like connection can be seen between the mates. It is presumably through this that the injection of the piece of chromosome takes place.)

Then what of the inability of the F⁺ donor to transmit λ-lysogeny to an F⁻ ly^- mate? This turned out to be a consequence of "zygotic induction," that is to say, whenever the λ prophage is transferred into a non-lysogenic cell, induction occurs, the prophage becomes a vegetative phage, lyses and destroys the zygote. Here is evidence that the prophage does not behave like a normal bacterial gene; under these circumstances it acts like a dominant lethal!

Since a bacterium can carry a considerable number of different prophages, provided they are unrelated, the next problem was to discover how the prophage loci were distributed on the bacterial chromosome. About 7 ultraviolet-inducible prophages and 7 that were non-inducible were selected as a sample for study. It became evident that all the representatives of the former group were located at various points in the segment between *gal* and *R,* whereas all the others lie outside of that segment. Most of them are in another segment marked by the maltose-mannitol-xylose markers, which certain other Hfr mutants inject into their mates in place of the *O-gal-λ-R* segment. It seems that ultraviolet-inducibility may be a property of a particular segment of the bacterial chromosome, and not an inherent property of individual phages. The order of the inducible prophages could readily be mapped in three independent ways: (1) by the frequency of recombination with *gal* in the cross of Hfr gal^+ ly^- S^s with F⁻ gal^- ly^+ S^r (where *ly* stands for the prophage being tested) ; (2) by the percentage of zygotic induction in the cross Hfr ly^+ with F⁻ ly^-; and (3) by noting the time required for the prophage to enter the F⁻ cell after the parents are mixed, this time of course varying directly with distance from *O-gal* along the segment toward *R.* The several methods agree perfectly in the deduced seriation of the prophage loci—and thereby demonstrate a perfection of mapping linked loci that even the correlation of 3-point crosses and salivary chromosome analyses in *Drosophila* can scarcely equal.

An even more significant question was the following: how is the prophage integrated with the bacterial chromosome? Is it synapsed alongside of a particular homologous region? Or has it actually been inserted into the continuity of the bacterial chromosome as a substitute for a particular part? Light was thrown on these alternatives by further studies with lambda. Lambda undergoes mutations, like other phages, which affect its plaque size, plaque type, or host range. By exposing the phage to small doses of ultraviolet radiation before infection, the amount of recombination within the lambda segment or locus may be increased. The results showed that all the lambda mutants lie within this segment and very closely linked to a *c* locus which determines the phage's capacity for lysogenization, its immunity pattern, and probably the specific location of the prophage on the bacterial chromosome. Among a sizable number of independently obtained c mutants all fell into three phenotypic classes according to the clearness of the plaques formed. Mutants of each c phenotype were found to form a cluster on the linkage map, the c_1 mutants, which have lost the ability to lysogenize, in the center; the c_3 mutants, with capacity reduced to about 1/100, on the left; the c_2 mutants, with capacity reduced to about 1/10, clustered on the right. The entire c segment comprises about 1/15 of the total genetic length of the lambda region. Two more points seem particularly significant. First, the c mutants of different types ($c_1 + c_2$, $c_1 + c_3$, $c_2 + c_3$) can cooperate in mixed infections to yield a rate of lysogenization equal to that of the wild-type. Second, in crosses between lambda and the other related phages, the mutant characters to right or left of the c locus can be transferred to yield recombinants; but no recombination takes place within the c locus. To all intents and purposes it *is* the identity of the phage. To illustrate, prophage 434 which has received the right and left portions of lambda marked by the mutants co_1 and co_2, respectively, but has its own c locus, remains 434 in immunological type and stays located at the 434 site, to the right of lambda.

A preliminary answer to the questions raised in the preceding paragraph has been obtained by studying the recombination within the lambda region in conjunction with that in the bacterial chromosome. By marking the latter to right and left of the lambda region, one would expect that if lambda is inserted in the chromosome, then every single crossover within the lambda region would result in a separation of the bacterial genetic markers to right and left. Actually, recombination within the lambda region was found to be relatively independent of any recombination of the bacterial markers. This implies that the prophage is in all probability not inserted into the bacterial chromosome, but attached to it in some other way. Further evidence can be derived from the effect of the decay of P^{32} introduced into the prophage. The latter can be inactivated by the P^{32} decay without any corresponding lethal effect upon the entire bacterial chromosome.

Jacob points out that in a number of cases the presence of a prophage in a bacterium modifies various, seemingly unrelated properties of the host. Particularly important is the association in *Corynebacterium diphtheriae* of lysogenicity, that is, the presence of a prophage, with the production of the characteristic deadly diphtheria toxin. The toxigenic character is passed from strain to strain by certain lysogenizing temperate phages.

An interesting speculation is whether the much-mooted "latent viruses," if they do exist in the cells and tissues of higher organisms, are not analogous to the bacterial prophages. One item that makes this idea seem rather plausible is the resemblance between the transmission of lysogeny and of maternally inherited traits in which a cytoplasmic element is involved. Lysogeny, as has been pointed out, can be transmitted only from the F⁻ parent, equivalent to a female parent because it contributes both cytoplasm and nuclear material to the progeny. The Hfr parent, equivalent to the male because it transmits only chromosomal substance to the progeny, never transmits lysogeny because of zygotic induction and its fatal consequences. This is remarkably like some cases of maternal inheritance in animals, particularly that of CO_2 sensitivity in *Drosophila*, which l'Héritier has shown to be of a viral nature. The relations which are now being disclosed between active phage, prophage, and bacterial host may eventually illuminate many hitherto mysterious relationships, such as that between viruses and cancer.

The Reconstitution of Virus from Nucleic Acids and Protein.

Reports in 1955 of the fractionation of tobacco mosaic virus into nucleic acid and protein portions which were without biological activity, and of their successful reconstitution into active tobacco mosaic virus created a great stir not only among scientists but also in the popular press. In their present contribution dealing with the extension of that work, Fraenkel-Conrat, Singer, and Williams first of all make it clear that subsequent investigation showed that the nucleic acid fraction was not devoid of all activity, as they had at first thought. Infectivity, as Gierer and Schramm independently pointed out, is a property of the nucleic acid itself. It nonetheless remains true that the reconstituted particles have a much higher activity than can be demonstrated in the nucleic acid fraction alone, although this is perhaps because the "unwrapped" nucleic acid is so much more labile and difficult to work with. In recent assays, according to Fraenkel-Conrat, the reconstituted particles, which like the native virus have a protein sheath around a core of RNA, have exhibited 10 to 25 per cent of the biological activity of the native tobacco mosaic virus, whereas the naked nucleic acid has only 1 per cent of the activity of native virus, or in relation to the nucleic acid of the latter, only 1/2000 of its activity. [According to Franklin, the RNA is not strictly speaking a "core" at all. From evidence derived from x-ray scattering when a heavy-atom derivative of the virus is utilized, the RNA lies at a radial distance of about 40Å from the axis of the tobacco mosaic virus particle, or about halfway out to the surface.]

The most significant development to grow out of the reconstitution experiments to date is the feasibility of putting together RNA and protein from different sources—making, one might say, artificial hybrids. These experiments, performed with six strain mixtures, clearly demonstrated that RNA is the main genetic material of the virus; for the symptoms of infection evoked with the artificial hybrids always corresponded to the source of the RNA, never to that of the protein. Using typical tobacco mosaic virus (TMV) and Holmes' ribgrass virus (HR) in most of the work, Fraenkel-Conrat and his coworkers found, for example, that HR nucleic acid + TMV protein yielded an infectious particle with all the characteristics of HR except that it not infrequently showed a higher specific infectivity, intermediate between those of TMV and HR. Conversely, TMV nucleic acid + HR protein yielded a particle with the characteristics of TMV, including its high specific infectivity. Virus progeny of the second generation retained the characteristics of those of the first generation hybrids.

Amino acid analyses of the hybrid virus progeny of HR nucleic acid + TMV protein seem to show some very slight deviations in content of some amino acids from the characteristic HR content, in particular, less lysine and more glycine. However, a mutant of this hybrid was found with appreciably higher infectivity, almost equal to that of tobacco mosaic virus, and with an amino acid makeup different from both parental strains. On some hosts its symptoms resembled the lesions produced by tobacco mosaic virus and on other hosts the lesions produced by HR. In preparing controls by separating the nucleic acid and protein of HR and then reconstituting them into infectious particles, another mutant with markedly different amino acid composition and producing a unique set of symptoms was discovered. It may well be, therefore, that the "unwrapping" of the nucleic acid and the reconstitution of virus particles render the nucleic acid particularly labile and subject to mutation.

Another type of experiment now made possible is that of mixing the nucleic acids from two different strains and then reconstituting entire particles. Typical TMV lesions and typical HR lesions, as well as lesions of an intermediate type, were obtained after mixing TMV and HR nucleic acids. However, since it proved possible to isolate both pure TMV and pure HR virus from the lesions of intermediate type, it is not clear whether or not true hybrid RNA particles can be produced in this manner.

Considerable labor has gone into the demonstration that the infectivity of the nucleic acid fractions (prior to reconstitution) is genuine and not a product of contamination with undissociated virus particles. In the case of TMV nucleic acid, it could be shown that the activity of the RNA fraction was at least 100 times greater than that of any tobacco mosaic virus that could be sedimented out by the ultracentrifuge, which can sediment tobacco mosaic virus almost quantitatively. Rabbit anti-TMV antibodies, highly effective against tobacco mosaic virus, do not inactivate the RNA derived from it; and on the other hand, the activity of the latter is very sensitive to salt and to ribonuclease, whereas native tobacco mosaic virus is not.

Contrary to the conclusions of Schramm (in the Discussion), who holds that the active RNA unit is of high molecular weight—corresponding to the entire nucleic acid core of a single virus particle, and therefore about 3×10^6—the Berkeley workers find that infectivity is associated with material of a low or average molecular weight, about 2 or 3×10^5. High ionic strength disturbs this "native" structure, but pH changes are less harmful to it.

Nucleic Acids—Chemical Composition and Structure

Chargaff's witty and penetrating skepticism served to illuminate many facets of this particular topic, to warn all workers of the danger of elevating theory into dogma, no matter how elegant the theory, and to caution against the glib application of language and concepts appropriate to one level to phenomena on an entirely different level of organization.

His remarks summarized certain salient regularities in the composition of nucleic acids. One of these is the limited number of purine and pyrimidine bases to be found in them. RNA (or PNA, pentose nucleic acid) is limited to adenine, guanine, cytosine, and uracil. DNA is not so strictly limited to adenine, guanine, cytosine, and thymine; for in plants to a considerable extent and in animals to a lesser degree, cytosine may be in part replaced by 5-methyl cytosine. This pyrimidine does not occur at all in microorganisms, but 5-hydroxymethyl cytosine occurs in the DNA of some of the coliphages. In a thymineless mutant of *E. coli* grown on medium lacking thymine, 6-N-methyladenine can be incorporated in its place; but that may not occur under usual circumstances.

In comparing the polynucleotides with polypeptides, Chargaff said one ought never to forget a certain fundamental difference between them. To insert a different amino acid in a polypeptide one must break peptide linkages, but the substitution of purine or pyrimidine bases in a polynucleotide would require only the cleavage of a glycosidic bond and would not affect the sugar-phosphate backbone of the structure. The definitive structure of DNA is by no means certain, even as respects the 5′:3′ phosphate bridges, or the presence of a terminal phosphate group. Nor is there really critical evidence that the sugar in DNA is always deoxyribose. The regularities applicable to all DNA are as follows (using A, G, C, T, and U for adenine, guanine, cytosine, thymine, and uracil respectively; 6-Am for the nucleotides with an amino group in position 6, namely, adenylic and cytidylic acids; and 6-K for the nucleotides with a 6-oxy group, namely, guanylic and thymidylic or uridylic acids):

(a) A = T
(b) G = C
(c) A + G = C + T, and
(d) A + C = G + T, or in other words 6-Am = 6-K

On the other hand, the ratio of A + T : G + C varies from 0.4 to 1.9.

In the pentose nucleic acids only one of these regularities holds good, namely, A + C = G + U, or 6-Am = 6-K; and even this does not apply to certain plant viruses. This basic property of all the nucleic acids has recently led Elson and Chargaff to speculate that the most satisfactory model to fit the facts would consist of two polynucleotide chains bonded to a polypeptide chain, by means of hydrogen bonds between the peptide carbonyl groups and the 6-amino groups of adenine or cytosine, and between the peptide amino groups and the 6-keto groups of guanine or uracil (or thymine). At any rate, the protein moiety of nucleoproteins ought not to be lightly dismissed as inconsequential.

Finally, Chargaff emphasized that "sequence cannot be the sole agent of biological information"—logically because that would be to neglect the third dimension which is of such general importance in bio-chemical relationships, and evidentially because of the ease with which transforming agents can be inactivated in a variety of ways. But in so far as sequence is concerned, Chargaff points to recent findings in his own laboratory that in both DNA and RNA the purine nucleotides tend to be next to purines and the pyrimidines next to pyrimidines more often than would be expected on a random basis.

New Light on the Structure of DNA.

The widespread attention which has been given to the Watson-Crick model of DNA structure, based on x-ray diffraction studies not only of DNA extracted from a wide variety of sources but also of intact DNA in sperm heads and in phages, makes it scarcely necessary to describe it in more than the very succinct terms which Crick used in the Symposium: "It consists of two polynucleotide chains running in opposite directions and twined round one another. The two chains are held together by hydrogen bonds between the bases, each base being joined to a companion base on the other chain. This pairing of bases is specific, adenine going with thymine, and guanine with cytosine."

According to Wilkins, the structure of the B form of DNA, derived from the A form by stretching or swelling it, is now firmly established. The original Watson-Crick model presented too large a diameter, and an improved model has been constructed with a reasonable fit to the x-ray data.

There is great difficulty, Crick stated, in reconciling with the data a paranemically coiled structure. Those who propose such a structure (Gamow; Linser) in order to obviate the difficulties of separating the coils after replication of the strands has taken place should realize that they are raising even greater difficulties with bond angles and distances than they hope to resolve.

Chemical evidence in favor of the model is that already given by Chargaff. Replacement of cytosine by methyl cytosine or hydroxy-methyl cytosine creates no problem; but the incorporation of large amounts of 6-aminopurine will do so. A solution may lie in the possi-bility that incorporation of that compound in place of thymine might not be a replacement at random. Like 5-methyl cytosine, which for the most part replaces cytosine only when next to guanine, the 6-amino-purine may not replace thymine at random. The simplest way to account for this would be if it were not incorporated singly, but as an element of a dinucleotide, for example, attached to thymidylic acid.

The physical-chemical evidence in favor of the double helix struc-ture of DNA comprises (1) the titration curve, which suggests that the bases do form hydrogen bonds within the structure; (2) the shape and size of the molecule, determined from light scattering, viscosity, and sedimentation data, and implying that the DNA molecule is extended in solution, although not quite straight, and has a diameter consonant with the model; and (3) the rates of inactivation by gamma rays, acid, or enzyme, which imply two strands that do not come apart until both strands are broken almost opposite one another. The postulated base pairing is the only satisfactory one that allows all four bases to occur in each helix. It ought not to be supposed, however, that all the DNA must be in this form, although a substantial part of it must be to yield the x-ray diffraction pictures. Moreover, the chains are probably folded at intervals in the living state.

Criticizing various schemes that have been offered with the desire of relating the double helical structure of DNA to replication and func-tion, Crick himself holds it obvious that the sequence of bases could best express itself as an information code by means of the patterns of sites for hydrogen bonding presented by the structure.

The work of Wilkins and his coworkers has begun to throw light on the structure of nucleoproteins. In nucleoprotamine, it seems, the protamine chain is wound helically around the DNA structure in the *smaller* of the two grooves between the polynucleotide chains. This might suggest Chargaff's speculative model, but Crick would connect the positively charged basic groups of the protamine chain alternately up and down to the negatively charged phosphate groups of the DNA backbone. To get around the difficulty that there would not be enough basic side-chains on the protamine (the ratio of arginine to phosphate groups is 1:1 and only $\frac{2}{3}$ of the protamine side-chains are basic), it is suggested that the protamine chain is folded whenever non-polar amino acids occur, as they sometimes do, in pairs. The work on nucleohistone has progressed only to the point of showing that the DNA structure is present in characteristic form, and that there is some large repeating unit in it.

To the evidence of chemical heterogeneity in DNA Butler and Shooter add evidence of physical heterogeneity. In a single specimen a very wide range of sedimentation constants has been observed, the range of which, however, depends on the preparative methods employed. The implication that there is considerable variety in the shapes or weights of the DNA particles cannot at present be clarified, although the formation of aggregates, or the formation of protein bridges between DNA molecules, or varying degrees of degradation might be involved. Schachman and Doty each find evidence that the polydispersity of DNA is related more to variation in weight than in shape, but the latter is not excluded. Schachman also reported that DNA isolated from phage is more homogeneous than that obtained from calf thymus, as well as being much larger (molecular weight of 25×10^6 compared to 6 or 7×10^6). Monty described evidence to support the view that protein bridges are of considerable importance. The DNA studied is actually in the form of a deoxyribonucleoprotein, the protein being a lipoprotein and not a histone. Mitochondria possess a hydrolytic enzyme system (probably DNAase I, according to Dounce), of great activity in breaking down the DNA-protein configuration. Some of the products of this hydrolysis are neither free peptides nor free nucleotides, but are units probably containing the original bond-points between the DNA and the protein. The bond is labile to heat in the presence of dilute acid or alkali, and thus may be a phosphoamide bond.

The Structure of RNA and Synthetic Polyribonucleotides.

The x-ray diffraction picture of RNA looks suggestively like that of DNA, except for poorness in quality. The work was discouraging, however, as Watson and Rich each reported, until the synthetic polyribonucleotides of Ochoa became available. The x-ray diagrams of poly-AU and poly-AGUC are identical to those obtained from natural RNA, and even those from mono-polymers (poly-A and poly-C) are similar and indicate highly ordered structures. Poly-G has not yet been obtained.

The evidence suggests a helical molecule with nucleotides spaced at 3.75Å and a fiber axis repeat of 15Å, or every four nucleotides. The size of the unit crystallographic cell indicates that more than one poly-nucleotide chain is present. Since three chains would require a density obviously greater than that measured, it is concluded that there are two chains. A satisfactory model has been made (for poly-A) with two intertwined chains, the sugar-phosphate backbones on the outside and the bases pointing toward the central axis and held together by hydro-gen bonds, as in the now famous DNA model. The molecule, according to this model, would have a diameter of about 8Å.

Watson expresses the belief that the RNA molecule is very similar to that of the artificial poly-A, for the following reasons: (1) fibers of both are negatively birefringent; (2) similar systematic meridional absences in the diffraction photographs imply a similar helical arrange-ment; (3) in both, the first obvious layer is at 15Å, and both patterns reveal a prominent non-meridional reflection about 45° from the meridian; and (4) both patterns show a strong reflection on or near the equator in the 5Å region. The two patterns clearly differ only in the fact that the RNA pattern has strong meridional reflections at 3.3Å and 3.8Å, whereas poly-A has only the one, at 3.75Å. Significantly enough, Poly-C, according to Rich, has the 3.3Å meridional and 5Å equatorial reflections. If evidence is thus growing to indicate a struc-ture for RNA very nearly parallel to that of DNA, nevertheless, as Watson points out, the RNA structure would have difficulty in forming hydrogen bonds with regularity, and the similarity may rest mainly upon the tendency of the sugar-phosphate backbones to coil together as in DNA.

Rich has added information in respect to poly-U and the reaction mixture of poly-A and poly-U. Unlike the fibers of poly-A or poly-AU, which are negatively birefringent, poly-U fibers are not birefringent. The x-ray diffraction pattern is amorphous and gives no sign of a repetitive structural organization. As already mentioned, the diffrac-tion pattern of poly-AU, made when adenosine and uridine disphos-phates are polymerized together, is very like that of natural RNA. On the contrary, when poly-adenylic acid and poly-uridylic acid are first made and then mixed in solution, the poly-A + poly-U spon-taneously forms a two-stranded helix similar to DNA. Upon mixing, the viscosity increases rapidly and very long, tough, strongly negative

birefringent fibers appear. If vigorously stretched, the sign of birefringence becomes positive, as is true of DNA and RNA fibers. The
x-ray diffraction pattern varies with humidity, the helical pitch changing from 32Å at low relative humidity to over 36Å at 100% humidity.
The number of residues per turn is about ten. Although in these respects
like DNA, the first layer line, here so strong, is weak in the DNA
pattern. This is most simply explained by assuming that in poly-A +
poly-U the backbone chains are parallel instead of anti-parallel as in
DNA, and that consequently an additional hydrogen bond can be
formed, between the hydroxyl group on ribose carbon 2 and the
oxygen of the opposite phosphate group. Alternatively, the chains may
be anti-parallel as in DNA, but the molecule larger in diameter.

A particularly pregnant comment is that made by Rich on the significance of this evidence that the extra hydroxyl group of ribose, as
contrasted with deoxyribose, obviously does not prevent the molecule
from assuming a configuration like that of DNA. Hence RNA may well
be able to duplicate itself by a mechanism identical to that of DNA—
whatever that may be.

D'Arcy Thompson would indeed have been delighted at this growing
recognition of the biological importance of helices, on the molecular
as well as the chromosomal and grosser morphological levels. Barbara
Low has pointed out in the Symposium that helical structures have
been discovered not only in DNA—and now in RNA—but also in
keratin, collagen, polyglycine, and some polypeptides of synthetic
origin. In all such structures the repeat unit of the backbone must be
precisely structurally equivalent, whereas the side-chain residues vary.
But where in polynucleotide helices the stabilizing hydrogen bonds link
the opposed nucleotides of the two backbone chains, in collagen and
other polypeptides the hydrogen bonds link separate amino acid residues of a single chain, the configuration of which is determined by the
steric relations of certain side-chains, arranged in an ordered and repeating sequence.

The α-helix is the most stable backbone-chain configuration. Its
stability and regularity may be disrupted by prolyl residues, which
cannot be fitted into the smooth sequence of the helix; or by cystine
disulfide cross-linkages. An example of the latter phenomenon is to
be seen in keratin, whose individual α-helices are themselves coiled
together into a ropelike structure. The individual chains are held to
one another by cystine disulfide linkages. If these were disposed at
random, the change to the stretched β-configuration could not take
place without rupture of the -S-S- linkages, and of this there is no
evidence. It would seem, therefore, that the cystine disulfide linkages

must be relegated to certain non-oriented portions interpolated in the helical peptide chain.

There is even evidence of a helical structure in some of the globular proteins of relatively low molecular weight, including insulin and possibly hemoglobin and ribonuclease. Polypeptide chains in the α-helix configuration and 25 to 30Å in length seem to be closely packed in cylindrical array, but with certain irregularities. For example, in insulin the distances between —SH groups on the pentapeptide residues 6 to 11 of the A chain are so far apart as necessarily to make the disulfide intrachain bond interfere with the formation of a continuous helix in this portion of the molecule, although the terminal portions of the A chain and the entire B chain may be coiled in an α-helix.

There is at present little or no way of relating the helical structure of such molecules as DNA, collagen, or keratin, or the helical portions of globular proteins, to the functions of these substances. We are still a long way from bridging the gap between the double helix of a DNA molecule and the functional unit of the genetic material in a chromosome or virus. Indeed, the latter may involve several helical units of DNA and maybe protein as well. Assuredly, there must be a close relation between the structure of the collagen molecule and the function of collagen in providing architectural support and some mechanical flexibility. But the functioning depends not only on the stereochemistry of the individual helical unit but also on the way in which these are packed together. Until the latter is known in detail, the precise role of the former must remain uncertain. Much the same may be said of keratin, with the additional limitation that appreciable regions of non-helical structure exist in this molecule, that the α-helix depends for its maintenance on the interchain disulfide bonds, and is not completely defined. While the α-helices provide the necessary mechanical stability, here again the way in which they are joined and packed together is essential to the picture. As Barbara Low graphically puts it, "The properties of a woven fabric depend both on the fiber used and on the weave."

In globular proteins the loss of a specific intramolecular configuration entails a loss of the protein's biological specificity, probably because reactive sites or groups on the molecule become altered or inaccessible. Denaturation occurs when covalent bonds or even an extensive number of hydrogen bonds are broken. A molecule that had been wholly or partially "opened up" might thereafter either refold into the original or into some new configuration, but would more probably interact with other molecules to form an aggregate. Intramolecular disulfide linkages protect against such denaturing influences and might be expected to increase the likelihood of refolding, and hence of reactivation, rather than aggregation, which denotes a permanent loss of biological function. Inasmuch as the α-helix provides the most stable backbone structure known, it may be supposed that if such coiled regions do exist in globular proteins they contribute significantly to its over-all stability. One may speculate, according to Barbara Low, that inasmuch as the globular protein has its reactive sites at the molecular surface, its internal structure is important chiefly in providing stability for the molecule as a whole, and in this provision α-helices may contribute very largely to the maintenance of configuration at the active sites.

Synthesis of Nucleotides and Nucleic Acids.

The reports of Ochoa on the successful synthesis of polyribonucleotides and of Kornberg on that of polydeoxyribonucleotides aroused the highest enthusiasm among the participants in the Symposium. Clearly these advances bring within reach not only the artificial synthesis of hereditary materials but open up breathtaking vistas down which one may glimpse the controlled synthesis of proteins and a full understanding of the mechanisms of genetics and enzymatic control over metabolism and growth. A major "breakthrough" has undoubtedly been achieved, perhaps the greatest in biochemistry since Edouard Büchner established the nature of enzymes.

As Kornberg pointed out in his comprehensive review of both nucleotide and polynucleotide synthesis, the steps to the successful synthesis of the latter first involved an understanding of the participation of ribose phosphates and purine and pyrimidine nucleotides, and their respective pathways of synthesis. Ribose-5-phosphate is the key pentose in these reactions. It can be formed in at least four ways, but the direct oxidative pathway from glucose-6-phosphate via ribulose-5-phosphate, and the anaerobic pathway from glucose-6-phosphate via fructose-6-phosphate are the principal competing routes. From ribose-5-phosphate comes, by means of the donation of a pyrophosphate group from ATP, the newly discovered activated sugar phosphoribosylpyrophosphate (PRPP), which is of widespread occurrence. It is able to react with pyrimidines or purines to form nucleotides directly; or it can react with glutamine to form 5-phosphoribosylamine, which is the ribotide precursor of purine nucleotides.

The synthesis of purine and pyrimidine nucleotides differs in a major respect. The pathway of purine nucleotide synthesis is commonly *de novo*, starting from ammonia, phosphate, and simple carbon sources, and not involving free purines or nucleosides. The latter may be utilized in some organisms in a "salvage" operation, but that use is secondary in significance compared to the pathway worked out by

Buchanan and by Greenberg and their coworkers, and reported in previous McCollum-Pratt Symposia. On the other hand, pyrimidine nucleotide synthesis proceeds principally via a free base, orotic acid, which is derived from aspartic acid to begin with and is converted by reaction with phosphoribosylpyrophosphate to a nucleotide that is in turn converted into uridine-5′-phosphate. Uracil itself is utilized in such organisms as *Lactobacillus* in salvage operations, i.e., it is derived most probably from the enzymatic hydrolysis of RNA.

Nucleotides are notoriously inert when it comes to participation in the synthesis of polynucleotides or coenzymes. Studies on the synthesis of coenzymes already led some years ago (see McCollum-Pratt *Symposium on Phosphorus Metabolism*, Vol. I) to the expectation that the diphosphate and triphosphate nucleoside forms are the active precursors of polynucleotides. Further work on uridine triphosphate (UTP) led to the discovery by Kornberg's group of a liver enzyme that phosphorylates uridylic acid (UMP) to the triphosphate level by the transfer of a pyrophosphate group from ATP, and later of an enzyme in yeast that transphosphorylates adenosine, guanosine, and uridine nucleosides. The several reactions may be summarized in the general form:

nucleoside-P + *nucleoside*-PPP ⇌ nucleoside-PP + *nucleoside*-PP
2 nucleoside-PP ⇌ nucleoside-P + nucleoside-PPP.
2 *nucleoside*-PP ⇌ *nucleoside*-P + *nucleoside*-PPP.

Other groups likewise demonstrated the existence of enzymes that transfer phosphate from ATP to GMP, UMP, or CMP, and from ADP to GDP, UDP, CDP, or IDP (see below for abbreviations).

Last year Ochoa's group galvanized biochemists and geneticists alike with the report that there had been isolated from the microorganism *Azotobacter vinelandii* and partially purified an enzyme which catalyzes the synthesis of highly polymerized ribonucleotides from 5′-nucleoside diphosphates, with release of inorganic phosphate. The enzyme has been named polynucleotide phosphorylase, and is already known to be widely distributed among bacteria, e.g., in *E. coli* and *Micrococcus lysodeikticus*. The reaction was shown to be reversible, and the linkages in the artificial polyribonucleotides formed were found to be 3′-5′ phosphoribose ester bonds just as in natural RNA. Thermodynamically, the reaction utilizes the energy of the pyrophosphate bond in the 5′-nucleoside diphosphates to form the diester bonds of the polynucleotide chain. The equilibrium favors the formation of the polynucleotide, but not very strongly.

Polymers composed wholly of a single kind of unit have been formed from adenosine (A), inosine (I), guanosine (G), uridine (U), and cytosine (C) diphosphates, respectively; and two mixed polymers have also been made, one from ADP and UDP in equimolar proportions, and the other from ADP, GDP, UDP, and CDP in molar proportions of 1: 0.5: 1: 1. The former is termed the AU polymer; the latter, the AGUC polymer.

The existence of enzymes that utilize 5'-diphosphates in the synthesis of polyribonucleotides led to a prompt search for the occurrence of the precursors within living cells. Potter and his colleagues were able to find not only the diphosphates, but also monophosphates and triphosphates of guanosine, uridine, and cytosine, in addition to the previously known ones of adenosine.

The synthetic polyribonucleotides terminate with a phosphate ester in the 5'-linkage. Action on the synthetic forms by enzymes that split natural RNA, e.g., snake venom phosphodiesterase, spleen phosphodiesterase, and pancreatic ribonuclease, is strictly analogous to the action on RNA. For example, the last-named of the three enzymes, which cleaves only pyrimidine nucleoside phosphodiester bonds distal to the 3'-linkage, will not split the poly-A synthetic compound at all, but cleaves the U, C, AU, and AGUC polymers as would be expected, viz., complete digestion of the poly-U ribonucleotide releases 3'-UMP.

By preparing the AU polymer with P^{32}-labeled ADP and unlabeled UDP and then digesting the synthetic polyribonucleotide with pancreatic ribonuclease or hydrolyzing it with alkali, it proved possible for Ochoa and his coworkers to determine the frequency with which various nucleotide sequences occur in the polymer. Of the adenylic acid residues in the polynucleotide, 53 per cent were preceded by uridylic acid. The distribution appears to be almost random. Thus, given sequences such as UU, UAU, UAAU, and UAAAU appear to be followed about equally often by either A or U. The average length of U sequences was 2.35, of A sequences 2.0.

When natural RNA is exhaustively digested with ribonuclease and then dialyzed against distilled water, a non-dialyzable core composed largely of purine nucleotides is left. The artificial polymer AGUC, when similarly treated, yields a similar core amounting to about 20 per cent of the total nucleotides. In the first poly-AGUC ribonucleotide made, the proportion of guanylic acid, in relation to the three other nucleotides, was about half that of natural RNA from *Azotobacter*, as might be expected from the molar proportions of 1: 0.5: 1: 1 which were used in the mixture of precursors. Later an equimolar proportion was used for preparing a second artificial RNA, and in this case the proportions of adenylic and guanylic acids were identical with those occurring in natural *Azotobacter* RNA (10 : 13), although there was a deficiency of uridylic acid (4.2 instead of 7.3) and an excess of cytidylic acid (11.1 instead of 9) over the expected proportions. This departure from the ideal result was attributed to the use of crude enzyme in the preparation, and the hope was expressed by Ochoa that use of the isolated pure enzyme would enable his group to prepare a polyribonucleotide identical with natural RNA in the proportions of its component nucleotides.

The forms of RNA isolated from *Staphylococcus aureus, Mycobacterium phlei,* and *Alcaligenes fecalis,* organisms which are rich in polynucleotide phosphorylase, differ significantly in some respects in the relative abundance of the four nucleotides. Thus it may be possible, by using the polynucleotide phosphorylases from different organisms, to construct artificial RNA's differing characteristically in composition.

The molecular weights of the synthetic polyribonucleotides fall into the range of molecular weights exhibited by natural RNA from various sources. Values calculated from sedimentation data cluster around 7×10^4, while those calculated from light-scattering data are higher (1.48×10^5 to 1.86×10^6). The molecular weights of the AGUC polymer and of natural *Azotobacter* RNA derived from the same kind of data (sedimentation) are the same, 7×10^4 and 6×10^4, respectively.

Average chain-lengths, as determined by end-group assays, yield far lower estimates of molecular weight. Thus, poly-AGUC was found to have an average chain-length of only 30 residues. But this is again in harmony with the values for natural RNA, e.g., yeast and turnip yellow mosaic virus RNA were found to have 12 and 53 residues, respectively, or molecular weights of 4000 and 16,000. These values, so much below those obtained from the physical measurements, are thought to be evidence that the weights obtained from the latter are the result of an aggregation of polynucleotide chains.

Is polynucleotide phosphorylase responsible for the synthesis of RNA within the living cell? To this question the answer remains somewhat doubtful, because of the low affinity of the enzyme for the 5'-diphosphate substrates. "One would have to assume," say Ochoa and Heppel, "that high local concentrations of nucleoside diphosphates might be available to the phosphorylase in the cell."

Many questions remain to be answered regarding the action and the role of polynucleotide phosphorylase. As to the reaction mechanism, for instance, does the enzyme require a nucleotide chain as a primer of the reaction to start with, or can it commence to form the polynucleotide simply with two nucleotide diphosphate molecules? Another important question to be answered, especially important in view of the enzyme's considerable lack of specificity, is whether the enzyme is actually a single entity or a mixture of enzymes. That the latter may be the case is possibly indicated by the failure of purified enzyme from *E. coli* or *M. lysodeikticus* to act on GDP as sole substrate. The

Azotobacter enzyme will do so, but only with difficulty, and utilizes it freely only when other nucleoside diphosphates are present. On the other hand, when several diphosphates are present together they compete with one another, and that fact argues for a single enzyme, and competition between the diphosphates for a single reactive site.

As for nucleotide sequence, which seems so essential to the specificity of different RNA's, there is still no clue to suggest how it is determined. It is hard to see how different sequences could be produced unless there are different RNA-synthesizing enzymes for each distinct kind of RNA; or alternatively, unless the specificity does not reside in the enzyme at all, but results from the performance of each existing sort of RNA as a template for the synthesis of the new polynucleotides. The generality of polynucleotide phosphorylase has by no means been established. Although it occurs widely in bacteria, and is also to be found in yeast, yet its presence in the higher plants in significant quantity is still uncertain; and the possibility of its presence in animal tissues is indicated only by the incorporation of AMP into RNA of pigeon liver and rat liver homogenates.

Further studies on this incorporation of labeled AMP into RNA in rat liver preparations were reported to the Symposium by Potter and his coworkers. An optimum balance must be maintained in the system between too little and too much ATP, for some ATP is required for the generation of the diphosphates, but too much ATP leads to phosphorylation of the end groups of the RNA chain and consequently puts an end to further lengthening. When microsomal RNA was labeled with orotic acid-6-C^{14} in a homogenate system free of both nuclei and whole cells, and the labeled RNA was then added to a fresh unlabeled system, delabeling at once began. But when RNA was similarly labeled in the whole animal and then taken out, the microsomal RNA was not delabeled under the same conditions. This contrast demonstrates that the terminal nucleosides may undergo exchange but that nucleotides away from the end positions do not. Further experiments with tissue slices from animals killed at varying times after the injection of the labeled orotic acid seem to show that in the presence of nuclei the incorporation of orotic acid into RNA comes to a halt long before the time when its incorporation into RNA, in a nucleus-free homogenate, would be diminished. The meaning of this nuclear control over the amount of labeling of pyrimidine nucleotides in RNA is not yet understood.

In spite of considerable search, no sign has yet been found of any deoxyribose analogue of PRPP. It therefore seems unlikely that deoxynucleotide synthesis depends on a pyrophosphoryl derivative of deoxyribose-5-phosphate. Deoxynucleosides, however, may be formed in bacteria and in animal tissues in a variety of ways. Both purine and pyrimidine deoxynucleoside phosphorylases occur, and will produce the nucleosides by coupling the bases and deoxyribose-1-phosphate. Moreover, in a number of bacterial species there is a deoxynucleoside transglycosidase that exchanges free purine or pyrimidine bases with those in deoxynucleosides without phosphorolysis or hydrolysis. The deoxynucleotides, formerly known only as products of DNA degradation, have now entered the realm of synthesis. Once Friedkin and others had shown that thymidine and deoxycytidine are incorporated into DNA, Kornberg and his coworkers found that in *E. coli* there is an enzyme capable of producing thymidine-5'-phosphate from thymidine and ATP. Thymidine di- and tri-phosphates are also formed, and the same enzyme phosphorylates deoxyuridine at a rate about one-third that of thymidine. Yet this nucleoside kinase is regarded by Kornberg as lying aside from the main route of deoxynucleotide synthesis, and as probably involved only in salvage.

A more significant pathway for the synthesis of thymidine-5'-phosphate was reported by Friedkin and Kornberg. Deoxyuridine-5'-phosphate will react, in the presence of an *E. coli* enzyme, either with serine or with hydroxymethyl tetrahydrofolic acid to form the thymidine nucleotide. Moreover, the *E. coli* enzyme that rapidly converts thymidine-5'-phosphate to the triphosphate (TTP) fails to carry out the parallel conversion of deoxyuridylic acid to deoxyuridine triphosphate. The extremely interesting suggestion is therefore made that this specificity may explain why thymine, and not uracil, is a component of DNA. It would appear that the deoxyuridylic acid must be methylated *before* it can be converted into a triphosphate and thereupon incorporated into DNA. The β-carbon of serine is transferred to tetrahydrofolic acid—making hydroxymethyl THFA—which then acts as a methyl donor to the pyrimidine. The same *E. coli* kinase that uses ATP to convert thymidylic acid to the triphosphate can also produce the respective nucleoside triphosphates from deoxycytidylic, deoxyadenylic, and deoxyguanylic acids. Only deoxyuridylic acid remains unaffected. These studies, which show that deoxyuridylic acid is methylated to form thymidylic acid, imply that the reduction of ribonucleotides to deoxyribonucleotides occurs as an earlier step in the synthesis of DNA.

By analogy with coenzyme synthesis, Kornberg arrived at the conception that the lengthening of a polynucleotide chain should occur by reaction with a nucleoside diphosphate or triphosphate. One mechanism would be that of additions of nucleotide units to the end of the polynucleotide chain terminating as a di- or tri-phosphate. In this case, inorganic phosphate or pyrophosphate would be displaced. (An alternative mechanism would be that of addition to the sugar end of the chain, with displacement of inorganic phosphate from ADP or of pyrophosphate from ATP.) While Kornberg was trying to use ribonucleoside triphosphates to synthesize polyribonucleotides, Grunberg-Manago and Ochoa demonstrated that it was the nucleoside diphosphate rather than the triphosphate which was the active component of the system. Kornberg was then enabled to purify an enzyme from *E. coli* that synthesizes nucleoside diphosphates into a polynucleotide chain. (Beers has likewise accomplished this result with an enzyme from *Micrococcus lysodeikticus.*) Kornberg has also found that in the *E. coli* system an "activator" is capable of producing a fourfold increase. The activator is non-dialyzable but heat-stable, and is neither RNA nor DNA.

Fractionation of the *E. coli* extracts permitted Kornberg and his coworkers to separate a number of enzymes that convert thymidine by steps (through thymidine-5'-phosphate, diphosphate, and triphosphate) to an acid-insoluble nucleic acid product which was part of a DNA or some closely related molecule. It was degraded by pancreatic deoxyribonuclease, but not much, if any, by ribonuclease, strong alkali, or weak acid. The purified system for the synthesis of this artificial DNA included TTP or TDP, ATP, a heat-stable DNA fraction regarded as a "primer," and two enzyme fractions, each of which has been purified more than 100-fold. The deoxynucleoside-5'-triphosphates of adenine, guanine, and cytosine were prepared and tested in the same system. They too were incorporated into the synthesized DNA at rates comparable to that of the TTP when the crude enzyme preparations were used, but at slower rates after the enzymes were highly purified. This fact may signify the presence of different enzymes for the several deoxyribonucleoside triphosphates. Mixtures of all four triphosphates showed better than additive rates of incorporation, so that polymerization is facilitated when all four are present. Even so, the "primer" was still necessary to obtain a maximal rate of synthesis. This "primer" upon analysis has proved to be composed of one fraction indistinguishable from DNA itself, and another fraction composed of a mixture of deoxycytidylic, deoxyadenylic, and deoxyguanylic acids. Clearly, all four deoxyribonucleoside triphosphates are actually needed for the synthesis. When this was seen to be true, the system could be considerably simplified. ATP was no longer needed, and one of the two enzymes could be dispensed with, since these were of value only to provide the missing triphosphates. Mg^{++} and DNA still proved to be essential.

Ochoa and his coworkers have likewise found enzymes in *A. vinelandii* that transfer phosphate from ATP (or ITP) to deoxyribosenucleoside-5'-monophosphates. Deoxyadenosine and deoxycytidine monophosphates are the most effective receivers of phosphate, thymidine monophosphate is a relatively poor one, and inosine triphosphate proved quite unable to convey phosphate to inosine monophosphate.

Kornberg's reaction is not readily reversible. With the simplified system, a net synthesis of DNA can be demonstrated, together with a release of inorganic pyrophosphate during the course of the reaction. Thymidine diphosphate could not effectively replace TTP—in other words, it is the deoxyribonucleoside *triphosphates* that are the immediate precursors of DNA, in contrast to the direct utilization of the ribonucleoside *diphosphates* in the synthesis of the polyribonucleotides and RNA.

With this achievement there now lies before us the dazzling prospect of synthesizing such units of heredity as a bacterial transforming factor or a "gene" of tobacco mosaic virus. But to do this we must first learn the way to control the sequence of nucleotides in a polynucleotide chain. That will be the next great step in the artificial synthesis of genetic material.

Seymour Cohen's contribution to the Symposium dealt with the chemical structure of the DNA of the T-even bacterial viruses (T2, T4, T6), with the interrelationships of protein synthesis, DNA synthesis, and RNA synthesis in infected *E. coli* cells, and with the intermediary metabolism of the nucleic acids, especially in regard to certain thymine-requiring mutants in which nuclear and cytoplasmic synthesis appear to be experimentally separable. A significant feature is that when a bacterium is infected with one of these phages, enzyme synthesis on the part of the host cell stops. It therefore seems likely that somehow the virus genes themselves can multiply and the virus protein be synthesized without requiring any synthesis of specific enzymes. If all enzyme synthesis can be bypassed in the analysis of phage replication, the problem would no doubt be greatly simplified.

When the now-famous phages exemplified by T2 infect a bacterium, the protein of the outer coat and of most of the tail, which is necessary for the phage's adsorption to and penetration of the host cell, remains outside. Pure DNA, with some 3 per cent of the total phage protein, is injected into the host cell. The multiplication of the virus requires only this genetic charge; thus "DNA not only supplies the information essential to its own duplication but also that necessary to encase the DNA in the differentiated proteins of the outer coat and tail."

The total DNA of a phage particle amounts to 2×10^{-16} g., of a molecular weight estimated by Schachman and Cohen from sedimentation and viscosity data to be about 25,000,000. This value is higher than that obtained by most other workers. The isolated nucleic acids of three mutant pairs of T2, T4, and T6 were all found to possess the same ratios of the four purine and pyrimidine bases. Wyatt and Cohen discovered a unique feature of these DNA's—they contain, instead of cytosine, a new pyrimidine, 5-hydroxymethyl cytosine (HMC). Successive treatment with deoxyribonuclease and phosphatase was not able to release the HMC nucleoside. Since infection of *E. coli* with a T-even virus rapidly activates a bacterial deoxyribonuclease that degrades the bacterial DNA, it was apparent that the refractoriness of the HMC nucleotide to DNAase might be what protects the virus DNA from destruction while the host DNA is broken down. The molecular basis of the resistance of the viral DNA to deoxyribonuclease was discovered independently by Volkin and Sinsheimer. It resides in the presence of glucose on the hydroxymethyl group of HMC. This protective glucosylation was found to be complete in the DNA of T4r^+ but to involve only 77 per cent of the HMC nucleotides of T2r^+. Correspondingly, as Streisinger and Weigle have found, the T4 stock has a high efficiency in producing plaques on certain host bacteria, while the T2 stock has a lower efficiency. A vast majority, if not all, of the T2 progeny of a T2 × T4 cross possess the high plating efficiency of the T4 parent.

Cohen and his coworkers have consistently found that the r (host-range mutant) phages have more glucose than the r^+ phages. In general, the resistance of the virus DNA to attack by DNAase is fairly well correlated with the glucose content. The new points thus established are that in the compulsion of a host bacterium to synthesize viral DNA, not only is it necessary for it to produce the right sequence of bases but also for it to determine whether or not glucose is to be added to the hydroxymethyl cytosine, as well as to choose between varieties of HMC nucleotides. Such choices are quite puzzling, in view of the fact that if glucose on the hydroxymethyl group of HMC prevents the action of phosphatase on the nucleotide phosphate bond, then the presence of phosphate ought, at the nucleotide level, to hinder the addition of glucose to the molecule. Or, conversely, the addition of glucose at the nucleoside level should hinder subsequent phosphorylation of the molecule.

In an infected bacterium protein continues to be synthesized without interruption. The first protein made goes into phage to the extent of barely 10 per cent, later-made protein up to 50-60 per cent. Nevertheless, the initial protein synthesis is also an essential part of phage production, for when it is inhibited by the amino acid analogue, 5-methyl tryptophan, the phage (T2) does not grow and net DNA synthesis in the host is halted. Even when the action of the inhibitor is limited to the period following the initial phase of protein synthesis, the synthesis of phage DNA can proceed without further protein synthesis, although eventually protein will be required to complete the formation of mature phage particles (Burton). Together with the finding of Stent and his collaborators that P^{32}-labeled cells infected with P^{32}-labeled virus and immediately after infection stored at $-190°$C. lose the ability to produce phage as a function of the radioactive decay, whereas similarly infected cells first allowed to commence phage development and then stored at the same temperature become independent of radioactive decay, this evidence raises the possibility that genetic specificity is transferred from DNA to protein, and seriously calls in question the validity of the Watson-Crick scheme of replication, in so far as viruses are concerned.

A net synthesis of DNA in an infected bacterial cell is observable only after a lag of 5 to 9 minutes. There is a reciprocal relation between the disappearance of cytosine from the bacterial DNA and the synthesis of viral 5-hydroxmethyl cytosine. Even in these experiments a requirement for protein synthesis prior to DNA synthesis might obtain.

Although it was long thought that within infected cells there is no synthesis of RNA, it has now been demonstrated by Volkin and Astrachan that in T2-infected *E. coli* there is some incorporation of P^{32} from labeled inorganic phosphate into RNA, in spite of the lack of any net synthesis of the latter. According to their Symposium report, the results differ in peptone broth medium and synthetic medium, the incorporation coming to a rapid standstill in the former but continuing at a linear rate in the latter. What is more interesting, over short periods of time the incorporation of P^{32} into RNA equalled and even greatly exceeded that into DNA, and the analysis of the mononucleotides showed that there was significantly more (about $1\frac{1}{2}$ to 2 times as much) P^{32} in the adenylic and uridylic acids than in the cytidylic and guanylic acids (30A: 30U: 22G: 18C). It is proposed that the RNA synthesized is thus of a unique type, differing from the typical bacterial RNA; and that the correspondence of the labeled RNA mononucleotides to the ratio of the bases in T2 DNA (32A: 32T: 18G: 18C) implies that this RNA is a precursor of the phage DNA. Although the function of this RNA as a precursor of phage DNA is certainly not conclusively demonstrated at the moment, the possible intervention of RNA as well as protein as intermediates between infecting DNA and new DNA certainly casts some doubt on the simple picture of a direct DNA replication as a sufficient explanation of the increase in the genetic material.

In considering the formation of the whole virus, Cohen emphasized the problems involved in getting the DNA inside the protein coat. The elegant experiments of Hershey and his coworkers have clearly shown, by virtue of the inhibition of protein synthesis with chloramphenicol, that DNA synthesis can proceed to the extent of forming a very large pool of virus DNA without extensive protein synthesis to accompany it; and that subsequently the synthesis of the protein still permits the encasement of the DNA within its coat. How it is possible for DNA to get folded up and packed into the covering? Is there in fact at least a very thin protein covering over the DNA from the moment of its synthesis?

Cohen also pointed to the possibility that the supposed metabolic inertness of DNA, deduced from its lack of apparent phosphorus turnover, might be an illusion. A considerable activity of the nucleotides might occur if the same phosphorus atom is reused to make the phosphodiester linkage after cleavage and exchange has occurred.

In studying the intermediary metabolism of the nucleic acids in a phage-infected bacterium, the prime difficulty arises from the abundance of alternative pathways which are demonstrable in cell-free systems. At present it appears that whereas in normal growing cells deoxyribose is formed chiefly from ribose that is derived from glucose via the oxidative phosphogluconate pathway, in infected cells, on the contrary, deoxyribose is formed chiefly by way of a different pathway, although the precise nature of this path is still undefined.

The discovery of hydroxymethyl cytosine in the DNA of the phage had led to the intriguing suggestion that it serves to entrap that pyrimidine, and that the consequent shortage of cytosine in the bacterial cell leads to its failure to produce its own DNA and RNA. This is borne out by the experimental fact that hydroxymethyl cytosine cannot serve as a substitute for cytosine in the nutrition of pyrimidine-requiring mutants of *E. coli*. It would necessarily follow that in a normal bacterial cell the formation of HMC must be suppressed. Another striking difference between the metabolic activity of the normal bacterium and the infected one is that in the normal cell thymine and thymidine are not utilized significantly, but in the synthesis of viral DNA in the infected cell thymidine is utilized, so that reactions at the nucleoside level, probably the methylation of precursor to thymine and the hydroxymethylation of deoxcytidine, must be of importance.

The study of Barner and Cohen of pyrimidine synthesis in infected cells has led to the isolation of 5-methyl deoxycytidine, which is deaminated to yield thymidine by the deoxycytidine deaminase of *E. coli*, and at an even faster rate than the deamination of deoxycytidine itself by the same enzyme. The postulated steps in the formation of the deoxyribosides of hydroxymethyl cytosine and thymine in the synthesis of viral DNA are shown in Fig. 2. Several dihydrouracil and dihydrocytosine derivatives have been synthesized, but seem to lack

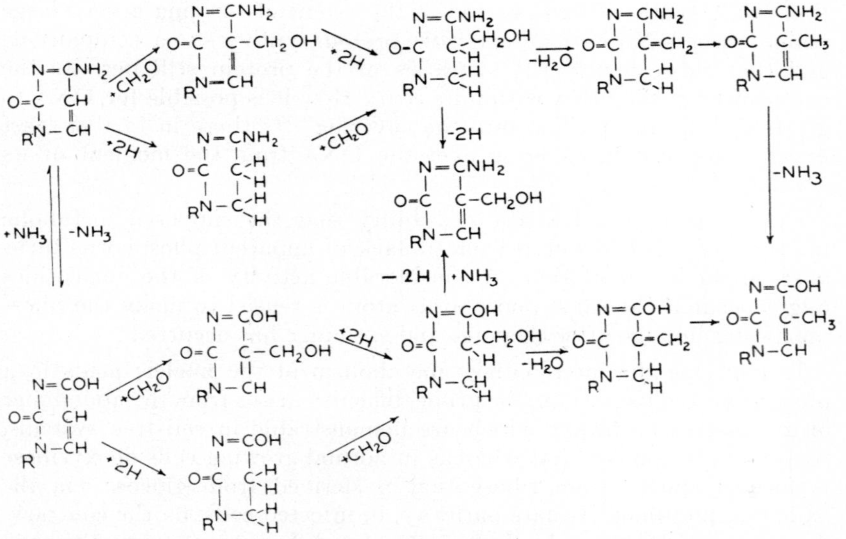

FIG. 2. Postulated steps in the formation of HMC and thymine deoxyribosides.
(From Cohen.)

biological activity. Cohen remains optimistic about the possible functioning of dihydro-hydroxymethyl derivatives as intermediates.

Cohen and his coworkers have been intensively studying the synthesis of nucleic acid in a thymine-requiring mutant strain of *E. coli* (15_T-). Infection of this strain with phage T2 restores its blocked thymine synthesis. Cultures may be synchronized in division by taking them off thymine for an initial period, during which DNA stops increasing but RNA and protein continue to be synthesized, and by then restoring thymine so that DNA synthesis is instantaneously resumed. In such cultures, it is apparent that DNA synthesis (but not RNA synthesis) is cyclic, stopping during actual cell division and resuming between divisions. In the case of a double mutant which also requires phenylalanine, protein synthesis and DNA synthesis can be separated. When thymine alone is supplied, only DNA synthesis occurs. When phenylalanine alone is supplied, no DNA is made, but RNA and protein increase almost as much as when both thymine and phenylalanine are supplied to the double mutant. The synthesis of RNA when phenylalanine alone is supplied is always greater than that of protein.

Folic acid deficiency, brought about by sulfanilamide or a folic acid analogue, will bring about a failure to synthesize thymine even in bacteria normally capable of this (*E. coli* B). The folic acid deficiency may be counteracted by a mixture of such compounds as thymine, methionine, histidine, or pantothenate, which are donors of essential one-carbon pieces. Omission from this mixture of particular compounds (with the exception of thymine) produces the typical bacteriostatic effect of sulfanilamide. When thymine is omitted, the effect is bactericidal instead, and the bacteria are unable after a period of unbalanced growth to resume normal division. Cohen has found that in the thymine-requiring mutant strain, bromouracil and thymine at more than a 3:1 ratio inhibit multiplication of the organisms after a single division, whereas bromouracil alone somewhat reduces the killing effect of a lack of thymine. In the former case, long filaments are produced, and it seems that some abnormal, pathological sort of DNA must be formed. At the nucleoside level bromouracil deoxyriboside is more lethal than bromouracil, a fact from which it may be inferred that in the mutant strain thymine is converted to thymidine before the nucleotide is formed. In other strains of *E. coli*, which do not incorporate free thymine into DNA, bromouracil deoxyriboside is without effect even in large amounts. An alternative pathway to the normal one must, then, exist for the synthesis of the thymine nucleotides in the thymine-requiring mutant, as in the infected cell synthesizing viral DNA (see above).

It is very interesting that the lethal effects produced by treatment with ultraviolet light, nitrogen mustards, or penicillin alike form a pathological pattern similar to that which results from a thymine deficiency. These agents may be suspected of resembling one another in that each blocks DNA synthesis at some point and so produces an unbalanced growth that ends in death.

Mutation, too, must be related to DNA synthesis if the mutations are, as some suppose, errors in the duplication process. Although the fact that mutations cannot be induced in isolated, inert virus preparations fits this view, the occurrence of both spontaneous and induced mutations in non-dividing cells is more difficult to explain on this basis. The evidence presented by Cohen and others that the genetic material is not necessarily inert in non-dividing cells—which may be growing or exchanging thymine with the medium—may be taken to strengthen the view that mutation consists in an error in duplication. It would follow that agents which inhibit the synthesis of DNA, and of thymine particularly, should be anti-mutagenic. Cohen and Barner, however, have observed in the thymine-requiring strain growing on a thymine-deficient medium mass-mutations, especially of the "leaky" type, to thymine independence. Cohen asks whether a thymine deficiency may itself be mutagenic. Possibly our anticipated power to produce specific mutations may unfold as we learn how, by means of nutritional techniques and metabolic reactions, to influence the structure or biosynthesis of DNA.

The Mechanism of Duplication

The replication of DNA—assuming the correctness of the Watson-Crick model of two helices wound around one another (i.e., plectonemically coiled) and in many turns—presents a grave topological difficulty to which much thought has been given. Stent points out that the "winding number" of such a duplex helix (i.e., the number of complete rotations made by a vector connecting two points at the same level in the opposite chains) is invariant no matter what distortion of the chains occurs, provided the ends be fixed. The winding number for DNA would be 150 per million molecular weight, or 900 for a molecular weight of 6 million, and 2750 for one of 25 million. So long as the winding number is greater than zero, the braid composed of the two interwound chains cannot be separated by combining them, but can be separated only if breaks occur. Even if a daughter duplex is formed on the parent double-helix without any separation of the strands of the latter, the topological difficulty still remains. It would be impossible to separate the parent from the daughter duplex without breaking them. The possibility that the duplex consists of short sections of alternating positive and negative winding numbers has been ruled out because stereochemically it seems impossible to construct a model with left-handed helices. The possibility that short sections of DNA alternate with short sections of non-DNA material wound in a complementary fashion is ruled out by the chemical evidence. And the possibility that the winding number is really zero (i.e., a paranemic coiling, as of two separate coils simply pushed into one another) is ruled out by the x-ray diffraction data.

It seems mechanically almost inconceivable that the strands could become separated by being pulled lengthwise in opposite directions. Other suggestions which have been offered are as follows: (1) the chains may separate by unwinding; (2) they may separate by enzymatic digestion; or (3) they may separate by breaks and reunions. The first method was thought to require too much energy until a recent study by Levinthal and Crane showed that the rotation required—one complete rotation for each turn to be unwound—actually would require only about 150 calories per mole of replicated chain link, or far less than the total energy required for the formation of the phosphate diester linkages of the polynucleotide chain. If the duplex rotates like a speedometer cable, without flopping, and if the untwisting proceeds pari passu with the replication itself, the Y-shaped configuration which would result would rotate as a whole in a clockwise direction. [An untwisting scheme conceived by Platt is even less simple.] The second method has not been worked out elaborately. According to an idea of Watson's, one chain of the parent duplex might be digested away, the remaining one then serving as a template for the formation of numerous single, either identical or complementary, replicas not interwound with the parent chain and readily separable from it. These in turn might synthesize complementary chains that would mature into "resting" duplexes. The break and reunion solution of the problem has been considered by Delbrück, who suggests that the breaks and rejoins occur pari passu with replication, in such a way that the broken terminal of each parent chain rejoins with the end of the daughter replica of corresponding polarity. The result would be that every chain would consist of short segments of old and new material in alternation.

Stent classifies the replication schemes, on the basis of their distribution of the parent material, into *conservative, semi-conservative,* and *dispersive* mechanisms. In the first, the integrity of the parent material is entirely preserved within a single one of the daughter duplexes. In the second mechanism, one chain in each daughter duplex is old, one new. In the last mechanism, the distribution of the old material is uniform throughout the four chains of the two daughter duplexes. Delbrück's scheme is obviously dispersive; Bloch's and Butler's schemes are conservative; and the original proposal of Watson and Crick was semi-conservative in nature. If unambiguous tests could be made of the distribution of the parent material in the daughter duplexes, a considerable reduction in number of the potential replication mechanisms might be made.

To complicate the issue, at least in bacteriophages, replication and genetic recombination cannot be separated experimentally. This impels Stent to classify recombination mechanisms into "fragmenting" and "non-fragmenting." Crossing over, according to the conventional concept, is of course fragmenting; "copy-choice" (a switch of the replica being formed from one template to another) might be either fragmenting or non-fragmenting, in terms of the distribution of parent material in the daughter duplexes. The experimental result would be unambiguous only if the integrity of the entire parent duplex, or of its two chains separately, was indefinitely preserved. But in the transfer of labeled DNA from a parent phage to its progeny only 35 to 50 per cent is recovered, and the unrecovered DNA is seemingly a random portion of the entire DNA of the parent, and no specific part.

The transfer experiments with bacteriophage made over the past six years by various workers agree in showing that about half the parental

DNA is transferred in big pieces and the remainder is more widely distributed. In experiments in which the distribution has been traced into the second generation, the large pieces do not undergo any further breakup. Thus Levinthal and Thomas, from an elegant extension of radioautographic technique to the molecular level, reported to the Symposium that in intact phage the first generation progeny carried $24 \pm 3\%$ of the P^{32} in uniformly labeled parent phage, and the second generation progeny carried $26 \pm 3\%$. Their method involves surrounding the radioactive particles with an electron-sensitive nuclear emulsion. The electron tracks formed by the decay of radioactive atoms in the particles radiate so as to form stars. Detection of the emission is virtually 100 per cent efficient, and the activity of a particle is detectable down to a level of 15 disintegrations per month. The number of tracks per star is the parameter of significance, since it varies with the random incorporation of the radioactive isotope into the material. From the results, Levinthal computes that the large piece of DNA which maintains its identity has in phages T2 and T4 a molecular weight of approximately 45 million. One such large piece is released from each phage particle by osmotic shock; and approximately half of the P^{32}-label of such a piece is transmitted to the first and second generation progeny intact. Levinthal is inclined to believe that this "big piece" is the chromosome of the bacteriophage. To test this a cross was made between labeled and unlabeled T2 phages distinguished by carrying different h alleles. At least 90 per cent of the particles that formed stars also carried the h^+ marker of the labeled parent, as would be expected if the labeled big piece of DNA is in fact the chromosome of the phage. This result, however, is at variance with that obtained by Sato and Stent, using a P^{32}-inactivation method, and the interpretation, therefore, remains uncertain.

The alternative experimental method just mentioned involves strongly labeling phage particles with P^{32}, the decay of which when incorporated into the DNA of the phage results in the killing of the virus (Hershey et al.). Fewer than 1 in 10^4 unlabeled virus particles grown in labeled bacteria living on labeled medium proved not to be subject to death from the decay of the P^{32}—whence it follows that the half-portion of the DNA of the parent phage particle which is transmitted to the phage progeny cannot very often be transmitted as a complete complement to any individual daughter particle. But in the converse experiment, Stent and Jerne found that although the progeny particles carried on the average 2% of the parental P^{32} per particle, the inactivation by P^{32} decay was less than 0.2% of that of the parent. It follows that most of the transferred P^{32} must be concentrated within a relatively few progeny particles. In a second-generation transfer experiment, Stent and his coworkers found that the amount of P^{32} which can be transferred from the first generation to the second diminishes from 50% to 25% as the exposure of the first generation to P^{32}-decay is prolonged. This is taken to mean that half of the radioactive DNA is transferred in big pieces that make the recipients unstable, half in pieces so small that the recipients are unaffected. Transfer from the second generation of phage to a third resembles kinetically the first-to-second generation transfer just described. These results thus strengthen the conclusions drawn by Levinthal from the radioautographic method. The recognition of the bipartite (big pieces; small pieces) nature of the transmitted DNA necessitates a complete reevaluation of the indications as to whether replication is conservative, semiconservative, or dispersive. If the two portions of the DNA are not equivalent in role, it must first be determined whether it is the big piece, or the small pieces, that constitute the genetic material and are responsible for the replication of the DNA. If, as Levinthal thinks, the big piece is the chromosome of the phage particle, then replication cannot be dispersive and recombination cannot be fragmenting. This is all that can be said at the moment.

Certainly the parental DNA is dispersed to a considerable degree in the course of replication and recombination, as the experiments of Garen and of Burgi show. When a cross is made between labeled and unlabeled phages differing in a genetic host-range marker, up to 65% of the P^{32} label may separate in one generation from the genetic marker with which it was introduced. But this could be due to unspecific transfer as well as to fragmenting recombination. Certainly the labeled DNA is not randomly distributed, for 20 to 30% of it tends to stay with the original associated marker gene. Yet the experiment of Sato and Stent showed that this portion of the DNA that "stayed true" was either not identical with the "big piece" or else was not linked equally to all loci. The issue is further complicated by the strange finding (Luria and Dulbecco; Doermann et al.) that phage particles irradiated with ultraviolet and rendered unable to infect host bacteria may nevertheless transmit marker genes to progeny if mixed with live phage particles which can infect the bacteria and "rescue" the inactivated phage. Such rescued markers may appear in the progeny independently of one another. It now turns out that much of the DNA from the irradiated parent particles turns up in progeny that are similarly "dead," i.e., unable to infect by themselves, whereas the rest of the DNA gets into live particles (Hershey). The number of "dead" progeny is no greater than the number of "dead" parents—hence no replication of the DNA in these particles seems to have occurred. The reverse cross shows that some 20 to 30% of the DNA from a live parent particle gets into "dead" progeny. Taken altogether, these results support the concept of the bipartite nature of phage DNA.

Another type of experiment conducted by Stent shows that bacterial nuclei of an initially unlabeled culture, after being grown on medium labeled with P^{32} for slightly more than a generation, almost all assimilate P^{32} and become subject to death from its decay. Labeled nuclei grown in non-radioactive medium experience a dilution of their P^{32} and become less subject to death from its decay. This experiment serves to eliminate the possibility that the DNA of the E. coli nucleus replicates by a conservative mechanism without fragmentation because of genetic recombination; but that is all it tells. Distribution experiments with plant chromosomes (Plaut and Mazia) are no more explicit. In short, says Stent, ". . . two fundamental difficulties have so far prevented us from drawing any unambiguous conclusions concerning the question whether DNA replication is conservative, semi-conservative, or dispersive. An observed *unequal* distribution of the parental atoms may be due to an unequal role in the duplication process of various fractions of the total DNA contained in the self-duplicating structure, while an observed equal distribution may only reflect the randomizing effect of some post-replication event like fragmentation by genetic recombination."

The biological activity of the DNA molecule seems able to survive the rupture of a large majority (95% or more) of its phosphate diester linkages, when these are broken by P^{32} decay or even by enzymatic digestion. This is hard to conceive if replication involves a separation by unwinding of the two strands of the duplex.

Most difficult of all in respect to the interpretation of the replication mechanism is the recent work by Stent and his coworkers on the apparent transfer of genetic information from parent DNA to progeny DNA through some intermediary substance. The observations are as follows. First, when P^{32}-labeled bacteria are infected with P^{32}-labeled phage, the ability of the infected cell to liberate infective progeny can no longer be suppressed by radioactive decay, soon after the development of the phage has begun, even though the parent DNA and all of its replicas are highly radioactive. It would seem that the genetic information may be transferred through some intermediate that is not subject to radioactive destruction. Second, it was found that replication of the phage DNA does not occur in infected bacteria if protein synthesis has been inhibited, in any of several ways. If, however, the inhibiting condition is delayed until DNA synthesis has already begun, then the inhibition of protein synthesis cannot halt the synthesis of DNA. The adopted interpretation is that some protein is necessary for the initiation of DNA synthesis, but that once a little of it has been provided, DNA replication can proceed.

If "copying choice" (transreplication) is the right explanation for genetic recombination in phages, then the "mating" of templates and the conditions controlling the switching of a growing replica from one to the other cannot be ignored in considering the replication mechanism in general. Except in the temperate phages, the rounds of mating and the rounds of replication are equal in number (e.g., T2, T4). As for the temperate phages (λ), it is possible that the phage may "mate" with a particular portion of the bacterial chromosome, so that the lack of correspondence is not critical; and this might even be true of the non-temperate phage T1, in which likewise the rounds of mating and replication are not equal.

In summary, says Stent, "no definite conclusions regarding replication can be drawn at the present moment." Nevertheless, the progress made in the definition of the problem and the unexpected discovery of the bipartite nature of the DNA of the phage particle have opened up fruitful avenues of future investigation. If, as Levinthal suggests, the "big piece" is the phage chromosome and if half its atoms remain together in a single particle in spite of many successive cycles of recombination and replication, it must be that one of the chains in the original double helix remains intact. Copying choice rather than crossing over by matched breakage and cross-reunion, and a semi-conservative type of replication would be in harmony with the evidence. The heterozygous phage particles discovered by Hershey and Chase could arise from the presence of two replicas each of which had switched from one parent strand to the other in the duplex, but at slightly different points. Meanwhile it may be kept in mind that such mechanisms and events operate at a very different level of organization than the chromosomal level studied by the cytologist and geneticist. We are still a long way from relating that level to the molecular level of DNA structure.

Other unresolved issues were stated by Lederberg in his final summation. What is the detailed structure of DNA? Beyond the Watson-Crick model, even if entirely correct, there lie numerous questions: how perfect is the pairing? do adjacent nucleotides interact? are there interruptions in the chains? are all linkages 3'-5' phosphate diester bonds? how can a complete analysis of the sequence of bases be achieved? can we analyze the "big piece" chemically? Next are the problems of DNA synthesis, where one would certainly like to know the biological specificity, if any, of the synthetic polymer, and whether the synthesis is a replication or a lengthening of the DNA required as a "primer." Thirdly, tests of the biological specificity of nucleic acids are urgently required, especially of DNA extracted from phage particles. Here Spiegelman's protoplast preparations may become very useful tools.

In spite of the brilliant studies already reported here, which may justify the optimistic view that "factorial descriptions are (about to be) replaced by chemical ones," it is still very clear that geneticists and biochemists are for the most part talking different languages that remain mutually unintelligible, while the biophysicists and crystallographers add to the babel with a third. The microbiologists are trying valiantly in this commotion to dispel semantic confusion, even at the risk of generating yet another terminology. Benzer's notable new terms, the *muton, recon,* and *cistron,* will undoubtedly become widely used because they so neatly distinguish the several operational concepts into which our onetime unit of heredity, the *gene,* has dissolved. [Less commendable is his application of formal taxonomic terms to the hierarchy of mutations, since that usage may create confusion, if taken seriously, in more areas than those where it might simplify exposition.] Stent's analysis of replication into conservative, semi-conservative, and dispersive mechanisms, and of recombination into fragmenting and non-fragmenting types, will clearly help to keep ideas in order and may in fact possess heuristic value by stimulating new and more critical experimentation. One must see the problem before the experiment can be conceived. In general, as Lederberg has emphasized, one must struggle to keep from regarding terms as facts, as geneticists have been prone to do; and one must in any case identify his own usage of each polyfaceted term.

INDEXES

AUTHOR INDEX

SUBJECT INDEX

A

Abortive transduction: 411; and motility, 414

Acetylornithinase: adaptive formation of, 276-289; adaptive phenomenon, 278

Acetylornithine: and arginine diphasic growth, 279; effect of cultivation conditions on, 282

Acricotopus lucidus: salivary gland chromosome of, 42

Adenine nucleotide: coenzyme synthesis from, 593

AGUC polymer: structure of, 624

Alanine-1-C^{14}: retention of incorporated in proteins, 215

Alanine-1-C^{14} incorporation: D- and L-alanine effect upon, 214; into different protein fractions of thymus, 227; into proteins of isolated nuclei, 203, 204; test for reversibility of, 224; sucrose concentration effect upon, 212; restoring in DNAase-treated nuclei, effect of different kinds of DNA, 219, 221, 222; by isolated nuclei, effect of benzimidazole derivatives, 208

Alleles, complementarity of: 17

Allelism: functional test for, 8; gene conversion and problems of, 114-122

Ameiurus, oocyte nuclei of: 40

Amino acid composition of tobacco mosaic virus: 507

Amino acid incorporation: into proteins of isolated nuclei, 203; specificity of nucleoside effect, 269

C^{14}-Amino acid incorporation by isolated calf thymus nuclei: 225; effect of anoxia on, 207

C^{14}-Amino acid uptake, DNAase effect on: 217

Amino acids, nucleotides effect on incorporation into protein: 268-274

Amphiuma; nucleus from spleen of, 44; oocyte nucleus of, 40, 49

Antigenic specificities: transmission of in Paramecium aurelia, 147; transmission of through conjugation, 148

B

Arbacia punctulata: 171; protein fraction of, 181; sedimentation patterns of, 181

Archoplasm, 178

Arginine, and acetylornithine, diphasic growth: 279

Ascospores, mutants from: 102

AU polymer: nucleotide sequences in, 624; ribonuclease digestion products of, 621; scheme of cleavage by alkali, 621; scheme of cleavage by pancreatic ribonuclease, 623

B

Bacterial recombination: 488

Bactericidal treatments, mode of action: 679

Bacteriophage: 13; transfer experiments with, 714

Balbiani rings: diagram of structure in, 53; in polytene chromosomes, 52

Benzimidazole derivatives, effect on alanine-1-C^{14} uptake by isolated nuclei: 208

5-Bromouracil-2-C^{14}, chromatographic fractionation of DNA containing, 378-385

C

Capsule transformations: limitations of classical system, 322; recovery of, 322

Caryonides, in *Tetrahymena pyriformis:* 158

Cell division, role of nucleus, nucleic acids and associated structures in: 168, 775

Cellular heredity: role of cytoplasm in, 141; three systems of in *Paramecium aurelia,* 154

Cell conjugation, sexual recombination, 421

Chemistry of mitosis, some problems in: 169-184

Chironomus, salivary chromosome in: 50

839